Pharmacology
FOR TECHNICIANS

Don A. Ballington
Mary M. Laughlin
Skye A. McKennon

Sixth Edition

PARADIGM
EDUCATION SOLUTIONS

St. Paul

Senior Vice President	Linda Hein
Managing Editor	Brenda M. Palo
Developmental Editor	Stephanie Schempp
Director of Production	Timothy W. Larson
Production Editor	Carrie Rogers
Copyeditor	Suzanne Clinton
Proofreader	Margaret Trejo
Cover and Text Designer	Dasha Wagner
Layout Designer	Dasha Wagner, Kristen Gobel
Illustrators	S4Carlisle Publishing Services
Indexer	Terry Casey
Vice President Sales and Marketing	Scott Burns
Director of Marketing	Lara Weber McLellan
Digital Projects Manager	Tom Modl
Digital Production Manager	Aaron Esnough
Web Developer	Blue Earth Interactive

Care has been taken to verify the accuracy of information presented in this book. However, the authors, editors, and publisher cannot accept responsibility for Web, e-mail, newsgroup, or chat room subject matter or content, or for consequences from application of the information in this book, and make no warranty, expressed or implied, with respect to its content.

Trademarks: Some of the product names and company names included in this book have been used for identification purposes only and may be trademarks or registered trade names of their respective manufacturers and sellers. The authors, editors, and publisher disclaim any affiliation, association, or connection with, or sponsorship or endorsement by, such owners.

Photo Credits: Following the index.

We have made every effort to trace the ownership of all copyrighted material and to secure permission from copyright holders. In the event of any question arising as to the use of any material, we will be pleased to make the necessary corrections in future printings. Thanks are due to the authors, publishers, and agents listed in the Photo Credits for permission to use the materials therein indicated.

978-0-76386-776-8 (Text)
978-0-76386-777-5 (eBook)

© 2017 by Paradigm Publishing, Inc., a division of EMC Publishing, LLC
875 Montreal Way
St. Paul, MN 55102
E-mail: educate@emcp.com
Web site: www.emcp.com

Printed in the United States of America

23 22 21 20 19 18 17 16   1 2 3 4 5 6 7 8 9 10

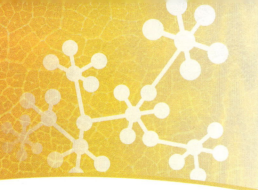

BRIEF CONTENTS

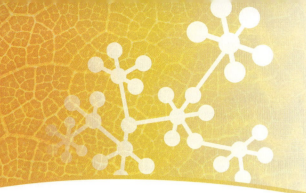

TABLE OF CONTENTS

Pharmacology for Technicians: What Makes This New Edition Exciting?

Pharmacology for Technicians, Sixth Edition is a cutting edge and up-to-date textbook designed to help students achieve success on the certification exam and in the workplace. Using an accessible and student-friendly approach, this textbook supports a comprehensive pharmacology course for students preparing to become pharmacy technicians. *Pharmacology for Technicians, Sixth Edition* helps students develop a commitment to the pharmacy field so that, as pharmacy technicians, they remain challenged by this swiftly changing field and motivated to continue to learn about the drugs that improve the lives of patients. The *Sixth Edition* features include:

- Alignment with new ASHP™ curriculum standards, covering accreditation topics in a logical order with easy-to-understand language.
- The web-based *Course Navigator* learning platform to assemble all student and instructor resources in one easy-access location.
- Expanded information about drugs, including side effects, contraindications, cautions and considerations, and drug interactions.

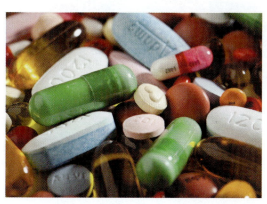

- All new margin features to help engage students and assist their learning.
- An all new section in each chapter exploring complementary and alternative therapies.
- Increased coverage of professionalism, soft skills, communication, and cultural awareness.
- An all-new workbook available in print or digital format.
- Additional practice with memorizing drugs and learning the basics of pharmacology.

Study Assets: A Visual Walk-Through

Print and eBook

1 **Learning Objectives**

establish clear goals to focus each chapter.

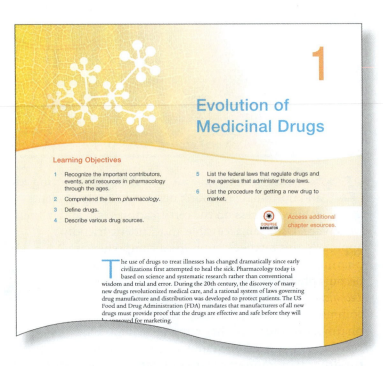

2 **Online Resource Icons**

callout digital resources.

Video **Web** **3-D**

3 **Attractive Margin Features**

spotlight important information.

 Practice Tip

Provides reminders about key elements of pharmacy practice.

Pharm Facts

Highlight interesting trivia and fun facts.

 Safety Alert

Serves as warnings to avoid problems in the field.

 Put Down Roots

Offers word origins to make terms memorable.

Work Wise

Gives advice on professionalism, and on-the-job scenarios.

Name Exchange

Reminds students about items with two names, such as brand and generic drugs.

Numerous Figures, Diagrams, Tables and Photographs

enhance visual learning, aid memory, and provide study tools.

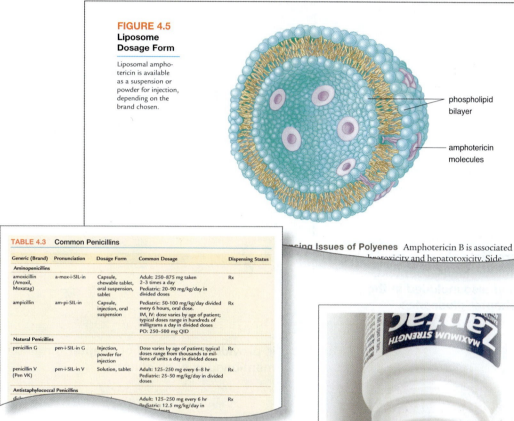

FIGURE 4.5
Liposome Dosage Form

Liposomal ampho-tericin is available as a suspension or powder for injection, depending on the brand chosen.

phospholipid bilayer

amphotericin molecules

sing Issues of Polyenes Amphotericin B is associated
...hrotoxicity and hepatotoxicity. Side

TABLE 4.3 Common Penicillins

Generic (Brand)	Pronunciation	Dosage Form	Common Dosage	Dispensing Status
Aminopenicillins				
amoxicillin (Amoxil, Moxatag)	a-mox-i-SIL-in	Capsule, chewable tablet, oral suspension, tablet	Adult: 250–875 mg taken 2–3 times a day Pediatric: 20–90 mg/kg/day in divided doses	Rx
ampicillin	am-pi-SIL-in	Capsule, injection, oral suspension	Pediatric: 50-100 mg/kg/day divided every 6 hours, oral dose. IM, IV: dose varies by age of patient; typical doses range in hundreds of milligrams a day in divided doses PO: 250–500 mg QID	Rx
Natural Penicillins				
penicillin G	pen-i-SIL-in G	Injection, powder for injection	Dose varies by age of patient; typical doses range from thousands to mil-lions of units a day in divided doses	Rx
penicillin V (Pen VK)	pen-i-SIL-in V	Solution, tablet	Adult: 125–250 mg every 6–8 hr Pediatric: 25–50 mg/kg/day in divided doses	Rx
Antistaphylococcal Penicillins				
dic...			Adult: 125–250 mg every 6 hr Pediatric: 12.5 mg/kg/day in...	Rx

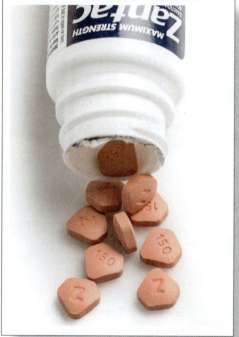

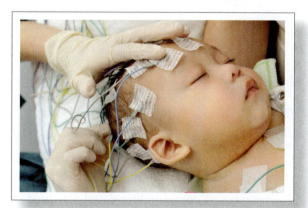

5 Chapter Summaries

reinforce key points in each chapter.

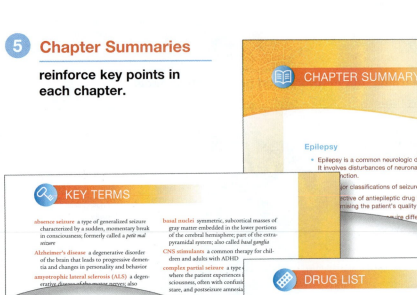

CHAPTER SUMMARY

Epilepsy

- Epilepsy is a common neurologic disorder defined as paroxysmal seizures. It involves disturbances of neuronal electrical activity that interfere with normal function.
- The major classifications of seizures are generalized and partial.
- The objective of antiepileptic drug therapy is to eliminate seizures without compromising the patient's quality of life because of adverse effects.
- ...require different drugs.
- ...therapeutic ranges. A slight dosage...

KEY TERMS

absence seizure a type of generalized seizure characterized by a sudden, momentary break in consciousness; formerly called a *petit mal seizure*

Alzheimer's disease a degenerative disorder of the brain that leads to progressive dementia and changes in personality and behavior

amyotrophic lateral sclerosis (ALS) a degenerative disease of the motor nerves; also

basal nuclei symmetric, subcortical masses of gray matter embedded in the lower portions of the cerebral hemisphere; part of the extrapyramidal system; also called *basal ganglia*

CNS stimulants a common therapy for children and adults with ADHD

complex partial seizure a type of seizure where the patient experiences impaired consciousness, often with confusion, blank stare, and postseizure amnesia

convulsion involuntary contractions or contortions of the...

6 Key Terms

are highlighted in bold, and defined in context, and also included in the chapter glossaries.

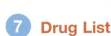

DRUG LIST

Anticonvulsants

carbamazepine (Epitol, Tegretol)
ethosuximide (Zarontin)
felbamate (Felbatol)
fosphenytoin (Cerebyx)
gabapentin (Neurontin, Horizant)
lacosamide (Vimpat)
lamotrigine (Lamictal)
levetiracetam (Keppra)

Amyotrophic Lateral Sclerosis (ALS), Multiple Sclerosis (MS), and Huntington's Disease

dimethyl fumarate (Tecfidera)
fingolimod (Gilenya)
glatiramer acetate (Copaxone)
interferon beta-1a (Avonex, Rebif)
interferon beta-1b (Betaseron, Extavia)
mitoxantrone (Novantrone)
natalizumab (Tysabri)
riluzole (Rilutek)
...amide (Aubagio)

7 Drug List

is provided at the end of chapter for all drugs mentioned in each chapter.

8 Index

provides a quick location guide for terms and topics.

✴ *Course Navigator*

Student Resources

- **Glossary Terms with Audio Pronunciations** aids with visual and auditory learning.
- **Digital Flash Cards** make it easy to study key terms, common brand and generic drugs, and all core content.
- **Study Games** make it fun to practice key chapter concepts.

- **End-of-Chapter Review Exercises** align with Bloom's Taxonomy of learning and include fact-based quizzes, critical thinking questions, higher-level applications, problem solving, and research activities:

> **Check Your Understanding** Check Your Understanding–multiple choice and true/false exercises (computer graded)
>
> **Diseases and Drug Therapies** short sentence answer questions that check synthesis of content (with instructor rubrics)
>
> **Dispensing Medications** short sentence answer questions that check synthesis of content (with instructor rubrics)
>
> **Pharmacology at Work** critical-thinking and application assignments (with instructor rubrics)
>
> **Reflecting on the Profession** short sentence answer questions that address professionalism and soft skills (with instructor rubrics)
>
> **Internet Research** short-essay writing/presentation projects (with instructor rubrics)
>
> **What Would You Do?** scenario-based short answer assignments (with instructor rubrics)

- **Supplemental Resources** include links to Top 200 Drug lists, Most Common Hospital Drugs, and other useful study resources from the most recommended pharmaceutical and medical websites.

- **Canadian Pharmacy Technician Supplement** addresses topics specific to Canadian pharmacy by Melissa Bleier, BscPharm, RPh. (For more information, see page xv.)

- **Practice Tests** provide computer-graded feedback, answers, and answer rationale.

- **Comprehensive Chapter Exams and Course Final Exam** test understanding of chapter topics and the complete course.

Instructor Resources

- **Alignment to ASHP Curriculum Goals and ASHP Accreditation Advice**

- **Course and Chapter Planning Tools** includes syllabus examples and chapter lessons and activities.

- **PowerPoint Slides** highlight key points of chapter content.

- **Computer-Graded Review Quizzes, Practice Tests, and Exams** have been developed by experts for preassembled and assemble-your-own quizzes and tests.

- **Simple, Adaptable Instructor Rubrics for Higher Level Learning Exercises** include presentations, discussions, short answer questions, and short essays.

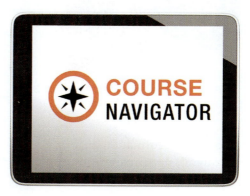

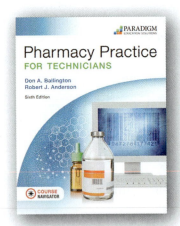

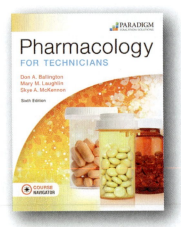

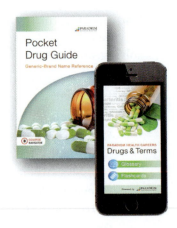

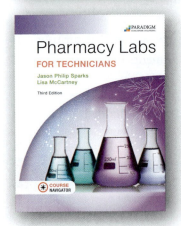

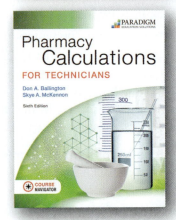

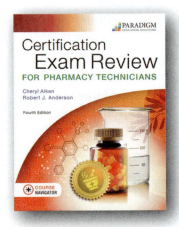

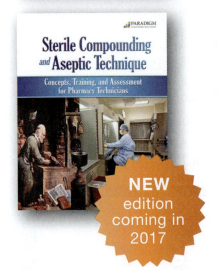

NEW edition coming in 2017

Paradigm's Comprehensive Pharmacy Technician Series

In addition to *Pharmacology for Technicians, Sixth Edition*, Paradigm Publishing, Inc. offers other titles designed specifically for the pharmacy technician curriculum:

- *Pharmacy Practice for Technicians, Sixth Edition*
- *Pocket Drug Guide: Generic Brand Name Reference* and *SmartPhone App**
- *Pharmacy Labs for Technicians, Third Edition*
- *Pharmacy Calculations for Technicians, Sixth Edition*
- *Certification Exam Review for Pharmacy Technicians, Fourth Edition*
- *Sterile Compounding and Aseptic Technique, Second Edition*

* For more information on Paradigm's new SmartPhone App on drugs and terms, see page xv.

Related Health Career Titles

Additional titles in Paradigm's Health Career line of courses are particularly useful for pharmacy technicians:

- *Medical Terminology: Connecting through Language*
- *Pharmacology Essentials for Allied Health*
- *What Language Does Your Patient Hurt In?: A Practical Guide to Culturally Competent Care, Third Edition*
- *Exploring Electronic Health Records*
- *Deciphering Procedural Coding*
- *Introduction to Health Information Management*

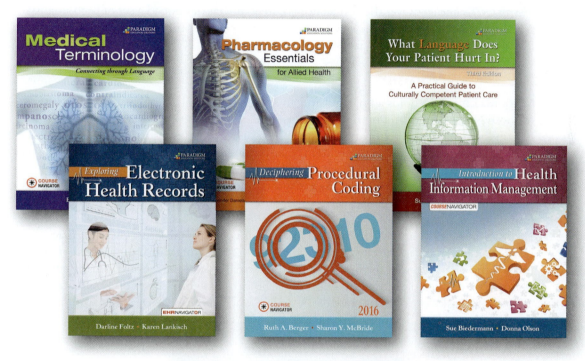

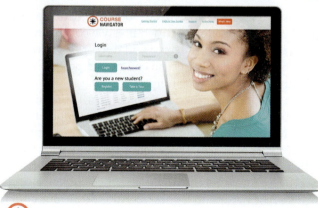

✳ *Course Navigator* resources accompany all new editions.

About the Authors

Don A. Ballington

Don A. Ballington, MS, has been a leader in the pharmacy technician profession. He was a founding member of the Pharmacy Technicians Educators Council (PTEC) and served as its president. As a dynamic professor and program director, he coordinated the pharmacy technician training program at Midlands Technical College in Columbia, South Carolina, for 27 years. In 2005, he received the Council's Educator of the Year Award. Mr. Ballington has conducted site visits for pharmacy technician accreditation and helped develop education curriculum standards with the American Society of Health-System Pharmacists (ASHP). He has also been a consulting editor for the *Journal of Pharmacy Technology*. Over the course of his career, he has developed a set of high-quality training materials for pharmacy technicians. These materials became the foundation for Paradigm's Pharmacy Technician series.

Mary M. Laughlin

Mary M. Laughlin holds a PharmD and an MEd. Dr. Laughlin has been an item writer for both North American Pharmacist Licensure Examination (NAPLEX) and the Pharmacy Technician Certification Exam (PTCE). Dr. Laughlin retired from her role as a PRN pharmacist for Walgreen's in Memphis, Tennessee, in 2010. Currently, she serves as a volunteer pharmacist at the Charitable Christian Clinic in Hot Springs, Arkansas. Previously, Dr. Laughlin has served as assistant director of the pharmacy at the Regional Medical Center in Memphis and assistant professor of pharmacology and pharmacoeconomics at the College of Pharmacy, located on the campus of the University of Tennessee Health Science Center in Memphis. She has been involved in initiating two pharmacy technician programs in the city of Memphis. In 2002, Dr. Laughlin and her team of pharmacy technicians received the Innovations in Pharmaceutical Care award, presented by the Pharmacy Technician Certification Board (PTCB). Dr. Laughlin serves on the Pharmacy Technician Task Force for the state of Tennessee, and on the advisory board for the pharmacy technician training program at the Tennessee Technology Center at Memphis.

Skye A. McKennon

Skye A. McKennon is a licensed pharmacist, board-certified pharmacotherapy specialist (BCPS), group exercise instructor, certified lifestyle coach, and preventionist. Dr. McKennon completed her bachelor's degree and doctor of pharmacy (PharmD) degree from Washington State University. She also completed postdoctoral residency training at Swedish Medical Center in Seattle, Washington.

Dr. McKennon has practice experience in the institutional and ambulatory pharmacy settings. Notably, she was instrumental in the development of a lipid management clinic at Evergreen Health. Her passion for teaching and education led her to faculty positions at the University of Washington School of Pharmacy and at the University of Utah College of Pharmacy. Courses designed and directed by Dr. McKennon include applied pharmacotherapeutics, institutional pharmacy practice, and diabetes prevention. She has been both an instructor and a guest lecturer of various courses for pharmacy and other health science students, including therapeutics, pharmacotherapy for older adults, global health brigades, and law and ethics.

Dr. McKennon has presented her work at international and national symposiums such as the Seventh International Conference on Interprofessional Practice and Education and the American Association of Colleges of Pharmacy annual meeting. She is also a contributor to her regional pharmacy community and regularly provides live and online continuing education.

Acknowledgements

The quality of this body of work is a testament to the many contributors and reviewers who participated in the creation of Pharmacology for Technicians, Sixth Edition. We offer a heartfelt thank-you for your commitment to producing high-quality instructional materials for pharmacy technician students.

Contributing Writers, Textbook Content

Tina Burke, PhD, CPhT
Front Range Community College

Andrea Iannucci, PharmD
Assistant Chief Pharmacist
Oncology and Investigational Drugs Services
UC Davis Medical Center
Sacramento, CA

Tanja B. Monroe, CPhT
Hematology/Oncology Clinical Pharmacy Technician III
Student Pharmacy Technician Internship Coordinator
University of California Davis Health System (UCDHS)
Sacramento, CA

Reviewers, Textbook Content

Andrea R. Redman, PharmD, BCPS
Walden University

Krystal Green, CPhT, MBA
Piedmont Virginia Community College

Contributing Writers, Digital Content

Kevin Hope, RPh, BCNP
Horry Georgetown Technical College

Laurisa McKissack, CPhT, RPhT, MBA
Virginia College

Andrea R. Redman, PharmD, BCPS
Walden University

Paradigm's Health Career Drugs and Terms App

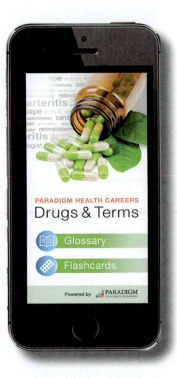

It identifies more than 3,000 drugs and terms. Students are able to:

- Search the terms database by drug class or body system.

- Use flashcards included in the app to review Schedule II drug classes and common medical terminology.

- Create their own flashcards to practice identifying drugs and terms.

This app also offers audio functionality to help students master pronunciation.

Canadian Pharmacy Technician Supplement

 This supplement assists Canadian students in understanding the differences between US and Canadian pharmacy practice. The supplement has four parts that can be read alongside specific chapters in this textbook:

- Part 1: Scope of Pharmacy Technicians in Canada (Chapter 1: The Profession of Pharmacy)

- Part 2: Drug Regulation in Canada (Chapter 2: Pharmacy Law, Regulations, and Standards)

- Part 3: Controlled Substances (Chapter 2: Pharmacy Law, Chapter 7: Community Pharmacy Dispensing, and Chapter 14: Medication Safety)

- Part 4: Top 100 Drugs Dispensed in Canadian Pharmacies (Chapter 4: Introducing Pharmacology)

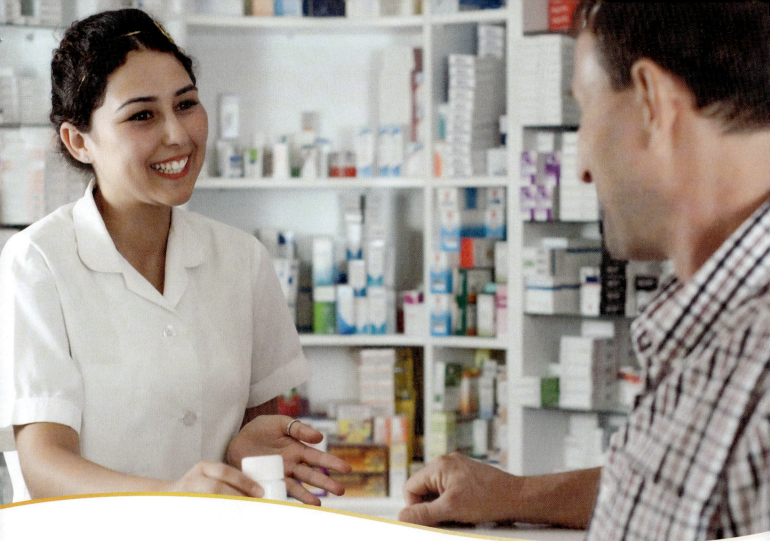

UNIT

1 Introduction to Pharmacology

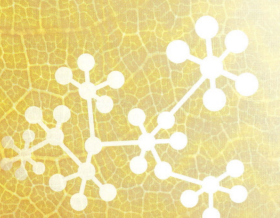

1

Evolution of Medicinal Drugs

Learning Objectives

1 Recognize the important contributors, events, and resources in pharmacology through the ages.

2 Describe the term *pharmacology*.

3 Define drugs.

4 Describe various drug sources.

5 List the federal laws that regulate drugs and the agencies that administer those laws.

6 List the procedure for getting a new drug to market.

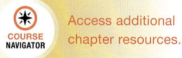

Access additional chapter resources.

T he use of drugs to treat illnesses has changed dramatically since early civilizations first attempted to heal the sick. Pharmacology today is based on science and systematic research rather than conventional wisdom and trial and error. The discovery of many new drugs during the 20th century revolutionized medical care, and a rational system of laws governing drug manufacture and distribution was developed. Today, laws and regulations protect patients and ensure that drugs are effective and safe before they are approved for the market.

History of Medicinal Drugs

Over the last few centuries, tremendous advances have been made in the understanding of the causes of diseases and their treatments with medicine. The study of ancient documents shows that people have been treating physical and mental ailments with medicines for thousands of years. Clay tablets from Babylonia, from the 18th century BCE, list more than 500 medicinal remedies.

Early humans believed the world was controlled by good and evil spirits. The sick were thought to be victims of evil forces or of a god's anger. Consequently, medical treatment was largely controlled by religious leaders who guarded their healing knowledge closely. At the same time, folk knowledge of the healing properties of natural substances slowly grew through trial and error.

Early Remedies

For thousands of years, the only materials that could treat illnesses were substances such as plants and minerals that were located nearby and easy to gather. With time and experience, ancient peoples learned to formulate practical recipes for various treatments. Over time, many of these ancient people began to document their recipes and remedies.

Plants and other naturally occurring substances were administered using some of the same methods used today: topically, orally, through inhalation, and rectally. The *Ebers Papyrus*, an Egyptian medical source compiled in approximately 1550 BCE, lists more than 700 different herbal remedies used by healers. These remedies consisted of botanical drugs drawn from the natural environment and used internally, such as castor bean, garlic, and poppy seed. The most common mixtures were laxatives and enemas. The concept of a **drug** (or a medication) appears in early Greek records as the word *pharmakon*, which also meant magic spell, remedy, or poison.

The Greek physician Hippocrates (c. 460–377 BCE) was the first to propose that disease was caused by natural rather than supernatural causes. Although he practiced herbal medicine like his contemporaries, he rejected unsupported theory and superstition in favor of observation and classification, or empirical learning. Hippocrates was also the first to dissect the human body to study the functions of specific organs.

Another Greek physician, Galen (c. 130–201 CE), lived in Rome and built on Hippocrates' ideas of empirical learning. Using concepts discussed by Hippocrates and the philosopher Aristotle, Galen believed disease was caused by an imbalance of one of four "humors"—blood, phlegm, black bile, and yellow bile. Illnesses were cured with an herbal compound of an opposing quality (moist, dry, cold, or warm). Galen's vast writings about these compounds, known as galenicals, influenced medical knowledge for more than 1,000 years. Greek physicians had such a profound effect on the field of medicine that knowledge of the Greek alphabet is vital to an understanding of many medical and pharmacologic terms. Table 1.1 features the Greek alphabet.

The text *De Materia Medica*, compiled by Dioscorides in the first century CE, was a major influence on European pharmaceutical knowledge until the 16th century. In it, Dioscorides scientifically described and classified 600 plants by substance rather than by the disease they were intended to treat.

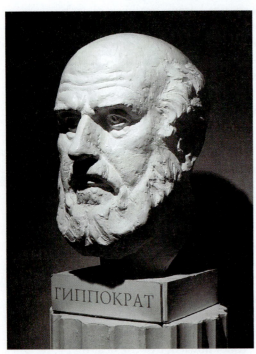

Hippocrates proposed that diseases came from natural rather than supernatural causes and he was the first to dissect the human body to study the functions of specific organs.

Chinese and Indian Medicine

The roots of Chinese traditional medicine rest on the extensive body of knowledge produced by Li Shizhen, a 16th-century Chinese physician who lived during the Ming Dynasty. Li Shizhen compiled a resource called *Bencao Gangmu (Compendium of Materia Medica)* that lists more than 1,000 plants and 8,000 recipes used in the treatment of illnesses. This work, which also describes the causes of various illnesses, is considered the most comprehensive text in traditional Chinese medicine.

In 1000 BCE, a Hindu surgeon named Sushruta wrote a medicinal work called *The Book of Life*. It is divided into 184 chapters and contains descriptions of 1,120 illnesses, 700 medicinal plants, 64 preparations from minerals, and 57 preparations from animal sources.

TABLE 1.1   Greek Alphabet

Capital	Lowercase	Greek Name	English
A	α	alpha	a
B	β	beta	b
Γ	γ	gamma	g
Δ	δ	delta	d
E	ε	epsilon	e
Z	ζ	zeta	z
H	η	eta	h
Θ	θ	theta	th
I	ι	iota	i
K	κ	kappa	k
Λ	λ	lambda	l
M	μ	mu	m
N	ν	nu	n
Ξ	ξ	xi	x
O	o	omicron	o
Π	π	pi	p
P	ρ	rho	r
Σ	σ	sigma	s
T	τ	tau	t
Y	υ	upsilon	u
Φ	φ	phi	ph
X	χ	chi	ch
Ψ	ψ	psi	ps
Ω	ω	omega	o

Drugs in the Middle Ages

During the Middle Ages, as the Christian church became a dominating cultural force, the practice of medicine and pharmacy passed again from lay practitioners to religious leaders. Monasteries became centers of treatment and intellectual studies. Monks wrote and copied medical texts and grew medicinal plants in herb gardens.

The Swiss physician Paracelsus (1493–1541) was the first to challenge the teachings of Galen. He denounced the philosophy of humors in medicine and advocated the use of individual drugs rather than mixtures or potions. He reasoned that treating diseases with individual drugs would make it easier to determine which agent helped, which made the patient worse, and how much of a drug was needed. This concept continues to be used in modern pharmacology.

In 1546, Valerius Cordis published the *Dispensatorium* in Nuremberg, Germany. This type of official listing is often referred to as a **pharmacopoeia**.

Drugs in the Modern Age

The 17th and 18th centuries saw several advances in pharmacy and chemistry. In 1618, London physicians compiled the first English pharmacopoeia. Some drug mixtures introduced at this time, such as tincture of opium, cocoa, and ipecac, are still used today.

In the 19th century, the French physiologist Claude Bernard (1813–1878) advanced the knowledge of how drugs work on the body when he demonstrated that certain drugs (such as curare) have specific sites of action within the body. His use of laboratory methods to study drugs led him to be credited as one of the founders of the field of experimental **pharmacology**, which is the science of drugs and their interactions with the systems of living animals.

Early North American Pharmacology

Early North American colonies had few medical personnel. As a result, early settlers had to rely on domestic or home remedies. As the colonies grew in the 18th century, they attracted a broader range of immigrants, including physicians and apothecaries. An **apothecary** was the forerunner of today's pharmacist.

Like their European counterparts, most colonial physicians owned a dispensary or pharmacy. They prescribed, prepared, and dispensed drugs imported from Britain. The American Revolution forced American physicians, druggists, and wholesale distributors of drugs to manufacture their own chemically based drugs and to make common preparations of crude drugs. In 1820, the first official listing of drugs in the United States, the *Pharmacopoeia of the United States,* known today as the **US Pharmacopeia (USP)**, was published by the Massachusetts Medical Society, with approval from a national convention of physicians.

During the 19th century, in both the United States and Europe, a division emerged between those medical practitioners who treated patients and those who were primarily interested in preparing medicines. It wasn't until after the American Civil War (1861–1865), however, that the boundaries between the professions of physician and pharmacist were clearly drawn. Practitioners who treated patients supported the growth of the pharmaceutical profession because it released them from the responsibility of compounding medicines and stocking a shop. In 1852, the American Pharmaceutical Association or APhA (now called the American Pharmacists Association) was formed, partly as a result of encroachment by other medical areas into pharmacy. Through this organization, pharmacists realized the opportunity for individual growth and increased professional stature.

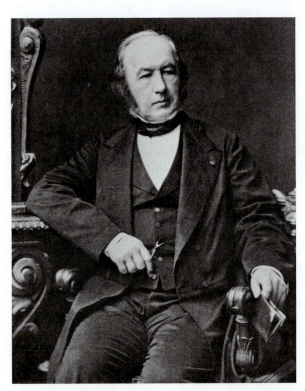

Claude Bernard used laboratory methods to study drugs and demonstrated that certain drugs have specific sites of action within the body.

19th- and 20th-Century Pharmacology

By the second half of the 19th century, pharmacology had become a scientific discipline. Following the lead of Oswald Schmiedeberg (1838–1921) at the University of Strasbourg in Germany, several European universities established departments of pharmacology.

Major breakthroughs in medical care came with the discovery of several important drugs. In 1847, Ignaz Semmelweis helped reduce deaths from puerperal fever by requiring those entering maternity wards to scrub their hands first in chlorinated limewater. In the 1860s, Joseph Lister introduced antiseptics into surgery with his use of carbolic acid for cleansing instruments and suture materials.

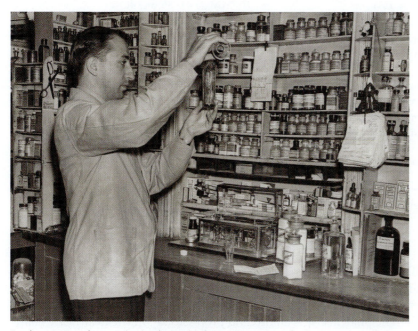

By the 1940s, pharmacies in the United States were employing many modern techniques and medications that are still in use today.

In 1907, Paul Ehrlich, a German bacteriologist, introduced arsphenamine, or Salvarsan, to treat syphilis. This rudimentary antimicrobial was the first chemical agent used to treat an infectious disease. In 1923, Sir Frederick Banting, a Canadian physiologist, and his assistant Charles Best successfully extracted the hormone insulin from the pancreas to create the first effective treatment for diabetes.

In 1935, the first sulfa drug, Prontosil, was introduced by the German Gerhardt Domagk. Ten years later, penicillin was discovered by the bacteriologist Sir Alexander Fleming at St. Mary's Hospital in London.

Contemporary Pharmacy Practice

Today's pharmacy practice continues to build on past knowledge. Scientists research new, innovative drug treatments for the disorders and diseases that affect the human body. **Contemporary pharmacy** is a science based on systematic research to determine the origin, nature, chemistry, effects, and uses of drugs. One key concept in pharmacology is that drugs do not create new functions in the body; they only affect existing functions. Thus, a critical component of understanding pharmacology is knowing the basic lab values of the medical field; these are presented in Table 1.2.

Though early drugs came from natural sources, most modern drugs are synthesized in the laboratory. Hence, the growth of present-day pharmacologic knowledge has been greatly stimulated by the development of synthetic organic chemistry, which has provided new tools and led to the development of many new therapeutic agents. As new drugs are introduced, it is essential that those who prescribe and dispense them also thoroughly understand them.

TABLE 1.2 Normal Laboratory Values*

Serum Plasma
- Albumin 3.2–5 g/dL
- Bicarbonate 19–25 mEq/L
- Calcium 8.6–10.3 mg/dL
- Chloride 98–108 mEq/L
- Creatinine 0.5–1.4 mg/dL
- Glucose 80–120 mg/dL
- Hemoglobin, glycosylated 4–8%
- Magnesium 1.6–2.5 mg/dL
- Potassium 3.5–5.2 mEq/L
- Sodium 134–149 mEq/L
- Urea nitrogen (BUN) 7–20 mg/dL

Cholesterol
- Total <200 mg/dL
- LDL 65–170 mg/dL
- HDL 40–60 mg/dL
- Triglycerides 45–150 mg/dL

Liver Enzymes
- ALT (SGPT) <35 IU/L
- AST (SGOT) <35 IU/L
- GGT
  - Male 11–63 IU/L
  - Female 8–35 IU/L

CBC
- Hematocrit (Hct)
  - Male 41–50 mL/dL
  - Female 36–44 mL/dL
- Hemoglobin (Hgb)
  - Male 13.5–16.5 g/dL
  - Female 12.0–15.0 g/dL
- WBC with differential 4,500–11,000 per microliter

ALT=aminotransferase alanine; AST=asparate aminotransaminase; CBC=complete blood cell count; GGT=gamma-glutamyl transferase; HDL= high-density lipoprotein; IU=International Unit; LDL=low-density lipoprotein; WBC=white blood cell count

*Values may vary slightly based on laboratory.

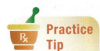

Practice Tip

The role of the pharmacist is evolving and states have varied pharmacy practice laws. For example, in some states a pharmacist can prescribe medication underneath a collaborative practice agreement with a physician. Other states allow pharmacists to administer drugs.

The Pharmacist and Pharmacy Technician

A **pharmacist** is licensed to prepare, sell, and dispense drugs and compounds; fill prescriptions; and advise patients and customers on proper usage. The primary responsibility of a pharmacist is to make sure that drugs are dispensed properly and used appropriately. The pharmacist is an integral professional on the healthcare team. Furthermore, as pharmacists are being asked increasingly to focus their expertise and judgment on direct patient care and counseling, responsibilities related to dispensing have shifted to the pharmacy technician.

The **pharmacy technician** is an important member of the healthcare team who works under the supervision of a licensed pharmacist to assist with activities not requiring the professional judgment of a pharmacist. Although pharmacy technicians legally cannot counsel patients, because doing so requires the judgment of a pharmacist, technicians are involved in all facets of drug distribution. Depending on state law, a pharmacy technician's responsibilities could include the following:

- receiving written prescriptions or requests for prescription refills from patients or their caregivers
- verifying that the information on the prescription is complete and accurate
- counting, weighing, measuring, and mixing medication
- preparing sterile IV and chemotherapy compounds
- preparing prescription labels and selecting appropriate containers
- establishing and maintaining patient profiles
- ordering and stocking prescription and over-the-counter (OTC) medications
- assisting with drug studies

- transcribing prescriptions over the telephone
- transferring prescriptions
- tracking and reporting errors
- checking another technician's work in the preparation of medicine carts
- educating healthcare professionals about pharmacy-related issues
- obtaining laboratory results for pharmacists
- helping patients with OTC drugs
- making sure patients are counseled by the pharmacist (the technician should always ask whether there are any questions for the pharmacist)
- overseeing and maintaining automated dispensing systems
- maintaining pharmacy records
- cleaning the pharmacy (because the pharmacy is a restricted area, this responsibility is always completed by pharmacy personnel)

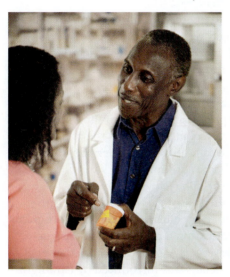

In addition to dispensing medications, the pharmacist plays an important role in instructing patients about side effects of medications, food and drug interactions, and dosing schedules.

These responsibilities vary tremendously from state to state. For example, in Tennessee a Certified Pharmacy Technician can legally take a prescription over the phone. In some states, a technician can check the work of another technician. Studies show that technicians who check each other's work—picking medications for unit dose carts—are just as accurate as pharmacists who check a pharmacy technician's work, if not more so.

One of the most efficient measures to prevent medication errors is patient counseling. Even though the technician cannot counsel per se, it is the duty of the technician to make sure the patient understands that the pharmacist is available for counseling. A patient should never leave the facility without being asked whether they have any questions regarding the drugs. Sometimes the technician can respond to these questions by reading information to the patient, but more often the technician will need to get the pharmacist to talk to the patient. One drug-related problem in the United States is **nonadherence**, or not following the prescription instructions. Patients who understand their medications and know why and how to take them are more likely to take them appropriately.

One responsibility that technicians are claiming across the country is that of overseeing the **automated dispensing process**, which may be a robot or a dispensing machine. As the pharmacy becomes more and more automated, someone must assume the responsibility of overseeing those machines. Technicians are now involved with complicated computer programs that ensure that safe and effective systems are in place to dispense drugs automatically.

Pharmacy Technician Certification

Five organizations—the American Pharmacists Association (APhA), the American Society of Health-System Pharmacists (ASHP), the Illinois Council of Health-System Pharmacists (ICHP), the Michigan Pharmacists Association (MPA), and the National Association of Boards of Pharmacy (NABP)—have joined to form the **Pharmacy Technician Certification Board (PTCB)** in order to maintain a national certification program. The PTCB develops standards and acts as the nationally recognized credentialing agency. To become a credentialed pharmacy technician, one must pass a certification exam. The exam tests an individual's knowledge and skills required to perform as a technician, and covers both hospital and retail pharmacy settings. Exams also cover pharmacy law, drug classes, dosage forms, common side effects, interactions, and indications. Practice tests are available from various sources.

Many states require certification by national examination. All states recognize the PTCB certification; other certifications are state specific. Several states recognize the Exam for the Certification of Pharmacy Technicians (ExCPT) certification. Most states require that technicians register with their state board of pharmacy in order to do background checks and track pharmacy personnel. Each state has different requirements, but all are raising standards and maintaining a system to track pharmacy technicians. Most states require pharmacy technicians to have a high school diploma or GED, be at least 18 years of age, and have no felony convictions. Each state has different standards regarding what a technician may and may not do, so technicians must be knowledgeable of the laws in the state in which they practice. Renewal requirements also differ in each state.

ASHP has assumed the responsibility of certifying technician-training programs. There are three national organizations for pharmacy technicians: the **American Association of Pharmacy Technicians (AAPT),** the **Pharmacy Technician Educators Council (PTEC),** and the **National Pharmacy Technician Association (NPTA)**.

AAPT was organized in 1979 to promote safe and cost-effective ways to dispense and distribute medications. It is run by volunteer pharmacy technicians and is quite influential in decisions made with regard to the profession. It presents the pharmacy technician as an integral part of the healthcare team and provides leadership in representing the interests of its members and the healthcare community.

PTEC was organized in 1989 by Don Ballington. The *Journal of Pharmacy Technology* was selected as its official journal. The purpose of this organization is to share information among those who are teaching in the pharmacy technician programs across the country. The focus is on curriculums, educational materials, and instructional techniques. In July 1998, at the national meeting in Aspen, Colorado, the very first pharmacology text written especially for technicians was introduced by Paradigm Education Solutions.

NPTA was founded in 1999 and is an association dedicated to advancing the value of pharmacy technicians and the vital roles they play in pharmaceutical care. The organization is composed of pharmacy technicians practicing in a variety of practice settings, such as retail, independent, hospital, mail-order, home care, long-term care, nuclear, military, correctional facility, formal education, training, management, sales, and many more. NPTA publishes the magazine *Today's Technician*.

Medicinal Drugs

Recall that a drug (or a medication) is a medicinal substance or remedy used to change the way a living organism functions. Drug action on a living system is known as **pharmacologic effect**. Drugs are often classified according to their use. A **therapeutic agent** relieves symptoms of a disease, whereas a **prophylactic drug** is used to prevent or decrease the severity of disease. Medications are indicated for numerous uses, such as relief of symptoms, replacement of missing natural chemicals, supplementation, diagnosis of disease, disease prevention, and healing.

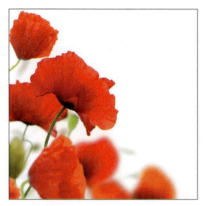

The opioid medication morphine is derived from the poppy.

Drug Origins and Sources

The study and identification of natural sources for drugs is called **pharmacognosy**. Drugs are derived from a variety of sources: plant parts or products, animals, fungi, minerals, chemicals, and recombinant deoxyribonucleic acid (rDNA).

Various parts of many plants can be used to make drugs. Examples of drugs that are derived from plants include ergotamine from rye fungi, digoxin from foxglove, and morphine from the opium poppy. Drugs from animal products include thyroid hormone, which is obtained from domestic animal sources. An example of a drug derived from a mineral is silver nitrate.

Many drugs are produced synthetically from chemical substances. Drugs made synthetically include sulfonamides, aspirin, sodium bicarbonate, and many others. Bioengineered drugs, produced by recombinant DNA technology, are some of the most expensive drugs available; such a drug is also called a **biopharmaceutical** or **biologic medical product**. Current examples include adalimumab (Humira) and etanercept (Enbrel). Table 1.3 provides examples of drug sources along with the corresponding drug names and therapeutic effects.

Pharm Facts

By law, the generic name of a drug must be at least half the size of the brand name on all product labels.

Drug Names and Classifications

Every drug has three names: a chemical name, a generic name, and a brand name. The **chemical name** describes the chemical makeup of the drug in detail, such as para-(N-acetyl) aminophenol. It is usually long and may be difficult to pronounce. The **generic name** is a shorter name that identifies the drug without regard to who in particular is manufacturing and marketing the drug, such as acetaminophen. Also referred to as a USAN (United States Adopted Name), the generic name is not protected by a trademark. It is often a shortened version of the chemical name or an indicator of the class of drug. The **brand name** or *"trade name"* is the name under which the manufacturer markets the drug, such as Tylenol. It is a trademark of a particular company, which has the exclusive right to use that brand name. It is also often referred to as the "proprietary name."

The generic name for a drug begins with a lowercase letter, as in pantoprazole, whereas the trade name usually begins with a capital letter, as in Protonix. Both terms refer to the same drug. Several different companies can manufacture the drug denoted by a given generic name, but they use different brand names.

Drug names are developed according to principles of safety, consistency, and logic, while considering the drug's intended use and existing trade names. The *USP Dictionary of USAN and International Drug Names* describes the process for giving a name

---

TABLE 1.3 **Drug Sources, Drug Names, and Their Therapeutic Effects**

Drug Source	Drug Name	Therapeutic Effect
Animal: hog or cow stomach	Pepsin	Digestive enzyme
Bioengineered: erythropoietin	Epoetin	Stimulator of red blood cell formation
Mineral: silver	Silver nitrate	Anti-infective
Plant: foxglove	Digoxin	Cardiac
Synthetic: omeprazole	Prilosec	Gastric acid inhibitor

to a specific chemical entity. General considerations include safety in using the name for prescribing, dispensing, ordering, and administering a drug as well as suitability of the name for use in health-related educational programs and publications. Another consideration is the ability to use the name for drug identification and exchange of information internationally. A request for a drug name is made after an Investigational New Drug (IND) Application has been submitted to the Food and Drug Administration (FDA).

Complementary and Alternative Medicine

Work Wise

Patients may ask technicians working in the community pharmacy setting to help them find herbal supplements. Try to familiarize yourself with how the supplements and herbs are organized. Sometimes they are arranged alphabetically and other times by body system.

Americans spend billions of dollars each year on many different types of alternative medicine. **Alternative medicine** is a term used to describe medical products and practices that are not part of standard care. It is used in place of conventional medicinal practices and standard care and may include homeopathy, herbs, supplements, and acupuncture. An example of alternative medicine could be using acupuncture to treat back pain from a muscle spasm.

Complementary medicine (or integrative medicine) employs similar methods to alternative medicine, but is used together with conventional practices. An example of complementary medicine is using an alternative strategy (acupuncture) with a conventional strategy (muscle relaxant medication) to treat back pain from a muscle spasm. However, pharmacy technicians should be aware that the terms "alternative" and "complementary medicine" may be used interchangeably. In fact, the abbreviation **CAM** stands for **Complementary and Alternative Medicine**.

More than 40% of Americans admit to using CAM. Reasons for popularity include greater availability of information on the Internet, increased contact with cultures that use alternative medicine, perceptions of greater safety, and distrust of conventional medicine.

Although interest in CAM is widespread, there are concerns about its use. First, scientific evidence to support the efficacy and safety of CAM is often scarce and usually does not mirror the strength of evidence available for drugs. Second, many healthcare providers (such as pharmacists and physicians) lack the training, knowledge, and confidence in CAM. Third, patients frequently do not disclose use of CAM therapies to their healthcare providers. This omission may be dangerous because interactions can occur between CAM (such as herbs) and prescribed drugs.

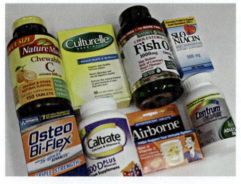

Manufacturers of dietary supplements are not permitted to make claims of curing or treating ailments. They may only state that the products are supplements to support health.

Last, many CAM products are unregulated, which can cause confusion. For example, if a product is made by two different manufacturers, there is no way to know whether one is as strong as the other.

Dietary Supplements

A **dietary supplement**, especially an herb, exerts a weak pharmacologic effect on the body similar to that of drugs. Glucosamine is an example of a dietary supplement that provides nutrients for bone cartilage to treat mild arthritic symptoms. Consequently, dietary supplements may cause side effects, adverse reactions, and drug interactions. As with OTC drugs, consumers can purchase dietary supplements without a prescription and should read the labels carefully.

Because dietary supplements are considered food supplements that maintain health, consumers should not exceed the recommended daily dose or serving size.

Pharmacy technicians should be aware that dietary supplements do not have the same stringent controls as prescription medications and are regulated by the Dietary Supplement Health and Education Act (DSHEA) of 1994. The FDA can only regulate dietary supplements when concerns for patient safety exist, as in the case of weight-loss drugs. Consumers should know that while many of these products are tested by independent consumer laboratories, their quality is questionable.

The use of herbs by patients poses a particular challenge to healthcare practitioners. Quite often, patients take herbal supplements and fail to disclose that information when asked about their current medications or medication history. As a result, some patients, particularly older adults, may have an adverse reaction when combining their herbal supplement and their prescription medications. Therefore, pharmacy technicians can help patients avoid adverse reactions by gathering and recording information about the patient's use of herbs or other dietary supplements.

Drug Facts

Active Ingredients .... Purpose

Conium maculatum 6X ....redness
Graphites 12X...dryness
Sulphur 12X .... tearing, burning

Uses:

According to homeopathic principles, the active ingredients in this medication temporarily relieve minor symptoms associated with styes, such as:

Homeopathic medications contain one or more ingredients in a diluted form to stimulate the immune system. Homeopathic medicines, like other OTC medications, must be labeled for specific uses that do not require a medical diagnosis or monitoring.

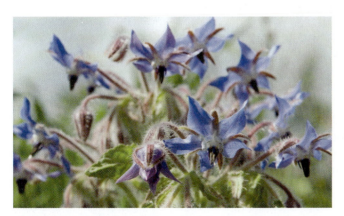

The flowers and leaves of the borage plant are used as a homeopathic remedy to treat fever, cough, and depression. The seed oil of the plant is used to treat skin conditions such as eczema and seborrheic dermatitis.

Homeopathy

Another group of products under FDA control is called homeopathic medications. The term **homeopathy** is derived from the Greek root words *homos*, meaning "similar," and *pathos*, meaning "suffering or disease." Homeopathic practice uses subclinical doses of natural extracts or alcohol tinctures in which the active ingredient is diluted from one part per ten (1:10) to more than one part per thousand (1:1,000), or even higher. The concept is that these small doses are sufficient to stimulate the body's own immune system to overcome the specifically targeted symptom.

Homeopathic medications are available over the counter. An OTC homeopathic medication is labeled for a self-limiting condition, or a condition that does not require medical diagnosis or monitoring, and is nontoxic. The use of homeopathic medications was popular in the United States in the early 19th century and remains popular in many areas of Europe today. These medications are sometimes considered "natural treatments," and the risk of side effects is usually minimal.

Drug Regulation

The manufacture, sale, and use of drugs are regulated by the US legal system. State and federal laws govern the development, prescribing, and dispensing of drugs; providing a rational system of checks and balances to ensure everyone's safety. These laws have been developed and refined over the past century.

The Food and Drug Administration

In 1906, the Federal Food and Drug Act, often referred to as the Pure Food and Drug Act, was passed as the first attempt by the US government to regulate the sale of drugs or substances that affect the body. In 1927, the Food, Drug, and Insecticide Administration was formed. In 1930, its name was changed to the **Food and Drug Administration (FDA)**. This agency of the federal government is responsible for ensuring that any drug or food product approved for marketing is safe when used as directed on the label. The FDA controls purity, labeling accuracy, and product safety.

The passage of the Food, Drug, and Cosmetic Act of 1938 initiated the current system of drug regulation in the United States. The act required all new drugs to be proven safe before being marketed. The basic definition of "safe" under this act is "non-toxic" when used in accordance with the conditions set forth on the label. This act also specifies that every new drug must have been the subject of an approved **New Drug Application (NDA)** before US commercialization. The NDA is the vehicle through which a **drug sponsor**, usually a pharmaceutical company, formally proposes that the FDA approve a new pharmaceutical for sale and marketing in the United States.

In 1951, the **Durham-Humphrey Amendment** established two classes of drugs. A **legend drug** is sold only by prescription and is labeled "Rx only." An **over-the-counter (OTC) drug** may be sold without a prescription.

The FDA has the responsibility of regulating both legend and OTC drugs as well as medical and radiological devices, food, cosmetics, biologics, and veterinary drugs. In Canada, the corresponding federal agency is Health Canada. The FDA does not test drugs itself although it does conduct limited research in the areas of drug quality, safety, and effectiveness. A company seeking to market a drug is responsible for testing it and submitting evidence that it is safe and clinically effective.

Medication Guides

The FDA requires that a **medication guide**, which features specific written information regarding a medication, be distributed to patients when certain drugs are dispensed from a retail pharmacy or upon discharge from the hospital. Many retail computer systems are set up to print the medication guide automatically when the drug label is printed. Medication guides may also be obtained from the FDA. Some medication guides are prepared for entire classes of drugs. Examples of such classes of drugs are nonsteroidal anti-inflammatory drugs (NSAIDs) and antidepressants. Other medication guides are prepared for specific drugs. Medication guides must be given to patients at *all* dispensings—not just the the first time the drug is dispensed to the patient.

The pharmacy technician plays a vital role in making sure that the patient receives the proper medication guide. The technician can also put the guide together with the drug for the pharmacist when the pharmacist verifies the drug. Many different systems

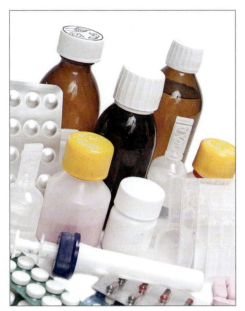

Medications come in many different forms, but all must pass the FDA approval process.

can be adopted to make this work. It is important for the pharmacist and technician to work together to make sure that the pharmacy is compliant with this federal regulation.

Drug Approval Process

The FDA requires that the manufacturer of any new drug provide evidence of its safety and effectiveness before the drug will be allowed to enter the US market. The drug must be shown to be safe through an intensive testing process that is undertaken by a drug sponsor, which is usually a pharmaceutical company. A drug sponsor must obtain permission from the FDA before testing any new drugs. Any hospital, physician, or researcher involved in experimental drug testing must also get FDA approval.

Drug sponsors are responsible for testing the efficacy and safety of their drugs on animals and, later, on human subjects through controlled clinical trials. Before the clinical testing begins, researchers analyze the main physical and chemical properties of the drug in the laboratory and study its pharmacologic and toxic effects in laboratory animals.

All test results are made available to the FDA through the NDA, which also specifies proposed labeling (indications for use, dosing, safety information, and more) for the new drug. The NDA contains details on the entire history of the development and testing of the drug. It documents results of the animal studies and clinical trials; describes components and composition of the drug; explains how the drug behaves in the body; and provides the details of manufacturing, processing, and packaging, with a special emphasis on quality control. The FDA also requires that the NDA include samples of the drug and its labels. A team of FDA physicians, statisticians, chemists, pharmacologists, and other scientists then reviews the contents of the NDA. If the drug is shown to be safe and effective, the team will likely recommend that the FDA approve it. Drugs sometimes may be used for purposes other than the ones approved by the FDA. This is called "off-label" use, and insurance companies may not pay for drugs used for these purposes.

Clinical Trials

If initial laboratory and animal model research on a particular drug is sufficiently promising, the developer will submit an application to the FDA requesting permission to begin testing the drug on humans. Human testing, referred to as a **clinical trial**, is used to determine whether new drugs or treatments are both safe and effective. Protocols for testing are typically developed by researchers and are subject to the approval of an FDA review board. These protocols describe what type of people may participate in the trial, the schedule of tests and procedures, medications and their dosages, and the length of the study. Throughout the trial phases, participants are monitored to determine the safety and efficacy of the drug. Only about 20% of the drugs that enter clinical trials are ultimately approved for marketing.

During clinical trials, patients are typically separated into two groups. The experimental group receives the drug to be tested, while the control group receives either a standard treatment for the illness or a placebo. A **placebo** is an inactive substance that the patient believes is a medication but that has no pharmacologic effect. In general, neither trial participants nor the study investigators know whether a particular participant is in the experimental or the control group. This type of study, which allows for greater objectivity on the part of the investigators, is referred to as a **double-blind study**. It is considered the gold standard of clinical trials.

Clinical trials of new drugs proceed through four phases:

- **Phase I** The drug is administered to a small group of healthy people (twenty to one hundred) to evaluate its safety, determine a safe dosage range, and identify side effects. Phase I studies assess the most common acute adverse effects and clarify what happens to a drug in the human body.

- **Phase II** The drug is studied in patients who have the condition the drug is intended to treat. At this point, it is determined whether the drug has a favorable effect on the disease state. Short-term placebo-to-drug comparisons are made in double-blind trials to determine the range and response of various doses.

- **Phase III** The drug treatment is compared to commonly used treatments. During this phase, study investigators collect information that will allow the drug to be used safely. This phase continues the double-blind, placebo-to-drug comparisons begun in Phase II or the comparison of the new drug to the standard of care. Dose escalations are used to determine the efficacy of the drug in treating the target disease.

- **Phase IV** Once the drug has been approved for marketing, Phase IV studies continue testing it as long as the drug is in clinical use to collect information about its effects in various populations and to identify any side effects associated with long-term use.

In the past, the entire FDA approval process for a drug took approximately 7 to 10 years. Recently, however, the FDA has taken steps to make urgently needed drugs available sooner. The Prescription Drug User Fee Act of 1992 instituted reforms that shortened the review process for new drugs. This act required that drug companies pay fees upon the submission of NDAs; these funds are used to hire an adequate number of reviewers. Now the FDA must act on standard applications for new drugs within 10 months and act on priority applications for drugs used to treat serious diseases within six months. Figure 1.1 illustrates the FDA review process.

A classification system helps to determine the order in which applications are reviewed. Priority is given to drugs with the greatest potential benefit. Drugs that offer a significant medical advantage over existing therapies for any given disease state are assigned priority status. Drugs for life-threatening diseases are considered first.

FIGURE 1.1
The Drug Review Process

After the government approves a manufacturer's IND application, a drug must pass through three phases of testing on human subjects before it is ready for final review by the FDA.

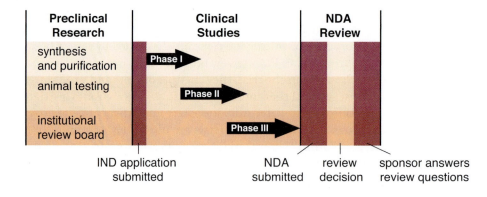

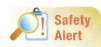
It is important to remember that no drug is absolutely safe. The FDA's approval is based on a judgment about whether the benefits of a new drug to users will outweigh its risks (risk-benefit analysis). The FDA will allow a product to present more of a risk when its potential benefit is great, especially if the product is used to treat a serious, life-threatening condition.

For example, drugs are not traditionally tested on pregnant women. Instead, the FDA uses all available information (mainly from animal studies) to assess the risks each drug marketed in the United States poses to pregnant and lactating women. The old FDA pregnancy categories (from safest to unsafe: A, B, C, D, and X) have been replaced with new labeling requirements. In the packaging information for each drug, the manufacturer must include the following three sections covering topics related to pregnancy: (1) Pregnancy, (2) Lactation, and (3) Females and Males of Reproductive Potential.

The new labeling system provides more helpful information about a medication's risks to the expectant mother, the developing fetus, and the breast-fed infant. In addition, contact information for registries that collect and maintain information regarding the effects of medication on pregnant women are provided. The third subsection includes information on pregnancy testing, birth control, and a medication's effect on fertility.

Postmarketing Surveillance

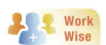
The consumer's well-being is the FDA's most important concern. Public health cannot be safeguarded without procedures to monitor the quality of drugs once they are marketed. The FDA's Office of Compliance oversees the drug manufacturing process, ensuring that manufacturers follow Good Manufacturing Practices (GMPs) as spelled out in FDA regulations.

In addition to demonstrating that a drug is safe and effective, a manufacturer must adhere to standards set by the US Pharmacopoeia–National Formulary (USP–NF) when manufacturing the drug. These standards ensure the strength, quality, effectiveness, and purity of the drug as well as its safety.

Some adverse reactions do not become apparent until after a drug has been approved and has been used by a large number of people. Therefore, postmarketing surveillance (Phase IV trials) is critical to ensure that drugs that pose serious safety threats are promptly removed from the market. Professionals and consumers can report serious adverse reactions to **MedWatch**, the FDA's Medical Products Reporting Program. The purpose of this program is to improve the postmarketing surveillance of medical products and to ensure that new safety information pertaining to drug use is rapidly communicated to the medical community, thereby improving patient care. If a drug poses a health risk, the FDA will remove it from the market even though it has already been approved.

Removing Drugs from the Market

A drug is considered safe if the FDA determines that the benefits of the drug outweigh the risks when the drug is used by patients for its approved purposes. The drug must also be labeled for use for the indications stated in the approval by the FDA, not for other uses. Any other use is considered unapproved.

Safe does not mean harmless, because every drug has risks. When the FDA receives reports of significant adverse events, it evaluates the events to determine their seriousness and the likelihood that they were drug related. Adverse drug events are sometimes so rare that they cannot be predicted. These rare events surface as the drug is prescribed for use with large numbers of people. At other times, a drug turns out to be more toxic than suggested by the clinical trials. When the FDA believes a drug no longer has a place in treatment, it will ask the manufacturer to withdraw the product from the market voluntarily.

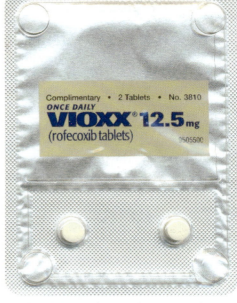

In 2004, Vioxx, a drug used to treat arthritis pain, was voluntarily withdrawn from the market because of a suspected link between the drug and increased heart attack risk.

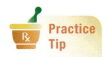

Practice Tip

Black box warnings are the sternest warnings put on drug labels. As you are learning pharmacology, you should make special note of these warnings.

Boxed or Black Box Warnings

For drugs that are on the market and have been found to be problematic but still provide therapy for specific conditions, a **Boxed (or black box) Warning** will be placed on the package insert (see Figure 1.2). This warning alerts prescribers to the known problems associated with the use of the drug. The prescriber must then weigh the advantages of using this drug against the associated risks. Thousands of drugs on the market have black box warnings. They are deemed safe enough to continue using, but they have known problems.

Controlled Substances

The Controlled Substances Act (Title II of the Comprehensive Drug Abuse Prevention and Control Act of 1970) was designed to combat escalating drug abuse. It promoted drug education and research into the prevention and treatment of drug dependence; strengthened enforcement authority; and designated schedules, or categories, for drugs with a high potential for abuse, according to their probability of abuse. A drug listed on one of these schedules is known as a **controlled substance**.

FIGURE 1.2
Black Box Warning

The FDA requires a specific format for a black box warning: The text must be in boldfaced type and have bullets or subheads that highlight the serious adverse effects of the drug.

> **WARNING: SUICIDAL THOUGHTS AND BEHAVIORS**
> *See full prescribing information for complete boxed warning.*
> - **Increased risk of suicidal thinking and behavior in children, adolescents, and young adults taking antidepressants (5.1).**
> - **Monitor for worsening and emergence of suicidal thoughts and behaviors (5.1).**
> *When using PROZAC and olanzapine in combination, also refer to Boxed Warning section of the package insert for Symbyax.*

The **Drug Enforcement Administration (DEA)** was established in 1973 as a branch of the US Department of Justice. The DEA is responsible for regulating the sale and use of specified drugs. It works at the national, state, and local levels. Individuals and institutions that handle or prescribe any controlled substances must be registered by the DEA. The prescriber's DEA registry number must be associated with the prescription when it is filled.

Controlled substances are divided among five categories, or schedules, each with its own set of restrictions imposed on the prescribing of such substances. For example, schedule I drugs have the highest potential for abuse and have no accepted medical use. They may be used solely for research purposes. Table 1.5 summarizes the five categories of controlled substance schedules and includes corresponding abuse potential,

TABLE 1.5 Schedules for Controlled Substances

Manufacturer's Label	Abuse Potential	Physical and Psychological Dependence	Medical Use	DEA Dispensing Instructions	Examples
C-I	Highest potential for abuse	Severe physical or psychological dependence	No accepted medical use in the United States.	For research only. Must have license to obtain.	Heroin, lysergic acid diethylamide (LSD), marijuana
C-II	High possibility of abuse, which can lead to severe psychological or physical dependence	Severe physical or psychological dependence	Drug has a currently accepted medical use.	Dispensing is severely restricted. Cannot be prescribed by phone except in an emergency. No refills on prescriptions.	Oxycodone, meperidine, hydromorphone, fentanyl, morphine, hydrocodone
C-III	Moderate potential for abuse and addiction	Moderate to low physical or high psychological dependence	Currently accepted medical use.	Prescriptions can be refilled up to five times within six months if authorized by a physician.	Codeine with aspirin, codeine with acetaminophen, anabolic steroids
C-IV	Low abuse potential; associated with limited physical or psychological dependence	Limited physical or psychological dependence	Currently accepted medical use.	Prescriptions can be refilled up to five times within 6 months if authorized by a physician.	Benzodiazepines, meprobamate, phenobarbital
C-V	Lowest abuse potential	Limited physical or psychological dependence	Currently accepted medical use.	Some sold without a prescription depending on state law; purchaser must be over 18 years and is required to sign a log and show a driver's license.	Liquid codeine preparations, pregabalin

*This table represents federal law. Each state may have laws that differ from federal law. Marijuana is considered a C-I substance by the DEA. However, there is growing support of marijuana's medical use. Many states now have laws that allow its use for medical purposes and some states have legalized marijuana's recreational use.

accepted medicinal uses, and examples of each category. Controlled substance product labels must indicate the schedule of the drug (see Figure 1.3).

The DEA mandates that C-III, IV, and V drugs may only be refilled five times, for a total of six fillings per prescription, within a six-month period. C-IIs are not allowed refills, but the length of time for which the prescription is good depends on the state. These drugs have the highest potential for abuse, and may be stored separately from other drugs in a locked location. When in doubt about the class of a drug, if it is in a locked location it is most likely a C-II. C-IIs are also high-alert medications because if they are involved in errors, they are more likely to result in patient harm. The pharmacy must have the original, signed prescription for a C-II drug. An exception is an e-prescription, which must be sent from a secure location and requires two identifiers from the sender before it will transmit.

Federal laws determine how medications are handled and scheduled. However, some states have stricter laws. The strictest law always takes precedence. States also vary on who may write prescriptions for controlled substances.

Inventory control is critical when dealing with C-IIs. They must be ordered using a form called **DEA Form 222**. The paper form is filled out in triplicate: the first and second copies are sent to the supplier, and the third is kept in the pharmacy. When the drugs arrive in the pharmacy, the pharmacy must document on the 222 exactly which and how many drugs were received—and this form must be kept for two years. The DEA also has a secure electronic ordering system that allows ordering of C-IIs without paper forms. When C-IIs have expired, DEA Form 106 must be completed to document the destruction of the supply, and there must be a witness to the destruction. The pharmacist usually receives (checks in) and destroys controlled substances.

FIGURE 1.3
Prescription Drug Label

Schedule II controlled substances, such as narcotics and amphetamines, have the highest potential for abuse, drug tolerance, and psychological or physical dependence among drugs with accepted medical use.

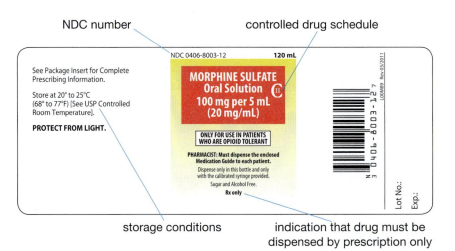

NDC number — controlled drug schedule

storage conditions — indication that drug must be dispensed by prescription only

Generic Drugs

At some stage in the drug development process, a drug sponsor will apply for patent protection. A **patent** protects the drug sponsor's investment in developing the drug by granting the sponsor the sole right to manufacture the drug while the patent is in effect. Under patent protection, the generic and brand names of a drug both belong to the drug sponsor. The manufacturer's proprietary right to the drug expires as soon as the patent expires, leaving other companies free to produce this drug as a nonproprietary, or generic, drug, possibly under their own brand name as well as the generic

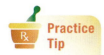
name. When this occurs, the price differential between the brand-name drug and the generic preparation is frequently substantial.

The substitution of generic drugs for more expensive brands is an important means of reducing healthcare costs, and many insurance companies require the use of generics before they will reimburse patients for drug costs. Some insurance companies provide a list of brand-name drugs that they will reimburse.

Drug companies must submit an **Abbreviated New Drug Application (ANDA)** to the FDA to obtain approval to market a generic product. In approving a generic drug, the FDA requires many rigorous tests and procedures to ensure that the drug is interchangeable with the innovator drug under all approved indications and conditions of use. The generic drug must meet the following requirements:

- It must contain the same active ingredients as the original brand-name drug.
- It must be identical in strength, dosage form, and route of administration.
- It must have the same use indications.
- It must meet the same batch requirements for identity, strength, purity, and quality.
- It must yield similar blood absorption and urinary excretion curves for the active ingredient.

When the above criteria are met, the generic drug should produce pharmacologic effects similar to the innovator drug (the original brand-name drug).

The FDA has devised an A/B rating system to establish the therapeutic equivalence of generic drugs. The rating indicates whether the agency has judged a drug to be therapeutically equivalent to the innovator drug by meeting the criteria of pharmaceutical equivalence, bioequivalence, labeling, and Good Manufacturing Practices. The FDA has also identified generics that are not therapeutically equivalent. (This information is published in an FDA book referred to as the *Orange Book*.) Although few drugs fall into this latter category, be aware that such drugs do exist.

Part of the responsibility of the healthcare practitioner is to lower costs without compromising the health of the patient. Healthcare costs have risen at an alarming rate in this country, but pharmaceutical costs have not increased at the same rate—primarily because of generic drugs. Billions of dollars are saved when generics are used.

Over-the-Counter Drugs

Many drugs used in the treatment of disease are OTC drugs. These drugs do not require a prescription. Drug companies recognize that consumers' instant recognition of OTC brand names has marketing value and sales potential. Consequently, companies are reluctant to change OTC brand names, even when the ingredients of the drugs change. Thus, drug companies commonly reuse brand names for products with different ingredients. Healthcare professionals are very concerned about this practice, but a loophole in the federal regulations allows it. The confusion created by this practice is potentially very dangerous. For example, Gaviscon, an OTC drug used for alleviating heartburn, previously contained alginic acid. Now it consists of aluminum hydroxide and a magnesium compound. Taking aluminum hydroxide can be very dangerous for a patient with renal impairment, because it could lead to aluminum toxicity. Patients taking this OTC medication may not know it contains aluminum.

This is one area where the pharmacy technician has tremendous responsibility and can play an important role. Reading the ingredients when helping patients select

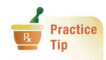

Practice Tip

The FDA's MedWatch can be found at: http://Pharmacology6e.ParadigmCollege.net/MedWatch. ISMP's site is found at http://Pharmacology6e.ParadigmCollege.net/ISMP.

Web

OTC products is essential. It is also very important to report product problems to the FDA's MedWatch or the Institute for Safe Medication Practices (ISMP). Both can be found online.

Whether ideal or not, the reality is that the pharmacy technician is the individual who ultimately guides patients to these drugs. Although pharmacy technicians cannot counsel nor recommend drugs, they certainly need to be able to inform patients what conditions these drugs are used to treat. In most pharmacies, OTC drugs are shelved in sections according to vague categories of ailments. For example, drugs for constipation and drugs for diarrhea are in the same section. Although the label contains information, patients are easily confused and often do not understand the medical terms or cannot read the very tiny print on the box. The technician is much better suited than the stock person to help patients find the drugs they are looking for and to describe the use for drugs. In no way could this be construed as counseling. Often it is as simple as reading from the box to an older patient who cannot possibly read the very small print on these labels. It is very important that the pharmacy technician is familiar with these drugs.

FDA Food Health Claims

Weighing risks against benefits is the primary objective of the FDA. By ensuring that food products and producers meet certain labeling standards, the FDA protects consumers and enables them to know what they are receiving.

In July 1999, the FDA authorized a new health claim that allows food companies to promote disease-fighting and cancer-fighting benefits of whole grains in various breakfast cereals. Manufacturers of whole grain foods that contain 51% or more whole grain ingredients by weight can now make the following claim: "Diets rich in whole grain foods and other plant foods and low in total fat, saturated fat, and cholesterol may reduce the risk of heart disease and certain cancers." In October 1999, the FDA authorized the use on food labels of health claims for the role of soy protein in reducing the risk of coronary heart disease. Consumers must realize that these products are not substitutes for prescribed medications but are to be used together with drug therapy.

CHAPTER SUMMARY

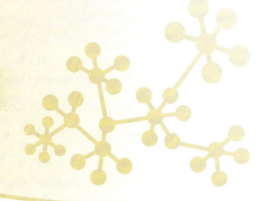

History of Medicinal Drugs

- Historically, humans have sought to find relief for their ailments.

- Humans have used drugs to gain increased control over their lives and to make their lives better and longer. Throughout history, drugs have held a special fascination for humans.

- Pharmacology is a broad term that includes the study of drugs and their actions on the body.

- The 20th century brought major breakthroughs in medical care.

Contemporary Pharmacy Practice

- Five organizations—the APhA, ASHP, ICHP, MPA, and NABP—joined to form the Pharmacy Technician Certification Board (PTCB) to maintain a national certification program.

- AAPT is composed of pharmacy technicians. This organization provides leadership, promotes the interests of its members, and represents them as members of healthcare teams.

- PTEC is an organization of educators that focuses on pharmacy technician training curriculums and networking to share ideas.

- PTCB maintains a national certification program for technicians.

- NPTA is another organization supporting pharmacy technicians. It advocates for pharmacy technicians to achieve their potential.

- Interactions between potent chemicals and living systems contribute to knowledge of biologic processes and provide effective methods for diagnosing, treating, and preventing many diseases. Compounds used for these purposes are called drugs.

- Drugs are derived from sources such as plants, animals, minerals, synthetic materials, and bioengineering advances.

- More patients each year use complementary and alternative medicine. However, there is very little governmental regulation over this industry. These medications can also interact with prescription medications.

Drug Regulation

- Laws govern the drug industry and protect patients' rights.

- Pharmacists must provide medical guides to patients when they dispense any drug that contains FDA-required specific information.

- A boxed or black box warning makes the prescriber aware of any serious problems that have occurred with a drug since it has been on the market.

- The FDA requires that all new drugs be proved effective and safe before they can be approved for marketing.

- Controlled clinical trials, in which results observed in patients receiving the drugs are compared to the results of patients receiving a different treatment or placebo, are the best way to determine the effects of a new drug.

- When the benefits outweigh the risks, the FDA considers a drug safe enough to be approved.

- Drugs are not tested on pregnant women, but, based on all available information, drugs are labeled to identify the risks each drug marketed in the United States poses to pregnant and lactating women.

- Federal law divides controlled substances into five schedules according to their potential for abuse and clinical usefulness: C-I (research only), C-II (dispensing is severely restricted); C-III (can be refilled up to five times in six months if authorized by the physician); C-IV (same restrictions as C-III); C-V (may, depending on state law, be sold without a prescription).

- Generic drugs must be equivalent to the brand-name drugs, and are given an A/B rating by the FDA.

- Pharmacy technicians can play an important role in helping patients identify ingredients in OTC medications, especially when it is possible that the ingredients of a previously purchased OTC medication have changed.

FDA Food Health Claims

- The FDA sets food labeling standards to ensure that consumers know what is in the food they are buying.

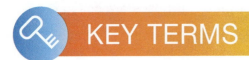 KEY TERMS

Abbreviated New Drug Application (ANDA) the application drug companies send to the FDA to market a generic product

alternative medicine use of medical products and practices that are not part of standard care

American Association of Pharmacy Technicians (AAPT) a national association of pharmacy technicians that promotes the interests of its members as well as general healthcare interests

apothecary forerunner of the modern pharmacists; a shop where medicines are gathered, stored, and compounded by skilled artisans using herbs and other natural ingredients

automated dispensing process a computerized drug storage device that automatically tracks drug distribution

biopharmaceutical (biologic medical product) a drug produced by recombinant DNA technology

black box warning information printed on a drug package insert to alert prescribers to potential problems with the drug

brand name the name under which the manufacturer markets a drug; also known as the *trade name* or *proprietary name*

C-I schedule I controlled substance; a drug with the highest potential for abuse, which may be used only for research under a special license

C-II schedule II controlled substance; a drug with a high potential for abuse, for which dispensing is severely restricted and prescriptions may not be refilled

C-III schedule III controlled substance; a drug with a moderate potential for abuse, which can be refilled no more than five times in six months and only if authorized by the physician for this time period

C-IV schedule IV controlled substance; a drug dispensed under the same restrictions as schedule III but having less potential for abuse

C-V schedule V controlled substance; a drug with a slight potential for abuse, some of which may be sold without a prescription depending on state law, but the purchaser must sign for the drug and show identification

chemical name a name that describes a drug's chemical composition in detail

clinical trial drug testing on humans, used to determine drug safety and efficacy

complementary and alternative medicine (CAM) medicine practices that are not part of standard care but are sometimes used in conjunction with standard practices

contemporary pharmacy a science based on systematic research to determine the origin, nature, chemistry, effects, and uses of drugs.

controlled substance a drug with potential for abuse; organized into five categories or schedules that specify the way the drug must be stored, dispensed, recorded, and inventoried

DEA Form 222 the form used to order C-II substances

dietary supplement a category of nonprescription drugs that includes vitamins, minerals, and herbs, which is not regulated by the FDA

double-blind study a clinical trial in which neither the trial participants nor the study staff know whether a particular participant is in the control group or the experimental group

drug a medicinal substance or remedy used to change the way a living organism functions; also called a *medication*

Drug Enforcement Administration (DEA) the branch of the US Justice Department that is responsible for regulating the sale and use of drugs with abuse potential

drug sponsor the entity, usually a pharmaceutical company, responsible for testing the efficacy and safety of a drug and proposing the drug for approval

Durham-Humphrey Amendment legislation that established distinctions between prescription drugs and nonprescription drugs

Food and Drug Administration (FDA) the agency of the federal government that is responsible for ensuring the safety of drugs and food prepared for the market

generic name a name that identifies a drug independently of its manufacturer; sometimes denotes a drug that is not protected by a trademark

homeopathy a system of therapeutics in which diseases are treated by administering minute doses of drugs that, in healthy patients, are capable of producing symptoms such as those of the disease being treated

legend drug a drug that requires a prescription; labeled "Rx only" on medication stock bottle

medication guide specific information about certain types of drugs that is required by the FDA to be made available to the patient

MedWatch a voluntary program run by the FDA for reporting serious adverse events, product problems, or medication errors; serves as a clearinghouse to provide information on safety alerts for drugs, biologics, dietary supplements, and medical devices, as well as drug recalls

National Pharmacy Technician Association (NPTA) a national organization promoting pharmacy technicians

New Drug Application (NDA) the vehicle through which drug sponsors formally propose that the FDA approve a new pharmaceutical for sale and marketing in the United States

nonadherence when patients do not follow the instructions for properly taking medication

over-the-counter (OTC) drug a drug that may be sold without a prescription

patent a government grant that gives a drug company the exclusive right to manufacture a drug for a certain number of years; protects the company's investment in developing the drug

pharmacist an individual who is licensed to prepare and sell or dispense drugs and compounds and to fill prescriptions

pharmacognosy the study and identification of natural sources of drugs

pharmacologic effect the action of a drug on a living system

pharmacology the science of drugs and their interactions with the systems of living animals

pharmacopoeia an official listing of medicinal preparations

pharmacy technician an individual working in a pharmacy who, under the supervision of a licensed pharmacist, assists in activities not requiring the professional judgment of a pharmacist

Pharmacy Technician Certification Board (PTCB) a national organization that develops pharmacy technician standards and serves as a credentialing agency for pharmacy technicians

Pharmacy Technician Educators Council (PTEC) an organization of instructors dedicated to developing and sharing pharmacy technician program curriculums, educational materials, and instructional materials, advocating for greater education, training, certification, and responsibilities for technicians across the states

pharmakon a Greek word meaning a magic spell, remedy, or poison that was used in early records to represent the concept of a drug

placebo an inactive substance with no treatment value

prophylactic drug a drug that prevents or decreases the severity of a disease

therapeutic agent a drug that relieves symptoms of a disease

US Pharmacopeia (USP) the independent, scientific organization responsible for setting official quality standards for all drugs sold in the United States, as well as standards for practice

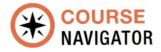 **COURSE NAVIGATOR**

Access interactive chapter review exercises, practice activities, flash cards, and study games.

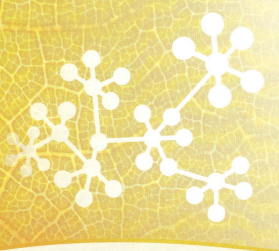

2

Basic Concepts of Pharmacology

Learning Objectives

1 Describe the role of receptors in the body.

2 Compare and contrast the meaning of agonist and antagonist in terms of pharmacology.

3 Describe the four processes of pharmacokinetics: absorption, distribution, metabolism, and excretion.

4 Define the terms used to describe the beneficial and harmful effects of drugs.

5 Describe the ways through which common drugs interactions occur.

COURSE NAVIGATOR Access additional chapter resources.

Pharmacology examines how drugs work in the body (drug action) and how the body responds to the drug (drug effect). The goal of drug therapy is to produce in the body a response that cures or controls a specific disease or medical condition. Drugs work via a series of processes, which can be described through the science of pharmacokinetics. An understanding of these processes enables safe and effective treatments to be developed for various diseases.

Drug Actions

Drugs work by a variety of chemical mechanisms. Although detailed understanding of these mechanisms involves an advanced knowledge of biochemistry (the chemistry of the molecules of living organisms) and is beyond the scope of this book, it is important for the pharmacy technician to have a basic understanding of these processes.

Homeostasis describes the body's constant effort to maintain a state of health and stability. Homeostasis is achieved by a system of control and feedback mechanisms that causes the body to keep its living processes in balance. When the body's own processes cannot maintain a healthy state, drugs can be used to help restore or maintain homeostasis. Many drugs exert powerful and specific actions in the body by working the same way as the chemical components the body itself uses for control and feedback.

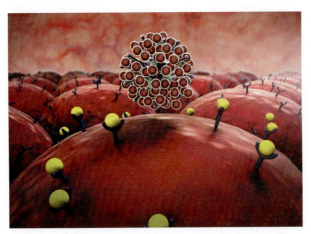

The receptors (in black) in this image are bound by yellow chemical messengers.

Messengers and Receptors

For the body to maintain healthy control over its processes, cells must perform various tasks and communicate with each other. The principal way in which cells communicate is through the action of chemical messengers. These messengers are chemical substances that cells produce and send out into the extracellular fluids of the body. Histamine, prostaglandin, and bradykinin are some important **endogenous chemical messengers** (ones that originate within the body). Once the messenger has been released, it can diffuse throughout the extracellular fluid and eventually reach its target cell. The messenger recognizes and communicates with the target cell via a specific protein molecule, or **receptor**, on the surface of or within the cell. When the messenger molecule binds with the receptor, some effect is produced in the target cell. That effect is the next step in the body's response to the condition that caused the messenger to be produced.

The various types of cells within the body contain different types of receptors, and only certain cell types possess the receptor required to combine with a particular chemical messenger. To bind with a specific cell type, the messenger must have a chemical structure (i.e., the specific geometrical arrangement of atoms) that is complementary to the structure of that cell's receptors. This property of a receptor site is known as **specificity**. For example, the cells involved in immune responses have receptors that are highly specific to molecules on the surfaces of bacteria, viruses, and some cancer cells. Receptors control many important body functions, such as blood clotting and smooth muscle contraction; they also play an important role in protecting the body against injury and infection.

The strength by which a particular messenger binds to its receptor site is referred to as its **affinity** for the site. Affinity is an important concept for understanding how drugs work in the body.

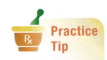

Practice Tip

Drugs that are classified as blockers (such as beta-blockers) are *antagonists*. This means beta-blockers prevent stimulation of certain beta-receptors.

Mechanisms of Drug Action

Drugs act like chemical messengers to perform their specific actions in the body. Some drugs bind to a particular receptor and trigger the same cellular response as the body's own chemical messenger does. Such a drug is termed an **agonist** of the messenger and enhances the natural reactions of the body.

Other drugs work via a competitive mechanism to block the action of the endogenous messenger. When two substances, such as an endogenous messenger and a drug, have an affinity for the same receptor, they compete for available receptor sites. The number of receptor molecules occupied by each substance depends on the relative concentrations of the two substances as well as their relative affinities for the receptor. A drug that has a similar structure to the endogenous messenger may have a high affinity for the receptor site. When the drug binds to the receptor site, it prevents the endogenous messenger from binding there. If the drug does not trigger the cell's response itself, it inhibits the natural reaction of the body to the messenger. Such a drug is termed an **antagonist** (seen in Figure 2.1).

Some drugs produce their effects not by interacting with specific receptors but by embedding themselves in cell membranes, which largely consist of chemically

FIGURE 2.1 Antagonist Drugs

Medications typically work as agonists (those that stimulate a receptor site) or antagonists (those that block a receptor site to prevent stimulation).

BEFORE DRUG

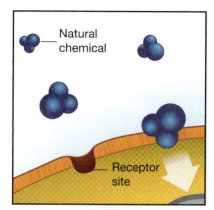

Normal cellular activity

AGONIST DRUG

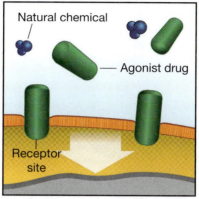

Enhanced cellular activity

ANTAGONIST DRUG

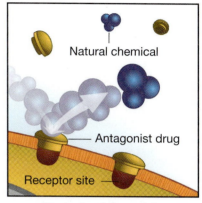

Blocked cellular activity

nonspecific lipids. A **lipid** is a fatty molecule, which is an important part of the cell wall. Lipids generally repel water. The effectiveness of these drugs is related to their lipid solubility. **Solubility** is the ability of a substance to dissolve in a fluid, whether a watery one such as blood or a fatty one such as membrane lipids.

Drugs can also combine with specific molecules in the body other than receptors, such as enzymes, transport proteins, and nucleic acids. Some antidepressants, for example, work by binding to the protein that removes the messenger serotonin from nerve terminals.

Other drugs act without any direct interaction with the cell. For example, drugs can work through an osmotic effect, meaning they can change the amount of water available to flow across a permeable barrier. Mannitol is such a drug. It interferes osmotically with water reabsorption by the kidneys.

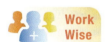

Work Wise

You may hear pharmacists and other healthcare providers use the term PK as an abbreviation for *pharmacokinetics*. *ADME* is another abbreviation used in pharmacokinetics. It stands for absorption, distribution, metabolism, and elimination.

Pharmacokinetics

The study of the activity of a drug within the body over a period of time is known as **pharmacokinetics**. Pharmacokinetic research enables scientists to understand how a drug works within the body to affect both normal physiology and disease. Pharmacokinetics involves a series of processes that produce specific effects.

Each drug's pharmacokinetics can be described in terms of four processes of interaction with the body: absorption, distribution, metabolism, and elimination. An understanding of these processes provides an important framework for researchers who are involved in developing drugs. Figure 2.2 presents a schematic model of these processes.

Absorption

Absorption is the process whereby a drug enters the circulatory system. That is, the chemical constituents of the drug are absorbed into the bloodstream. The absorption of a drug depends on its route of administration, its solubility in blood or other bodily fluids, and other physical properties. The form of the drug is an important factor in

FIGURE 2.2
The Pharmacokinetic Process

The main phases of drug/body interactions are absorption, distribution, metabolism, and elimination (ADME).

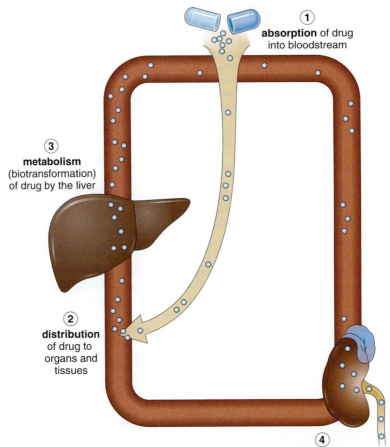

① **absorption** of drug into bloodstream

③ **metabolism** (biotransformation) of drug by the liver

② **distribution** of drug to organs and tissues

④ **elimination** of drug in liquid waste by kidney and solid waste by intestine

Practice Tip

Absorption of certain drugs depends on food. Some drugs are absorbed better by the body on an empty stomach. Others are better absorbed with food. As a pharmacy technician, you can help patients by placing auxiliary labels on drugs that require special attention to food.

controlling its solubility. For example, drugs in liquid solution are already dissolved, so they are absorbed more readily than those in solid form.

The most common route of administration is oral. Other routes include intramuscular, subcutaneous, rectal, sublingual, transdermal, inhalation, and epicutaneous (topical) routes. Intravenous and intra-arterial administration do not require time for absorption because the drug is immediately present in the systemic blood circulation.

Disintegration and dissolution depend on the physical properties of the drug and its dosage form. Oral medications in the form of tablets or capsules must first disintegrate to release the drug into the gastrointestinal (GI) tract where it is dissolved; therefore, the rate of absorption is slower with tablets and capsules than with oral solutions. Factors that affect dissolution include the chemistry of the drug as well as manufacturing variables such as the surface area of the drug particles released from the tablet or capsule. Some drugs interact with gastric contents such as food. This effect can reduce the amount of drug available for absorption or, more often, increase the amount of time it takes the drug to be absorbed.

Because of its large surface area, the small intestine is the primary site of absorption for many drugs, just as it is the site of absorption for food. The degree of movement within the GI tract also affects absorption of oral drugs. The faster the rate of gastric emptying, the more rapid the absorption rate of a drug because it reaches the vast absorptive surface of the small intestine more quickly.

In the small intestine, the drug must cross the cell membranes of the epithelial cells. Membranes are composed of lipids, proteins, and carbohydrates. Pores are small openings or empty spaces in the membrane through which low-weight molecules pass freely. Lipid-soluble molecules, small hydrophilic (water-soluble) molecules, and ions readily pass through cell membranes. Some drugs may be metabolized by enzyme action within the epithelial cells before they reach systemic blood.

Distribution

Distribution is the process by which a drug moves from the bloodstream into other body fluids and tissues and ultimately to its sites of action. Blood flow is the most important rate-limiting factor for distribution of a drug. Three additional factors affect the rate and degree of distribution.

Binding to Plasma Proteins The biological activity of a drug relates to the concentration of unbound or "free" drug in circulation. If a drug molecule binds to a protein in blood plasma, that drug molecule is essentially inactive. An unbound drug molecule, however, can reach its site of action. Disease states can also affect protein binding. Renal failure, for example, may cause a loss of plasma proteins (with less available for binding) or accumulation of metabolic wastes that could potentially displace some bound drugs. Liver disease may also decrease the number of plasma proteins to transport drugs. These conditions can therefore increase both the therapeutic and the toxic effects of a drug.

Binding to Cellular Constituents Drugs can bind to proteins other than those in blood plasma, such as proteins in tissues. This type of binding usually occurs when the drug has an affinity for some cellular constituent.

Blood-Brain Barrier The capillaries in the central nervous system (CNS) are enveloped by glial cells, which present a barrier to many water-soluble compounds. This **blood-brain barrier** prevents many substances from entering the cerebrospinal fluid (CSF) from the blood. Therefore, many drugs cannot get to the CNS because they are unable to pass through the blood-brain barrier. Pathologic states such as inflammation will reduce this resistance, and the barrier can become more permeable under such conditions. For example, though general anesthetics easily penetrate this barrier, penicillin cannot penetrate the CNS unless the meninges are swollen.

Metabolism

The process of **metabolism** converts drugs to other biochemical compounds and then excretes them through metabolic pathways. The converted substance is called a **metabolite** of the drug, and the sequence of chemical steps that convert a drug to a metabolite is called a **metabolic pathway**.

Many factors can alter metabolism and elimination. Disease states, age, and genetic predisposition all affect the way the body metabolizes drugs. Two processes are important to drug metabolism are **induction** and **inhibition**, both of which can control specific enzymes.

Induction Drugs, foods, and smoking can affect the concentration of a particular enzyme. Drugs that increase these enzymes can decrease the pharmacologic response to other agents (e.g., phenobarbital increases the metabolism and therefore decreases the effect of warfarin) or to themselves (e.g., carbamazepine can stimulate self-metabolism).

Inhibition Some agents can slow or block enzyme activity, which impairs the metabolism of drugs and may increase their concentration and toxic or pharmacologic effects. For example, alprazolam is a benzodiazepine that can be used for anxiety. When combined with a drug that inhibits its metabolism (such as the antifungal drug ketoconazole), alprazolam concentrations increase. This can lead to undesirable effects such as respiratory depression.

In addition, if given together, two drugs may decrease or enhance each other's metabolism. Some drugs decrease the metabolism of other drugs by **competitive inhibition** of a particular drug-metabolizing enzyme; this can generally be overcome by increasing the dosage. **Noncompetitive inhibition**, on the other hand, cannot be overcome, and will lead to **complete inhibition**.

Elimination

Elimination, the removal of a drug or its metabolites from the body, occurs primarily in the kidneys (through urine) and the liver (through feces), but other routes exist. Drugs may be exhaled by the lungs or excreted in perspiration, saliva, and breast milk. The rate at which a drug is eliminated from a specific volume of blood per unit of time is referred to as its **clearance**.

Pharmacokinetic Parameters

An understanding of the pharmacokinetic processes enables researchers to determine regarding how a particular drug should be administered to the patient to obtain a specific response. Safe and effective drug therapy requires that a drug is delivered to its target sites in concentrations that will treat the disease state for which it is intended without producing a state of toxicity.

A **dose** is the quantity of a drug administered at one time. **Dosage** refers to the administration of a specific amount, dose number, and dose frequency of drug. As greater dosages of a drug are given, a greater response will occur, but eventually a point will be reached when either no improved clinical response occurs, or the adverse effects outweigh the beneficial effects. This limitation is called the **ceiling effect**. Figure 2.3 illustrates the typical **dose-response curve**. Increased dosing beyond the ceiling may result in toxicity, leading to side effects or even death.

FIGURE 2.3
Dose Response Curve

As greater doses of a drug are given, a greater response is noted until a point is reached when the response no longer improves with increased dosing. This is known as the ceiling effect.

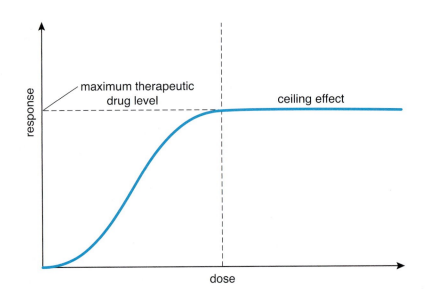

Many dosages are fairly universal from patient to patient. In some cases, however, dosage must be individualized to the patient because of variables such as age, size, weight, sex, race, nutritional state, disease state, kidney function, and pregnancy, as well as other drugs the patient may be taking. A determination of individual patient dose and dosing intervals can be made, if necessary, based on the testing of drug concentrations in body fluids such as blood, plasma, and urine. Typically, only a portion of the dose administered becomes biologically active in the body. The fraction of the administered dose that is available to the target tissue is an expression of the drug's **bioavailability** (see Figure 2.4). Drugs taken orally must pass through the intestinal wall and traverse the liver before entering the blood and

FIGURE 2.4
Furosemide Labels

Oral furosemide is approximately 50% bioavailable. Therefore, only half of the ingested amount is available to the target tissue. Nearly all of a dose of intravenous furosemide is bioavailable. The intravenous furosemide label shown below is 20 mg and the oral label shown above is 40 mg. Due to the bioavailability of each dosage form, these doses are roughly equivalent in terms of physiologic effect.

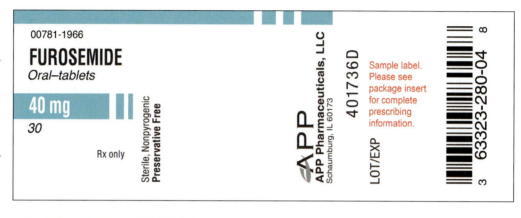

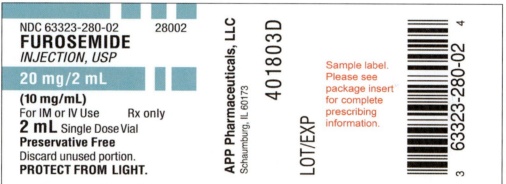

FIGURE 2.5
Therapeutic Range

An optimum dosage range yields beneficial effects without causing toxic effects, whereas underdosing has little benefit on the healing process, and overdosing can lead to toxicity and death.

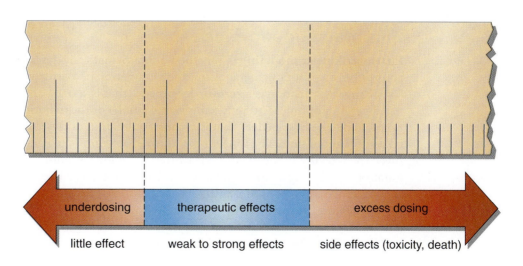

reaching systemic sites. Metabolism in the liver before a drug reaches the systemic circulation is referred to as the **first-pass effect** (or first-pass metabolism). If a drug undergoes considerable first-pass metabolism, its bioavailability will be decreased when it is administered orally. Some drugs have such a substantial first-pass effect that they essentially must be administered by injection, thereby bypassing the liver.

The **therapeutic range**, also called the therapeutic window, is the range of serum concentrations for a particular drug that provides the optimum probability of achieving the desired response with the least probability of toxicity. Figure 2.5 illustrates the concept of therapeutic range. A defined therapeutic range provides the best chance for successful therapy. Some patients may require concentrations of drug below or above the usual therapeutic range.

Doses and dosing intervals are determined by results from clinical trials but may need to be adjusted on an individual basis. Adjustment is often determined based on a blood sample and is particularly beneficial for attaining the desired concentration for a drug with a narrow therapeutic range. When the amount of drug in a patient's blood gives the desired response, it is said to be at the **therapeutic level**. The length of time a drug is at this level is referred to as its **duration of action**. This concept is illustrated by the curve in Figure 2.6.

The time required to achieve therapeutic levels of a drug can be shortened by the administration of a **loading dose**—an amount of a drug that will bring the blood concentration rapidly to a therapeutic level. When the drug concentration reaches a therapeutic level, the patient receives a **maintenance dose** at regular intervals to keep the drug at a therapeutic level. The rate of clearance of the drug is important for calculating the maintenance dose.

FIGURE 2.6
Duration of Action

Plasma drug concentration must reach a minimum therapeutic level before physiologic activity is noted.

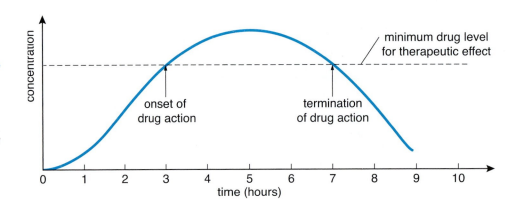

Pharmacokinetic Modeling

Pharmacokinetic modeling is a method of mathematically describing the process of absorption, distribution, metabolism, and elimination of a drug within the body. For some drugs, elimination is a **zero-order** process; that is, a fixed quantity of drug is eliminated per unit of time. The best example is alcohol. For the majority of drugs, elimination is said to be **first-order**. That is, a constant fraction of the remaining drug is eliminated per unit of time. The time it takes the body to eliminate half of such a drug is called the **half-life** of the drug and is written $t_{1/2}$. A longer half-life implies a longer duration of the drug action. It takes about five to seven half-lives to consider the drug "removed" from the body—meaning that only 1%–3% remains. If the $t_{1/2}$ of a drug is two hours, then the drug will be gone in 10 to 14 hours. If the $t_{1/2}$ is 30 hours, then it will take 150 to 210 hours, or six to nine days, to eliminate the drug. A drug with a long half-life may produce effects for days or even weeks after being discontinued.

Drug Effects

The pharmacokinetics described above provide critical insight for predicting the effects of each specific drug. Some effects are beneficial while others can be detrimental or dangerous. Just as each person is different, each person's reaction to a drug may be different. Thus, monitoring patients closely helps to ensure their response to the drug is appropriate.

Beneficial Responses

The desired action of a drug in the treatment of a particular disease state or symptom is referred to as a **therapeutic effect**. The therapeutic effect is the action for which the drug is prescribed. Drugs can act locally or they can act on the body as a whole. A **local effect** is confined to a specific part of the body (e.g., using lidocaine to numb an area for stitches). A **systemic effect**, on the other hand, is a generalized, all-inclusive effect on the entire body (e.g., using lisinopril to lower blood pressure).

Sometimes drugs are prescribed to prevent the occurrence of an infection or disease. In this case, the drug effect is referred to as **prophylaxis**. Patients who will be undergoing surgery often receive prophylactic antibiotics, which aim to prevent the occurrence of infections.

In selecting a drug for an individual patient, the healthcare practitioner considers its medically accepted uses and situations in which it should or should not be given. A disease, symptom, or condition for which a drug is known to be of benefit is termed an **indication** for the drug; that is, if the patient has the condition, use of the drug may be beneficial. A disease, symptom, or condition for which the drug will not be beneficial and may do harm is termed a **precaution**. When a disease, symptom, or condition precludes the use of a drug due to harm, it is called a **contraindication**.

Adverse Effects or Side Effects

An adverse effect or **side effect** is a secondary response to a drug other than the primary therapeutic effect that the drug was intended to produce. On occasion, drugs can be prescribed for their side effects. For example, many antihistamines cause drowsiness, and therefore they are found in many over-the-counter (OTC) insomnia preparations. Sometimes two drugs are prescribed together because the combination has fewer or more easily tolerated side effects than a high dose of either. Nausea, rash, and constipation are the most common side effects and are usually fairly benign. Others can be very bothersome and even serious.

Allergic Responses

An **allergic response** is a local or general reaction of the immune system to an otherwise harmless substance. A substance that produces an allergic response is known as an **allergen**. In general, a molecule that stimulates an immune response, whether allergic or not, is known as an **antigen**.

The first exposure to an allergen generally produces little or no observable response. Rather, what is critical about the initial exposure is the resulting "memory storage" that characterizes active immunity. Upon a subsequent exposure, the body recognizes ("remembers") the antigen and responds with a more potent antibody response. This response can elicit reactions that range from uncomfortable to life threatening. Some responses start within minutes of exposure; others may be delayed.

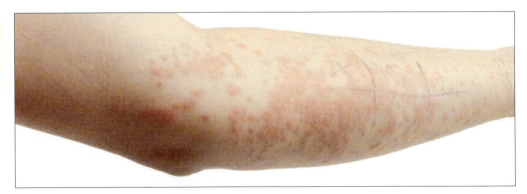

Rashes are often caused by an allergic reaction.

Exposure to the allergen may cause mild, moderate, or, in some cases, severe inflammation. Some common allergic reactions to drugs include nasal secretions, swelling, wheezing, an excessively rapid heart rate, **urticaria** (hives), **pruritus** (itching), **angioedema** (abnormal accumulation of fluid in tissue), **wheals** (red, elevated areas on body), and, in rare cases, even death.

An **anaphylactic reaction** is a severe allergic response resulting in immediate, life-threatening respiratory distress, usually followed by vascular collapse and shock and accompanied by hives. An **idiosyncratic reaction** is an unusual or unexpected response to a drug that is unrelated to the dose given.

Other Responses to Drugs

Drug **dependence** is a state in which a person's body adapts physiologically and psychologically to a drug and cannot function without it. Dependence should not be confused with **addiction**, which is a dependence characterized by a perceived need to use a drug to attain the psychological and physical effects of mood-altering substances. One sign of addiction is a decrease in psychological well-being and social or vocational functioning. Patients who are being treated for various disease states may become dependent on medications without exhibiting the signs of addiction.

Drug abuse is the use of a drug for purposes other than those prescribed and/or in amounts that were not directed. Abusive use of drugs can be, but is not always, linked to addiction.

When patients have been taking a drug over a significant period, they may begin to develop a decreased response to the drug. This decrease in response to the effects of a drug with continued administration is referred to as **tolerance**. As tolerance develops, the dosage of the drug may need to be increased to maintain a constant response.

Drug Interactions

Another reaction to drugs involves **interaction**. One drug can have an effect on the action of another. Foods, herbal supplements, and other substances such as alcohol and nicotine can also interact with drugs. A common mechanism in which a substance can interact with a drug is by inducing or inhibiting enzymes that metabolize the drug, as described previously. A system of enzymes called **cytochrome P-450** contributes to many drug interactions because it plays a key role in oxidizing drugs and other substances.

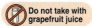

Grapefruit provides an example of a food-drug interaction. Grapefruit juice contains certain chemicals that inhibit a form of cytochrome P-450 that is found primarily in the intestines. Because of this inhibition, less of the drug undergoes first-pass metabolism, so more active drug is absorbed into the bloodstream, increasing the risk of overdose. The effect of grapefruit juice on intestinal enzymes is partially irreversible; thus, enzyme levels do not return to normal immediately after the juice is cleared from the intestines. Absorption of drugs from the intestines may be affected for up to a day following ingestion of grapefruit juice.

It is important that prescribers and pharmacists have a complete list of all prescription drugs, OTC medications, vitamins, and herbal remedies that a patient is taking so that potential interactions can be recognized and appropriately handled. The pharmacy technician should routinely ask patients for this information.

Table 2.1 describes a number of common drug relationships.

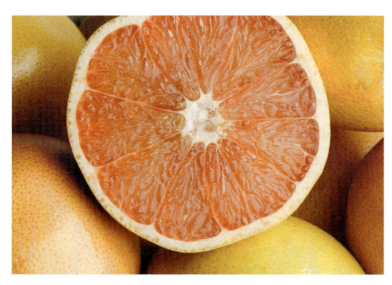

Grapefruit and grapefruit juice interfere with proper absorption of several common drugs.

TABLE 2.1 Common Drug Relationships

Drug Relationship	Description
Addition	The combined effect of two drugs is equal to the sum of the effects of each drug taken alone.
Antagonism	The action of one drug negates the action of a second drug.
Potentiation	One drug increases or prolongs the action of another drug, and the total effect is greater than the sum of the effects of each drug used alone. If one drug prescribed alone cannot produce the desired effect, another drug can be prescribed to increase the first drug's potency. This term is used when one of the drugs has little or no action when given alone, and the second drug increases the potency of the first drug.
Synergism	The combined effect of two drugs is more intense or longer in duration than the sum of their individual effects. Drugs that work synergistically are usually prescribed together.

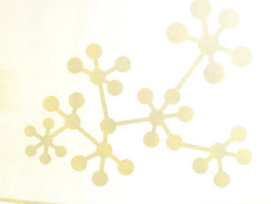

CHAPTER SUMMARY

Drug Actions

- A receptor is a molecule on the surface of or within a cell that recognizes and binds with specific molecules, producing some effect in the cell.

- By binding to receptors on or within body cells, drugs can mimic or block the action of chemical messengers to exert powerful and specific actions in the body.

- One drug can compete with another drug for its intended receptor.

- Pharmacokinetics is the study of the time course of absorption, distribution, metabolism, and elimination of drugs and their metabolites in relation to the time they are present in the body.

- The pharmacokinetic process is sometimes referred to as ADME.

- The primary sites of elimination are the kidneys and the liver. Drugs may also be exhaled by the lungs or excreted in perspiration.

- Body fluids can be tested over a period of time to examine how the body handles a specific drug.

Drug Effects

- Drug effects include therapeutic effects and side effects.

- Drugs can interact with other drugs, herbs, food, and the patient's own body.

- Two drugs may be prescribed together because the combination has fewer or more tolerable side effects than a high dose of either.

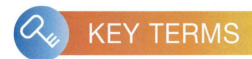 KEY TERMS

absorption the uptake of essential nutrients and drugs into the bloodstream

addiction a dependence characterized by a perceived need to take a drug to attain the psychological and physical effects of mood-altering substances

affinity the strength by which a particular chemical messenger binds to its receptor site on a cell

agonist a drug that binds to a particular receptor site and triggers the cell's response in a manner similar to the action of the body's own chemical messenger

allergen a substance that produces an allergic response

allergic response an instance in which the immune system overreacts to an otherwise harmless substance

anaphylactic reaction a severe allergic response resulting in immediate life-threatening respiratory distress, usually followed by vascular collapse and shock and accompanied by hives

angioedema swelling under the skin that can be a life-threatening allergic reaction, manifested by a swelling of the tongue, lips, or eyes

antagonist a drug that binds to a receptor site and blocks the action of the endogenous messenger or other drugs

antigen a foreign substance or toxin introduced into the body that stimulates an immune response

bioavailability the fraction of drug made available at the site of physiological activity

blood-brain barrier a barrier that prevents many substances from entering the cerebrospinal fluid (CSF) from the blood; formed by glial cells that envelope the capillaries in the central nervous system (CNS), presenting a barrier to many water-soluble compounds although they are permeable to lipid-soluble substances

ceiling effect a point at which no clinical response occurs with increased dosage of a drug

clearance the rate at which a drug is eliminated from a specific volume of blood per unit of time

competitive inhibition a process whereby a drug blocks enzyme activity and impairs the metabolism of another drug; can usually be overcome by increasing the dosage of the drug

complete inhibition a state in which a drug cannot be metabolized by a person's body, regardless of the dosage

contraindication a disease, condition, or symptom for which a drug will not be beneficial and may do harm

cytochrome P-450 a system of enzymes that plays a key role in oxidizing drugs and other substances

dependence a state in which a person's body has adapted physiologically and psychologically to a drug and cannot function without it

distribution the process by which a drug moves from the blood into other body fluids and tissues to its sites of action

dosage the specific amount, dose, number, and dose frequency of an administered drug

dose the quantity of a drug administered at one time

dose-response curve the visual chart of how a drug reaches a point where a larger dose reaches its ceiling effect

drug abuse the use of a drug for purposes other than those prescribed and/or in amounts that were not directed

duration of action the length of time a drug gives the desired response or is at the therapeutic level

elimination removal of a drug or its metabolites from the body by excretion

endogenous chemical messengers chemical messengers that originate within the body

first-order depending directly on the concentration of the drug; elimination of most drugs is a first-order process in which a constant fraction of the drug is eliminated per unit of time

first-pass effect the extent to which a drug is metabolized by the liver before reaching the systemic circulation

half-life the time necessary for the body to eliminate half of the drug in the body at any time; written as $t_{1/2}$

homeostasis stability of the organism

idiosyncratic reaction an unusual or unexpected response to a drug that is unrelated to the dose given

indications the common intended uses of the drug to treat specific diseases, symptoms, or conditions

induction the process whereby a drug increases the concentration of certain enzymes that affect the pharmacologic response to another drug

inhibition the process whereby a drug blocks enzyme activity and impairs the metabolism of another drug

interaction a change in the action of a drug caused by another drug, a food, or another substance such as alcohol or nicotine

lipid a fatty molecule, that is an important constituent of cell membranes; includes natural oils, waxes, and steroids

loading dose amount of a drug that will bring the blood concentration rapidly to a therapeutic level

local effect an action of a drug that is confined to a specific part of the body

maintenance dose amount of a drug administered at regular intervals to keep the blood concentration at a therapeutic level

metabolic pathway the sequence of chemical steps that convert a drug into a metabolite

metabolism the process by which drugs are chemically converted to other compounds

metabolite a substance into which a drug is chemically converted in the body

noncompetitive inhibition a process whereby a drug blocks enzyme activity and impairs the metabolism of another drug, leading to complete inhibition

pharmacokinetic modeling a method of mathematically describing the process of absorption, distribution, metabolism, and elimination of a drug within the body

pharmacokinetics individualized doses of drugs based on absorption, distribution, metabolism, and elimination of drugs from the body

precaution a disease, symptom, or condition for which the drug will not be beneficial and may do harm

prophylaxis effect of a drug in preventing infection or disease

pruritus itching sensation

receptor a protein molecule on the surface of or within a cell that recognizes and binds with specific molecules, thereby producing some effect within the cell

side effect a secondary response to a drug other than the primary therapeutic effect for which the drug was intended

solubility a drug's ability to dissolve in body fluids

specificity the property of a receptor site that enables it to bind only with a specific chemical messenger; to bind with a specific cell type, the messenger must have a chemical structure that is complementary to the structure of that cell's receptors

systemic effect the distribution of a drug that has a generalized, all-inclusive effect on the body

therapeutic effect the desired action of a drug in the treatment of a particular disease state or symptom

therapeutic level the amount of drug in a patient's blood at which beneficial effects occur

therapeutic range the optimum dosage, providing the best chance for successful therapy; dosing below this range has little effect on the healing process, while overdosing can lead to toxicity and death

tolerance a decrease in response to the effects of a drug as it continues to be administered

urticaria hives, itching sensation

wheals slightly elevated, red areas on the body surface

zero-order not depending on the concentration of the drug in the body; elimination of alcohol is a zero-order process in which a constant quantity of the drug is removed per unit of time

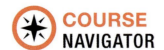

COURSE NAVIGATOR

Access interactive chapter review exercises, practice activities, flash cards, and study games.

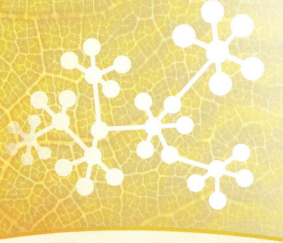

3

Dispensing Medications

Learning Objectives

1   Describe the components of a prescription.

2   State commonly used prescription abbreviations.

3   Explain the "rights" of correct drug administration.

4   Recognize common dosage forms.

5   Describe the routes of administration and dosage forms.

6   Recognize factors that influence the effects of drugs, particularly in older adults and pediatric populations.

7   Describe the role of the pharmacy technician in medication safety.

COURSE NAVIGATOR

Access additional chapter resources.

P harmacy technicians play a key role in the dispensing of pharmacologic agents. This role requires a thorough understanding of the components of the prescription and the responsibilities of pharmacy personnel. The prescription includes all the information necessary for the pharmacist to fill the prescription with the correct dosage form and for the patient to take the medication correctly. Two age groups of patients—older adults and children—have special needs that must be considered in dispensing drugs.

The Prescription

A **prescription** is a written or oral direction for medication to be dispensed to a patient. A physician or other licensed practitioner issues a prescription, and it is filled by a pharmacist. When a prescription is issued and dispensed in an **institutional setting** (or facilities that assume total care of patients such as hospitals or long-term care facilities) it is called an **order** or a *medication order*. The term *prescription* is used in **noninstitutional settings.**

Prescription requirements may vary by state but typically should contain all of the following:

- the patient's name
- the date the prescription was written
- the **inscription**, which states the name of the drug, dose, and quantities of the ingredients
- the **signa**, often referred to as the "sig," which provides directions to be included on the label for the patient to follow in taking the medication
- an indication of the number of refills allowed, or "no refills" if that is the case
- the signature (handwritten, or electronic if from an e-prescription, but not stamped) and address of the prescribing physician
- an indication of whether generic substitution is permitted

If the prescription is for a controlled substance, as discussed in Chapter 1, the Drug Enforcement Agency (DEA) number of the prescribing physician must be on the prescription.

Figure 3.1 is an example of a prescription with the essential elements labeled. Figure 3.2 is an example of an e-prescription. The symbol at the top of the form, ℞ or Rx, is the symbol for prescription. If a medication has this symbol on the container, the medication may not be dispensed unless a prescriber writes an order or prescription for it. It cannot be sold over the counter (OTC).

Pharmacy technicians should always double-check a prescription for accuracy and to ensure that all of the legal requirements have been met. Depending on state laws, the label on the medication container given to the patient must include the patient's name, the date the prescription was filled, the inscription, the signa, the number of refills, the expiration or beyond use date, the prescriber's name, the Rx number, and the phone number and address of the pharmacy.

FIGURE 3.1
The Essential Elements of a Prescription

The pharmacy technician should always check these elements.

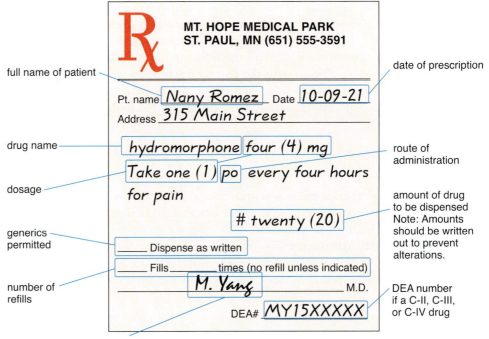

FIGURE 3.2
E-prescription

E-prescriptions contain the essential elements of a prescription in an electronic format.

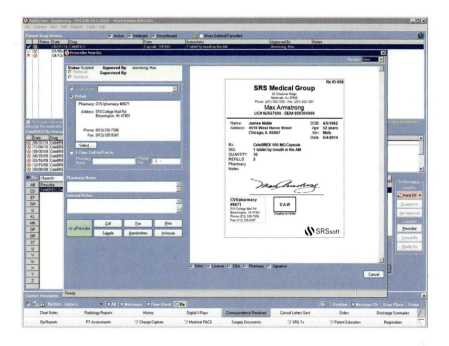

TABLE 3.1   Abbreviations Used in Writing Prescriptions

Abbreviation	Translation	Abbreviation	Translation
ac	Before meals	NKA	No known allergy
am	Morning	NKDA	No known drug allergy
bid	Twice a day	npo	Nothing by mouth
c̄	With	pc	After meals
cap	Capsule	po	By mouth
DAW	Dispense as written	prn	As needed
D/C	Discontinue	q	Every
g	Gram*	qh	Every hour
gr	Grain	q2h	Every 2 hours
gtt	Drop	qid	Four times a day
h or hr	Hour	qs or qsad	A sufficient quantity
IM	Intramuscular	stat	Immediately
IV	Intravenous	tab	Tablet
L	Liter	tid	Three times a day
mcg	Microgram	ud	As directed
mEq	Milliequivalent	wk	Week
mL	Milliliter		

* The abbreviation gm is sometimes used for gram.

Note: Some prescribers may write abbreviations using capital letters or periods. However, periods should not be used with metrics or medical abbreviations, because they can be a source of medication errors.

 Put Down Roots

Many of the abbreviations used in writing prescriptions come from Latin. For example, the abbreviation "*ac*" is from the Latin words *ante cibum* and translates to "before meals."

Per os is Latin for "by mouth," hence the abbreviation *po*.

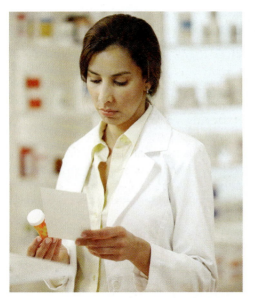

Carefully checking prescriptions is an important responsibility of the pharmacy technician.

To fill the prescription safely, the pharmacy technician should be familiar with common abbreviations used in prescriptions, listed in Table 3.1. Although these abbreviations are standard usage for prescribers, pharmacists, and their technicians, the instructions to the patient are not abbreviated but spelled out in full and phrased as simply as possible to ensure proper use of the medication. There is strong evidence to show that abbreviations are the source of many medication errors. When taking a verbal order or prescription, it is recommended that abbreviations *not* be used.

The abbreviations in Table 3.2 have been identified as the cause of many errors and should never be used. Additional dangerous abbreviations are listed at the Institute for Safe Medication Practices (ISMP) website. Even though these abbreviations are unapproved, the technician will frequently see them and will need to be able to interpret them in order to fill a prescription.

Most pharmacies give the patient an information sheet with additional details regarding the proper way to take the medication (especially in regard to food intake), possible side effects, and situations in which the prescribing physician should be consulted. Limiting the number of refills allowed without another physician consultation is a way to prevent the patient from encountering severe side effects from the medication.

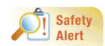

Safety Alert

Check the ISMP website at http://Pharmacology6e.ParadigmCollege.net/ISMP for dangerous abbreviations and dose designations.

Web

Work Wise

Many drugs look alike in spelling or packaging, such as azaTHIOprine and azaCITIDine. Other drugs sound alike, such as Celexa and Zyprexa. To help prevent errors, the ISMP publishes a list of Confused Drug Names. Many of these are also discussed in Appendix A.

TABLE 3.2 Official "Do Not Use" List of Abbreviations

Do Not Use	Potential Problem	Use Instead
U, u (unit)	Mistaken for 0 (zero), the numeral 4 or cc	Write "unit"
IU (International Unit)	Mistaken for IV (intravenous) or the numeral 10	Write "International Unit"
Q.D., QD, q.d., qd (daily)	Mistaken for each other	Write "daily"
Q.O.D., QOD, q.o.d, qod (every other day)	Period after the Q mistaken for "I" and the "O" mistaken for "I"	Write "every other day"
Trailing zero (X.0 mg)*	Decimal point is missed	Write X mg
Lack of leading zero (.X mg)		Write 0.X mg
MS	Can mean morphine sulfate or magnesium sulfate	Write "morphine sulfate"
MSO4 and MgSO4	Confused for one another	Write "magnesium sulfate"

*A "trailing zero" may be used only where required to demonstrate the level of precision of the value being reported, such as for laboratory results, imaging studies that report size of lesions, or catheter/tube sizes. It may not be used in medication orders or other medication-related documentation.

Correct Drug Administration "Rights"

Work Wise

If something seems strange about a prescription (like a dose), speak up. As a pharmacy technician, you are a valuable asset to your pharmacist. Your pharmacist will be glad you expressed your concern.

The "rights" of medication administration, illustrated in Figure 3.3, offer useful guidelines when filling prescriptions for patient medications. The healthcare professionals who are involved in the process from prescribing through administration use these concepts to avoid medication errors. A drug complication can occur whenever they are not followed correctly. Six of these rights are overviewed below.

- **Right Patient** Always verify the patient's name before dispensing medication. Always use at least two patient identifiers (name plus room number, address, birthdate, phone number, or other data).

- **Right Drug** Always check the medication against the original prescription and the patient's disease state. The medication label contains important information about the drug that will be dispensed to the patient. Figure 3.4 provides an example of a medication label.

- **Right Strength** Check the original prescription for this information, and pay attention to the age of the patient.

FIGURE 3.3
"Rights" for Correct Drug Administration

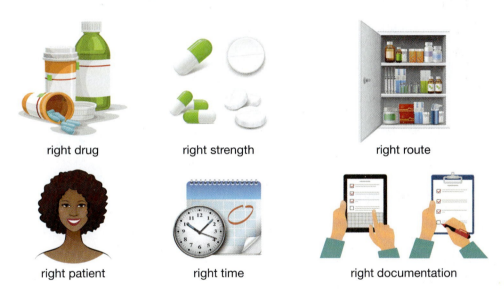

right drug

right strength

right route

right patient

right time

right documentation

FIGURE 3.4
Medication Label on a Dispensing Container

Important information, such as the drug name, dosage form, dosage strength, precautions, and usual dosage and frequency of administration will be provided on the medication dispensing container.

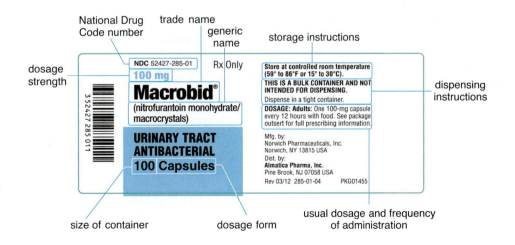

- **Right Route** Check that the physician's order agrees with the drug's specified route of administration. Many medications can be given by a variety of routes, and the route of administration can affect the medication's absorption.
- **Right Time** Check the prescription to determine the appropriate time for the medication to be administered. Some medications must be taken on an empty stomach (one hour before or two hours after a meal), while others should be taken with food. Sometimes, a certain time span is needed between doses to maintain a therapeutically effective blood level.
- **Right Documentation** You must accurately record that the correct patient has been given the correct medication with the right strength, route, and time.

Dosage Forms and Routes of Administration

A medicinal agent may be administered in many different forms for convenient and efficacious treatment of disease. The route and dosage form are determined by many factors, including the disease being treated, the area of the body that the drug needs to reach, and the chemical composition of the drug itself. Each drug has its own characteristics related to absorption, distribution, metabolism, and elimination. Drugs are prepared for administration by many conceivable routes, but the primary routes are oral, parenteral, and topical. Table 3.3 lists a few examples of these routes. Examples of the common drug forms associated with the three primary administration routes are presented in Table 3.4.

The age and condition of the patient often determine the dosage form that will be used. Pediatric and older adult populations frequently have special needs. These two groups often need liquid dosage forms. Convenience may also play a role in the

TABLE 3.3 Common Routes of Administration

Route	Example
Peroral (po, by mouth)	Buccal (dissolves in the cheek) Oral (swallowed) Sublingual (under the tongue)
Parenteral (not through the alimentary canal, but by injection through some other route)	Epidural (fibrous membrane of spinal cord) Intra-arterial (artery) Intracardiac (heart) Intramuscular (muscle) Intraspinal/intrathecal (spinal fluid) Intrasynovial (joint-fluid area) Intravenous (vein) Subcutaneous (beneath the skin)
Topical (applied to surface of skin or mucous membranes)	Inhalation (lung) Intranasal (nose) Ophthalmic (eye) Otic (ear) Rectal (rectum) Transdermal (skin surface) Urethral (urethra) Vaginal (vagina)

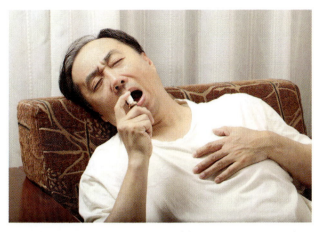

Nitroglycerin, a medication commonly used in patients with chest pain, is administered sublingually.

selection of the appropriate dosage form. Drugs with distinctive sizes, shapes, and colors are inherently easier to identify. Dosage forms that reduce the frequency of administration without sacrificing efficacy are often advantageous and improve patient **adherence** (the patient's adherence to the dose schedule and other particular requirements of the specific drug regimen).

Peroral Routes

The **peroral (po)** route is the most economical and most convenient way to give medications. The term po comes from the latin *per os*, meaning, "by opening." This route is commonly referred to as the **oral** route. The term *oral* means that the medication is given by mouth either in solid (such as a tablet or capsule) or in liquid form (such as a solution or syrup). Once the medication enters the mouth, it must be swallowed to reach the stomach. Then it must pass to the area of absorption, most commonly the small intestine, although some medications are absorbed in the stomach.

The absorption process takes time and is affected by several factors, including the presence of food (which slows the process) or digestive disorders. It is important to

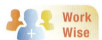 **Work Wise**

All drugs come with a package insert from the manufacturer. The package insert contains important information, such as administration directions. The package insert can tell you if a medication should be taken with or without food, or without regard to food.

TABLE 3.4   Common Dosage Forms

Route	Primary Dosage Forms
Peroral (po, by mouth)	Capsules
	Elixirs
	Gels
	Powders
	Solutions
	Suspensions
	Syrups
	Tablets
	Troches/lozenges
Parenteral	Solutions
	Suspensions
Topical	Aerosols
	Creams
	Emulsions
	Enemas
	Gels
	Inhalants
	Lotions
	Ointments
	Pastes
	Powders
	Sponges
	Sprays
	Suppositories
	Transdermal patches

refer to a reliable drug reference guide to determine whether the medication should be given with or without food and whether any specific assessments should be done before dispensing it.

Sublingual (under the tongue) and **buccal** (between the cheek and gum) routes of administration are used when a rapid action is desired, or when a drug is specifically designed to be easily absorbed into blood vessels. The medication enters the bloodstream directly from the richly vascularized mucous membrane of the mouth and produces its effects more quickly than drugs that are swallowed. This dosage form cannot obtain the same effect if swallowed.

When taking medication by the sublingual route, the patient should hold the tablet under the tongue until it dissolves completely. For buccal administration, the patient should place the tablet between the cheek and gums, close the mouth, and hold the tablet there until it is dissolved. It is important to remind the patient not to drink water or swallow excessively until the tablet is completely absorbed.

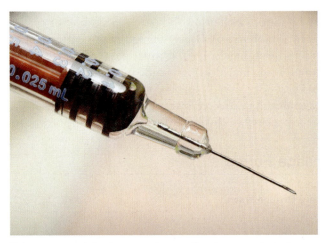

Subcutaneous injections require needles that are relatively shorter, as pictured above. Intramuscular injections require longer needles.

Parenteral Routes

Administration of drugs by injection is referred to as the **parenteral** route (meaning "outside of the intestines"). Injections can be painful, and there is a risk of infection at the site of puncture, but parenteral administration may be necessary for several reasons. Some drugs, such as insulin, are inactivated in digestive juices, so swallowing them would be ineffective. Other medications would be inactivated by first-pass metabolism, described in Chapter 2, if they had to pass through the liver before entering the bloodstream, so they are injected directly into the tissues of the body. Parenteral routes also offer the potential for quick absorption of injected medication into the bloodstream and a rapid effect (especially for the intravenous route). Parenteral products also offer an alternative during times when the patient cannot tolerate oral medications, such as during severe vomiting.

Often the prescriber forgets to write a prescription for the needle to inject these drugs. You may need to call the prescriber to clarify which needle is needed, because different medications need different size needles. For example, it can be dangerous to inject heparin intramuscularly (IM), so the prescription should indicate a subcutaneous (SC, or Subcut) needle. If the prescription for the appropriate needle is in the patient profile, a lot of pain and confusion can be prevented. Drugs may be injected into

- muscle: **intramuscular (IM)**
- vein: **intravenous (IV)**
- skin: **intradermal**
- tissue beneath the skin: **subcutaneous (SC, SQ, or Subcut)**
- spinal column: **intraspinal** or **intrathecal**

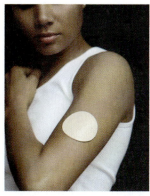

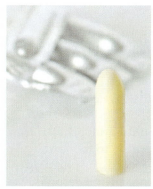

A nicotine patch is a topical medication that a patient can use to quit smoking. The effect of a nicotine patch is systemic in that it delivers nicotine to the entire body.

Rectal suppositories are usually packaged in foil and require refrigeration.

Topical Routes

Topical medications are applied to the surface of the skin or mucous membranes. The desired effect can be **local** (affecting only a small area of the body) or **systemic** (affecting the body as a whole). Other topical routes are inhalation, ophthalmic, otic, nasal, rectal, and vaginal.

The **inhalation** route delivers medications to the respiratory system. These medications are usually intended for one or more of the following purposes: to alter the condition of the mucous membranes, to alter the character of the secretions in the respiratory system, to treat diseases and infections of the respiratory tract, or to produce general anesthesia.

Medications can be administered via the **ophthalmic** route by **instillation** (administration of a medication drop by drop), of drops of a liquid preparation into the conjunctival sac of the eye, or by application of a cream or ointment.

Drugs administered by the **otic** route, into the ear, are used locally to treat inflammation or infection of the external ear canal or to remove excess cerumen (wax) or foreign objects from the canal. Eardrops come in **solutions** (where the active drug is dissolved in liquid) and **suspensions** (where the active drug particles are mixed, but not dissolved, in liquid). If the patient has a tube in the ear, a suspension rather than a solution should be used. When a prescription for ear drops is dispensed, the technician should always ask whether the patient has an ear tube.

Medications can be administered via the **nasal** route. Nasal administration can result in local and/or systemic drug effects. Examples of intranasal drugs that are used for local effect include corticosteroids (used for rhinitis) and decongestants (used for congestion). Nasal drugs that are used for systemic effect include hormone products, migraine medications, and nicotine replacement. Nasal products are typically available as a spray or drops for instillation.

Medications that are administered by the rectal route are most commonly in the form of a **suppository** or an **enema** (a liquid that is injected in the rectum). Suppositories are soft, rounded pieces of cocoa butter, glycerin, or a synthetic base. When inserted into the rectum, they melt at body temperature and release the medication to be absorbed through the walls of the large intestine. The primary advantage of rectal administration is that the medication does not depend on the digestive system to be absorbed into the bloodstream. Therefore, this route is frequently used to treat nausea and vomiting. Suppositories can also be used for local effect to treat constipation. Additionally, the rectal route is ideal for treating fever in infants and young children.

Medications given by the **vaginal** route can be used to treat a **local infection** (restricted to or pertaining to one area of the body) caused by either bacteria or fungi. There can also be some systemic absorption (absorption into the bloodstream) through this route, enabling the medication to circulate and affect other parts of the body.

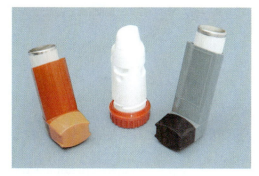

Inhalers, as pictured above, deliver medications to the respiratory system topically.

Factors That Influence Drug Action

A variety of factors can influence the effects of drugs and may require dosage adjustment. Ensuring that patients receive the correct medication at the correct dosage, and that a newly prescribed medication does not adversely interact with other drugs that a patient is taking are all of paramount importance. Several procedures are in place to help ensure medication safety, and the pharmacy technician plays a role in following these procedures.

Children and older adults may require a reduced dose because of alterations in metabolism of drugs and reductions in excretion or elimination from the body. In these instances, if the dosage is not decreased, it may have toxic effects on the patient. The prescriber can use a variety of formulas when prescribing medications for pediatric or older adult patients.

Patients with specific diseases may be unable to absorb, metabolize, or excrete certain medications. Impaired gastrointestinal (GI) function may affect absorption, impaired liver function may affect metabolism, and impaired kidney function may affect elimination. Inadequate nutritional intake may also adversely affect the metabolism of drugs. Therefore, the patient's disease state must be evaluated before medications can be prescribed.

Physicians also consider psychological and genetic factors when prescribing medications. The mental state of a patient can influence the body's ability to release chemical substances needed to absorb or metabolize a drug properly. Genes can also control the release of chemicals and the way the body absorbs or metabolizes various medications. Unfortunately, these factors are less predictable than age, gender, and disease state.

Before prescribing medications, healthcare practitioners must evaluate all patients for immune responses and document any allergic responses to foods or medications in the patient chart. Each time a new medication is dispensed, the pharmacy technician should ask whether the patient has had any additional allergic responses so that the records can be kept up to date.

Special Considerations in Older Adults

Older adults have special needs in relation to their medications. Aging affects both the chemical reactions that administered drugs undergo in the body (pharmacokinetics) as well as how the body reacts to the drugs (pharmacodynamics). In addition, older adults have more chronic diseases than the young and also tend to use more drugs—both prescription and nonprescription. Four out of five older individuals have at least one chronic disease, and many in this age group take numerous medications, three to four times daily. For some older adults, medication can support their independence and help them lead independent lifestyles. As a result, geriatric medicine has emerged as a new and important medical specialty of the healthcare system.

Changes in Physiologic Function

Aging can involve declines in both mental function (ability to continue to meet the demands of daily life) and physiologic well-being (normal functioning of the body). Physiologic changes do not occur at the same rate for all individuals, and many changes are not always predictable. Successful aging is characterized by losses in physiologic function that are **nonpathologic** (not related to disease). Impaired aging represents **pathologic** (manifestations of disease) changes with greater physiologic loss than in average persons of the same age group.

The following is a list of some of the changes that body systems may undergo with aging:

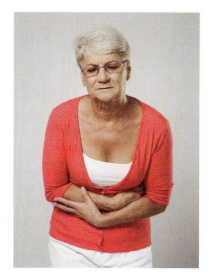

Constipation is a common GI change in older adults.

- **Visual Changes** As the lenses of the eye become less elastic, more dense, and yellow, visual acuity is compromised; this can often be improved with corrective lenses. Macular degeneration and cataracts become a problem.

- **Auditory Changes** Hearing loss occurs in all sound frequencies, but especially in the high ranges. Impairment of sound localization and loudness perception is a problem for many older adults. A delay in central processing of auditory messages results in an increase in the time it takes for the person to respond to a question.

- **Gastrointestinal Changes** These changes create many problems, including decreases in saliva production, esophageal motility, hydrochloric acid secretion, absorptive surface, and rate of gastric emptying. Constipation may be a complaint.

- **Pulmonary Changes** Many older adults have chronic obstructive pulmonary disease (COPD). Aging brings on increased rigidity of the chest wall, decreased vital capacity (maximum intake and exhalation), decreased response to **hypoxia** (reduced oxygen in the blood), and hypercapnia (increased carbon dioxide in the blood). If an older adult patient also has cardiac disease, these functions are further compromised.

- **Cardiovascular Changes** Hypertension and coronary artery disease are major issues to address. Age-related cardiovascular changes are less appreciable at rest. Decreased cardiac response to exertion, however, is more noticeable. Cardiac output often decreases in older adults.

- **Renal Changes** Changes pertaining to the fluid excreted by the kidneys can result from a decrease in the number of functioning **nephrons** (units of the kidney) and in renal blood flow. Older adults have a higher incidence of renal insufficiency (reduced capacity to filter blood). **Incontinence** (inability to retain urine in the bladder) is often a problem; with these individuals, adult diapers or pads become a necessity. Instability of the bladder muscle, overflow, and sphincter weakness are the causes. Diuretics, often necessary medications to treat an existing illness, may aggravate this condition. Urinary retention may result from prostate hypertrophy, malignancies, kidney stones, anticholinergic drug intake, or urinary tract infections.

- **Hormonal Changes** Functional changes pertaining to the endocrine system are a natural consequence of aging.

- **Body Composition Changes** The proportion of total body weight composed of fat increases with age while lean body mass and total body mass decrease. Albumin (the main blood plasma protein) production decreases with aging,

Pharm Facts

Normally, blood flow (as measured per minute) decreases about 1 percent per year as an individual ages, beginning at about age 35 (40 percent from ages 35 to 75).

possibly because of poor nutrition, hepatic disorders, or other disease states. Loss in bone density (osteoporosis) causes some loss of height. Arthritis also takes its toll on the skeletal system.

Altered Drug Responses

Age-related changes in organ function and body composition can alter the response to medication. The following factors play an important part in selecting a drug and its dosage:

- **Absorption Changes** Changes in GI function with aging may affect the rate of drug dissolution, breakdown of enzymes, and drug ionization. Reduction in the rate of gastric emptying may delay intestinal absorption of some drugs. For most patients, the rate and extent of absorption are determined by passive diffusion during contact with the surface area of the gut. Reduction in absorptive surface decreases absorption. GI fluid secretion also decreases.

- **Distribution Changes** Alterations in body composition, such as protein binding (less protein means more free drug in plasma), affect the distribution of drugs. If a drug is highly protein-bound, it may have enhanced pharmacologic or toxic effects in older adults. Other factors that affect distribution are decreases in total body water, lean body mass, and cardiac output.

- **Metabolism Changes** During metabolism, a drug is transformed biochemically to a more water-soluble compound. Older adults may have impaired metabolism, which decreases clearance and allows the drug to accumulate, sometimes to toxic levels. Decline in liver metabolism results from reductions in both enzyme activity and blood flow.

- **Elimination Changes** Elimination by the kidneys decreases because of reduced filtration rate, blood flow, and tubular secretion. The result of decreased kidney elimination of drug products is an increased half-life that may require a reduction in dose of a drug.

As mentioned, older patients are more likely than younger patients to have chronic diseases requiring long-term treatment. Many take from 3 to 12 or more medications, and they tend to have a disproportionate number of **adverse drug reactions** (**ADRs**; see Table 3.5). Maintaining accurate medication profiles is important in these cases. Many ADRs are attributable to antithrombotic, diuretic, and nonsteroidal anti-inflammatory drugs. The pharmacy technician must take special care when dispensing these drugs and double-check the dose and compare it to the patient profile.

A group of drugs that are especially important to monitor for older adult patients is included in the Beers Criteria (commonly called the **Beers List**). This list, which was originally published to provide information on potentially problematic drugs for patients in long-term care facilities, is now useful for older adult patients in other settings. The Beers Criteria continues to grow and is periodically revised. Computer

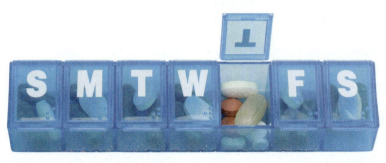

Using tools such as this pillbox will help patients who must take medications daily to remember to take them. The pharmacy technician can help inform patients about such medication management strategies.

TABLE 3.5 Common Adverse Reactions Potentiated in Older Adults

- Central nervous system (CNS) changes (often misdiagnosed as disease manifestations)
- Constipation
- Dermatitis
- Diarrhea
- Drowsiness
- Falls
- GI upset
- Incontinence
- Insomnia
- Rheumatoid symptoms
- Sexual dysfunction
- Urinary retention
- Xerostomia (dry mouth)

databases commonly contain warnings attached to these drugs. A warning does not mean that the patient should not take the drug but rather that drugs on this list should be closely monitored in the older adult population. There is a corresponding Canadian list of drugs that require careful monitoring when used in older adults. Drugs on both lists include amitriptyline (Elavil), reserpine, dipyridamole (Persantine), thioridazine (Mellaril), chlorpromazine (Thorazine), clorazepate (Tranxene), diazepam (Valium), chlordiazepoxide (Librium), and indomethacin (Indocin). There are others, but these are especially important to monitor.

Polypharmacy is the term often used to describe concurrent use of multiple medications. ADRs often result from overprescribing. When many drugs are prescribed for a patient, especially when the patient sees more than one physician, the potential for drug interactions or other problems is high. Owing to the slowing of drug metabolism with aging, older adults can often obtain the desired pharmacologic effect with a much lower dose than is normally prescribed, but this can be difficult to prevent if the patient uses different pharmacies or does not disclose all of their conditions and medications.

Aging can also affect cognitive abilities. An inadequate understanding of the need for the medication and the dosage directions for the medication (e.g., whether it is to be taken with or without food) can lead to failure to take the drug, unintentional overdosing, taking the medication for the wrong reason, or taking drugs prescribed for another person. This failure to adhere to the appropriate drug regimen is referred to as **nonadherence** and is especially prevalent among older adults. Pharmacy technicians can provide invaluable services in this area. They can make sure the patient gets written information and provide aids to dosing and ways to remember to take medication.

The older adult population presents a special challenge for the pharmacy technician and will constitute much of the pharmacy practice. As people age, they may need more drugs to maintain a healthy lifestyle. Patients visit a pharmacy not because they feel well, but rather because they have health problems. They can no longer function as they did when they were younger, and it is the technician who often has to deal with this frustration. Technicians must develop skills that enable them to empathize and effectively communicate with older adults. Successful pharmacy technicians treat older adult patients with respect and understanding.

Special Considerations in Children

Providing drug therapy to children presents a unique set of challenges. As they grow, children undergo profound physiologic changes that affect drug absorption, distribution, metabolism, and elimination. Failure to understand these changes and their effects can lead to underestimating or overestimating drug dosage, with the resultant potential for failure of therapy, severe adverse reactions, or perhaps fatal toxicity.

Age may be the least reliable guide to drug administration in children because of the wide variation in the relationship between age and degree of organ-system development. Height correlates better with lean body mass than does weight. Body surface area may be the best measure because it correlates with all body parameters; however, it is not easily determined. Body weight is most commonly used because of its ease of calculation. Children who are small for their age should receive conservative doses, but larger children may require a dose recommended for the next higher age bracket.

Pediatricians often prescribe an OTC medication for a child without telling the parent how to dose the drug, or they think the dosing instructions will be on the package. A caretaker may purchase the medication only to find that the drug is intended for use in an older child and that appropriate dosage information for a younger or smaller child is not provided with the medication. The pharmacist may have to determine the child's dose for the caretaker. The pharmacy technician should always refer these questions to the pharmacist.

The following considerations are important when dosing children:

- The dosage should be appropriate for the child's age. A dose appropriate for a full-term infant may not be appropriate for a premature infant or a toddler.
- Calculations should be double-checked by the pharmacist and possibly by another pharmacy technician.
- All dosages should be reevaluated at regular intervals.

Allergic Response

An **allergy** is a state of hypersensitivity of the immune system induced by exposure to a particular substance. Many of these substances, called **allergens**, occur naturally in the environment; some are seasonal, some are found in food, whereas others occur in pharmaceutical products. In response to an allergy, the body releases chemicals such as **histamine**, which produces symptoms commonly known as the *allergic reaction*—red, watery eyes; sneezing; urticaria; rash; and bronchiolar constriction—when exposed to these substances. A histamine that causes such symptoms is designated as H_1 and is treated with antihistamines. Gastric mucosal cells release a different type of histamine, known as H_2, which is treated with the H_2 blockers nizatidine (Axid), famotidine (Pepcid), cimetidine (Tagamet), and ranitidine (Zantac) (see Chapter 10). Both antihistamines and H_2 blockers are sold over the counter. Most allergic reactions are not serious, and these drugs can be self-prescribed and administered. However, some allergic reactions can be life-threatening.

The pharmacy technician must be keenly aware that dangerous allergic reactions are a possibility for some medications. One of the most important tasks for the technician is to screen patients for allergies. Allergies must be a part of the patient's medical record, and the technician must always make sure this issue has been addressed before any drugs are dispensed. If the patient has no allergies, the technician enters "NKA" (no known allergies) or "NKDA" (no known drug allergies) into the record. Under no circumstances should this field be left blank either in the computer or on the patient chart.

Teaching Patients Medication Management

The pharmacy technician can play an important role in helping patients learn how to manage medications. If the drug does not enter the body or enters it incorrectly, it will not work as desired. The pharmacy technician can positively affect patient adherence by providing clearly written instructions and aids to implement the process.

Federal law requires that the pharmacy collect the patient's history regarding drugs prescribed as well as side effects and adverse reactions experienced by the patient. The pharmacy technician can positively affect patient drug therapy by accurately collecting and recording the patient's medication history in the patient's profile. The pharmacist filling the prescription is responsible for providing information about the prescription drugs ordered and their proper administration to the patient. The pharmacist can help the patient understand the administration instructions as well as any precautions. The following are specific instructions to emphasize:

- methods for administering the drug
- how to make swallowing easier
- times and time intervals for administration and what to do if a dose is missed
- whether a medication can or should be taken with or without food
- possible side effects and which ones should be reported to the physician
- how long the medication should be taken

It is important that the pharmacy technician explain to patients that the pharmacist is available to answer questions or provide instructions. Also, the technician is allowed to read to the patient the label, medication guide, or educational materials dispensed with the drug—this is *not* counseling and can be very helpful to the patient. However, technicians should read the exact wording of the written information and should bear in mind that they must not offer advice to patients.

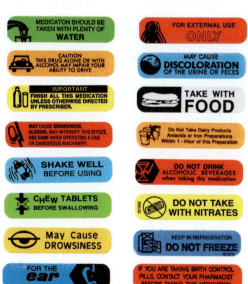

When a patient receives a prescription, it will sometimes include labels that provide instructions for how to self-administer the medication properly. These labels, referred to as *auxiliary labels*, use color and symbols to communicate their message.

Technicians can ensure that patients understand how to read medication labels. Important items to look for include the trade name and/or generic name, the dosage strength, frequency and route of administration, precautions and warnings, and potential interactions. It is important to remember, however, that technicians cannot—by law—counsel patients. Figure 3.5 provides an example of a doctor's prescription and the corresponding medication label that should be affixed to the drug container. The label provides directions that the patient needs to understand and follow. By federal law, many prescriptions require a medication guide, which is an explanation of how the drug works and its potential side effects. Pharmacists must dispense the guide with the drug.

Many drugs that are now available over the counter previously required a prescription. This change occurred because the drugs were found to help with common, uncomplicated problems and carry a relatively low risk of adverse effects. However, it is important that patients read the information provided with these drugs to understand their action, interactions, cautions, and possible side effects. OTC drugs can also interfere with the desired effects of prescription drugs ordered by the prescriber.

FIGURE 3.5
Medication Label Information

The information on a prescription, as shown in

(a), is translated for the patient as instructions on the medication label, as shown in

(b). This label also includes the physician's name and the date the prescription was filled, the drug name, the number of refills, and the pharmacy's address and phone number.

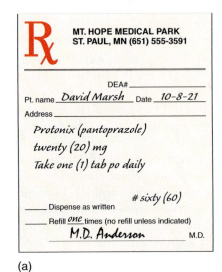

(a)

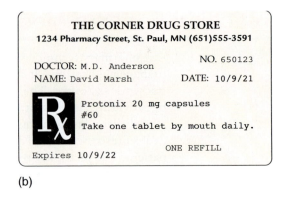

(b)

That is why it is important to obtain information about the patient's OTC drug use as well as information about prescription medications.

A medication regimen can be effective only if the patient or caregiver follows the directions for administration. A care plan may include modifying the patient's lifestyle and keeping medical appointments for follow-up care.

When a patient does not adhere to instructions, there may be a relapse or aggravation of the disease. Hospitalization may then be required, causing healthcare costs to rise. The end result may even be the death of the patient.

Reasons why a patient does not adhere to a care plan can be varied and often complex. They include side effects that cause discomfort, failure to understand the disease, confusion caused by cognitive impairment or the complexity of the regimen, and simple forgetfulness. In general, teenagers and older adults have the highest rates of nonadherence.

Side effects are a common reason for nonadherence. If a medication produces discomfort, the patient may discontinue its use. Although side effects of some medications subside as the drugs are continuously used, others may persist. It is important to educate patients about the importance and benefits of medication and potential side effects in order to promote adherence. Patients may be willing to tolerate some side effects if they are aware of them and understand that they will experience relief over the long term. For this reason, side effects should be addressed initially. The pharmacist should inform patients of potential side effects, the importance of correct dosing, what to do if an adverse effect occurs, and how to monitor treatment.

Lack of reliable information regarding disease states or medication treatments can be another barrier to adherence. Patients who do not understand how a drug may improve their disease state will be at a higher risk of nonadherence than patients who have some understanding of drug action and can see how the treatment will affect their disease. Patients lacking sufficient knowledge of their disease and the drug therapy for the disease may not understand the importance of consistent use. Thus, healthcare professionals should educate patients about their disease so that they will understand the drug therapy required. This education should include information about the assumed benefits of the drug regimen, side effects, and the consequences of failing to follow the drug regimen.

Adherence decreases as the number of daily medications and the complexity of the regimen increase. Multiple medications, multiple instructions regarding medications, and drugs that have to be taken at a certain time of the day or several different times of the day, and with (or without) food may all confuse the patient, resulting in poor adherence. The result may be missed doses and a less-than-desired therapeutic response, or an increased risk of ADRs and hospitalization. With a simpler regimen, there is a greater chance of patient adherence. Consequently, pharmacists and prescribers should evaluate therapeutic alternatives that ensure patient adherence. Patients with cognitive impairment that affects their ability to understand and follow directions concerning their drugs will be at a higher risk of nonadherence.

Forgetfulness is another reason for lack of adherence. Pharmacy technicians can encourage patients to use various kinds of reminders to aid their memory. Reminders may include taking medications at the time certain daily tasks are performed, placing colored stickers on the calendar after the medication is taken, using pillboxes with daily compartments, setting watches with alarms, using pill bottle cap alarms or other electronic devices, and using technology such as mobile device reminders and applications.

Above all, patients need to monitor their own medication regimens. Pharmacists and pharmacy technicians are in a position to build a trusting relationship in which the patient is generally willing to accept recommendations to promote adherence.

Medication Safety

Ensuring that patients receive the correct medication at the correct dosage and that a newly prescribed medication does not adversely interact with other drugs that a patient is taking are extremely important. Several procedures are in place to help ensure medication safety, and the pharmacy technician plays a role in these.

The FDA is authorized to require drug manufacturers to have **Risk Evaluation and Mitigation Strategy (REMS)** programs. The goal of REMS programs is to ensure that the benefits of a drug outweigh its risks. These REMS programs may be as simple as dispensing a medication guide to a patient, or they may involve special dispensing and/or prescribing requirements. REMS programs may require prescribers and dispensing pharmacists to complete training regarding certain drugs, and technicians may need to take special steps when dispensing the drug. REMS programs may vary from state to state, but the technician needs to be aware of REMS programs and the goals behind them.

Technician Role

Technicians are an integral part of the medication dispensing process, and pharmacists rely heavily on them to prevent and catch errors. Properly trained and educated technicians can make a tremendous difference in the quality of care a patient receives. Technicians must verify the patient's address, date of birth, phone numbers, allergies, and conditions such as pregnancy. Another role of the technician is to make sure the patient gets proper counseling from the pharmacist. This counseling process is very important in minimizing errors.

E-Prescribing

E-prescribing is a method of prescribing medications electronically. A prescriber enters a prescription into a computer program that communicates directly with a computer program at a designated pharmacy. E-prescribing eliminates the need for a written prescription and can potentially reduce errors and improve patient safety by

TABLE 3.6 Drugs That Should Be Dispensed in Original Containers

Brand Name	Generic Name
Accolate	zafirlukast
Afinitor	everolimus
Aggrenox	dipyridamole and aspirin
Atripla	efavirenz, emtricitabine, tenofovir
Augmentin—chewable and oral suspension	amoxicillin-clavulanate
Creon, Pancrease, Zenpep, Viokase	pancrelipase
Crixivan	indinavir
Edarbi	azilsartan—and any combination of this drug
Effient	prasugrel
Ella	ulipristal
Hepsera	adefovir
Horizant	gabapentin
Intelence	etravirine
Kuvan	sapropterin
Mephyton	phytonadione
Nitrostat	nitroglycerin
Norvir	ritonavir
Pradaxa	dabigatran
Procardia	nifedipine
Sandimmune, Neoral, Gengraf	cyclosporine—capsules and oral solution
Tekturna	aliskiren—and any combination of this drug
Treximet	sumatriptan and naproxen
Trileptal	oxcarbazepine
Truvada	emtricitabine, tenofovir
Tyzeka	telbivudine
Viread	tenofovir

Note: Drugs such as those that come in blister packs, drugs packaged in 30- or 90-day supplies, and powdered drugs to which water must be added, are not included in this list.

eliminating illegible prescriptions and automatically checking for allergies, interactions, dosing errors, and therapeutic duplications. Accidental selection of the wrong drug, dose, or dosage form in the computer program by the prescriber could, however, create a new source of errors. E-prescribing is also costly because of the expense of installing appropriate computer programs.

Physician Order Entry

In hospitals, where physicians enter prescriptions into a database or electronic health record, a decrease in errors has been documented. This is called **computerized physician order entry (CPOE)** or prescriber order entry, and is different from e-prescribing. In physician order entry, the prescriber (physician or other qualified prescriber) personally enters drug orders (as opposed to pharmacists or other professionals) that are then verified and dispensed by pharmacy personnel.

Dispensing Cautions

For safety reasons, some medications must be dispensed in their original containers. Most of these drugs are affected by light or moisture or can only be stored in glass containers. Patients cannot receive a partial prescription of any of these medications, because this would require them to be repackaged—and doing so might affect the drug. In some cases, the pharmacist or pharmacy technician should not handle the drugs. Table 3.6 lists these medications.

Tamper-Resistant Pads

Prescribers who file for Medicaid reimbursement must use tamper-resistant pads for written prescriptions. If a tamper-resistant pad has not been used, the technician must call and verify the prescription. The technician then documents the date and time of the call, the name of the person who verified it, and the technician's initials on the prescription. This regulation is intended to encourage the use of e-prescribing.

Medication Reconciliation

One critical goal for community and hospital pharmacies is to share information from patient profiles—a process known as **medication reconciliation**. Such sharing of health information is allowed under the privacy provisions in Title II of the Health Insurance Portability and Accountability Act (HIPAA) and is part of the continuum of care and the effort to improve patient safety as patients move from one level of care to another. Studies show that patients are most vulnerable during transitions of care from one level of care to another when many medication errors occur. This applies to transitions that occur between hospitals, between hospital and community, and within a hospital, a rehabilitation center, an assisted living facility, or other healthcare facility. Hospitals should communicate drug regimen information to the patient's next care setting. In the future, retail pharmacies will receive greater numbers of calls from providers who need this information. Pharmacy technicians play a major role in making these transitions safer.

Understanding the Profession

So now you've explored the history of pharmacology, its basic theories and practices, and the process of filling prescriptions. Are you ready to commit to this career?

The remainder of this book and course will introduce you to the various body systems and the diseases and conditions that can negatively affect a person, as well as the medications that can cure or lessen the severity of those conditions.

Along the way, you will also be presented with opportunities to stretch your understanding of medical topics and to realize what it means to be a member of the profession. Through the questions and activities on the Course Navigator, you will explore ethical decisions, the demands of effective communication, cultural differences, interpersonal relationships, and more.

As you pursue your studies, keep in mind your ultimate goals, one of which is obtaining certification as a pharmacy technician. Another is securing employment in your profession. This book and its accompanying online content are designed to help you reach those goals as well as understand your potential for career advancement. Be sure to check with your instructor about the variety of materials available with this textbook that are related to career preparation and professionalism as a pharmacy technician. Also, familiarize yourself with the Pharmacy Technician Certification Board (PTCB), the American Association of Pharmacy Technicians (AAPT), and the National Pharmacy Technician Association (NPTA). These organizations offer highly informative websites for the pharmacy technician as well as other resources you will likely find helpful as you advance in your chosen career.

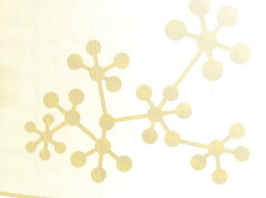

CHAPTER SUMMARY

The Prescription

- A request for the dispensing of medication to a patient is called an *order* in a hospital setting; outside the hospital setting it is called a *prescription*.

- To fill a prescription or order, the pharmacy technician must understand the meanings of abbreviations. Certain abbreviations should not be used on prescriptions or instructions because there is extensive evidence to document them as the source of medication errors.

Correct Drug Administration "Rights"

- The "rights" for correct drug administration are the right patient, the right drug, the right strength, the right route, the right time, and the right documentation.

Dosage Forms and Routes of Administration

- The three primary routes of administration are oral, parenteral, and topical. The pharmacy technician must be familiar with each dosage form. The most common are:

oral (po)	parenteral	topical
capsules	epidural injections	creams
solutions	intramuscular (IM) injections	gels
suspensions	intravenous (IV) injections	inhalants
syrups	subcutaneous injections	lotions
tablets		ointments
		patches
		suppositories

Factors That Influence Drug Action

- Altered drug responses in older adults are due to age-related changes in organ function and body composition. These physiologic changes include visual, auditory, gastrointestinal, pulmonary, cardiovascular, renal, hormonal, and body composition alterations.

- Some special problems of older adults are poor nutrition, adverse drug reactions, and poor adherence with drug regimens.

- Body surface area is the best measure to use in determining dosage for children, but it is difficult to ascertain; consequently, weight is most frequently used.

- Allergic reactions are a dangerous possibility for some medications, and are thus a vital piece of information in the patient's record.

- An important role for the pharmacy technician is recording patient allergies.

Teaching Patients Medication Management

- Patient adherence with the dose schedule and the specific requirements of a drug regimen is important.

- A pharmacy technician can positively influence patient drug therapy by accurately collecting and recording the patient's medication history in the patient profile.

- Pharmacy technicians can help patients understand how to read medication labels.

- Patients should read the information provided with OTC drugs to understand their action, interactions, cautions, and possible side effects.

- Pharmacy technicians cannot counsel patients about their medications and regimens, but they can recommend pharmacist counseling and explain the materials that accompany a medication.

Medication Safety

- E-prescribing helps eliminate errors related to poorly written prescriptions.

- Hospitals that use physician order entry have documented a decrease in errors.

- Medication reconciliation, a national patient safety goal, will prevent many errors by increasing accuracy of medication history as patients transition between care settings.

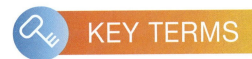 KEY TERMS

adherence a patient's compliance with the dose schedule and other particular requirements of the specified regimen

adverse drug reaction (ADR) an unexpected negative consequence from taking a particular drug

allergens particular substances that cause allergies

allergy a state of heightened sensitivity as a result of exposure to a particular substance

Beers Criteria a list of drugs for which monitoring is especially important in older adult patients; Beers List

buccal administration route via the mucous membrane between the cheek and the gums

computerized physician order entry (CPOE) a database entry for prescriptions records

enema a liquid that is injected in the rectum

e-prescribing the process of transmitting an electronic prescription directly from prescriber to pharmacy

histamine a chemical produced by the body that evokes the symptoms of an allergic reaction

hypoxia reduction of oxygen in the blood

incontinence the inability to retain urine in the bladder

inhalation administration of a medication through the respiratory system

inscription part of a prescription that identifies the name of the drug, the dose, and the quantities of the ingredients

instillation administration of a medication drop by drop

institutional setting facilities that assume total care of patients

intradermal injected into the skin

intramuscular (IM) injected into a muscle

intraspinal injected into the spinal column

intrathecal see intraspinal

intravenous (IV) administration of a medication through a vein, thereby avoiding the first-pass effect

local infection an infection restricted to or pertaining to one area of the body

medication reconciliation the process of obtaining a complete and accurate drug profile for a patient at each transition of care

nephrons glomerulotubular unit that is the working unit of the kidney

nonadherence the failure to adhere to a drug regimen

noninstitutional settings facilities such as clinics or community pharmacies that offer same day patient care

nonpathologic not related to disease

ophthalmic to be administered through the eye

oral see peroral (po)

order a prescription issued in an institutional setting; also referred to as a *medication order*

otic administered in the ear

parenteral administered by injection rather than by way of the alimentary canal

peroral (po) administration of a medication by mouth in either solid form, as a tablet or capsule, or in liquid form, as a solution or syrup; often referred to as *oral route*

polypharmacy the concurrent use of multiple medications

prescription a direction for medication to be dispensed to a patient, written by a physician or a qualified licensed practitioner and filled by a pharmacist; referred to as an *order* when the medication is requested in a hospital setting

Risk Evaluation and Mitigation Strategy (REMS) FDA-mandated programs for prescribing, dispensing, or taking certain drugs in order to manage associated risks

Rx the symbol for a drug prescription

signa part of a prescription that provides directions to be included on the label for the patient to follow in taking the medication

solution an active drug that is dissolved in liquid

subcutaneous (SC, SQ, Subcut) injected into the tissue just beneath the skin

sublingual administration route via mucous membrane under the tongue

suspension active drug particles that are mixed, but not dissolved, in liquid

systemic pertaining to or affecting the body as a whole

topical applied to the surface of the skin or mucous membranes

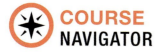
COURSE NAVIGATOR

Access interactive chapter review exercises, practice activities, flash cards, and study games.

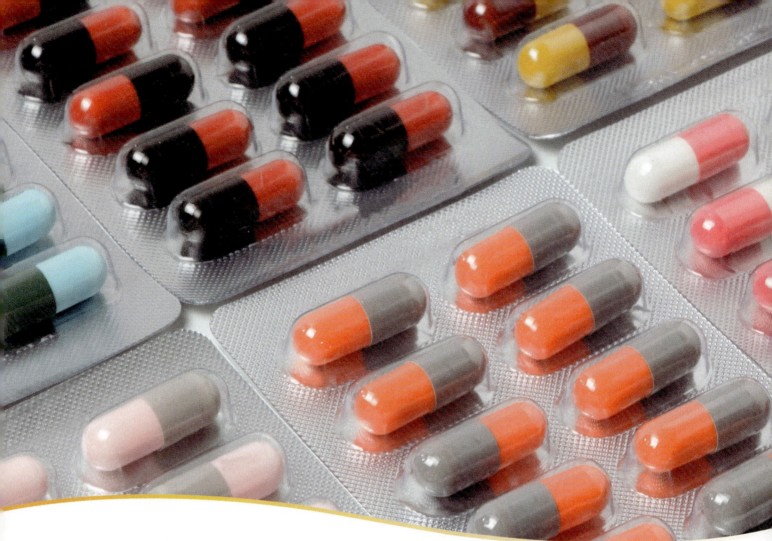

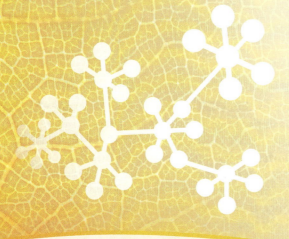

4

Antibiotics and Antifungals

Learning Objectives

1 Describe the differences between bacteria and fungi.

2 Identify the major types of antibiotics by drug class.

3 Determine which auxiliary labels to use when dispensing major types of antibiotics and antifungals.

4 Define therapeutic effects, side effects, contraindications, and administration routes of major antibiotics and antifungals.

5 Utilize appropriate antibiotic and antifungal general drug terminology in written and oral communication.

6 Describe treatments for common sexually transmitted infections.

7 Discuss storage requirements of liquid antibiotics.

8 List common ophthalmic antibiotics.

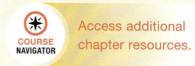

COURSE NAVIGATOR Access additional chapter resources.

The immune system is a complex network of barriers, organs, and molecules that has evolved over millions of years to work in concert to defend the body against invading pathogens. Before the 20th century, infection was the most common cause of death in the United States. The development of antibiotics and vaccines have helped treat and prevent infection.

The purpose of this chapter is to describe the immune system and explain the use of antimicrobial agents in treating bacterial infections that commonly afflict this system. Various bacteria are described along with the typical infections they cause. The number of antimicrobial drugs is large and varied, making this a long chapter. However, knowing these drugs will be useful because pharmacy technicians work with such medications in hospital and community pharmacy settings. Antibiotics are frequently dispensed for community-acquired infections, which account for more outpatient visits to physicians than any other medical condition. They are also used for infections acquired in hospital or institutional setting (nosocomial infections).

Fighting Bacterial Infections

Bacteria are single-celled organisms that live in almost all environments. For example, many bacteria can be found on the skin and in the bowels at all times. These skin and bowel organisms only cause disease when they either grow out of control or gain entry to the blood. Other bacteria are harmful (**pathogenic**) whenever they invade the body.

Sometimes, pathogenic bacteria produce toxins that cause many of the signs and symptoms experienced when infection is present. When bacteria penetrate body tissues, they sometimes establish an **infection**, in which their presence or toxins can cause tissue damage. The body's immune system fights back to destroy the bacteria, usually resulting in fever and inflammation. The body can overcome many simple infections, but more serious infections often require the assistance of antibiotics to kill the invaders.

Although infectious diseases have been known to exist for thousands of years, it was not until the 19th century that a major cause—bacteria—was identified through the work of Louis Pasteur and other scientists. By the early 20th century, the organisms that cause cholera, syphilis, bubonic plague, gonorrhea, leprosy, and other illnesses had been isolated and identified.

In 1907, German physician Paul Ehrlich patented the drug arsphenamine as a treatment for syphilis. Although this drug marked a breakthrough in eradicating a major infectious disease, it was not until 1936 that the first true antibiotic, sulfanilamide (a sulfonamide), was discovered. When penicillin became widely available in the 1940s, physicians finally had a powerful weapon to use against several common infections, including strep throat, pneumonia, and syphilis. Today, a wide variety of antibiotics are used to combat bacteria-caused infections. Each drug is effective against specific kinds of bacteria.

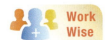

Work Wise

Many times bacteria names are abbreviated in the workplace. For example, you may hear *Streptococcus pneumoniae* called "Strep. pneumo." *Clostridium difficile* can be called "C. diff" and *Escherichia coli* is often referred to as "E. coli."

Types of Bacteria

Determining the appropriate antibiotic to use against a specific bacterium requires laboratory testing. A sample of material obtained from the infected area is stained, observed under the microscope, and classified according to characteristics that help determine the drug to prescribe.

Bacteria are either **aerobic**, which means they need oxygen to live, or **anaerobic**, meaning they can survive in an environment void of oxygen. Bacteria are also classified by their shape (see Figure 4.1) and arrangement of growth. If bacterial cells grow in chains or lines, their name begins with "strep." If they grow in clusters, their name begins with "staph." If they grow in pairs, their name begins with "diplo." For instance, *Staphylococcus aureus*, a common bacterium found on the skin, is round and grows in clusters like grapes. See Table 4.1 for more information.

FIGURE 4.1
Characteristic Bacterial Shapes

Spherical bacteria (a) are called *cocci*. Rod-shaped bacteria (b) are called *bacilli*. Spiral-shaped bacteria (c) are *spirochetes*. *Streptococcus pyogenes*, the bacteria that cause strep throat, is round and grows in chains.

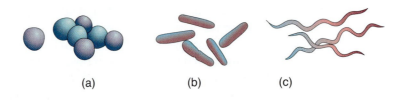

(a)   (b)   (c)

Finally, bacteria are said to be either *Gram-positive* or *Gram-negative*. This classification comes from a staining technique named after its developer, Hans Christian Joachim Gram. In this technique, a purple stain called crystal violet is applied to the

TABLE 4.1   Common Bacteria and Infections

Gram Stain	Shape	Bacteria	Associated Infection(s)
Aerobic			
Positive	Cocci	*Streptococcus pneumoniae*	Respiratory tract infection (RTI) and/or pneumonia
		Streptococcus pyogenes (Group A)	Strep throat
Positive	Cocci	*Staphylococcus aureus and other Staphylococcus spp.*	Skin infection Endocarditis
Positive	Cocci	*Enterococcus faecalis, faecium*	Intestinal infection, urinary tract infection (UTI)
Positive	Bacilli	*Bacillus anthracis*	Anthrax
Positive	Bacilli	*Gardnerella vaginalis Lactobacillus spp.*	Vaginal infections
Positive	Bacilli	*Listeria monocytogenes*	Meningitis
Positive	Bacilli	*Clostridium tetani* *Clostridium perfringens* *Clostridium botulinum* *Clostridium difficile*	Tetanus Gangrene Botulism Intestinal infection
Positive	Bacilli	*Corynebacterium diphtheriae*	Diphtheria
Negative	Cocci	*Neisseria meningitidis* *Neisseria gonorrhea*	Meningitis Gonorrhea
Negative	Bacilli	*Escherichia coli* *Klebsiella spp.* *Proteus spp.* *Enterobacter spp.* *Shigella spp.*	Intestinal infection
Negative	Bacilli	*Salmonella typhi*	Typhoid fever
Negative	Bacilli	*Yersinia pestis*	Plague
Negative	Bacilli	*Pseudomonas aeruginosa*	Various difficult-to-treat infections
Negative	Bacilli	*Haemophilus influenzae*	RTI
Negative	Bacilli	*Vibrio cholerae*	Cholera
Negative	Coccobacilli	*Bordetella pertussis*	Pertussis
Negative	Coccobacilli	*Helicobacter pylori*	Stomach ulcers
Anaerobic			
	Cocci	*Peptococcus, Streptopeptococcus*	Dental infection
	Bacilli	*Bacteroides fragilis*	Abdominal infection Sepsis
Miscellaneous			
Spirochetes		*Treponema pallidum* *Borrelia burgdorferi*	Syphilis Lyme disease
Atypical		*Mycoplasma pneumonia* *Legionella spp.*	RTI and/or pneumonia

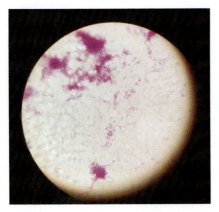

This photo shows Gram-positive bacteria through a microscope.

bacteria, and then they are viewed under a microscope. **Gram-positive bacteria** have a thick cell wall that absorbs this stain and appears purple. **Gram-negative bacteria** have a thin cell wall that does not absorb this stain.

Symptoms of Bacterial Infections

The general signs that an infection may be of bacterial origin are a fever of 101°F or higher and an increased number of white blood cells (>12,000/mm^3). The onset of fever alone, however, is not diagnostic of a bacterial infection. A fever may also be caused by a self-limiting viral illness or by some types of malignancy and auto-immune disorders. In many situations, localizing symptoms or physical findings are necessary to explain the fever.

Antibiotic Treatment and Action

An **antibiotic** is a chemical substance with the ability to kill or inhibit the growth of microorganisms. In developing antibiotics, the challenge is to find a way to kill the invading organism without harming the patient receiving treatment. This mission is easier to accomplish with bacteria than with other kinds of pathogens because many biological processes are unique to bacteria and not shared by humans. Antibiotics work by gaining access to the inside of the bacterial cell and interfering with these unique biological processes in one of six ways:

- preventing folic acid synthesis (sulfonamides)
- impairing cell-wall formation (penicillins and cephalosporins)
- blocking protein formation (macrolides, tetracyclines, and aminoglycosides)
- interfering with deoxyribonucleic acid (DNA) formation (quinolones)
- disrupting cell membranes (daptomycin)
- disrupting DNA structure (metronidazole)

Physicians and other healthcare providers prescribe antibiotics based on the type of pathogen that is suspected to be causing the infection, the antibiotic's spectrum of activity, and the location of the pathogen. An antibiotic's **spectrum of activity** is the range of bacteria against which it is effective. For example, penicillin can cover Gram-positive, aerobic bacteria, so it could be used for infections caused by Gram-positive, aerobic bacteria, such as *Streptococcus pyogenes* (strep throat). To identify the bacteria and facilitate the choice of drug treatment, a sample or swab of the bacteria is taken from the patient and grown in culture in the laboratory. Then, various antibiotics are tested on the culture to determine which drug has the best effect on the pathogen. This laboratory test is called a **culture and sensitivity (C&S)** test. The amount of drug needed to inhibit growth of

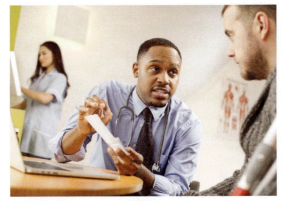

A physician informs his patients of the risk of developing antibiotic resistance.

the bacteria is called the **minimum inhibitory concentration (MIC)**, a result often reported along with the C&S results.

When a patient has a serious or life-threatening infection, an antibiotic treatment must begin immediately. In this situation, the patient is given a **broad-spectrum antibiotic**, which is effective against multiple organisms. This is referred to as **empirical treatment**.

Nosocomial infections, or healthcare-associated infections, are those that are acquired while in a hospital or nursing home and are often drug resistant and difficult to treat. In these cases, the common first choice of therapy cannot be used because the bacteria are already known to be resistant. Because these infections can be serious and even life-threatening, aggressive antibiotics may be warranted. In these cases, more powerful drugs would be started empirically and therapy would be modified based on C&S results.

The choice of route of administration (e.g., oral, intravenous [IV], intramuscular [IM]) for antibiotic therapy depends on the site and severity of the infection as well as the bacteria suspected to be causing it. In most cases, antibiotics are best given at even intervals throughout the day. In children, antibiotics are often dosed for an entire day, based on the child's weight, but are given in divided doses. Doses provided in this text are presented as general guides for recognizing when a prescribed dose is out of the ordinary. Always refer to the package insert or other reliable sources to verify proper dosing and double-check dose calculations for children.

An antibiotic may be either a **bactericidal agent**, which kills the invading organisms, or a **bacteriostatic agent**, which inhibits the growth or multiplication of bacteria. Preferably, antibiotic treatment is started after the bacteria have been identified by culturing. The outcome of antibiotic treatment can be evaluated in two ways: (1) the clinical response, meaning the signs and symptoms disappear, or (2) the microbiologic response, meaning the organism is completely eradicated. Bacterial infections are contagious until antibiotics have been administered for 24 to 48 hours. Viral infections are not treated by antibiotics.

Side Effects and Dispensing Issues of Antibiotics

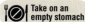

The parenteral forms of antibiotics should be mixed exactly as directed by the manufacturers. If mixed inappropriately, the drugs can be ineffective or may cause tissue or vein irritation, renal failure, or even death. When dispensing oral forms of these drugs, it is important to swab the counting tray with alcohol before placing a new drug on the tray to prevent cross-contamination, especially with penicillin and sulfa drugs. For example, if a tray used to dispense sulfa is not wiped down before another drug is placed on the tray, sulfa particles could stick to the new drug, potentially resulting in an adverse reaction if the drug is given to a patient who is allergic to sulfa.

Some antibiotics can cause extreme gastrointestinal (GI) upset, and the manufacturer may recommend that these drugs be taken with food. For most antibiotics, however, taking with food slows absorption of the drug. Therefore, the technician should not make this recommendation or place a "take with food" sticker on an antibiotic unless prompted to do so by the computer or patient handouts.

Another important piece of information about antibiotic agents is that they can interfere with the action of birth control pills and reduce the effectiveness of this contraceptive. The patient should be made aware of this and be warned to use backup contraception while taking the antibiotic.

To maintain consistent drug serum levels, ideally antibiotics should be administered around the clock. An IV administration route can facilitate around-the-clock dosing for very ill patients. Otherwise, spacing the dosage evenly throughout the day will suffice to maintain a relatively constant drug serum level.

Antimicrobial Resistance

When choosing appropriate drug therapy, the prescriber must also take into account **antibiotic resistance**. Bacteria have the ability to develop defense mechanisms that resist or inactivate antibiotics used on them. For instance, many bacteria that cause common respiratory tract infections (RTIs) are now resistant to the most frequently used drugs, like **amoxicillin**. Antibiotic resistance is a growing problem as we use more and more of these common drugs. If a patient were to develop an infection that was resistant to the most powerful antibiotics, no therapy would exist to treat the infection, a grim situation that could cause death. To help prevent antibiotic resistance, prescribers must be mindful of using appropriate antibiotics only when necessary.

The pharmacy technician's role in preventing overuse of antibiotics is to ensure that all antibiotic prescriptions display an auxiliary label on the bottle that advises the patient to take all of the medication. Because prescriptions for antibiotics have begun to stipulate **dose loading** on the front end, the patient will be instructed that, after the initial dose, successive doses will be smaller. In any event, it is important that the patient complete the prescribed course of medication and not save or share any of the medication.

Major Classes of Antibiotic Drugs

Before 1935, systemic bacterial infections could not be effectively treated with drugs. An infection could be attacked topically with an **antiseptic** (a substance that kills or inhibits the growth of microorganisms on the outside of the body) or a **disinfectant** (an agent that destroys infectious organisms on nonliving objects), but these chemicals could not be used systemically because they were not safe enough. With the discovery of sulfonamides in 1935, a new era began. Since that time, several additional classes of antibiotics have been discovered. All drugs in each class of antibiotics have some similarities in their molecular structure.

Sulfonamides and Nitrofurantoin

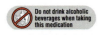

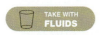

Sulfonamides, or sulfa drugs, are one of the oldest antibiotics on the market and are effective against a broad spectrum of microorganisms. Sulfonamides are bacteriostatic and work by blocking bacteria from making folic acid, an essential substance for survival. Although humans can absorb folic acid from food, bacteria cannot, and thus must make folic acid. Table 4.2 lists the most commonly used sulfonamines.

Sulfa drugs are used most often to treat urinary tract infections (UTIs). The most common sulfa drug is a combination containing **sulfamethoxazole and trimethoprim**. This combination is especially good for UTIs caused by *Escherichia coli*. Sulfa drugs are also used to treat community-acquired methicillin-resistant *Staphylococcus aureus* (MRSA) skin infections and as

FIGURE 4.2
Macrobid Label

Nitrofurantoin is sold under several names, one of them being Macrobid

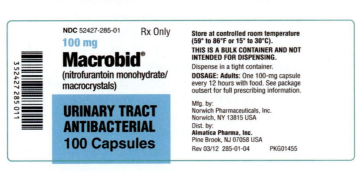

prophylaxis against *Pneumocystis carinii* pneumonia, a common deadly lung infection in patients who have end-stage acquired immunodeficiency syndrome (AIDS).

Like sulfa drugs, nitrofurantoin is used to treat UTIs (see Figure 4.2). Its mechanism of action is not well understood, but its spectrum of activity is similar to that of sulfonamides. It works best if taken with food and plenty of fluids. Table 4.2 lists dosing information for common sulfonamides and nitrofurantoin. Nitrofurantoin may be an appropriate alternative in patients with UTI that are unable to use sulfa drugs.

TABLE 4.2 Commonly Used Sulfonamides and Nitrofurantoin

Generic (Brand)	Pronunciation	Dosage Form	Dispensing Status	Common Dosage
nitrofurantoin (Macrobid, Macrodantin)	nye-troe-fyoor-AN-toyn	Capsule, oral liquid	Rx	Adult: 50–100 mg 1–4 times a day Pediatric: 5–6 mg/kg/day in divided doses
sulfamethoxazole-trimethoprim (Bactrim, Bactrim DS, Septra, Septra DS)	sul-fa-meth-OX-a-zole trye-METH-oh-prim	IV, oral suspension, tablet	Rx	Varies depending on age and infection treated

Therapeutic Uses Sulfonamides are commonly used for the following illnesses and some specific bacteria:

- UTIs
- otitis media (middle ear infection), especially in children
- lower respiratory tract infections
- prophylaxis in *Pneumocystis carinii* pneumonia in immunocompromised patients.

Side Effects and Dispensing Issues Sulfa drugs in use today cause fewer allergic reactions than older sulfa drugs did. The most common side effect is a rash. Other side effects include nausea, drug fever (often confused with a recurrent fever from the infection), vomiting, jaundice, blood complications (acute hemolytic anemia, agranulocytosis, and aplastic anemia), and kidney damage. **Stevens-Johnson syndrome**—a reaction that can be fatal, marked by large red blotches on the skin—can occur from use of sulfas.

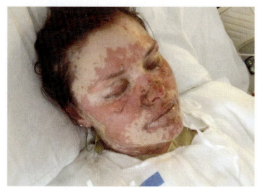

Stevens-Johnson syndrome, a potentially fatal reaction, can occur with the use of sulfa drugs.

If a rash occurs, the patient should stop taking the drug immediately. Sulfa drugs should have a label warning patients to avoid the sun, which can cause severe skin rashes. Sulfonamides can crystallize in the urine and deposit in the kidneys, resulting in a painful, dangerous condition. To reduce this risk, it is important that a patient taking sulfa drugs maintain an adequate fluid intake of at least six to eight glasses a day. The technician should always place an auxiliary label on sulfonamides and related drugs reminding the patient to drink lots of water or other fluids.

Because of the incidence of sulfa drug allergies, technicians should be careful to wipe down counting trays containing sulfa in an effort to prevent cross-contamination of the next drug used on the tray.

Nitrofurantoin use may also cause nausea or vomiting. A unique side effect is urine discoloration (nitrofurantoin makes the urine appear brown). Nitrofurantoin may cause false urine glucose tests.

Contraindications **Sulfamethoxazole-trimethoprim** is contraindicated in patients with a history of drug-induced immune thrombocytopenia; in megaloblastic **anemia** (a below-normal concentration of erythrocytes or hemoglobin in the blood) due to folate deficiency; in infants younger than two months of age; and in marked liver or kidney dysfunction.

Contraindications to nitrofurantoin include anuria (producing no urine), oliguria (having little urine), or significant impairment of kidney function; previous history of jaundice or hepatic dysfunction associated with prior nitrofurantoin use; pregnant patients at term, during labor and delivery, or when the onset of labor is imminent; and in neonates younger than one month of age.

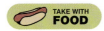

Cautions and Considerations Taking sulfa drugs with food can help alleviate the common side effects of nausea and vomiting. Sulfa allergy is common, so pharmacy technicians should always inquire about drug allergies when dispensing a sulfa drug.

Administering nitrofurantoin with food may improve absorption and decrease side effects. Nitrofurantoin turns urine brown. Patients should be alerted to this harmless but sometimes alarming effect.

Drug Interactions Sulfamethoxazole-trimethoprim may cause a condition called **long QT syndrome** (or **QT prolongation**) when combined with other drugs that lengthen the QT interval. Long QT syndrome is a heart rhythm disorder that can cause life-threatening cardiac **arrhythmias** (irregular heart beat). Drugs that prolong QT interval and increase risk include antiarrhythmic agents (such as amiodarone, bretylium, disopyramide, dofetilide, procainaide, quinidine, and sotalol), chlorpromazine, cisapride, dolastron, droperidol, mefloquine, moxifloxacin, tacrolimus, and ziprasidone. Sulfamethoxazole-trimethoprim may decrease the effectiveness of live vaccines (discussed later in this chapter) when coadministered.

Nitrofurantoin use may decrease the effectiveness of the antibiotic norfloxacin. Concurrent alcohol use should be avoided because of the risk of central nervous system (CNS) depression.

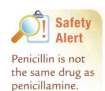

Safety Alert

Penicillin is not the same drug as penicillamine.

Penicillins

Penicillins were one of the first groups of antibiotics used in the treatment of bacterial infections and are obtained from the mold *Penicillium chrysogenum*. There are many different types of penicillins, and they mainly treat infections caused by Gram-positive bacteria (see Table 4.1 on page 69). These antibiotics kill bacteria by inhibiting the formation of their cell wall, and the weakened cell wall allows an excessive amount of water to enter the bacterium through osmosis. The cell increases in size and lyses (bursts), as the cell membrane cannot contain the cell contents. Human cells do not have rigid cell walls; therefore, they are not affected by penicillins. Some bacteria, however, are resistant to penicillins because the pathogens produce an enzyme called **beta-lactamase**, which destroys the beta-lactam ring present in the molecular structure of all penicillins. This action renders the drug inactive. For this reason, some penicillin products are available as a combination of penicillin with a **beta-lactamase inhibitor**. Table 4.3 lists commonly used penicillins.

Safety Alert

Up to 10% of patients in the United States report penicillin allergies. Although true penicillin allergies are serious and can be life-threatening, many self-reported allergies are in fact adverse drug reactions and not an allergic reaction. If you are taking a patient history, specifically ask what his or her reaction is to the offending agent. If a patient reports mild stomach upset or diarrhea, common side effects of penicillins, you may want to investigate the allergy claim.

Therapeutic Uses of Penicillin Penicillin is most active against growing and reproducing bacteria—generally Gram-positive aerobes and anaerobes. Penicillin and penicillin derivatives are among the drugs of choice for the following illnesses and some specific bacteria listed in Table 4.3:

- abscesses
- beta-hemolytic streptococcus
- meningitis
- otitis media
- pneumonia
- respiratory tract infections
- Strep pharyngitis
- tooth and gum infections
- sexually transmitted infections (STIs; syphilis and gonorrhea)
- endocarditis (heart valve infection) due to streptococci

Penicillin and other antibiotics have also been shown to reduce risk of disease or death for patients with subacute bacterial endocarditis, an inflammation of the lining of the heart and its valves. These patients are at risk any time a body cavity is invaded.

Preventative dosing, or prophylaxis, with penicillins may be recommended when a patient with certain conditions undergoes any kind of surgical procedure, including higher risk dental procedures. Amoxicillin is often used for patients who can use oral medication. In the case of penicillin allergy, cephalexin, clindamycin, azithromycin, or clarithromycin may be used.

Side Effects and Dispensing Issues Common side effects of penicillins include stomach upset and diarrhea. Taking them with food can help with these side effects; however, this may decrease absorption. Other rare but more severe side effects include mental disturbances, seizures, kidney damage, and bleeding abnormalities. These particular side effects tend to occur more often at higher doses and when the doses are administered by IV infusion.

Contraindications Most penicillin contraindications are associated with hypersensitivity. If a person has a true hypersensitivity to one type of penicillin, use of the others is contraindicated. **Amoxicillin-clavulanate** is contraindicated in patients with liver dysfunction and severe renal impairment.

Cautions and Considerations **Penicillin G benzathine** carries a black box warning that says it is not for IV use. Cardiopulmonary arrest and death have occurred, and the product should only be administered by deep IM injection.

Many patients who are allergic to penicillin may also be allergic to cephalosporins, another class of antibiotics that inhibits cell-wall formation. Therefore, pharmacy technicians should always inquire about all drug allergies when taking a patient's medication history or when preparing to administer penicillins or cephalosporins.

Oral penicillins work best when taken on an empty stomach, but if stomach upset occurs, they can be taken with food. Advise patients to avoid taking these medications with acidic beverages such as fruit juice or carbonated drinks such as cola products because the acid in these beverages can deactivate the drug. Instruct patients to shake oral suspensions well before every dose. Most of these suspensions must also be refrigerated. Suspensions prepared with water are good for only 14 days from the mixing date. Any medication left over after treatment should be disposed of properly.

TABLE 4.3 Common Penicillins

Generic (Brand)	Pronunciation	Dosage Form	Common Dosage	Dispensing Status
Aminopenicillins				
amoxicillin (Amoxil, Moxatag)	a-mox-i-SIL-in	Capsule, chewable tablet, oral suspension, tablet	Adult: 250–875 mg taken 2–3 times a day Pediatric: 20–90 mg/kg/day in divided doses	Rx
ampicillin	am-pi-SIL-in	Capsule, injection, oral suspension	Pediatric: 50-100 mg/kg/day divided every 6 hours, oral dose. IM, IV: dose varies by age of patient; typical doses range in hundreds of milligrams a day in divided doses PO: 250–500 mg QID	Rx
Natural Penicillins				
penicillin G	pen-i-SIL-in G	Injection, powder for injection	Dose varies by age of patient; typical doses range from thousands to millions of units a day in divided doses	Rx
penicillin V (Pen VK)	pen-i-SIL-in V	Solution, tablet	Adult: 125–250 mg every 6–8 hr Pediatric: 25–50 mg/kg/day in divided doses	Rx
Antistaphylococcal Penicillins				
dicloxacillin	dye-klox-a-SIL-in	Capsule	Adult: 125–250 mg every 6 hr Pediatric: 12.5 mg/kg/day in divided doses	Rx
nafcillin	naf-SIL-in	Injection	1000–2000 mg every 4 hr	Rx
oxacillin	ox-a-SIL-in	Injection, solution	Adult: 500–2,000 mg every 4–6 hr Pediatric: 50–100 mg/kg/day in divided doses IV: dose varies by age of patient; typical doses range in hundreds of milligrams a day in divided doses	Rx
Extended-Spectrum Penicillins				
piperacillin	pi-PER-a-sil-in	Injection	Varies depending on route, patient age, and type of infection treated; usually given multiple times a day	Rx
ticarcillin	tye-kar-SIL-in	Injection	Varies depending on route, patient age, and type of infection treated; usually given multiple times a day	Rx
Combination Penicillins				
amoxicillin-clavulanate (Augmentin)	a-mox-i-SIL-in klav-yoo-LAN-ate	Chewable tablet, oral suspension, tablet	Adult: 250–500 mg every 8–12 hr Pediatric: 20–45 mg/kg/day in divided doses	Rx
ampicillin-sulbactam (Unasyn)	am-pi-SIL-in sul-BAK-tam	Injection	Adult: 1.5–3 g every 6 hr Pediatric: 100–200 mg/kg/day in divided doses	Rx
piperacillin-tazobactam (Zosyn)	pi-PER-a-sil-in ta-zoe-BAK-tam	Injection	Adult: 3.375 g every 6 hr Pediatric: varies by age and weight of patient; usually given multiple times a day	Rx
ticarcillin-clavulanate (Timentin)	tye-kar-SIL-in klav-yoo-LAN-ate	Injection	Varies by age of patient; typical doses range in hundreds of milligrams a day in divided doses	Rx

Although IV preparations are often used in conjunction with other antibiotics (such as aminoglycosides, for difficult infections), they should not be mixed in the same IV bag.

Some bacteria have become resistant to **methicillin**, an older penicillin used for difficult staphylococcal infections. The antistaphylococcal penicillins (also called *penicillinase-resistant*) have largely replaced it in practice. **Methicillin-resistant Staphylococcus aureus (MRSA)** infections are resistant to all antistaphylococcal penicillins and, consequently, few drugs can treat them. Special precautions are used to protect against the spread of this bacteria to other patients. For instance, access to the affected patient's hospital room is restricted, and anyone who enters must don protective gear such as a gown, mask, and gloves.

Drug Interactions of Penicillins Antibiotics such as penicillins may reduce the efficacy of oral contraceptives. While rare, contraceptive failure may occur and patients should use backup contraception during therapy. Penicillins may increase the risk of bleeding when used with anticoagulants such as heparin and warfarin. Live vaccine effectiveness may be decreased with penicillin use and coadministration should be avoided.

Cephalosporins

Antibiotics of the **cephalosporin** family have a mechanism of action similar to penicillins, but they differ in their antibacterial spectrum, resistance to beta-lactamase, and pharmacokinetics. Research now suggests that of persons reporting a penicillin allergy, only 10-15% have evidence of a skin test-confirmed allergy. In those with a positive penicillin skin test, only 2% have evidence of a skin test-confirmed allergy to cephalosporin. Most computerized drug profile systems place penicillin and cephalosporin in the same category; therefore, if someone has an allergy to either, the computer system will indicate that the patient is allergic to both. Cephalosporins are divided into five groups, called **generations**. In general, first-generation cephalosporins work best on Gram-positive bacteria. Activity against Gram-negative bacteria increases through the subsequent generations (see Table 4.4).

The first-generation cephalosporins are similar to the penicillinase-resistant penicillins. They are used for mild to moderate **community-acquired** (not acquired in the hospital) infections in ambulatory patients. They can all be taken by mouth, except **cefazolin (Ancef)**, which is only administered IV or intramuscularly (IM; injected deep into the tissue of the muscle). IM and IV injections require longer needles than subcutaneous (SC; under-the-skin) injections.

Second-generation cephalosporins have increased activity, especially against *Haemophilus influenzae*, an important pathogen in the pediatric group. Second-generation cephalosporins are used for otitis media in children and for respiratory and urinary tract infections. They can all be dosed orally; **cefuroxime (Ceftin, Zinacef)** also has IV and IM forms.

The most recently developed third-generation cephalosporin drugs are active against a wide spectrum of Gram-negative organisms and are used in severe infections. They are manufactured in a mixture of dosage forms. Because of their long half-life, the agents are also used in ambulatory patients, especially children, with dosing done before and after school. Orally active third-generation cephalosporins include **ceftibuten (Cedax), cefdinir (Omnicef), cefditoren (Spectracef), cefixime (Suprax)**, and **cefpodoxime (Vantin)**. **Cefotaxime (Claforan), ceftazidime (Fortaz, Tazicef)**, and **ceftriaxone (Rocephin)** are available only in injectable forms. Injection of ceftriaxone may be painful, so it is often mixed with lidocaine to diminish the discomfort. It is used frequently in emergency room settings, and is also used to treat sexually transmitted infections (STIs).

Safety Alert

Alert the pharmacist and prescriber if a patient who is allergic to penicillin is prescribed a cephalosporin. Even if the prescriber wants the drug dispensed, it is important to document this communication in case the person does have a cross-reaction.

TABLE 4.4 Common Cephalosporins

Generic (Brand)	Pronunciation	Dosage Form	Common Dosage	Dispensing Status
First Generation				
cefazolin (Ancef)	sef-AZ-oe-lin	Injection	250 mg to 1 g taken every 6, 8, or 12 hr (dosing depends on type of infection being treated); also given before or during surgical procedures	Rx
cephalexin (Keflex)	sef-a-LEX-in	Capsule, oral suspension, tablet	Adult: 250–750 mg every 6 hr Pediatric: 25–50 mg/kg/day in divided doses	Rx
Second Generation				
cefaclor (Ceclor)	SEF-a-klor	Capsule, chewable tablet, oral suspension, tablet	Adult: 250 mg every 8 hr or 375–500 mg every 12 hr Pediatric: 20–40 mg/kg/day divided every 8–12 hr	Rx
cefotetan (Cefotan)	SEF-oh-tee-tan	Injection	500 mg–3 g every 12 hr	Rx
cefoxitin (Mefoxin)	SEF-ox-ih-tin	Injection	1–2 g every 6–8 hr; also given before or during surgical procedures	Rx
cefuroxime (Zinacef)	se-fyoor-OX-eem	Injection, oral suspension, tablet	IM/IV: 750 mg to 1.5 g every 8 hr; also given before or during surgical procedures PO: Adult: 250–1,000 mg twice a day Pediatric: 20–30 mg/kg/day divided twice a day	Rx
Third Generation				
cefdinir (Omnicef)	SEF-di-neer	Capsule, oral suspension	Adult: 300–600 mg every 12–24 hr Pediatric: 7 mg/kg every 12 hr or 14 mg/kg every 24 hr	Rx
cefditoren (Spectracef)	sef-de-TOR-en	Tablet	200–400 mg twice a day	Rx
cefixime (Suprax)	SEF-icks-eem	Oral suspension	Adult: 400 mg/day Pediatric: 8 mg/kg/day	Rx
cefotaxime (Claforan)	sef-oh-TAX-eem	Injection	Pediatric dose: 50–224 mg/kg/day divided every 4-6 hours IM: 0.5–1 g single dose IM/IV: 1–2 g every 4–12 hr depending on severity of infection	Rx
cefpodoxime (Vantin)	Sef-poe-DOX-eem	Oral suspension, tablet	Adult: 100-200 mg twice a day Pediatric: 10 mg/kg/day divided every 12 hours	Rx
ceftazidime (Fortaz, Tazicef)	SEF-tay-zi-deem	Injection	Adult: 1–2 g every 8–12 hr Pediatric: 30–50 mg/kg/dose every 8–12 hr	Rx
ceftibuten (Cedax)	sef-TYE-byoo-ten	Capsule, oral suspension	Adult: 400 mg once a day Pediatric: 9 mg/kg/day	Rx
ceftriaxone (Rocephin)	sef-trye-AX-one	Injection	Adult: 1–2 g once or twice a day Pediatric: 50–75 mg/kg/day once or twice a day	Rx
Fourth Generation				
cefepime (Maxipime)	SEF-e-peem	Injection	Adult: 1–2 g every 8–12 hr Pediatric dose: 50 mg/kg/dose every 8-12 hours	Rx
Fifth Generation				
ceftaroline (Teflaro)	SEF-tare-oh-leen	Injection	600 mg every 12 hr	Rx

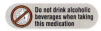

Cefepime (Maxipime) is an injectable fourth-generation cephalosporin and is considered to have broad-spectrum coverage. It is used for treating pneumonia, urinary tract infections, and **sepsis** (inflammatory response to infection resulting from blood-borne infections) caused by Gram-negative organisms. Cefepime is considered as effective as the third-generation cephalosporin ceftazidime (Fortaz), but it is more cost-effective because cefepime is given twice daily, whereas ceftazidime is dosed two or three times daily. Because of their activity against *Pseudomonas*, both are used for hospital-acquired infections.

Ceftaroline (Teflaro) is a fifth-generation cephalosporin. Ceftaroline has activity similar to ceftriaxone, with the benefit of being effective against MRSA.

Therapeutic Uses Cephalosporins are among the drugs of choice for the following conditions:

- dental work, oral infections—oral first and second generation
- heart and pacemaker procedures (surgical prophylaxis)—cefazolin
- neurosurgical operations (surgical prophylaxis)—cefazolin
- obstetric/gynecologic (OB/GYN) procedures and surgery (surgical prophylaxis)—cefazolin
- orthopedic surgery (surgical prophylaxis)—cefazolin
- upper respiratory tract and sinus infections—oral second generation
- urinary tract infections (UTIs)— parenteral third generation
- meningitis—parenteral third generation
- intra-abdominal infections—cefoxitin, cefotetan

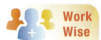

Work Wise

The IV forms of cephalosporin drugs can usually be mixed in either normal saline or a 5% dextrose solution. These solutions are generally placed in either a 50-mL or 100-mL bag and administered over 30 minutes.

Side Effects and Dispensing Issues Cephalosporins share the same side effects as penicillins; a few have also been known to initiate unique toxic reactions. They generally are associated with a lower frequency of toxicity than many other antibiotics. Use of the specific drugs should be gauged by sensitivity testing of the microorganism isolated from the patient.

Common side effects of cephalosporins include nausea, vomiting, diarrhea, headache, and dizziness. Most of the time, these effects are tolerable. Other rare but more severe side effects include mental disturbances, seizures, heart palpitations, and bleeding abnormalities. These particular side effects tend to occur more frequently at higher doses and when the drugs are administered IV. Some of the more serious side effects can be worsened by alcohol intake, so patients should avoid alcohol while taking a cephalosporin.

Several of the cephalosporin drugs have noteworthy dispensing issues. Patients with diabetes who are prescribed cefdinir in oral suspension form must be informed of its high sugar content (2.86 g per teaspoonful). Cefpodoxime is an oral suspension. With the exception of cefdinir and cefixime, which may be stored at room temperature, oral suspensions of cephalosporins must be refrigerated following reconstitution. A dropper, spoon, or oral syringe with milliliter and teaspoon markings should be dispensed with these drugs.

NDC 0143-9665-10
20 g

Cefazolin®
Bulk package
20 g • IV

Cefazolin is a first-generation cephalosporin that is injectable and can be administered intravenously or intramuscularly.

Safety Alert

All of the cephalosporins look alike when written in the generic form. Watch for dosing and indications for use.

Contraindications The cephalosporins are contraindicated in patients with a hypersensitivity to other cephalosporins. Ceftriaxone should not be used in neonates with elevated bilirubin levels or in neonates who are receiving IV calcium-containing

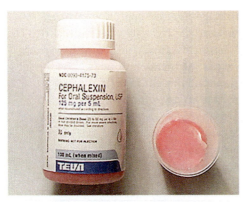

Most oral liquid forms of cephalosporins are available as suspensions and should be shaken well before use.

Work Wise

In addition to penicillins, other antibiotics such as cephalosporins, monobactams, and carbapenems also contain a beta-lactam ring. Therefore, you may hear healthcare practitioners refer to these antibiotics as "beta-lactams."

products. Cefditoren is contraindicated in patients with milk-protein hypersensitivity or carnitine deficiency. Cefepime is contraindicated in patients with penicillin or beta-lactam hypersensitivity.

Cautions and Considerations Allergic reactions to cephalosporins are common. Many patients who are allergic to penicillin may also be allergic to cephalosporins. Therefore, you should always inquire about all drug allergies when taking a patient's medication history or when preparing to administer either cephalosporins or penicillins.

Some cephalosporins should be taken with food, and others should be taken on an empty stomach. For example, cefditoren should be taken with food but not with antacids. Refer to the package insert to verify proper instructions with regard to food.

Most cephalosporin oral liquid dosage forms are suspensions and should be shaken well before every dose. This is because the active drug granules have a tendency to settle to the bottom of the bottle. Shaking will also provide even dosing throughout the regimen. These drugs are reconstituted in the pharmacy. Most cephalosporin suspensions must also be refrigerated. Cefdinir and cefixime are of the few suspensions that do not have to be refrigerated after reconstitution. When a suspension is prepared with water, it usually expires 14 days after mixing. Any medication left over after treatment should be disposed of properly.

Some of the products in this class can be taken twice a day instead of three times a day. This feature may be advantageous for parents with children in daycare or school, when it may be difficult to administer medications in the middle of the day.

Drug Interactions of Cephalosporins Warn patients against drinking alcohol with or within 72 hours of cephalosporin use because it can cause acute alcohol intolerance. Cephalosporins may increase the activity of the anticoagulant warfarin. Loop diuretics (such as furosemide) should be used with caution in patients taking cephalosporins because of an increased risk of **nephrotoxicity** (ability to damage the kidneys). Ceftriaxone should not be used in neonates receiving any calcium-containing products. Ceftriaxone use may also increase cyclosporine levels.

Carbapenems and Monobactams

The drug classes carbapenems and monobactams are grouped together here because they differ only slightly in their molecular structure from penicillins and cephalosporins. These drug classes kill bacteria by inhibiting the formation of the cell wall. **Carbapenems** are used for mixed infections that have both Gram-positive and Gram-negative bacteria; **monobactams** are used only for Gram-negative bacterial infections. Both drug classes are used in special situations for serious healthcare-associated infections (HAIs). Carbapenems include ertapenem, imipenem, and meropenem. Aztreonam is a monobactam. Table 4.5 provides more information on the carbapenems and monobactams.

Imipenem-cilastatin (Primaxin) is a carbapenem drug with excellent in vitro and in vivo activity against Gram-positive and Gram-negative bacteria. Side effects are similar to those of other beta-lactams except that seizures seem to occur more frequently. The carbapenem **meropenem (Merrem I.V.)** has similar coverage, but meropenem is less likely to cause seizures. It is approved for bacterial meningitis and intra-abdominal infections.

TABLE 4.5 Most Commonly Used Carbapenem, and Monobactam Drugs

Generic (Brand)	Pronunciation	Dosage Form	Common Dosage	Dispensing Status
Carbapenems				
doripenem (Doribax)	dore-i-PEN-em	Injection	500 mg every 8 hr	Rx
ertapenem (Invanz)	er-ta-PEN-em	Injection	1,000 mg once daily	Rx
imipenem-cilastatin (Primaxin)	i-mi-PEN-em sye-la-STAT-in	Injection	250–1,000 mg every 6–8 hr	Rx
meropenem (Merrem I.V.)	mer-o-PEN-em	Injection	500-1,000 mg every 8 hr	Rx
Monobactam				
aztreonam (Azactam)	AZ-tree-oh-nam	Injection, oral inhalation product	500–2,000 mg every 6–12 hr	Rx

Doripenem (Doribax) inhibits cell-wall synthesis and kills bacteria. It is indicated for intra-abdominal infections and UTIs. For injection, 500 mg is reconstituted with 10 mL of NS or sterile water and shaken gently. It is then added to 100 mL of NS or **dextrose solution (D_5W)** and shaken gently again. Doripenem is stable for 12 hours in NS and four hours in D_5W at room temperature after mixing. It is good for 72 hours (when reconstituted with NS) and 24 hours (when reconstituted with D_5W) if stored in the refrigerator. As with the other carbapenems, patients must be watched for seizures.

Ertapenem (Invanz) is an injectable (once-daily) carbapenem approved for severe community-acquired infections.

A monobactam, **aztreonam (Azactam)**, is also being used to treat serious infections, including sepsis, intra-abdominal infections, peritonitis, skin and soft tissue infections, and infections of the urinary tract. Aztreonam is active only against Gram-negative bacilli. The advantage of this drug is an unlikely cross-allergenicity with other beta-lactams. It is used against aerobic Gram-negative infections. Patients should notify their physician immediately if skin rash, redness, or itching develops.

Therapeutic Uses Carbapenems and monobactams are among the drugs of choice for the following conditions:

- intra-abdominal infections
- complicated skin/skin structure infections
- complicated UTIs

Side Effects and Dispensing Issues Side effects of carbapenems include skin rash, headache, anemia, and pain. Aztreonam inhalation can cause sore throat, cough, nasal congestion, wheezing, fever, and chest discomfort. The IV form of aztreonam may cause neutropenia, increased liver enzymes, and skin rash.

To make a common dose of doripenem, you reconstitute 500 mg with 10 mL of NS or sterile water for injection and gently shake to create a suspension. Next, you inspect the suspension visually for any foreign matter. Then you withdraw the suspension using a syringe and needle and add it to an infusion bag containing 100 mL of NS or D_5W. The expiration of doripenem in an NS infusion bag is 12 hours at room temperature and 72 hours under refrigeration. Doripenem in a D_5W infusion bag expires after four hours at room temperature and 24 hours refrigerated.

Contraindications Hypersensitivity to one carbapenem contraindicates use of other agents in the class. IM use of ertapenem is contraindicated in patients with a hypersensitivity to amide-type anesthetics. Aztreonam does not have contraindications.

Cautions and Considerations Seizures have been reported during treatment with carbapenems. These reactions occurred most commonly in patients with central nervous system (CNS) disorders such as a history of seizures and in patients with renal impairment. Carbapenems require dosage adjustment in patients with kidney dysfunction. Aztreonam has rare cross-allergenicity to penicillins, cephalosporins, or carbapenems and should be used with caution in patients with a history of beta-lactam hypersensitivity. Aztreonam requires dosage adjustment in patients with renal impairment.

Drug Interactions The CNS side effects of carbapenems may be potentiated by concurrent cyclosporine use. Ganciclovir when used with carbapenems may result in seizures. Carbapenems may decrease levels of the antiseizure medication valproic acid.

Vancomycin

A single drug in a class by itself is **vancomycin (Vancocin)**. Its mechanism is not fully understood, but it probably works by inhibiting cell-wall formation. Vancomycin has antimicrobial activity against Gram-positive bacteria and is used primarily to treat MRSA infections; in fact, it is the drug of choice. Unfortunately, some enterococci are resistant to vancomycin; these are called vancomycin-resistant *Enterococcus* (VRE). Table 4.10 provides more information on vancomycin.

Vancomycin is most frequently administered intravenously because the oral form is poorly absorbed into the bloodstream (see Figure 4.3). The oral dosage form is used, therefore, only for infections that are localized within the intestines. Intravenous doses range between 500 mg and 2 grams a day in divided doses.

FIGURE 4.3
Medication Label for Vancomycin

The name *vancomycin* was derived from the word *vanquish*, meaning "to defeat." When this drug was originally discovered in the 1950s, it was used to combat penicillin-resistant *Staphylococcus aureus*. Today, vancomycin is used to treat MRSA and is most frequently administered via the IV route.

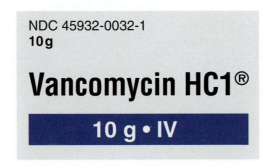

NDC 45932-0032-1
10g

Vancomycin HC1®

10 g • IV

Therapeutic Uses Vancomycin is among the drugs of choice for:

- MRSA infections
- endocarditis
- *Clostridium difficile* infections

Side Effects and Dispensing Issues Vancomycin may cause **nephrotoxicity** (kidney damage) and **ototoxicity** (hearing loss). With proper monitoring of blood levels and laboratory tests, these effects can be avoided or minimized. However, these side effects limit vancomycin's use to the treatment of difficult infections.

Vancomycin is typically administered intravenously. One gram of vancomycin for IV use is usually diluted in at least 250 mL of fluid. Even though the drug-to-diluent ratio is 1 gram to 200 mL, it is always best to mix this drug in a larger amount of fluid than the minimum required. This tactic will prevent the drug from being infused too quickly and the patient from experiencing red man syndrome (a syndrome associated with vancomycin infusion that results in flushing and redness in the neck and face, rash, and hypotension).

Contraindications Vancomycin does not have contraindications.

Cautions and Considerations Vancomycin must be administered slowly (usually over 60 minutes or more) to avoid red man syndrome.

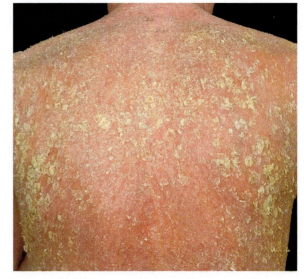

This photo shows a patient with red man syndrome.

Drug Interactions Vancomycin may decrease the effectiveness of live vaccines. Oral vancomycin should not be coadministered with bile acid sequestrants because of diminished vancomycin effect.

Lincosamides and Macrolides

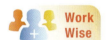

Work Wise

The azithromycin Z-Pak is an example of a drug that is supplied in a dose pack but can be dispensed from a bottle. The 250-mg and 500-mg tablets can be dispensed in a bottle or as a package. Just put the same instructions on the label and use the same strength of the drug that is in the package.

Lincosamides and **macrolides** work by blocking bacteria's ability to produce needed proteins for survival. At low doses, these drugs are bacteriostatic, but at high doses, they can be bactericidal.

Clindamycin (Cleocin) is the most commonly prescribed lincosamide and is used to treat infections caused by various organisms including anaerobes, *Staphylococcus aureus*, *Streptococcus pneumoniae*, and *Streptococcus pyogenes*. Clindamycin is used for bone and joint infections, gynecologic infections, intra-abdominal infections, sepsis, and skin and soft tissue infections.

Macrolides have a broad spectrum of activity: they work against some Gram-positive and Gram-negative bacteria. Macrolides are used mainly to treat respiratory tract infections and pneumonia. They are also used with other drugs to treat infection caused by *Helicobacter pylori*, the bacteria found in association with stomach ulcers.

Clarithromycin (Biaxin) is one such drug. The duration of therapy for one macrolide, **azithromycin (Zithromax)**, is unusually short but convenient (typically 3 to 5 days) relative to other antibiotics (usually 7 to 14 days). See Table 4.6 for additional dosing information. An azithromycin Z-Pak is dispensed differently than most antibiotics. On the first day, the patient takes a **loading dose** of 500 mg. Maintenance doses of 250 mg once daily are then taken on days 2 through 5 although this regimen can vary depending on the type of infection. There is also a three-pack of 500-mg tablets that should be taken once a day over a three-day period. Z-Max is an extended-release powder for oral suspension that delivers a full treatment in one dose. It comes in 1-gram and 2-gram packages and is approved to treat community-acquired pneumonia. Most of the azithromycin liquids are banana flavored.

TABLE 4.6 Common Lincosamides and Macrolides

Generic (Brand)	Pronunciation	Dosage Form	Common Dosage	Dispensing Status
Lincosamide				
clindamycin (Cleocin)	klin-da-MYE-sin	Cream, foam, gel, injection, lotion, oral solution, suppository, tablet, topical solution	IM, IV: 600–2,700 mg/day in divided doses PO: Adult: 150–300 mg every 6 hr Pediatric: 8–20 mg/kg/day in 3–4 divided doses Topical: varies depending on product; usually given 1–2 times a day	Rx
Macrolides				
azithromycin (Zithromax, Z-Pak, Z-Max, Zithromax Tri-Pak)	aye-ZITH-roe-mye-sin	Injection, ophthalmic solution, oral suspension, tablet	IV: 500 mg daily for 2–10 days depending on type of infection PO: Adult: 250–500 mg daily for 3–5 days Pediatric: varies by age and weight of patient as well as type of infection	Rx
clarithromycin (Biaxin)	kla-RITH-roe-mye-sin	Oral suspension, tablet	Adult: 250–500 mg every 12 hr Pediatric: 15 mg/kg/day divided every 12 hr	Rx
erythromycin (EES, EryC, EryPed, Ery-Tab, Erythrocin, Pediazole)	eh-rith-roe-MYE-sin	Capsule, gel, injection, ophthalmic ointment, oral suspension, pledget, solution, tablet	Varies depending on age of patient and type of infection; usually given 3–4 times a day	Rx

Safety Alert

Erythromycin and azithromycin can be misread, but the different doses should help identify the intended drug.

Therapeutic Uses Lincosamides are among the drugs of choice for:

- acne
- dental work
- anaerobic pneumonia
- bone infections
- bowel infections
- female genital infections
- intra-abdominal infections

Macrolides are among the most commonly prescribed drugs for the following illnesses and other specific bacteria:

- sexually transmitted infections
- group A beta-hemolytic streptococcus
- influenza
- Legionnaires' disease
- Mycoplasma pneumonia
- Streptococcus pneumonia

NDC 52584-870-21
9,000 mg / 60 mL

Cleocin Phosphate®

Bulk package

150 mg / mL • IM or IV

Clindamycin (Cleocin) has injectable (as pictured), oral, and topical dosage forms.

Side Effects and Dispensing Issues Common side effects of lincosamides and macrolides include stomach upset, nausea, vomiting, heartburn, abdominal pain, and diarrhea. To reduce these effects, patients should take lincosamides and macrolides with food. If abdominal pain or diarrhea is severe, the patient should seek medical attention immediately because such pain could indicate a serious problem.

Liver toxicity has also occurred with the use of erythromycin. Patients with prior liver problems should not take this medication. If **jaundice** (yellowing of skin and eyes) occurs with erythromycin use, medical attention should be sought immediately.

Clindamycin is available in oral, IV, and topical forms. When used for acne, clindamycin is often dispensed topically.

Azithromycin is available in several prepackaged forms.

Contraindications Clindamycin is contraindicated in patients with a hypersensitivity to other lincosamides.

Hypersensitivity to one macrolide contraindicates use of all other macrolides. Azithromycin and clarithromycin are contraindicated in patients with liver dysfunction associated with prior use. Other contraindications to clarithromycin include a history of QT prolongation or ventricular cardiac arrhythmia; concomitant use with cisapride, pimozide, ergotamine, dihydroergotamine, simvastatin, lovastatin, or astemizole; and concomitant use with colchicine in patients with liver or kidney impairment. Erythromycin is contraindicated with patients who are taking pimozide, cisapride, ergotamine or dihydroergotamine, astemizole, lov-astatin, or simvastatin.

Cautions and Considerations Oral suspension products should be shaken well before every dose. Most of these suspensions must also be refrigerated. Any of these suspensions prepared with water are good for only 14 days from mixing. Any medication left over after treatment should be disposed of properly.

Clindamycin has a black box warning because it can cause severe and possibly fatal colitis. Its use should be reserved for treatment of serious infections for which use of other antimicrobials is inappropriate.

Drug Interactions Macrolides, especially erythromycin and clarithromycin, have many drug interactions. Some of the effects caused by these interactions can be severe. For example, macrolides should not be given with QT prolonging agents such as antiarrhythmics and tricyclic antidepressants due to QT prolongation. Diltiazem should not be used with macrolides. Methadone and macrolides may lead to life-threatening arrhythmias. Clarithromycin interacts with several HIV medications including protease inhibitors (covered in Chapter 5). Concurrent use increases clarithromycin levels and decreases the protease inhibitor level. Efavirenz and etravirine should not be used with clarithromycin. Clarithromycin and proton pump inhibitors interact, and monitoring for increased adverse reactions should occur. Clarithromycin should not be used with alpha-adrenergic blockers. Azithromycin should not be administered with antacids due to decreased absorption.

Clindamycin should not be used concurrently with erythromycin (erythromycin effectiveness decreases). Clindamycin may increase the neuromuscular blocking effects of mecamylamine.

Aminoglycosides

A class of drugs called **aminoglycosides** kills bacteria by blocking their ability to make essential proteins for survival. Aminoglycosides are often used in conjunction with other antibiotics (e.g., penicillins, cephalosporins, and vancomycin). Aminoglycosides work synergistically with these other drug classes. **Synergistic drug therapy** is when two or more drugs are used together because they employ different mechanisms of action (in this case, the inhibition of protein synthesis [aminoglycosides] and cell-wall lysis [penicillins, cephalosporins, and vancomycin]) that work better together than either drug works alone. The aminoglycosides gentamicin and tobramycin are used to treat eye infections in patients with immuno-deficiency.

Many healthcare institutions have instituted pulse dosing, whereby aminoglycosides are given once a day instead of multiple times a day. Because the side effects of aminoglycosides can be serious, less exposure to the drug during the day seems to help reduce its toxic effects. Special nomograms (dosing algorithms) are used for dosing in these situations. Table 4.7 includes common aminoglycosides and their routes of administration.

Therapeutic Uses Aminoglycosides are commonly used for:

- life-threatening infections due to Gram-negative aerobes
- sepsis (a systemic inflammatory response to infection resulting from blood-borne infections)
- infections in patients with a compromised immune system
- peritonitis

Side Effects and Dispensing Issues Side effects of aminoglycosides can include nephrotoxicity (kidney damage) and ototoxicity (tinnitus, hearing loss, and balance problems). With proper monitoring of blood levels and laboratory tests, these effects can be avoided or minimized. However, these side effects limit the use of aminoglycosides to the treatment of difficult infections.

Aminoglycosides are often dosed based on weight or therapeutic drug levels. Because of this, pharmacy technicians preparing these drugs should be aware that doses will vary.

Contraindications Cross-sensitivity may exist among aminoglycosides; therefore, hypersensitivity to one aminoglycoside contraindicates the use of others.

TABLE 4.7 Common Aminoglycosides

Generic (Brand)	Pronunciation	Dosage Form	Dispensing Status
amikacin	am-i-KAY-sin	Injection	Rx
gentamicin (Garamycin, Gentak)	jen-ta-MYE-sin	Injection, ophthalmic ointment, ophthalmic solution	Rx
tobramycin (TOBI, Tobrex)	toe-bra-MYE-sin	Injection, ophthalmic ointment, ophthalmic solution, solution for nebulizer inhalation	Rx

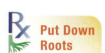

NDC 6332-3017-302
20 mg / 2 ml

Gentamicin®
Pediatric

IM or IV • 2 ml single-dose vial

Gentamicin is an aminoglycoside that is used in pediatric and adult patients.

℞ Put Down Roots

It is easy to recognize aminoglycosides by looking at their names. The aminoglycosides end in the suffix –cin.

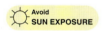

Cautions and Considerations Aminoglycosides carry boxed warnings. One warning is for toxicities associated with use (nephrotoxicity and ototoxicity). Another warns that patients using aminoglycosides should be carefully monitored by healthcare personnel. Aminoglycosides should be avoided in pregnancy due to increased risk of fetal harm. Aminoglycosides have been known to cause neuromuscular blockade in some cases. If a patient complains of muscle weakness, difficulty breathing, numbness, tingling, twitching, or seizures, the drug should be discontinued. Patients with muscular disorders, such as myasthenia gravis or Parkinson's disease, should not be given aminoglycosides. Caution must be used if aminoglycosides are given after surgery because they may interact with neuromuscular blockers, a class of drugs used in many surgical procedures.

Although aminoglycosides are often used in conjunction with other antibiotics such as cephalosporins or penicillins, they should not be mixed in the same IV infusion bag. Ophthalmic preparations should be kept as sterile as possible. Patients should be instructed not to touch the tip of the applicator to the eye or other surfaces during medication administration.

Drug Interactions The risk of kidney toxicity increases when aminoglycosides are used concurrently with nonsteroidal anti-inflammatory drugs (NSAIDs). Coadministration with loop diuretics may increase the risk of ototoxicity.

Tetracyclines

Another class of drugs for bacterial infections is **tetracyclines**, which are bacteriostatic drugs that inhibit protein synthesis within bacterial cells. Consequently, they require a functioning immune system to cure an infection. Tetracyclines are broad-spectrum, and more information can be found in Table 4.8.

Therapeutic Uses of Tetracyclines Tetracyclines are among the drugs of choice for:

- acne
- anthrax
- chronic bronchitis

TABLE 4.8   Commonly Used Tetracyclines

Generic (Brand)	Pronunciation	Dosage Form	Common Dosage	Dispensing Status
doxycycline (Vibramycin, Oracea, Adoxa)	dox-i-SYE-kleen	Capsule, injection, oral liquid, tablet	100–200 mg twice a day	Rx
minocycline (Minocin, Solodyn)	mi-noe-SYE-kleen	Capsule, injection	100 mg every 12 hr	Rx
tetracycline (Sumycin)	te-tra-SYE-kleen	Capsule, oral liquid, tablet	250–500 mg 2–4 times a day	Rx

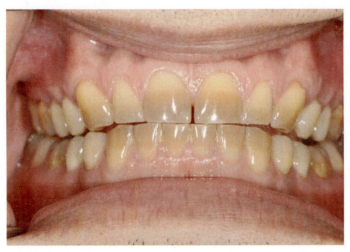
This photo shows permanent discoloration due to tetracycline use.

- Lyme disease
- *Mycoplasma pneumoniae* infection (walking pneumonia)
- *Rickettsia* infection (Rocky Mountain spotted fever)
- some sexually transmitted infections, such as chlamydia

Side Effects and Dispensing Issues

Common side effects of tetracyclines include stomach upset, nausea, and vomiting. Tetracyclines can be taken with food (but not dairy products or antacids [see Cautions and Considerations]) to reduce these effects. Tetracyclines also cause photosensitivity. Patients should be informed that their skin will burn faster when exposed to the sun and a skin rash may develop. When taking a tetracycline, patients should apply sunscreen and other protection (sun-protective clothing) when spending time outside.

When most drugs reach their expiration date, they usually lose effectiveness. Tetracyclines are unique in that once expired, they can degrade to toxic substances and may cause kidney failure. Therefore, the pharmacy technician should always diligently check expiration dates on tetracyclines. Patients should be alerted to complete drug courses, and if any drug remains, they should dispose of them and not save for future use.

Contraindications Hypersensitivity to one tetracycline contraindicates the use of other tetracyclines.

Cautions and Considerations Tetracyclines chelate (or bind) with metals and ions, such as calcium, aluminum, and magnesium. When this occurs, these medications cannot be absorbed into the bloodstream. As stated earlier, patients should avoid food, drink, and other products that contain these substances (such as cheese, milk, antacids, or laxatives).

With this drug class, recall that patients should be warned to avoid the sun because the drugs can cause photosensitization.

Tetracyclines also accumulate in teeth and bones and can cause permanent discoloration and enamel hypoplasia. Consequently, children younger than eight years of age and pregnant or lactating women cannot use tetracyclines because of possible permanent damage to teeth.

Tetracycline breaks down over time to become toxic. Therefore, expired tetracycline should be discarded properly and never saved for future use.

Drug Interactions As discussed above, tetracyclines should not be administered with aluminum-, calcium-, magnesium-, or zinc-containing products (such as antacids) due to decreased absorption. Tetracyclines should not be used with retinoids (such as isotretinoin) due to increased risk of pseudomotor cerebri. Digoxin levels may increase when it is used concurrently with tetracyclines. Adverse reactions of theophylline may be increased with concurrent tetracycline use.

Fluoroquinolones or Quinolones

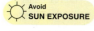

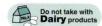

The class of drugs known as **fluoroquinolones** (also called **quinolones**) kills bacteria by inhibiting the enzyme that helps DNA to coil. If DNA cannot coil, it is rendered useless and the cell dies because it cannot function. Quinolones have strong, rapid bactericidal activity against Gram-negative bacteria and some Gram-positive bacteria. Table 4.9 lists the most commonly used quinolones.

Therapeutic Uses of Fluoroquinolones or Quinolones   Quinolones are among the drugs of choice for the following conditions:

Safety Alert

Cipro can be mistakenly read as Ceftin (cefuroxime).

- bone and joint infections
- eye infections
- serious RTIs
- serious UTIs

Quinolones also have a special use as treatment for anthrax, a potential bio-terrorism agent.

Because of overprescribing, resistance to quinolones has developed. Therefore, their use is discouraged in ordinary and frequently seen infections. Quinolones should be reserved for more serious and difficult-to-treat Gram-negative bacterial infections.

Safety Alert

"Ciprofloxacin" and "cephalexin" can look very much alike, depending on the handwriting.

Side Effects and Dispensing Issues   Common side effects of quinolones include nausea, vomiting, dizziness, diarrhea, and a bitter or unpleasant taste in the mouth. If the patient cannot tolerate these effects, different antibiotics will need to be chosen. Taking quinolones with food does not necessarily reduce these effects. These drugs also cause photosensitivity, so patients should wear sunscreen when outside. Less common but serious side effects include liver toxicity and alterations in glucose metabolism. Prolongation of the QT interval on electrocardiography has occurred with quinolone use. QT prolongation is a syndrome associated with an increased risk of life-threatening cardiac arrhythmia. Consequently, drugs that prolong the QT interval (such as quinolones) may not be the best choice for patients with heart problems.

Quinolones are available in oral and IV forms. If a patient is switched from oral to IV, dose adjustments must be made if the patient is using ciprofloxacin. For example, a 250-mg oral dose of ciprofloxacin would correspond to a 200-mg IV dose. The doses of levofloxacin and moxifloxacin are usually the same, regardless if given orally or intravenously. Quinolone drugs must be dispensed with a **medication guide**.

TABLE 4.9   Commonly Used Quinolones

Generic (Brand)	Pronunciation	Dosage Form	Common Dosage	Dispensing Status
ciprofloxacin (Cipro)	sip-roe-FLOX-a-sin	Injection, oral liquid, ophthalmic drops and ointment, otic, tablet, topical	IV: 200–400 mg every 12 hr PO: Adult: 250–750 mg every 12 hr Pediatric: 6–20 mg/kg every 8–12 hr	Rx
levofloxacin (Levaquin)	lee-voe-FLOX-a-sin	Injection, oral liquid, tablet	250–750 mg daily	Rx
moxifloxacin (Avelox)	mox-i-FLOX-a-sin	Injection, ophthalmic solution, tablet	IV and PO: 400 mg daily Ophthalmic: Instill 1 drop 2–3 times daily	Rx

The FDA mandates that medication guides must be issued with certain drugs to make certain information is communicated to prevent adverse effects, ensure patients are making informed decisions about serious side effects of a product, or communicate essential adherence instructions.

Contraindications Quinolones should not be used during pregnancy. Ciprofloxacin is contraindicated with concurrent administration of tizanidine.

Cautions and Considerations Quinolones carry boxed warnings for the risk of tendon inflammation and rupture and for increased muscle weakness in patients with myasthenia gravis. Changes in mental function and seizures have been reported with quinolones, especially ciprofloxacin. If a patient is exhibiting confusion, agitation, dizziness, hallucinations, insomnia, nightmares, or paranoia, use of the drug should be stopped and the patient should seek medical attention immediately. Quinolones are associated with joint malformation and usually should not be used in children. Quinolones are associated with photosensitivity and patients should avoid excessive sun exposure.

Drug Interactions Pharmacy technicians should be aware that many drugs interact with quinolones. For example, quinolones may inhibit clearance of caffeine and theophylline, leading to increased blood levels. Quinolones may prolong QT intervals and may enhance QT-prolonging effects of other drugs. Quinolones should not be taken with antacids, dairy products, or calcium-fortified juices because their absorption will be reduced.

Metronidazole

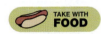

The drug **metronidazole (Flagyl)** is an antibiotic in the **nitroimidazole** class that is effective against fungi and protozoa as well as bacteria. Such capability is unusual, because the cells of fungi and protozoa are much more similar to those of humans than to those of bacteria. Table 4.10 includes more information on metronidazole.

Therapeutic Uses Metronidazole is among the drugs of choice for:

- amebic dysentery
- bacterial vaginosis
- *Clostridium difficile*
- *Giardia* infection
- *Helicobacter pylori* ulcers
- intestinal infections
- rosacea
- sexually transmitted infections, *Trichomonas*

Side Effects and Dispensing Issues The most common side effects of metronidazole are headache, anorexia, vomiting, diarrhea, and abdominal cramps. Taking metronidazole with food can help alleviate these effects. Metallic taste and urine discoloration may also occur.

The dosage forms of metronidazole are capsules, IV, tablets, topical, and vaginal. The topical and vaginal forms are easily confused. The vaginal form has an applicator. Check to be sure which form the prescriber wants if there is any doubt.

Contraindications Metronidazole is contraindicated in a hypersensitivity to nitro-imidazole derivatives. This medication is also contraindicated in the first trimester of pregnancy, use of disulfiram within the past two weeks, and use of alcohol during therapy or within three days of therapy discontinuation.

Cautions and Considerations Metronidazole carries a boxed warning for possible carcinogenicity. Because of this, unnecessary use should be avoided.

One of the most important things to remember about metronidazole is that it interacts with alcohol to cause a severe reaction. Patients can become quite ill with nausea, vomiting, flushing, sweating, and headache if they ingest any alcohol while taking metronidazole and for three days after stopping the medication. Some cough medicines and other over-the-counter (OTC) products have alcohol in them. Patients should be warned not to consume these products (in addition to alcoholic beverages) when taking metronidazole.

Drug Interactions Carbocisteine should be avoided in patients using metronidazole because of enhanced adverse effects. Metronidazole should be avoided, when possible, when patients are using QT-prolonging agents. Mebendazole and ritonavir may enhance the toxic effects of metronidazole. Metronidazole may increase the serum concentrations of warfarin, and increased monitoring should occur when the two are used together.

Linezolid

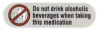

Linezolid (Zyvox), the first oxazolidinone approved by the FDA, inhibits bacterial protein synthesis. The drug must be protected from light. The dosage forms are IV, oral liquid, and tablet. The IV form comes in an IV bag. It should be administered alone and not given through a line that is administering other drugs. Linezolid is not suitable for simultaneous administration because it has many physical incompatibilities and may precipitate in the line. More information on linezolid can be found in Table 4.10.

Therapeutic Uses Linezolid may be used to treat the following:

- MRSA
- VRE
- other Gram-positive infections

Side Effects and Dispensing Issues Side effects associated with linezolid include headache, diarrhea, decreased hemoglobin, leukopenia, and thrombocytopenia.

Contraindications Linezolid should not be used with or within 14 days of taking monoamine oxidase inhibitors (MAOIs).

Cautions and Considerations Myelosuppression (such as anemia) has been reported in patients using linezolid. Caution should be exercised in patients with pre-existing myelosuppression or those using other drugs that cause myelosuppression. Optic neuropathy has been reported in patients treated for longer than 28 days. Serotonin syndrome may occur when linezolid is used with other serotonergic drugs.

Drug Interactions Linezolid may increase the toxic effects of alcohol, which should not be used concurrently. MAOIs should be avoided because of increased adverse effects. Linezolid may decrease the metabolism of the triptan medications used for migraine. The effectiveness of live vaccines decreases with linezolid use, and vaccine use should be postponed until 3 days after linezolid cessation.

TABLE 4.10 Miscellaneous Antibiotics

Generic (Brand)	Pronunciation	Dosage Form	Common Dosage	Dispensing Status
daptomycin (Cubicin)	DAP-toe-mye-sin	Injection	6–10 mg/kg once a day	Rx
linezolid (Zyvox)	li-NE-zoh-lid	Injection, oral liquid, tablet	600 mg every 12 hr	Rx
metronidazole (Flagyl)	me-troe-NYE-da-zole	Capsule, injection, tablet, topical	250–750 mg every 8–24 hr	Rx
vancomycin (Vancocin)	van-koe-MYE-sin	Capsule, injection	500–1,000 mg every 6–12 hr	Rx

Daptomycin

Daptomycin (Cubicin) is classified as a **cyclic lipopeptide** and works by binding to bacterial membranes and causing cell membrane depolarization, ultimately leading to an inhibition of DNA and RNA synthesis. Bacterial death follows. More information on daptomycin can be found in Table 4.10.

Therapeutic Uses Daptomycin may be used for the following conditions:

- complicated skin and skin structure infections
- *Staphylococcus aureus* blood infections

Side Effects and Dispensing Issues The most common side effects reported with daptomycin use include anemia, diarrhea, vomiting, and constipation. Chest pain, peripheral edema, skin rash, and respiratory side effects may also occur.

Daptomycin comes as a powder in a vial for reconstitution. Daptomycin should not be reconstituted with dextrose-containing solutions (such as D_5W). Instead, use NS or lactated Ringer's solution.

Contraindications Daptomycin does not have contraindications.

Cautions and Considerations Daptomycin use may result in eosinophilic pneumonia, and use must be discontinued immediately if it develops. Anaphylaxis has been reported with use. Daptomycin may be associated with myopathy and peripheral neuropathy. Use cautiously in patients with kidney dysfunction.

Drug Interactions HMG-CoA reductase inhibitors (commonly called statins) may enhance the adverse effects of daptomycin.

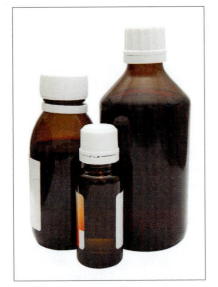

Liquid medications require extra attention because some must be refrigerated and others must not.

Storage of Liquid Antibiotics

After powdered antibiotics (also known as *lyophilized* antibiotics) are mixed, some need refrigeration and some may be stored at room temperature. This is important information the technician may pass onto the patient or caregiver. It is *not* counseling, and no professional judgment is required. Drug storage does not require one to make a decision—the drug is either refrigerated or stored at room temperature—and it is a valuable and necessary piece of information for the patient to have. Because there are many medications that do not require refrigeration and an equal amount that do, patients are often confused. Manufacturers have made an effort to minimize the number of drugs that do need refrigeration. Table 4.11 is provided to simplify this issue for the pharmacy technician.

The flavors of these liquid drugs may be changed to suit the patient's taste. It is usually the pharmacy technician who makes this suggestion and changes the flavors. This feature has made a big difference in adherence in the pediatric population.

TABLE 4.11 **Flavors and Storage of Liquid Antibiotics**

Drug	Brand Name	Refrigerate?	Flavor Additive
amoxicillin		Yes	Mixed berry
amoxicillin-clavulanate	Augmentin	Yes	Orange
ampicillin		Yes	Bubble gum
azithromycin	Zithromax	No	Cherry
cefaclor	Ceclor	Yes	Strawberry
cefdinir	Omnicef	No	Strawberry
cefixime	Suprax	No	Strawberry
cephalexin	Keflex	Yes	Berry
ciprofloxacin	Cipro	No	Strawberry
clarithromycin	Biaxin	No	Fruit
clindamycin	Cleocin	No	Fruit
doxycycline	Vibramycin	No	Raspberry
erythromycin		Depends on formulation	Orange
erythromycin-sulfisoxazole	Pediazole	Yes	Cherry-berry
linezolid	Zyvox	No	Orange
penicillin		Yes	Fruit
sulfamethoxazole-trimethoprim	Bactrim, Septra	No	Grape or Cherry
tetracycline	Sumycin	No	Fruit

Ophthalmic Antibiotics

Some of the antibiotics discussed in this chapter have an ophthalmic (eye) dosage form. In contrast, there are very few antibiotics that have an otic (ear) form, because the ophthalmic forms are also often used for ear conditions. However, otic (ear) medications are never used in the eye, since this would be extremely painful for the patient. This is because otic medicines are not manufactured with the same **pH** (acidity/alkalinity) as those for the eye. Table 4.12 lists antibiotic ophthalmic medications.

TABLE 4.12 Ophthalmic Dosage Forms

Generic (Brand)	Pronunciation	Dosage Form	Dispensing Status
azithromycin (AzaSite)	az-ith-roe-MYE-sin	Drops	Rx
bacitracin (AK-Tracin)	bas-I-TRAY-cin	Ointment	Rx
ciprofloxacin (Ciloxan)	sip-roe-FLOX-a-sin	Drops, ointment	Rx
erythromycin (Ilotycin)	e-rith-roe-MYE-sin	Ointment	Rx
gatifloxacin (Zymar)	gat-i-floks-a sin	Drops	Rx
gentamicin (Gentak, Genoptic)	jen-ta-MYE-sin	Drops, ointment	Rx
moxifloxacin (Vigamox)	moks-i-FLOKS-a-sin	Drops	Rx
ofloxacin (Ocuflox)	oh-FLOKS-a sin	Drops	Rx
sodium sulfacetamide (Bleph-10)	SOE-dee-um-sul-fa-SEE-ta-mide	Drops, ointment	Rx
tobramycin (Tobrex)	toe-bra-MYE-sin	Drops, ointment	Rx

Because the medication must have the same pH as the eye and because of the extreme sterility demanded in the manufacturing process of ophthalmics, eye drops are very expensive—especially the newer ones. They are often rejected by insurance companies, and a less expensive one must be used. The technician will need to let the prescriber know what is available and which ones the insurer will most likely cover.

Sexually Transmitted Infections

Most genital system infections are transmitted by sexual activity and are, therefore, called sexually transmitted infections (STIs), formerly known as *STDs* and *venereal diseases*. The best way to avoid STIs is to either abstain from sexual contact or to be in a long-term, mutually monogamous relationship with a partner who has been tested and is known to be uninfected. One of the most severe STIs, acquired immunodeficiency syndrome (AIDS), is caused by human immunodeficiency virus (HIV). HIV/AIDS and other viral STIs are discussed in Chapter 5. STIs of bacterial origin are discussed in the following sections.

Chlamydia

If untreated, an infection by *Chlamydia trachomatis* can progress to serious reproductive and other health problems with both short-term and long-term consequences. Chlamydia is known as the "silent" disease, because many people with chlamydia have no symptoms. It can occur in the rectum from anal intercourse and in the throat from oral sex. Chlamydial infections frequently occur with gonorrhea. Partners are frequently reinfected if their sex partners are not treated. It can be easily treated and cured with antibiotics.

Gonorrhea

Gonorrhea was first described by the Greek physician Galen in 150 A.D. It is caused by *Neisseria gonorrhoeae*. The organism attaches to mucosal cells in the oropharyngeal area, eye, joints, rectum, and male and female genitalia. Infection sets up inflammation, with leukocytes moving into the area and resultant pus production. Incubation is several days. Males experience painful urination and pus discharge. Complications can cause urethral scarring with partial blockage of the urethra. Blockage of the ductus deferens results in sterility. The female disease is more insidious. It may cause abdominal pain due to pelvic inflammatory disease (PID), which involves extensive infection of the uterus, cervix, fallopian tubes, and ovaries. Scarring in the fallopian tubes may block movement of the ovum; if the blockage is total, an ectopic pregnancy or sterility may result.

In either sex, untreated infections can cause a systemic infection involving the heart, meninges, eyes, pharynx, and joints (arthritis). The eyes of newborns can become infected, and blindness can result. In most states, erythromycin or silver nitrate solution is applied to the eyes of newborns as a prophylactic. If the mother is known to be infected, the infant is given penicillin intramuscularly.

Gonorrhea infection can be acquired at any point of sexual contact, including the pharynx and anus. Recovery does not confer immunity, and reinfection is possible. Penicillin was once frequently used for gonorrhea, but due to resistance a combination of a cephalosporin (such as cetriaxone) and a macrolide (such as azithromycin) is now common. The *Chlamydia trachomatis* microorganism is commonly found with gonorrhea.

Syphilis

Syphilis, which first appeared in Europe in the 15th century, is caused by the spirochete *Treponema pallidum*, a kind of bacterium that moves with a corkscrew-like action. A long incubation time allows sexual partners to be traced and treated before symptoms are apparent. Incubation averages three weeks, appearing somewhere between two weeks and several months following infection. The course develops in three stages.

Primary-Stage Infection

A primary-stage syphilis infection produces a small, hard-based, usually painless ulcer known as a **chancre** at the site of infection. Usually, the lesion heals in a few weeks. Females may be unaware of the infection if the chancre is on the cervix. In males, the chancre may be in the urethra. Fluids from the sore are highly infectious. Bacteria enter the bloodstream and lymphatic system.

Secondary-Stage Infection

A secondary-stage syphilis infection produces skin rashes, patchy hair loss, malaise, and mild fever. Lesions on mucous membranes contain organisms and are highly infectious. Symptoms subside after a few weeks, and the disease becomes latent. After two to four years of latency, the disease is usually no longer infectious.

Late or Tertiary-Stage Infection

A tertiary-stage syphilis infection usually occurs after an interval of at least 10 years. Lesions appear as a rubbery mass of tissue in many organs and sometimes the skin. There may be extensive damage, including deafness, blindness, CNS lesions, or perforation of the roof of the mouth resulting from a hyperimmune reaction to the remaining spirochetes. Because symptoms in the first two stages are not disabling, patients often enter the latent period without receiving medical attention.

Congenital Syphilis

Congenital syphilis occurs in newborns as a result of infection crossing the placenta into the fetus. Neurologic damage to the fetus results if pregnancy occurs during the tertiary stage. Pregnancy during the primary or secondary stage is likely to produce a stillborn child.

Other Sexually Transmitted Infections

Two other sexually transmitted infections, nongonococcal urethritis and vaginitis, play a major role in public health. Nongonococcal urethritis (NGU) may be caused by catheters or chemical agents; some of the cases are acquired sexually. Symptoms are often mild in males, but serious in females. Symptoms include genital discharge, burning while urinating, and itching. In women, it may also cause abdominal pain, abnormal bleeding, and the infection can progress to PID.

Vaginitis is characterized by vaginal discharge and odor. It can be caused by several bacteria. Infection due to *Gardnerella vaginitis* results from interaction between the organism and an anaerobic bacterium in the vagina, neither of which alone can produce the disease. It is characterized by a frothy discharge with fishy odor and a vaginal pH of 5 to 6. Vaginitis may also be caused by *Trichomonas vaginalis*, an organism normally found in both sexes. *T. vaginalis* causes an infection if vaginal acidity is disturbed. Leukocytes infiltrate the site and result in a profuse, yellowish or light cream-colored discharge with a disagreeable odor. It causes irritation and itching.

TABLE 4.13 Most Commonly Used Agents for Sexually Transmitted Infections

Generic (Brand)	Pronunciation	Dosage Form	Dispensing Status
Antibacterial			
azithromycin (Zithromax)	az-ith-roe-MYE-sin	Injection, oral liquid, tablet	Rx
ceftriaxone (Rocephin)	sef-trye-AX-one	Injection	Rx
doxycycline (Doryx, Vibramycin)	dox-i-SYE-kleen	Capsule, injection, oral liquid, tablet	Rx
erythromycin (many salts)	er-ith-roe-MYE-sin	Capsule, injection, oral liquid, tablet, topical	Rx
metronidazole (Flagyl)	me-troe-NYE-da-zole	Capsule, injection	Rx
penicillin G benzathine (Bicillin L-A)	pen-i-SIL-in G BENZ-a-theen	Only IM injection	Rx
tetracycline (Sumycin)	te-tra-SYE-kleen	Capsule	Rx

Agents for Treating Sexually Transmitted Infections

Table 4.13 presents the most commonly used agents for sexually transmitted infections. Many of these medications are also discussed in Chapter 5.

Azithromycin (Zithromax) is provided by the manufacturer in several forms. The powdered form is approved to be administered as a one-time dose to treat some sexually transmitted bacterial infections. For chancroid (syphilis lesion) in men and chlamydia in women, a 1 g dose is used. For gonococcal infections in either sex, a one-time dose of 2 g is administered.

Ceftriaxone (Rocephin) is used frequently, especially against penicillinase-producing bacteria.

Tetracycline (Sumycin) is commonly used to control *Chlamydia trachomatis*, which frequently occurs with gonorrhea. Tetracycline and **erythromycin (Ilotycin)** are both effective against chlamydia.

Penicillin G benzathine (Bicillin L-A) is used to treat syphilis. It is especially effective during the primary stage, and it is the only agent active against growing bacteria. Penicillin is administered in low concentration, but it is appropriate treatment because the spirochete grows slowly. It is effective for approximately two weeks.

**Doxycycline (Doryx, Vibramycin*)* is used to treat lymphogranuloma venereum.

Metronidazole (Flagyl) is used to treat *Gardnerella vaginitis* (formerly called *Haemophilus vaginalis*) infections. It is important that the patient complete the full course of treatment.

Fungi and Fungal Diseases

A **fungus** is a single-cell organism similar to an animal cell and to a green plant cell. All three are **eukaryotic** (having a defined nucleus), in contrast to bacteria, which are **prokaryotic** (lacking a defined nucleus). Fungi (plural of fungus, pronounced FUN-jye) include mushrooms, yeasts, and molds. They are distinguished from green plants by the absence of chlorophyll (the substance that gives plants their green color) and the fact that they reproduce by spores. Fungi cells are distinguished from animal cells and bacterial cells by the presence of a unique rigid cell wall. All eukaryotic cells have similar molecular machinery for performing life functions such as making proteins, replicating DNA, and storing and releasing energy. This machinery is different from the corresponding machinery in prokaryotic cells. Therefore, the antibiotics discussed earlier in this chapter that work so well against bacteria do not work against fungi, and a drug that can kill a fungus is likely to be toxic to a human as well. Still, there are some differences between human and fungal cells that can be used as the basis for antifungal drugs. For example, human cell membranes contain **cholesterol** (a type of lipid found in animal cells that is a key constituent of cell membranes and precursor to hormone production); the cell membranes of fungi contain **ergosterol**, another lipid unique to fungi.

Fungal Diseases

Usually, fungal infections are topical and mild. **Dermatophytes**, fungi of the skin, cause some of the most frequent and ordinary infections, such as athlete's foot and ringworm. *Candida* is another common fungus that causes vaginal yeast infections and oral thrush. However, when a fungus gains entry to the bloodstream or cannot be destroyed because of immunodeficiency, it can cause serious systemic infections. Table 4.14 lists common fungi and related infections.

TABLE 4.14 Examples of Fungal Organisms and the Resulting Infections

Organism	Fungal Infection	Description of Infection
Aspergillus	Aspergillosis	Inflammation in the skin, lungs, or bones
Blastomyces	Blastomycosis	Infection begins from inhalation through the lungs; produces tumors in the skin and other body tissues
Candida (yeast)	Candidiasis	Usually a superficial infection of the mucous membranes, but sometimes systemic
Coccidioides	Coccidioidomycosis	Known as Valley fever and endemic to the western United States, Mexico, and South America; an acute but benign self-limiting respiratory tract infection in its primary form, but a virulent, severe disease of the viscera, CNS, and lungs in its secondary form; sometimes misdiagnosed as lung cancer
Cryptococcus	Cryptococcosis	Invasion of CNS most commonly seen in immunocompromised patients
Histoplasma	Histoplasmosis	Usually asymptomatic infection resulting from inhalation of spores, but can cause acute pneumonia

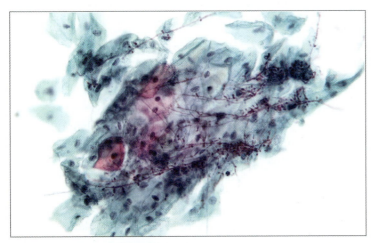

Fungi, such as these *Candida*, are unicellular organisms responsible for several systemic diseases.

Systemic fungal diseases are most likely to develop in patients whose immune systems, are depressed by disease, drug therapy (for example, the use of corticosteroids or antineoplastics), or poor nutrition. Patients at risk for fungal infections include those who have recently received transplants and are receiving immunosuppressive medications, patients with IV catheters, and those with some cancers or human immunodeficiency virus (HIV). Fungi can also cause systemic infections of the body organs and tissues such as the lungs, brain and central nervous system (CNS), and blood.

Put Down Roots

Many antifungal names end in –*zole* so if the generic form of the drug ends in –*zole* (especially –*conazole*), there is a good chance it is an antifungal.

Antifungal Medications

Some antifungal agents prevent the synthesis of ergosterol, a building block for fungal cell membranes. Because human cell membranes use cholesterol instead of ergosterol, they are affected minimally by antifungals. Other antifungal agents act by inhibiting fungal cytochrome P-450, which is different from human cytochrome P-450, so these medications have little effect on human cells but destroy the cells of the fungi. Some antifungals are available in topical dosage forms and are now available OTC. These topical agents will be discussed in Chapter 15.

Pulse dosing for fungal nail infections is sometimes used. Each pulse dose is usually one week per month. Because the drug persists in the nail for several months, this regimen works as well as continuous daily dosing. Because patients take much less drug, treatment is safer and costs less.

Antifungal drugs are dispensed as topical, IV, and systemic agents. Even though the topical agents seem relatively mild compared to other antifungal agents, serious side effects have been reported. Close attention to the dosing regimen is needed to avoid overdosing. Table 4.15 lists the most commonly used antifungals.

Polyenes

The **polyene** antifungal class includes **amphotericin B** and nystatin. Amphotericin B interferes with cell-wall permeability (the ability of a material to allow molecules or ions to pass through it), allowing electrolytes and other substances to leak out. Amphotericin B is an antifungal drug that is particularly toxic to the liver and kidneys. Thus, its use is reserved for the most serious and life-threatening fungal infections. Nystatin is an antifungal that can be used topically and systemically.

- **Abelcet**, **AmBisome**, and **Amphotec** are lipid complex injectable forms of amphotericin B that are associated with less kidney toxicity. These drugs are administered by IV infusion. They are indicated for treating aspergillosis or any type of progressive fungal infection in patients unresponsive to or intolerant of amphotericin B. A wide range of side effects similar to those of amphotericin B has been reported.

- **Nystatin (Mycostat)** is most often used in liquid form to swish and swallow. It is given commonly to patients with **oral candidiasis**, a yeastlike fungi causing infection in the mouth.

TABLE 4.15 Commonly Used Antifungals

Generic (Brand)	Pronunciation	Dosage Form	Common Dosage	Dispensing Status
Oral Thrush Agents				
clotrimazole (Mycelex)	kloe-TRIM-a-zole	Lozenge	Dissolve in mouth 5 times a day	Rx
nystatin (Mycostatin)	Nye-STAT-in	Oral suspension, powder, tablet	500,000–1 million units 3 times a day	Rx
Skin and Nail Agents				
butenafine (Lotrimin Ultra, Mentax)	Bew-TEN-a-feen	Topical cream	Once a day for 2 weeks	OTC, Rx
ciclopirox (Loprox, Penlac)	sye-KLO-pie-rox	Cream, gel, lotion, nail lacquer, shampoo, topical suspension	Depends on dosage form and site of infection but can take up to 12 weeks for cure	Rx
clotrimazole (Desenex, Lotrimin AF)	kloe-TRIM-a-zole	Cream, ointment, topical solution	Twice a day for 2–4 weeks	OTC
clotrimazole-betamethasone (Lotrisone)	kloe-TRIM-a-zole bay-ta-meth-a-sone	Cream, lotion	Twice a day for 4 weeks	Rx
griseofulvin (Grifulvin V, Gris-PEG)	gri-see-oh-FUL-vin	Oral suspension, tablet	Varies depending on age and weight of patient (4 weeks for athlete's foot, 4–6 months for nail infections)	Rx
ketoconazole (Nizoral)	kee-toe-KON-a-zole	Cream, foam, gel, shampoo	200–400 mg a day for 2–4 weeks	Rx

Generic (Brand)	Pronunciation	Dosage Form	Common Dosage	Dispensing Status
miconazole (Micatin, Neosporin AF)	mye-KON-a-zole	Lotion, powder, ointment, solution, spray, topical cream	Twice a day for 2 weeks	OTC
nystatin (Nyamyc, Nystop)	nye-STAT-in	Cream, ointment, powder	Twice a day until lesions heal	Rx
terbinafine (Lamisil AT)	TER-bin-a-feen	Cream, gel, spray	Once a day for 1–2 weeks	OTC
Systemic Agents				
amphotericin B	am-foe-TER-i-sin B	Powder for injection	Varies by patient and disease being treated	Rx
caspofungin (Cancidas)	kas-poe-FUN-jin	Powder for injection	70 mg as initial dose followed by 50 mg/day	Rx
fluconazole (Diflucan)	floo-KON-a-zole	Oral suspension, oral tablet, injection	IV: varies depending on infection being treated PO: 150 mg in 1 dose for vaginal infections, 200-800 mg/day for systemic infections	Rx
flucytosine (Ancobon)	floo-SYE-toe-seen	Capsule	50–150 mg/kg/day in divided intervals every 6 hr	Rx
itraconazole (Sporanox)	i-tra-KON-a-zole	Capsule, oral solution	200–400 mg/day	Rx
ketoconazole (Nizoral)	kee-toe-KON-a-zole	Tablet	200–400 mg/day	Rx
liposomal amphotericin B (Abelcet, Amphotec, AmBisome)	lye-poh-sohm-al am-foe-TER-i-sin B	Oral suspension, powder for injection	Varies by patient and disease being treated	Rx
micafungin (Mycamine)	mye-ka-FUN-gin	Powder for injection	Preventive therapy: 50 mg/day Active treatment: 150 mg/day	Rx
posaconazole (Noxafil)	poe-sa-KON-azole	Oral suspension, injection, tablet	100–400 mg twice or three times a day	Rx
voriconazole (Vfend)	vor-i-KON-a-zohl	Oral suspension, powder for injection, tablet	IV: 4–6 mg/kg every 12 hr PO: 200 mg every 12 hr	Rx
Vaginal Agents				
butoconazole (Gynazole-1)	bew-toe-KON-a-zole	Vaginal cream, vaginal suppositories	Once a day for 1–3 days	OTC, Rx
clotrimazole (Gyne-Lotrimin)	kloe-TRIM-a-zole	Vaginal cream and suppository	Once a day for 3–7 days	OTC
miconazole (Monistat)	mye-KON-a-zole	Vaginal cream	1,200 mg at bedtime for 1 day 200 mg/day for 3 days 100 mg/day for 7 days	OTC
tioconazole (Vagistat-1)	tee-oh-KON-a-zole	Vaginal ointment	1 applicator at bedtime for 1 day	OTC

Side Effects and Dispensing Issues of Polyenes Amphotericin B is associated with bothersome side effects in addition to nephrotoxicity and hepatotoxicity. Side effects are fever, chills, shaking, and headache. Prophylaxis with acetaminophen and/or an antihistamine such as diphenhydramine is often necessary to alleviate or prevent infusion-related side effects. A common, serious side effect is renal toxicity. Potassium, calcium, and magnesium stores are often depleted. Anemia (a below-normal concentration of erythrocytes or hemoglobin in the blood) is also common.

Amphotericin should be infused slowly or fever, chills, nausea, vomiting, and headache can occur. Amphotericin B is also available in an IV liposome dosage form (see Figure 4.5), which surrounds the drug molecules with a fat/oil layer. This protective layer decreases the drug's ability to come into direct contact with body tissues and thus reduces its toxic effects. Amphotericin B should not be mixed or "piggybacked" with other drugs. To avoid precipitation, it should not be mixed with **normal saline (NS)**. It is usually mixed in D_5W and stored in the refrigerator and must be infused within six hours of being mixed. Antiemetic substances (agents that prevent or eliminate nausea and vomiting; covered in Chapter 10), can reduce the severity of nausea and vomiting. If the patient does not have a central venous catheter, the IV site should be changed frequently, as phlebitis (inflammation of a vein) is common with administration of this drug.

Oral nystatin is associated with diarrhea, nausea, stomach pain, and vomiting. Topical nystatin is associated with hypersensitivity reactions. Because nystatin is available in oral and topical formulations, it is important to ensure the correct product is selected.

Contraindications of Polyenes Amphotericin B and nystatin do not have contraindications.

Cautions and Considerations for Polyenes Reports of anaphylaxis are associated with amphotericin B use, and infusions should be supervised. If patients exhibit signs of anaphylaxis, administration should be discontinued immediately.

Drug Interactions of Polyenes Amphotericin should not be used with foscarnet. Nystatin diminishes the effects of the probiotic *Saccharomyces boulardii*.

FIGURE 4.5
Liposome Dosage Form

Liposomal amphotericin is available as a suspension or powder for injection, depending on the brand chosen.

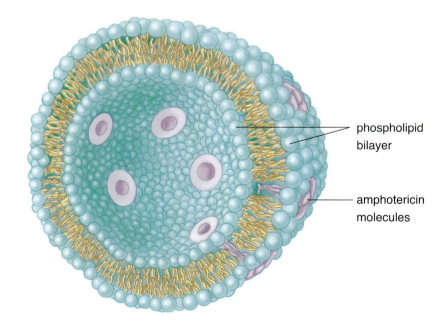

phospholipid bilayer

amphotericin molecules

Azoles

Antifungals ending in the suffix –*azole* are in the **azole** family and are generally well tolerated. Members of the azole family interfere with cytochrome P-450 and inhibit the formation of the fungal cell wall.

- **Clotrimazole (Mycelex)**, supplied as a troche (a small lozenge), is especially effective against oral candidiasis. It is also available topically for skin and nail infections (**Desenex, Lotrimin AF**) or vaginally (**Gyne-Lotrimin**).

- **Ketoconazole (Nizoral)** has the same side effect profile as most of the other antifungal agents. Side effects are dose dependent and include nausea, anorexia, and vomiting. Oral ketoconazole comes in tablet dosage form. It is also available topically.

- **Fluconazole (Diflucan)** is metabolized through the cytochrome P-450 system. The oral form is used for vaginal or oral candidiasis, whereas the IV form should be reserved for patients unable to tolerate oral therapy. The most common side effects are headache, rash, and GI upset.

- **Itraconazole (Sporanox)** is especially useful for fungal infections of the nails. The capsule should be taken with a fatty meal, but should not be taken within two hours of taking antacids or histamine-2 (H_2) receptor blockers. Because itraconazole can be toxic to the liver, patients should report any unusual nausea, vomiting, jaundice, or changes in the stool to the healthcare provider immediately. Capsules should not be substituted for the oral solution because the solution is more readily absorbed.

- **Posaconazole (Noxafil)** has different uses, depending on its dosage form. The tablet and intravenous forms are used for invasive *Candida* and *Aspergillus* infections. The suspension form, which is cherry flavored, may be used for oropharyngeal infections or for systemic infections. Oral dosage forms should be administered with a full meal.

- **Voriconazole (Vfend)** is an alternative to amphotericin B for life-threatening fungal infections. It can be started intravenously and switched to an oral dose. Voriconazole has serious side effects such as liver toxicity and blurred vision. Patients taking this drug should not drive at night.

Side Effects and Dispensing Issues When ingested orally, nausea, vomiting, abdominal pain, and diarrhea are the most frequently reported side effects. Itraconazole and ketoconazole are particularly likely to cause stomach symptoms. Voriconazole is associated with transient vision changes (such as seeing flashes of light or having sensitivity to light), visual hallucinations, alopecia, nail changes or loss, and skin rash. Topically applied azoles are associated with application-site reactions such as burning, discomfort, edema, and pain.

Itraconazole is available in capsules and oral solution. Capsules should not be substituted for oral solution because the solution is more readily absorbed. Patients should take itraconazole capsules with acidic food or drink to improve absorption. Posaconazole should be taken with food.

Voriconazole is available orally and intravenously. IV voriconazole must be infused over one to two hours and should not be infused simultaneously with any other products. Voriconazole must be reconstituted and used immediately.

Contraindications Azoles are contraindicated with concurrent use of quinidine; benzodiazepines such as alprazolam, chlordiazepoxide, clonazepam, diazepam, and triazolam; dofetilide; pimozide; and statins such as lovastatin, simvastatin, and atorvastatin.

Miconazole is contraindicated in patients with milk-protein allergy.

Cautions and Considerations Ketoconazole carries black box warning for hepatotoxicity and QT prolongation. Itraconazole carries two different boxed warnings. One warns that itraconazole should not be used with methadone, disopyramide, dofetilide, dronedarone, quinidine, ergot alkaloids, ergotamine, methylergometrine, irinotecan, lurasidone, oral midazolam, pimozide, triazolam, felodipine, nisoldipine, ranolazine, eplerenone, cisapride, lovastatin, simvastatin, ticagrelor, colchicine, fesoterodine, telithromycin, and solifenacin. Itraconazole's other boxed warning deals with heart failure and avoiding administration for fungal nail infections.

Fluconazole may cause QT prolongation, and caution should be exercised when using it with other medications that can cause arrhythmia.

Drug Interactions Azole antifungals are associated with multiple drug-drug interactions. Please see the contraindication section for a listing of drug interactions. Azole antifungals decrease the activity of the probiotic *Saccharomyces boulardii*.

Echinocandins

Protect medication from exposure to light

The generic names of the **echinocandin** class of antifungals end in the suffix *-fungin*. Echinocandins include caspofungin and micafungin. Echinocandins work by inhibiting the synthesis of D-glucan, which is an integral component of the fungal cell wall.

- **Caspofungin (Cancidas)** was the first echinocandin commercially available. It is only available in IV form for the treatment of invasive *Aspergillosis* and *Candida* in patients who are unresponsive to other therapies such as amphotericin B and itraconazole. It seems to cause fewer hypersensitivity reactions than the other drugs in this class.
- **Micafungin (Mycamine)** is used to treat patients with *Aspergillosis* and *Candida*.

Side Effects and Dispensing Issues The echinocandins are injectable and may result in infusion and hypersensitivity reactions including rash, redness, **hypotension**, and—in some cases—angioedema. Injection-site pain is another potential side effect.

Micafungin should be reconstituted and mixed with either NS or D_5W. After the diluent is injected into the vial, it should be gently swirled but not shaken. Once reconstituted, the micafungin preparation is good for 24 hours at room temperature and must be protected from light.

Contraindications Micafungin and caspofungin do not have contraindications.

Cautions and Considerations The echinocandins are associated with anaphylaxis and histamine-related reactions. Use should be discontinued immediately if anaphylaxis occurs.

Drug Interactions Echinocandins decrease the activity of the probiotic *Saccharomyces boulardii*. Cyclosporine may increase toxic effects of caspofungin. Rifampin may decrease the concentrations of caspofungin. Micafungin may increase drug levels of pimozide, and concurrent use is not recommended.

Miscellaneous Antifungals

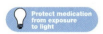
Protect medication from exposure to light

Other antifungals include the topical products **butenafine (Lotrimin Ultra, Mentax), ciclopirox (Loprox, Penlac),** and **terbinafine (Lamisil AT). Flucytosine (Ancobon)** and **griseofulvin (Grifulvin V, Gris-PEG)** are systemic.

Side Effects and Dispensing Issues Butenafine is associated with burning, contact dermatitis, erythema, irritation, pruritus, and stinging. Ciclopirox, which is applied topically, is associated with acne, alopecia, contact dermatitis, dry skin, skin burning, eye pain, and headache. Terbinafine may cause headache, skin rash, diarrhea, dyspepsia, and nasopharyngitis.

Flucytosine is associated with rash; leukopenia; thrombocytopenia; GI symptoms such as nausea, diarrhea, and vomiting; and hepatic side effects. Side effects of griseofulvin include dizziness, fatigue, skin rash, photosensitivity, and diarrhea. Griseofulvin may enhance toxic effects of alcohol. Concurrent use is not recommended. Contraceptive failure is possible with griseofulvin use and alternative nonhormonal contraception should be used. Griseofulvin liquid should be protected from light.

Contraindications Griseofulvin is contraindicated in patients who are pregnant or have liver failure or porphyria. Butenafine, ciclopirox, flucytosine, and terbinafine do not have contraindications.

Cautions and Considerations Flucytosine carries a black box warning to use extreme caution in patients with renal dysfunction. The agent should be used only in combination with other antifungals to prevent development of resistance. Patients with bone marrow depression, hematologic disease, or those undergoing therapy that suppresses the bone marrow should use flucytosine with caution.

Griseofulvin should be discontinued if granulocytopenia occurs. There is a potential cross-reaction between penicillin hypersensitivity and griseofulvin hypersensitivity. Severe skin reactions have been reported with griseofulvin use; it is recommended that patients discontinue therapy and seek emergency medical care if severe skin reactions occur.

Depression has been reported with terbinafine use. Patients should contact their healthcare practitioners immediately if they experience any signs and symptoms of depression.

Drug Interactions Systemic antifungals may diminish the therapeutic effect of *Saccharomyces boulardii*, and concurrent use should be avoided. Butenafine and ciclopirox do not have known drug interactions.

Terbinafine may increase serum concentrations of pimozide and thioridazine, and concurrent use should be avoided. It may decrease levels of tamoxifen.

Flucytosine may increase adverse or toxic effects of clozapine and dipyrone, and coadministration is not recommended. Gimeracil may increase the concentrations of flucytosine, and the use of the two agents together should be avoided.

Complementary and Alternative Therapies

Some complimentary and alternative therapies that may be used for infections include echinacea and zinc. Patients who are using complimentary and alternative should tell their healthcare providers, pharmacists, and pharmacy technicians. **Echinacea** (*Echinacea purpurea*) is an herb some patients use to treat the common cold, RTIs, and even vaginal yeast infections. It has been found to reduce the severity

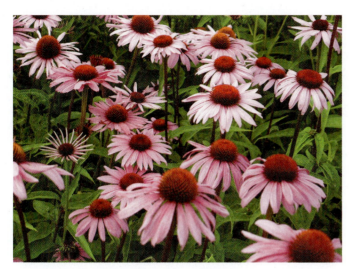

Echinacea comes from the purple coneflower plant and may be used to help treat the common cold.

and length of symptoms. Echinacea does not cure infections, but it may be used to augment drug therapy. Echinacea increases phagocytosis, the process by which the immune system cells "eat up" foreign cells such as bacteria. It also enhances lymphocyte activity. Echinacea products contain various concentrations of this herbal remedy. A standard dose has not been established. However, for echinacea to be effective, patients must use it multiple times a day and initiate its use at the very first signs of infection. Dosing is heaviest during the first 5 days of infection and continues for up to 10 days.

Topical zinc formulations have been used to treat and prevent infections for thousands of years. Zinc may be used to enhance wound healing and prevent wound-associated infections. Fungal infections of the scalp may also be treated with zinc. Others use zinc as prevention for respiratory tract infections. There is not a well-established dose for zinc. Side effects may include increased heart rate, agitation, vomiting, and nausea. Intranasal zinc has been associated with loss of smell.

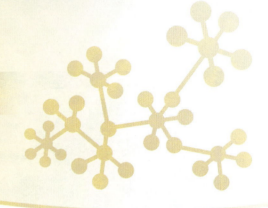

CHAPTER SUMMARY

Fighting Bacterial Infections

- Bacteria are single-celled organisms that occur in almost all environments. They can penetrate body tissues and set up areas of infection.

- An infection is an invasion of the body by pathogens, resulting in tissue response to organisms and toxins.

- Bacterial infections are contagious until antibiotics have been taken for 24 to 48 hours.

- Bacteria can be classified by oxygenation needs (aerobic or anaerobic), shape and arrangement of growth, and Gram-stain result (positive or negative). Classification directs antibiotic selection.

- General signs of infection that suggest a bacterial origin are fever (101°F or greater) and an increased number (>12,000/mm^3) of white blood cells. The onset of fever alone is not diagnostic of bacterial infection.

- The outcome of antibiotic treatment is measured in two ways: (1) the clinical response, meaning the signs and symptoms disappear, or (2) the microbiologic response, meaning the organism is completely eradicated.

- An antibiotic works in one of six ways: (1) preventing folic acid synthesis, (2) inhibiting cell-wall formation, (3) blocking protein formation, (4) interfering with DNA formation, (5) disrupting the cell membrane, or (6) disrupting DNA structure.

- A bactericidal agent kills bacteria.

- A bacteriostatic agent inhibits growth or multiplication of bacteria.

- Antibiotics may interfere with the effectiveness of contraceptives, and other drugs.

Major Classes of Antibiotic Drugs

Sulfonamides

- The sulfa drugs are the oldest antibiotics on the market, so the technician needs to know both the brand names and generic names of these drugs.

- Nitrofurantoin may be an acceptable alternative to sulfa drugs for UTIs.

- Sulfas are used in the treatment of UTIs, otitis media, GI infections, lower respiratory tract infections, and prophylaxis of *Pneumocystis carinii pneumonia* in immunocompromised patients.

- Patients taking sulfonamides should be told to drink six to eight glasses of water a day to keep the urine dilute and avoid crystallization of the drug in the urine. They should be told to avoid exposure to sunlight and to notify the healthcare practitioner if a rash appears (the most common side effect of the sulfas).

Penicillins

- Penicillin has many therapeutic uses and is usually used for the treatment of Gram-positive infections.

- Penicillin is bactericidal in that it kills bacteria by preventing them from forming the rigid wall needed for survival. Human cells do not have cell walls and are, therefore, uninjured by penicillin.

- Some bacteria are resistant to penicillins because they produce an enzyme called *beta-lactamase*. Beta-lactamase renders penicillins ineffective.

- Penicillin should be taken with water because the acids in fruit juices or colas could deactivate the drug. The most common side effect of the penicillins is diarrhea.

Cephalosporins

- Cephalosporins have a mechanism of action similar to penicillins but a broader spectrum of coverage.

- A patient allergic to penicillin may also be allergic to cephalosporins, and vice versa. The pharmacy technician will find both allergies in the computer because most systems enter the drugs under penicillin-cephalosporin allergy.

- The first-generation cephalosporins are similar to the penicillinase-resistant penicillins, with limited Gram-negative coverage. The second-generation cephalosporins have broader coverage, especially against *H. influenzae*. The third generation is active against a wide spectrum of Gram-negative organisms. The fourth-generation cephalosporin is considered "broad spectrum" with both Gram-negative and somewhat less Gram-positive coverage. The fifth generation cephalosporin, ceftaroline, has coverage against MRSA.

- Cephalosporins are probably the most commonly used antibiotics because they cover a very wide range of organisms and have lower toxicity than other antibiotics with the same coverage.

Carbapenems and Monobactams

- Carbapenems and monobactams are drugs that are structurally similar to penicillins and cephalosporins. They kill bacteria by inhibiting cell-wall synthesis.

- Carbapenems are used for mixed Gram-positive and Gram-negative infections. Monobactams, in contrast, are use primarily for Gram-negative bacteria.

- Carbapenem use is associated with seizures.

Vancomycin

- Vancomycin is an antibiotic with activity against Gram-positive bacteria and is used primarily to treat MRSA infections.

- Vancomycin can cause ototoxicity and nephrotoxicity. Many times, therapeutic drug levels are drawn and used or monitored to maximize effectiveness and minimize adverse reactions.

- Vancomycin is usually administered intravenously and must be diluted before use.

Lincosamides and Macrolides

- Lincosamides and macrolides can be bacteriostatic (at low doses) and bactericidal (at high doses) and work by blocking the bacteria's ability to produce needed proteins for survival.

- Clindamycin, a lincosamide, carries a black box warning because it can cause severe and possibly fatal colitis. Its use should be reserved for treatment of serious infections for which use of other antimicrobials is inappropriate.

- Azithromycin is a commonly used macrolide and is available in various formulations.

- Macrolides, in particular clarithromycin, have many drug interactions. It is important for the pharmacy technician to help the pharmacist maintain an accurate drug list for patients using them.

Aminoglycosides

- Aminoglycosides are used to treat very serious infections. They work by blocking a bacteria's ability to make essential proteins for survival.

- Nephrotoxicity and ototoxicity are concerns with aminoglycoside use. Drug blood levels and other laboratory measurements are used to minimize these potentially harmful effects.

Tetracyclines

- Tetracyclines are bacteriostatic and inhibit protein synthesis within bacterial cells.

- Patients taking tetracycline should be warned to avoid the sun, dairy products, and antacids and to take the drug on an empty stomach.

- Children and pregnant women should not take tetracyclines.
- Always watch the expiration date on tetracyclines. It can be dangerous to dispense one of these drugs if it is out of date.

Fluoroquinolones or Quinolones

- Fluoroquinolones or quinolones are antibiotics with strong, rapid bactericidal activity against Gram-negative bacteria and some Gram-positive bacteria and work by interfering with DNA formation.
- They are often used for bone and joint infections, eye infections, and serious RTIs and UTIs.
- Quinolones should not be used during pregnancy.

Metronidazole

- Metronidazole is unique in that it is effective against bacteria, fungi, and protozoa.
- Metronidazole use is associated with a metallic taste and urine discoloration.
- Metronidazole interacts significantly with alcohol to cause a severe reaction. Patients can become quite ill with nausea, vomiting, flushing, sweating, and headache if they ingest any alcohol while taking metronidazole and for three days after stopping the medication.

Linezolid

- Linezolid works by inhibiting bacterial protein synthesis and is used for MRSA, VRE, and other Gram-positive infections.
- Linezolid may increase the toxic effects of alcohol and should not be used concurrently.

Daptomycin

- Daptomycin works by inhibiting bacterial DNA and RNA synthesis and is used for complicated skin and skin structure infections and *Staphylococcus aureus* blood infections.
- Daptomycin comes as a powder for reconstitution and should not be mixed with dextrose-containing solutions.

Storage of Liquid Antibiotics

- After reconstitution, some antibiotics need to be stored in the refrigerator, whereas others may be kept at room temperature.
- The pharmacy technician may give the patient the information about whether the drug needs to be refrigerated—it is not counseling.

Ophthalmic Antibiotics

- Ophthalmic dosage forms may be used in the ear, but otic dosage forms should never be put in the eye.

- Ophthalmic antibiotics are very expensive because of stringent manufacturing requirements. The technician often needs to know which antibiotic is less expensive in order to advise the prescriber.

Sexually Transmitted Infections

- Sexual activity causes many genital system diseases.

- Chlamydia, gonorrhea, syphilis, nongonococcal urethritis, and vaginitis can all be treated with antibiotics.

Fungi and Fungal Diseases

- A fungus is a single-celled organism that has similarities to both animal and green plant cells.

- Drugs that fight bacterial infections are generally not effective for fungal infections.

- Fungal disease can range from topical and mild to systemic and severe.

Major Classes of Antifungals

Polyenes

- Examples of polyene antifungals include amphotericin B and nystatin.

- Amphotericin B is injectable and can be toxic to the liver and kidneys and is reserved for serious fungal infections.

- Nystatin can be used topically and systemically.

Azoles

- Azoles inhibit the formation of the fungal cell wall.

- When used orally, common side effects of azoles include nausea, vomiting, abdominal pain, and diarrhea.

- Drug interactions are a concern when patients are using azoles with other medications.

Echinocandins

- Caspofungin and micafungin are echinocandins that are used to treat patients with Aspergillosis and Candida.

- Echinocandins are associated with hypersensitivity reactions.

Complementary and Alternative Therapies

- Patients may use echinacea and zinc to prevent and treat infections.

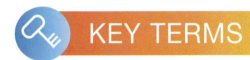

KEY TERMS

aerobic needing oxygen to survive

aminoglycoside a class of antibiotics that inhibits bacterial protein synthesis by binding to ribosomal subunits; commonly used to treat serious infections

anaerobic capable of surviving in the absence of oxygen

anemia a below-normal concentration of erythrocytes or hemoglobin in the blood

antibiotic a chemical substance with the ability to kill or inhibit the growth of bacteria by interfering with bacteria life processes

antibiotic resistance when bacteria develop defense mechanisms that resist or inactivate antibiotics used on them

antiseptic a substance that kills or inhibits the growth of microorganisms on the outside of the body to reduce the possibility of infection, sepsis, or putrefaction

arrhythmia variation in heartbeat, irregular heartbeat

bacteria small, single-celled microorganisms that exist in three main forms: spherical (i.e., cocci), rod shaped (i.e., bacilli), and spiral (i.e., spirilla)

bactericidal agent a drug that kills bacteria

bacteriostatic agent a drug that inhibits the growth or multiplication of bacteria

beta-lactamase an enzyme that destroys the beta-lactam ring present in the molecular structure of all penicillins

beta-lactamase inhibitor an agent that inhibits beta-lactamase

broad-spectrum antibiotic an antibiotic that is effective against multiple organisms

Candida a common fungus that causes vaginal yeast infections and oral thrush

carbapenems a class of drugs used for mixed infections that have both Gram-positive and Gram-negative bacteria

cephalosporin a class of antibiotics with a mechanism of action similar to that of penicillins, but with a different antibacterial spectrum, resistance to beta-lactamase, and pharmacokinetics; divided into first-, second-, third-, and fourth-generation agents

chancre a painless ulcer at the site of an infection

cholesterol a type of fatty acid or lipid found in animal cells that is a key constituent of cell membranes and precursor to hormone production

community-acquired contracted outside of the hospital

culture and sensitivity (C&S) the test to see which antibiotics have the best effect on a pathogen culture

cyclic lipopeptide a class of drug that binds to bacterial membranes, causing cell membrane depolarization

dermatophytes fungi that can cause infection of the skin

dextrose solution dextrose 5% in water (D_5W)

disinfectant a chemical agent such as rubbing alcohol used on inanimate surfaces and objects to destroy fungi, viruses, and bacteria, but not necessarily their spores

Echinacea (*Echinacea purpurea*) an herb some patients use to treat the common cold, RTIs, and vaginal yeast infections

empirical treatment broad treatment begun before a definite diagnosis can be obtained

ergosterol a lipid unique to fungi

eukaryotic having a defined nucleus

fluoroquinolones a class of drugs that kills bacteria by inhibiting the enzyme that helps DNA coil

fungus a single-cell organism that is similar to an animal cell and to a green plant cell

generations groups that organize cephalosporins

Gram-negative bacteria have a thick cell wall that absorbs Gram stain and appears purple

Gram-positive bacteria have a thin cell wall that does not absorb Gram stain

hypotension low blood pressure

infection a condition in which bacteria grow in body tissues and cause tissue damage to the host either by their presence or by toxins they produce

jaundice yellowing of skin and eyes

lincosamides drugs that block bacteria's ability to produce proteins for survival

loading dose amount of a drug that will bring the blood concentration rapidly to a therapeutic level

long QT syndrome (or QT prolongation) a heat rhythm disorder

macrolide a class of bacteriostatic antibiotics that inhibit protein synthesis by combining with ribosomes

minimum inhibitory concentration (MIC) the amount of drug needed to inhibit growth of the bacteria

methicillin-resistant *Staphylococcus aureus* (MRSA) a bacteria that causes infections that is resistant to certain drugs

monobactam a class of drugs used for Gram-negative bacterial infections

nephrotoxicity ability to damage the kidneys

nitroimidazole a class of drug effective against fungi, protozoa, and bacteria

normal saline (NS) a sterile IV or irrigation solution containing a concentration of 0.9% sodium chloride in water

nosocomial infections an infection acquired by patients in the hospital

oral candidiasis yeastlike fungi causing infection in the mouth

ototoxicity ability to damage the organs of hearing

pathogenic causing or capable of causing disease or infection

penicillin a class of antibiotics obtained from *Penicillium chrysogenum*; kill bacteria by preventing them from forming a rigid cell wall, thereby allowing an excessive amount of water to enter through osmosis and cause lysis of the bacterium cell

pH a measurement of acidity or alkalinity. pH 7 is neutral; a solution with a pH above 7 is alkaline; a solution with a pH below 7 is acidic; the pH of blood is approximately 7.4

polyene a class of drugs that interferes with cell-wall permeability

prokaryotic lacking a defined nucleus

pulse dosing dosing that produces escalating antibiotic levels early in the dosing interval followed by a prolonged dose-free period

quinolones a class of antibiotics with rapid bactericidal action against most Gram-negative and many Gram-positive bacteria; work by causing DNA breakage and cell death

sepsis a systemic inflammatory response to infection resulting from blood-borne infections

spectrum of activity the range of bacteria against which an agent is effective

Stevens-Johnson syndrome a sometimes fatal form of erythema multiforme (an allergic reaction marked by red blotches on the skin)

sulfonamides sulfa drugs; a class of bacteriostatic antibiotics that work by blocking a specific step in the biosynthetic pathway of folic acid in bacteria

synergistic drug therapy when two or more drugs are used together because they employ different mechanisms of action that work better together than either drug works alone

tetracyclines a class of broad-spectrum bacteriostatic antibiotics that are produced by soil organisms and inhibit protein synthesis by binding to bacterial ribosomes

vancomycin a class of drugs that probably works by inhibiting cell-wall formation

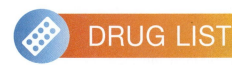

DRUG LIST

Sulfonamides and Related Drugs

nitrofurantoin (Macrobid, Macrodantin)
sulfamethoxazole-trimethoprim (Bactrim, Bactrim DS, Cotrim, Cotrim DS, Septra, Septra DS)

Penicillins

amoxicillin (Amoxil, Moxatag)
amoxicillin-clavulanate (Augmentin)
ampicillin
ampicillin-sulbactam (Unasyn)
dicloxacillin (Dycill)
methicillin
nafcillin (Unipen)
oxacillin
penicillin G (various)
penicillin V (Veetids)
piperacillin
piperacillin-tazobactam (Zosyn)
ticarcillin (Ticar)
ticarcillin-clavulanate (Timentin)

Cephalosporins

cefaclor (Ceclor)
cefazolin (Ancef)
cefdinir (Omnicef)
cefditoren (Spectracef)
cefepime (Maxipime)
cefixime (Suprax)
cefotetan
cefotaxime (Claforan)
cefpodoxime (Vantin)
ceftaroline (Teflaro)
ceftazidime (Fortaz , Tazicef)
ceftibuten (Cedax)
ceftriaxone (Rocephin)
cefuroxime (Ceftin, Zinacef)
cephalexin (Keflex)

Carbapenems

doripenem
aztreonam
ertapenem (Invanz)
imipenem-cilastatin (Primaxin)
meropenem (Merrem I.V.)

Monobactam

aztreonam (Azactam)

Vancomycin

vancomycin (Vancocin)

Macrolides

azithromycin (Zithromax, Z Pak, Zmax,
    Zithromax Tri-Pak)
clarithromycin (Biaxin)
clindamycin (Cleocin)
erythromycin (EES, EryC, EryPed, Ery-Tab,
    Erythrocin, Pediazole)

Aminoglycosides

amikacin
gentamicin (Garamycin, Gentak)
tobramycin (TOBI, Tobrex)

Tetracyclines

doxycycline (Adoxa, Doryx, Oracea,
    Vibramycin)
minocycline (Minocin, Solodyn)
tetracycline (Sumycin)

Quinolones

ciprofloxacin (Cipro)
levofloxacin (Levaquin)
moxifloxacin (Avelox)

Nitroimidazoles

linezolid (Zyvox)
metronidazole (Flagyl)
oxazolidinone

Cyclic Lipopeptide

daptomycin (Cubicin)

Lincosamides and Ophthalmics

azithromycin (AzaSite)
bacitracin (AK-Tracin)
ciprofloxacin (Ciloxan)
erythromycin (Ilotycin)
gatifloxacin (Zymar)
gentamicin (Gentak, Genoptic)
moxifloxacin (Vigamox)
ofloxacin (Ocuflox)
sodium sulfacetamide (Bleph-10)
tobramycin (Tobrex)

Agents for Treating STIs

azithromycin (Zithromax)
ceftriaxone (Rocephin)
doxycycline (Doryx, Vibramycin)
erythromcin (many salts)
metronidazole (Flagyl)
penicillin G benzathine (Bicillin L-A)
tetracycline (Sumycin)

Polyenes

amphotericin B
butenafine (Lotrimin Ultra,
    Mentax)
butoconazole (Gynazole-1)
caspofungin (Cancidas)
ciclopirox (Loprox, Penlac)
clotrimazole (Desenex, Lotrimin AF)
clotrimazole (Gyne-Lotrimin)
clotrimazole (Mycelex)
clotrimazole-betamethasone
    (Lotrisone)
fluconazole (Ancobon)
griseofulvin (Grifulvin V, Gris-PEG)
itraconazole (Sporanox)
ketoconazole (Nizoral)
liposomal amphotericin B (Abelcet,
    Amphotec, AmBisome)
micafungin (Mycamine)
miconazole (Micatin, Neosporin AF)
miconazole (Monistat)
nystatin (Mycostatin)
nystatin (Nyamyc, Nystop)
posaconazole (Noxafil)
terbinafine (Lamisil AT)
tioconazole (Vagistat-1)
voriconazole (Vfend)

Echinocandins

caspofungin (Cancidas)
micafungin (Mycamine)

Azoles

clotrimazole (Mycelex)
ketoconazole (Nizoral)
fluconazole (Diflucan)
itraconazole (Sporanox)
posaconazole (Noxafil)
voriconazole (Vfend)

Black Box Warnings

clindamycin (Cleocin)
flucytosine (Ancobon)
ketoconazole
metronidazole (Flagyl)
penicillin G
benzathine

Medication Guides

ciprofloxacin (Cipro)
levofloxacin (Levaquin)
moxifloxacin (Avelox)
ofloxacin (Ocuflox)

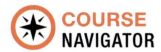
COURSE NAVIGATOR

Access interactive chapter review exercises, practice activities, flash cards, and study games.

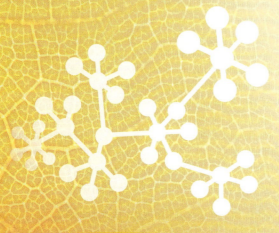

5

Viral Infection Therapy and Acquired Immunity

Learning Objectives

1 Explain the differences among bacteria, fungi, and viruses, and why the drugs used to treat them must have very different mechanisms of action.

2 Differentiate antiviral and antiretroviral drugs by their indications, therapeutic effects, side effects, dosages, and administration.

3 Use antiviral and antiretroviral terminology correctly in written and oral communication.

4 Identify drugs used for HIV and understand their synergism.

5 Describe the importance of immunization.

6 Identify common vaccines and their side effects.

COURSE NAVIGATOR

Access additional chapter resources.

Viruses are often confused with bacteria and fungi, but they are vastly different entities. Viruses are treated with drugs with markedly different mechanisms of action. Viral infections, if left untreated, may be harmful or even deadly.

Preventive strategies are preferred for infectious diseases (such as viruses) that are difficult to treat. The administration of vaccines provides prophylaxis for diseases that are associated with high risks of mortality or that result in significant illness. Vaccination, or immunization, is a way to boost the immune system in advance of exposure to disease-causing pathogens that impact public health and productivity.

Viruses and Viral Infections

A **virus** is a minute infectious agent that is much smaller than a bacterium. Viruses are not whole-cell organisms like bacteria, which can reproduce on their own and often survive in multiple environments. Instead, viruses consist only of segments of genetic material (DNA or RNA) surrounded by a capsule or protein coating. Viruses require host cells to reproduce. After attaching to the host cell, the virus alters the cell's function so that it starts producing more viral particles. The cell's normal function is halted and it dies, releasing newly formed viruses that invade other cells.

This process continues as the infection spreads. A virus can infect a spectrum of cells including animal, plant, or bacterial cells. In humans, viruses are among the most common infectious agents and are spread by one of the following routes:

- direct contact
- ingestion of contaminated food and water
- inhalation of airborne particles
- exposure to contaminated body fluids and/or contaminated equipment

The individual virus particle, a **virion**, consists of a core of genetic material, either deoxyribonucleic acid (DNA) or ribonucleic acid (RNA), and a protein shell, known as a **capsid**, that surrounds and protects the nucleic acid. Depending on the virus, the capsid may be covered with a membrane called an **envelope**, carrying surface proteins that attach to the host cell's receptors. A virus without an envelope covering the capsid is called a **naked virus**.

Stages of Viral Infection

Within the body, viral infection takes place at the cellular level in the following stages:

1. The virus attaches to cell receptors.
2. The virus penetrates the cell as the cell membrane indents and closes around the virus (endocytosis).
3. The virus escapes into the cytoplasm.
4. The virus sheds its covering (a process called **uncoating**) and presents its DNA or RNA to the cell nucleus.
5. The virus converts the nuclear activity in the cell to viral activity and rapidly produces new viral particles. (It uses the energy of the host cell to infect the cell and make more viruses.)

When viruses take over host-cell nuclear activity, they synthesize viral nucleic acid and protein, which leads to production of more virus particles. The infected host cell may be so damaged that it disintegrates, releasing bursts of mature virions. If the host cell is not destroyed, the virions are released slowly. If the virus is not a naked virus, the virion acquires its envelope from the nuclear or cell membrane of the host during the release process. All virus-infected cells have some cellular characteristics that differ from those of uninfected cells. These differences provide opportunities to target and block viral division with medications without affecting normal cells.

Influenza, hepatitis B, and human immunodeficiency virus (HIV) are common and significant illnesses caused by viral infections. **Influenza** (commonly referred to as the flu) is an example of a common viral infection; it is caused by the influenza virus. Symptoms are usually more severe than those of the common cold and include a rapid onset of malaise (vague discomfort and tiredness), myalgia (muscle pain), headache, chills, and fever. Patients with shortness of breath, wheezing, purulent (consisting of pus) or bloody sputum, fever persisting for more than seven days, or severe muscle pain should be advised to seek medical attention. Patients at high risk for complications secondary to influenza include elderly persons; patients with cardiovascular disease, renal disease, diabetes, or asthma; and **immunocompromised** patients, or those individuals who have a deficient immune system response. Immunocompromised patients include patients with HIV or who have recently received organ or tissue transplants. Annual vaccinations for these patient populations are recommended.

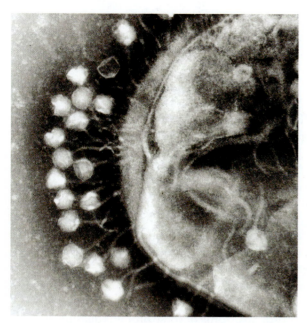
A virus does not have all the components of a cell and requires the metabolic and genetic resources of a living cell to replicate itself.

Hepatitis, an inflammation of the liver, has various forms referred to as A through G. It can range from a very benign disease to a serious illness leading to death. Hepatitis is a viral infection and will be discussed in Chapter 10. However, some of the drugs presented in this chapter are also used to treat hepatitis B.

The treatment of HIV has been impacted tremendously by new drugs. Although an HIV diagnosis used to usually indicate an early death, today it is viewed as a chronic disease that has to be managed. In treating HIV patients, the pharmacy team must be vigilant about checking for drug interactions. Most regimens include at least three drugs and a complicated dosing schedule. Manufacturers have combined some of these drugs to decrease the number of pills a patient must take.

Classification of Viral Infections

Viral infections are classified in several ways. One classification scheme uses the duration or length of time the viral particles have been in a body and the severity of the symptoms or illness that they cause. Another classification measures the extent of the infection within the body or the parts of the body that are affected. Viral infections can also be classified by the size and shape of the viral particles, genetic makeup (DNA or RNA), host, and induced pathogenic characteristics.

Viral Duration and Severity

Within the classification of viral duration and severity, there are three categories: acute, chronic, and slow. An **acute viral infection** quickly resolves with no latent infection. Examples include the common cold, influenza, and various other respiratory tract viruses. A **chronic viral infection** has a protracted course with long periods of remission interspersed with reappearance; a herpes virus infection is an example. A **slow viral infection** maintains a progressive course over months or years, with cumulative damage to body tissues, ultimately ending in the host's death. HIV is an example of a slow viral infection.

Extent of Viral Infection

When evaluating the extent of a viral infection, it must be determined whether the infection is local or generalized. A **local viral infection** affects tissues of a single system, such as the respiratory tract, eye, or skin. A **generalized viral infection** has spread or is spreading to other tissues by way of the bloodstream or tissues of the central nervous system (CNS).

Latent Viruses

Even after the symptoms of the acute stage of an infection have ceased, it is possible for a virus to lie dormant and undetectable in a cell. This is known as **latency**. Later, under certain conditions and possibly years after the initial breakout or transmission of infection, the virus may reproduce and again behave like an infectious agent, causing cell damage. Herpesviruses and HIV can both behave in this manner. Some viruses of this kind can transform normal cells into cancer cells.

Virus and Host Cell Interaction

A virus can have several damaging effects on a host cell. It can alter the structure of the host cell; incorporate itself into the genetic material of the host cell, thus becoming part of its nucleic acid pool; divide when the host cell divides; or kill the host cell.

Most viruses possess several antigens on their surfaces that stimulate host cells to produce immunoglobulins. An **immunoglobulin** is a type of antibody that is produced mainly by white blood cells (WBCs) called B lymphocytes. An immunoglobulin that matches a viral protein may prevent the virus from attaching to a cell receptor and may destroy the virus. T lymphocytes may also become sensitive to viral antigens, at which time they release chemicals to kill the virus or stimulate other cells, such as macrophages, to destroy the virus or virus-infected cells.

A significant response of some virus-infected cells is the production of **interferons**, which exhibit antiviral activities that are host-specific but not virus-specific. Interferons induce production of hundreds of other proteins. Some of these proteins disrupt various stages of viral replication, including synthesis of viral RNA. Other proteins help prevent viral spread to neighboring uninfected cells. Although interferons are produced in response to viral infection, they are encoded in the host cell's DNA. Therefore, interferons are host cell–specific; that is, interferon molecules made by human cells will work only in human cells.

Vaccination

Preventing viral infections by providing immunity is the purpose of **vaccination**. Vaccination exposes the patient to a component of a virus or an altered viral strain that does not produce infection. The exposure of the body to these foreign (though harmless) materials promotes the growth of B lymphocytes that produce antibodies specific to the designated virus. Later, if the vaccinated patient encounters the actual virus, the infection cannot develop because the patient's natural defenses are already primed from the vaccine. Because the discovery, testing, production, and implementation of vaccines are very complicated, **vaccines** are available for only a small number of viruses.

The difficulty of producing effective vaccines is increased by mutations in a virus's genetic material that change the structure and composition of its surface proteins. Previously effective vaccines may no longer recognize the virus as foreign and may, therefore, be useless. Influenza is such a virus. Every year, a new influenza vaccine is developed according to the genetic changes that are predicted to occur the following year. Because influenza viruses change from year to year, annual vaccinations are needed. The vaccine is only as good as its match to the infecting strain of influenza. The vaccine usually becomes available in September and is given throughout the flu season. It is recommended for all individuals age 6 months or older and is especially important for high-risk populations, such as healthcare workers (including pharmacists and pharmacy technicians), people in contact with patients who have influenza, nursing home residents, public safety workers, individuals age 65 years or older, and immunocompromised individuals. The vaccine is made from viral particles that are raised in poultry eggs and then inactivated or killed. For this reason, a healthcare practitioner must confirm that a patient is not allergic to eggs before giving the vaccine. In certain situations, an antiviral medication (oseltamivir or amantadine) may be prescribed to patients who cannot receive the vaccine or who have already been exposed to influenza.

Antiviral Agents (Nonretroviral)

Bacterial infections are easier to treat with medication than are viral infections. Because antibiotics often disrupt a cellular process unique to the invading strain, the medication can be administered without harming the patient. In contrast, because viruses use the host's own cellular processes to function and replicate, medications that block the life cycle of a virus are often toxic to the patient, much more so than antibiotics and in much the same way as chemotherapy agents for cancer. Thus, **antiviral drugs** have been formulated to seek out the virus and prevent its replication in body fluids or in host cells without interfering with normal cell function. Table 5.1 gives an overview of the most commonly used antiviral agents. HIV and antiretroviral drugs are discussed later in this chapter.

Therapeutic Uses of Antiviral Agents

Antiviral agents are the best option for treating the following viral infections:

- herpesvirus infections
    - ~ herpes simplex virus type 1 (HSV-1)
    - ~ herpes simplex virus type 2 (HSV-2)
    - ~ varicella-zoster
    - ~ cytomegalovirus (human herpesvirus type 5)
- influenza
- respiratory syncytial virus (RSV)

Antiherpes Agents

There are more than 100 various strains of herpesvirus; however, only a small proportion are regularly found in humans. The most common herpesvirus infections in humans are caused by HSV-1, HSV-2, and varicella-zoster virus. HSV-1 and HSV-2 are associated with oral and genital herpes, respectively. Oral herpes outbreaks are referred to as cold sores or fever blisters. Genital herpes may appear as sores below the waist, most commonly around the genitals or rectum. Varicella-zoster virus causes chicken pox (varicella) and shingles (herpes zoster). Antiviral agents for herpesvirus are commonly used to prevent and treat outbreaks.

Acyclovir

Acyclovir (Zovirax) acts by interfering with viral DNA synthesis. It is used to treat **genital herpes** in certain patients, herpes zoster (shingles), and varicella (chicken pox). The intravenous (IV) form is considered the drug of choice for herpes encephalitis. The dosage regimen changes depending on the type of infection being treated and the patient's status. Both short- and long-term side effects have been reported. Acyclovir can be used for suppression of herpes in patients who have had multiple outbreaks.

TABLE 5.1 Commonly Used Antiviral Drugs

Generic (Brand)	Pronunciation	Dosage Form	Common Dosage	Dispensing Status
Antiherpes Agents				
acyclovir (Zovirax)	ay-SYE-kloe-veer	Capsule, injection, ointment, oral suspension, tablet	Chicken pox (pediatric): PO: Children ≥2 years and ≤40 kg: 20 mg/kg 4 times a day; children >40 kg: 800 mg 4 times a day Topical: Varies by age, product, and indication Genital herpes (acute): IV: 5 mg/kg/dose 3 times a day for 5–7 days, followed with oral therapy for a minimum of 10 days total treatment PO: 200 mg 5 times a day or 400 mg 3 times a day for 7–10 days Genital herpes (chronic suppression): PO: 400 mg twice a day for 1 year Herpes zoster (shingles) and chicken pox (adult): IV: 10 mg/kg/dose 3 times a day for 7–10 days PO: 800 mg 5 times a day for 7–10 days	Rx
famciclovir (Famvir)	fam-SYE-kloe-veer	Tablet	Genital herpes (acute): 1,000 mg twice a day for 1 day Genital herpes (chronic suppression): 250 mg twice a day for 1 year Herpes labialis (cold sores): 1,500 mg single dose Herpes zoster (shingles): 500 mg every 8 hrs for 7 days	Rx
valacyclovir (Valtrex)	val-ay-SYE-kloe-veer	Tablet	Genital herpes (acute): 1 g twice a day for 10 days Genital herpes (chronic suppression): 1 g a day Herpes labialis (cold sores): 2 g every 12 hr for 1 day Herpes zoster (shingles): 1 g 3 times a day for 7 days	Rx
valganciclovir (Valcyte)	val-gan-SYE-kloh-veer	Oral liquid, tablet	Cytomegalovirus treatment: 900 mg twice daily for 21 days initially, 900 mg a day for maintenance Cytomegalovirus prophylaxis post-transplant: 900 mg a day	Rx
Anti-Influenza Agents				
amantadine (Symmetrel)	a-MAN-ta-deen	Capsule, syrup, tablet	Influenza (adult): 100 mg twice a day or 200 mg a day Influenza (pediatric): varies by age and weight of patient	Rx
oseltamivir (Tamiflu)	oh-sel-TAM-i-veer	Capsule, oral suspension	Influenza (adult): 75 mg twice a day for 5 days Influenza (pediatric): varies by age and weight of patient	Rx
rimantadine (Flumadine)	ri-MAN-ta-deen	Tablet	Influenza (adult): 100 mg twice a day Influenza (pediatric): 5 mg/kg a day	Rx
zanamivir (Relenza)	zan-AM-e-veer	Powder for inhalation	Influenza: 2 inhalations twice a day (duration of therapy varies)	Rx
Other Antiviral Agents				
ribavirin (Virazole, various brands)	rye-ba-VYE-rin	Capsule, oral solution, inhalation, tablet	RSV: Continuous aerosolization: 6 g administered over 12 to 18 hrs per day for 3 to 7 days Intermittent aerosolization: 2 g over 2 hrs 3 times daily for 3 to 7 days	Rx

Side Effects Acyclovir is associated with CNS side effects, such as confusion, hallucinations, and seizures.

Contraindications Acyclovir is contraindicated in patients with a hypersensitivity to valacyclovir.

Cautions and Considerations Use of acyclovir in older adults should be done with caution due to the aforementioned CNS side effects.

Drug Interactions Acyclovir use may diminish the therapeutic effect of varicella and herpes zoster vaccines. Foscarnet may enhance the nephrotoxic effect of acyclovir.

Famciclovir

Famciclovir (Famvir) is used to manage acute herpes zoster (shingles), to treat recurrent herpes simplex in immunocompromised patients, and to treat genital herpes. The primary side effects are nausea and headache. The advantage of this drug is that it can be dosed less frequently than acyclovir. It is a **prodrug**, which is a compound that must be metabolized in the body to form the active pharmacologic agent. The active compound after biotransformation is penciclovir.

Side Effects Famciclovir use is associated with headache, nausea, diarrhea, and fatigue.

Contraindications Famciclovir is a prodrug (a compound that is chemically converted to another active compound after administration) of penciclovir; therefore, penciclovir allergy contraindicates famciclovir use.

Cautions and Considerations Famciclovir contains milk products and should be used prudently by patients with milk product sensitivities.

Drug Interactions Famciclovir may diminish the therapeutic effect of varicella and herpes zoster vaccines.

Valacyclovir

Valacyclovir (Valtrex) is used to treat herpes zoster in immunocompetent adults and to treat genital herpes. It should be taken with plenty of water and within 48 hours of the onset of the zoster rash. It shortens the duration of postherpetic neuralgia. It is better absorbed than acyclovir, and once absorbed, it is converted to acyclovir in the liver and digestive tract. The end result is higher levels of acyclovir in the blood. Prescriptions for valacyclovir generally are for shorter periods and require fewer pills per day than with acyclovir.

Side Effects Valacyclovir has CNS side effects, such as confusion, hallucinations, and seizures. Other side effects include nausea, vomiting, diarrhea, and constipation.

Contraindications Valacyclovir is a prodrug for acyclovir and should not be used in patients with a hypersensitivity to acyclovir.

Cautions and Considerations Valacyclovir should be used with caution in older adults because of the aforementioned CNS side effects.

Drug Interactions Foscarnet may enhance the nephrotoxic effects of valacyclovir, and the combination should be avoided. Valacyclovir may decrease the effectiveness of live vaccines.

Valganciclovir

Valganciclovir (Valcyte) is an oral prodrug for **ganciclovir (Vitrasert)**. When working with valganciclovir, it is important to follow precautions appropriate for chemotherapy drugs (see Chapter 16). Do not handle broken or crushed tablets. As with chemotherapy drugs, damaged tablets should be disposed of in special containers. Valganciclovir has a black box warning regarding its mutagenic properties. Therefore, pregnant women should not handle this drug.

Side Effects Side effects associated with valganciclovir include hypertension, headache, insomnia, diarrhea, vomiting, tremors, fever, and increased serum creatinine.

Contraindications Valganciclovir is a prodrug for ganciclovir and should not be used in those patients with ganciclovir hypersensitivity.

Cautions and Considerations Valganciclovir has two black box warnings. The first warning is related to reports of severe leukopenia, neutropenia, anemia, thrombocytopenia, pancytopenia, bone marrow aplasia, and aplastic anemia. Patients with certain low levels of neutrophils, platelets, or hemoglobin should not use valganciclovir. Immuno-suppressed patients also should not use valganciclovir.

The other boxed warning concerns its effects on reproduction. Valganciclovir may temporarily or permanently impair fertility in men and women. It is also associated with birth defects and cancer. Women should use effective contraception during and for 30 days after valganciclovir treatment. Men should use barrier contraception during treatment and for 90 days after therapy. Pregnant pharmacy technicians should avoid directly handling valganciclovir.

Drug Interactions Valganciclovir may enhance the toxic effects of the antibiotic imipenem, including an increased seizure risk. It may also enhance the toxic effects of reverse transcriptase inhibitors (with the exception of stavudine).

Anti-Influenza Agents

Influenza, or flu, is a contagious viral infection of the respiratory system. There are different types of influenza, with type A and type B being the most common. Type A and type B cause seasonal flu, which affects up to 20% of Americans annually. Common symptoms include fever, fatigue, aches, and chills. For most people, influenza infections self resolve. However, in others, it can be deadly. Young children, older adults, residents of nursing homes, pregnant women, and those individuals with chronic illness are all at an increased risk for developing complications of influenza. Anti-influenza agents are used to prevent or treat influenza in high-risk patients.

Amantadine

Amantadine (Symmetrel) prevents absorption of viral particles into the host cell by inhibiting uncoating, which is the removal of the virus capsid proteins to expose the nucleic acid. Amantadine is used in the prophylaxis and treatment of influenza type A. Sufficient blood levels of the drug are necessary to prevent infection. If administered after infection has begun, amantadine still may reduce the severity of symptoms.

Side Effects Side effects are rare and primarily affect the CNS. Dizziness, headache, and weakness may occur with use. Because of its action on the CNS, amantadine also has some therapeutic effect on Parkinson's disease.

Contraindications Amantadine does not have contraindications.

Cautions and Considerations Older adults are at a higher risk for such side effects and should use caution when taking this drug.

Drug Interactions Alcohol and other depressants may enhance the CNS depressant effects of amantadine. Amisulpride and antipsychotic agents may decrease the anti-parkinsonian benefits of amantadine. Amantadine may prolong the QT interval, and use with other agents that have the same effect is not recommended. Live influenza vaccine effectiveness decreases with concomitant amantadine use.

Oseltamivir

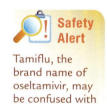

Safety Alert

Tamiflu, the brand name of oseltamivir, may be confused with FluMist, the nasal influenza vaccine.

Oseltamivir (Tamiflu) is an oral inhibitor of the enzyme neuraminidase, which is carried on the surface of the influenza virus. This drug is indicated for the treatment or prevention of influenza type A and type B. Therapy must be initiated within 48 hours of symptom onset. Food generally improves tolerance, so it is best to take oseltamivir orally at breakfast and dinner. Oseltamivir has been shown to decrease the duration of the flu by up to three days.

Side Effects Oseltamivir may cause vomiting, nausea, abdominal pain, and diarrhea. Less common side effects include nosebleeds and eye infections. Oseltamivir is used for the treatment and prophylaxis of influenza. Oseltamivir is ideally administered within 48 hours of symptom onset. If you are out of stock of this medication, it is best to help the patient find another pharmacy that has stock.

Contraindications Oseltamivir does not have contraindications.

Cautions and Considerations Oseltamivir should be used cautiously in patients with cardiovascular disease, hepatic impairment, and renal impairment.

Some oseltamivir formulations contain benzyl alcohol, which has been associated with toxic reactions (potentially fatal) in neonates. Avoid use of these formulations in the neonatal population.

The oral suspension contains sorbitol, which may cause diarrhea.

Drug Interactions Live influenza vaccine effectiveness decreases with concomitant oseltamivir use.

Rimantadine

Rimantadine (Flumadine) is indicated for prophylaxis and treatment of infections caused by influenza type A virus strains.

Side Effects The most frequent side effects involve the gastrointestinal (GI) tract and CNS. CNS side effects include dizziness, headache, and weakness.

Contraindications Rimantadine is contraindicated in patients with a hypersensitivity to drugs of the adamantine class.

Cautions and Considerations Use rimantadine with caution in patients with hepatic impairment, renal impairment, psychosis, or seizures. Older adults are at higher risk for such side effects and should use caution when taking these drugs.

Drug Interactions Antihistamines and caffeine increase neurotoxicity associated with rimantadine. Live influenza vaccine effectiveness decreases with concomitant rimantadine use.

Zanamivir

Zanamivir (Relenza) is indicated for the treatment and prophylaxis of influenza type A and type B. Therapy with zanamivir must be initiated within 48 hours of the onset of symptoms. If you are out of stock of this medication, you should help the patient find another pharmacy that has stock.

The drug is inhaled using a breath-activated plastic device called a Diskhaler. The recommended dosage is two inhalations daily, administered at 12-hour intervals, for five days. If the patient is also using a bronchodilator, the patient should be instructed to use the bronchodilator immediately prior to the administration of zanamivir. Zanamivir is sometimes prescribed as a prophylactic, especially in nursing homes and other group settings.

Side Effects Headache, throat/tonsil discomfort, and cough are side effects of zanamivir use.

Contraindications Zanamivir is contraindicated in patients with a hypersensitivity to milk protein.

Cautions and Considerations Zanamivir contains milk products and should be used prudently by patients with milk product sensitivities.

Drug Interactions Live influenza vaccine effectiveness decreases with concomitant zanamivir use.

Other Antiviral Agents

RSV causes acute respiratory illness in patients. RSV is the most common cause of lower respiratory tract infections in infants. Pediatric patients with RSV often present with difficulty breathing, bronchitis, or pneumonia. Adults with RSV have similar symptoms. While other therapies such as bronchodilators and corticosteroids are traditionally used first, the antiviral agent ribavirin may also be used.

Ribavirin

Ribavirin (Virazole) is useful in treating viral infections and may be useful in treating patients with RSV. Ribavirin comes in multiple dosage forms and is usually used by inhalation for RSV; it can be used orally for other indications. Ribavirin is absorbed systemically from the respiratory tract following inhalation. Absorption of the inhaled form depends on respiratory factors and the drug delivery system.

Side Effects Ribavirin has a serious side effect of hemolytic anemia, which may worsen underlying cardiac disease and lead to fatal and nonfatal heart attacks. Patients with heart disease should avoid using ribavirin. The most common side effects are fatigue, headache, and insomnia. Nausea and anorexia can also occur.

Contraindications Ribavirin is contraindicated in women who are pregnant, men whose female partners are pregnant, patients with hemoglobinopathies, patients with autoimmune hepatitis, and patients who are also taking didanosine.

Cautions and Considerations Ribavirin has several black box warnings. When used orally, ribavirin may cause hemolytic anemia, which may worsen underlying cardiac disease. When used for hepatitis C, ribavirin should not be used as monotherapy. In pediatric patients, ribavirin use may result in sudden respiratory deterioration.

Another black box warning exists for pregnant women because of its significant teratogenic and embryocidal effects. Avoid use in women who are pregnant; and women whose male partners are undergoing ribavirin therapy should use two contraceptive methods. Pregnant pharmacy technicians should avoid directly handling ribavirin. Lastly, the inhaled product also carries a boxed warning. The inhalation product should be used cautiously in patients using mechanical ventilation because there is a risk that ribavirin could precipitate in the respiratory equipment.

Drug Interactions Ribavirin may increase serum concentrations of azathioprine. Ribavirin may enhance the toxic effects of didanosine, so the combination should be avoided. Live influenza vaccine effectiveness decreases with concomitant ribavirin use.

HIV/AIDS and Antiretroviral Agents

Safety Alert

One of the biggest problems when treating HIV is non-adherence with the drug regimen because of problematic side effects and complex dosing.

A **retrovirus** is a virus that uses RNA as its genetic material. Retroviruses use an enzyme called **reverse transcriptase** to become part of the host's DNA, which allows replication of the virus.

Human immunodeficiency virus (HIV) is a retrovirus that attaches to receptors on the surface of **CD4 cells** (important cells underlying the immune response in the body). HIV then fuses with the CD4 cell membrane, which allows HIV to enter the host cell. Once inside the CD4 host cell, HIV releases and uses reverse transcriptase to convert its genetic material from RNA to DNA. HIV also releases **integrase**, an enzyme that integrates HIV DNA into the DNA of the host CD4 cell. In other words, HIV genetic material combines with the host cell's genetic material and is able to replicate along with the host cell. Newly formed immature HIV pushes out of the host CD4 cell and releases protease (an enzyme that promotes assembly of viral parts into intact HIV and allows HIV virions to be infectious). Figure 5.1 details this process. Patients with advanced and severe forms of HIV are said to have **acquired immunodeficiency syndrome (AIDS)**. In AIDS, even simple infections that normally would not cause any problems can become deadly.

The cadre of **antiretroviral** drugs used against HIV and AIDS saves lives, but these agents have numerous severe side effects and drug interactions, making them difficult medications to tolerate. These drugs can be combined into therapy, called a **cocktail**, to take advantage of the effects of synergistic drug therapy. By attacking the viral replication process in multiple stages, more viruses can be destroyed. Although these medications can reduce the number of viruses in the body to almost undetectable levels, patients must continue to take the drugs throughout their lives to prevent progression of the illness and death and must follow medication instructions carefully to receive optimal effect.

Different classes of drugs are used to treat HIV, including nucleoside reverse transcriptase inhibitors (NRTIs), nucleotide reverse transcriptase inhibitors (NtRTIs), non-nucleoside reverse transcriptase inhibitors (NNRTIs), protease inhibitors (PIs), and integrase inhibitors.

A patient with HIV generally takes a combination of three or more antiviral drugs from the different classes, such as one NNRTI plus two NRTIs or a PI combined with ritonavir and two NRTIs. Some of these cocktails are available packaged in a single tablet (e.g., Atripla, Stribild, and Truvada). Patients who are new to treatment may start with one of those combination pills. Over time, the virus develops resistance to the different antiviral agents, so patients will change drug treatments periodically throughout the course of the disease. Table 5.5 identifies commonly used HIV drugs. Table 5.7 identifies common HIV treatment combinations.

FIGURE 5.1 The HIV Life Cycle

Drugs for the treatment of HIV work at various phases of the HIV life cycle.

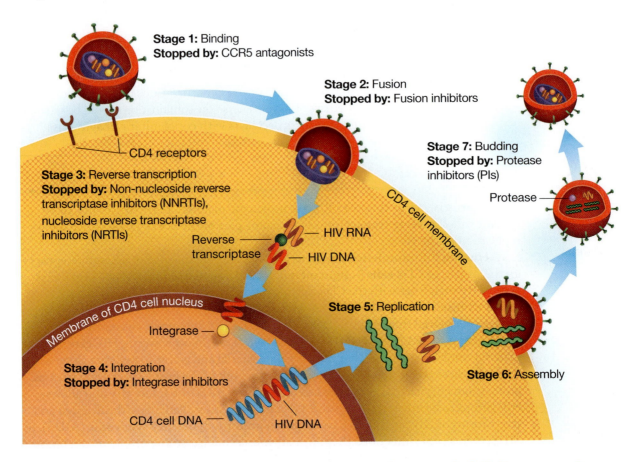

Stage 1: Binding
Stopped by: CCR5 antagonists

Stage 2: Fusion
Stopped by: Fusion inhibitors

CD4 receptors

Stage 3: Reverse transcription
Stopped by: Non-nucleoside reverse transcriptase inhibitors (NNRTIs), nucleoside reverse transcriptase inhibitors (NRTIs)

Reverse transcriptase

HIV RNA

HIV DNA

Stage 7: Budding
Stopped by: Protease inhibitors (PIs)

Protease

CD4 cell membrane

Membrane of CD4 cell nucleus

Integrase

Stage 5: Replication

Stage 4: Integration
Stopped by: Integrase inhibitors

CD4 cell DNA

HIV DNA

Stage 6: Assembly

Nucleoside Reverse Transcriptase Inhibitors and Nucleotide Reverse Transcriptase Inhibitors

Nucleoside reverse transcriptase inhibitors (NRTIs) and **nucleotide reverse transcriptase inhibitors (NtRTIs)** work by inhibiting reverse transcriptase. This action prevents the formation of a DNA copy of viral RNA, thus preventing the virus from multiplying or hiding itself. Figure 5.1 illustrates where NRTIs and NtRTIs work in the HIV life cycle. Table 5.2 provides an overview of the NRTIs and NtRTIs in current use. These drug classes commonly cause GI distress (nausea, diarrhea, abdominal pain), which usually improve within the first two weeks of therapy. More permanent side effects include lactic acidosis with hepatic steatosis (degeneration of the liver). Both drug classes carry black box warnings for liver problems.

NRTIs and NtRTIs, with the exception of didanosine, can be taken with or without food and generally do not interfere with other drugs. These agents are usually administered in two to three doses per day.

Abacavir

Abacavir (Ziagen) is an NRTI and one of the few HIV drugs that penetrate the CNS. This characteristic makes abacavir an invaluable therapeutic weapon because HIV

TABLE 5.2 Commonly Used Nucleoside Reverse Transcriptase Inhibitors (NRTIs) and Nucleotide Reverse Transcriptase Inhibitors (NtRTIs)

Generic (Brand)	Pronunciation	Dosage Form	Common Dosage	Dispensing Status
abacavir (Ziagen)	a-BAK-a-veer	Oral solution, tablet	600 mg a day	Rx
abacavir-lamivudine (Epzicom)	a-BAK-a-vir la-MIV-ue-deen	Tablet	600 mg/300 mg a day	Rx
abacavir-lamivudine-zidovudine (Trizivir)	a-BAK-a-vir la-MIV-ue-deen zye-DOE-vyoo-deen	Tablet	300 mg/150 mg/300 mg a day	Rx
didanosine (Videx)	di-DAN-oe-seen	Capsule, powder for oral solution	PO (capsule): 125–200 mg twice a day or 250–400 mg once a day PO (solution): 125–250 mg twice a day	Rx
efavirenz-emtricitabine-tenofovir (Atripla)	e-FAV-er-enz em-trye-SYE-ta-bean ten-OE-foe-veer	Tablet	600 mg/200 mg/300 mg a day	Rx
emtricitabine (Emtriva)	em-trye-SYE-ta-bean	Capsule, oral solution	PO (capsule): 200 mg a day PO (solution): 240 mg a day	Rx
emtricitabine-tenofovir (Truvada)	em-trye-SYE-ta-bean ten-OE-foe-veer	Tablet	200 mg/300 mg a day	Rx
lamivudine (Epivir)	la-MIV-yoo-deen	Oral solution, tablet	100 mg a day	Rx
lamivudine-zidovudine (Combivir)	la-MIV-ue-deen zye-DOE-vue-deen	Tablet	150 mg/300 mg twice a day	Rx
stavudine (Zerit)	STAV-yoo-deen	Capsule, powder for oral solution	30–40 mg every 12 hr	Rx
tenofovir disoproxil fumarate (Viread)	te-NO-fo-veer dye-soe-PROX-il FUE-ma-rate	Oral powder, tablet	300 mg a day	Rx
zidovudine (Retrovir)	zye-DOE-vyoo-deen	Capsule, injection, syrup, tablet	PO: 600 mg a day in divided doses IV: 1 mg/kg/dose infused over 1 hr, given 5–6 times a day	Rx

itself is able to penetrate and proliferate within the CNS. The use of alcohol will increase abacavir's toxicity, and patients must be instructed to avoid alcohol completely. Patients should also be cautioned about side effects that could signal an adverse and potentially life-threatening reaction to the drug. Fifty percent of patients experience hypersensitivity to abacavir, a state of altered reaction that generally occurs in the first six weeks. These side effects include rash, nausea, abdominal pain, malaise, or respiratory symptoms. The patient must be instructed to contact the prescriber, who will usually stop the medication. Hypersensitivity to a drug contraindicates its use.

Drug Interactions Ganciclovir and valganciclovir may enhance adverse effects of abacavir. Protease inhibitors may decrease the serum concentration of abacavir. Ribavirin may enhance side effects related to liver toxicity.

Didanosine

Didanosine (Videx) an NRTI, is always combined with two other antiretroviral agents. Patients should allow for an interval of at least two hours between the administration of didanosine and any drug that requires gastric acidity for digestion. For optimal tolerability and absorption, didanosine should be taken on an empty stomach 60 minutes before or 2 hours after meals. The pediatric solution must be reconstituted with purified US Pharmacopeia (USP) water to an initial concentration of 20 mg/mL, then further diluted with an antacid suspension to a final mixture of 10 mg/mL. A "shake well" auxiliary label must be affixed to the bottle.

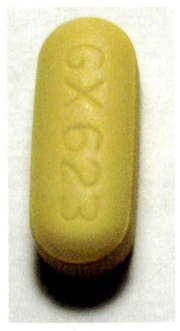

Abacavir has become a key medication in the treatment of HIV because it is able to penetrate the barriers to the CNS.

Contraindications Didanosine is contraindicated in patients currently using allopurinol or ribavirin.

Cautions and Considerations Didanosine must be taken on an empty stomach to work properly, and it cannot be taken with members of its own class (e.g., stavudine).

Drug Interactions Alcohol consumption may increase the risk of pancreatitis. Patients should not drink alcohol while taking didanosine. Allopurinol, febuxostat, and ribavirin may increase body concentrations of didanosine, and concurrent use should be avoided. Hydroxyurea may enhance the adverse effects of didanosine; didanosine may enhance the adverse effects of hydroxyurea. Tenofovir may diminish the effects of didanosine.

Emtricitabine and Lamivudine

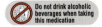
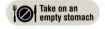
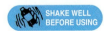

Emtricitabine (Emtriva) and lamivudine (Epivir) are NRTIs that behave similarly. They can simplify drug regimens because they are often taken once daily. Both drugs are well tolerated. Emtricitabine may discolor the skin (such as hyperpigmentation on the palms or soles). Lamivudine may precipitate pancreatitis. These medications can be taken without regard to meals.

Contraindications Emtricitabine and lamivudine do not have contraindications.

Cautions and Considerations Lamivudine is indicated to treat HIV and chronic hepatitis B. When used for hepatitis B, lamivudine has several black box warnings. The first warning is about product selection. The hepatitis B product should not be used to treat HIV. The second warning is about medication discontinuation. After therapy stops, patients should be monitored closely for hepatitis exacerbations. The third warning addresses HIV resistance. Providers need to be aware that HIV resistance may emerge when hepatitis B patients with undiagnosed HIV infection use lamivudine.

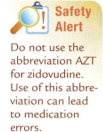
Emtricitabine has a black box warning stating it should not be used for the treatment of hepatitis. Emtricitabine and lamivudine may cause fat redistribution. Both drugs should be used cautiously in patients with renal dysfunction.

Drug Interactions Emtricitabine and lamivudine should not be used together. Ganciclovir, valganciclovir, and ribavirin may enhance the toxic effects of emtricitabine and lamivudine.

Stavudine

Stavudine (Zerit), an NRTI, is typically well tolerated. Adverse effects (peripheral neuropathy, pancreatitis, dyslipidemia, hepatic steatosis [fatty liver], and lactic acidosis) generally limit use. When available, other options are used before trying stavudine.

Contraindications Stavudine does not have contraindications.

Cautions and Considerations Stavudine has a black box warning for pancreatitis if it is used in combination with didanosine. If the patient develops pancreatitis or it is suspected, suspend therapy and discontinue any other agents that may cause pancreatitis. Patients with peripheral neuropathy should use stavudine with caution.

Drug Interactions Zidovudine may decrease the effectiveness of stavudine.

Tenofovir

Tenofovir disoproxil fumarate (Viread) is an NtRTI that can be dosed once daily without regard to food. Tenofovir disoproxil fumarate's limiting toxicity is kidney related. Other side effects include dizziness, depression, skin rash, and dyslipidemia.

Contraindications Tenofovir disoproxil fumarate does not have contraindications.

Cautions and Considerations Kidney toxicity is a concern with tenofovir disoproxil fumarate use, so patients should avoid other drugs that are toxic to the kidneys. Use should be discontinued in patients who experience renal function decline.

Drug Interactions Adefovir may decrease the effectiveness of tenofovir disoproxil fumarate. Tenofovir disoproxil fumarate may increase levels of adefovir. Concomitant use is not recommended.

Zidovudine

Zidovudine (Retrovir), an NRTI, was one of the first drugs developed specifically for the treatment of HIV. With the exception of stavudine, zidovudine can be combined with any of the other NRTIs. The combination of zidovudine with lamivudine, with or without a protease inhibitor, is recommended for the prevention of HIV after a needle-stick or sexual exposure. The most common side effects of zidovudine are headache, anorexia, diarrhea, GI pain, nausea, rash, and anemia.

Contraindications Zidovudine does not have contraindications.

Cautions and Considerations Zidovudine has a black box warning for hematologic toxicity (neutropenia and anemia). Use with caution in patients with compromised bone marrow function.

Another boxed warning is present because zidovudine use is associated with myopathy and myositis.

Drug Interactions Adverse effects of clozapine may be enhanced by zidovudine use. Zidovudine may decrease the efficacy of stavudine.

Non-Nucleoside Reverse Transcriptase Inhibitors

A **non-nucleoside reverse transcriptase inhibitor (NNRTI)** inhibits the action of HIV reverse transcriptase, by obstructing the enzyme's mechanical action rather than by mimicking a DNA building block. See Figure 5.1 for an illustration of where NNRTIs work in the HIV life cycle. Table 5.3 gives an overview of the most commonly used NNRTIs.

Delavirdine

Delavirdine (Rescriptor) is a cytochrome P-450 inhibitor, so in contrast to nevirapine and many other NNRTIs, it can increase the serum levels of some protease inhibitors. Side effects include central obesity/weight gain and Stevens-Johnson syndrome. This drug is also associated with rash, but at a lower frequency than nevirapine.

Contraindications Contraindications to delavirdine include concurrent use of alprazolam, astemizole, cisapride, ergot alkaloids, midazolam, pimozide, rifampin, or triazolam.

Cautions and Considerations Delavirdine should not be taken with any antacid. Patients should be instructed to avoid the ingestion of antacids for one hour before and one hour after the administration of delavirdine.

Drug Interactions Because delavirdine is a cytochrome P-450 inhibitor, it has many drug interactions. Combining delavirdine with the drugs listed in the section below should be avoided.

- Delavirdine inhibits cytochrome P-450 3A4 and may increase the serum concentrations of bosutinib, domperidone, ibrutinib, ivabradine, lomitapide, naloxegol, olaparib, pimozide, simeprevir, suvorexant, tolvaptan, trabectedin, and ulipristal.
- Delavirdine also inhibits cytochrome P-450 2D6 and may increase the serum concentrations of mequitazine, pimozide, and thioridazine.
- Delaviridine may enhance the effects of astemizole, efavirenz, and rilpivirine.
- Delavirdine may decrease serum concentrations of carbamazepine and etravirine.
- Fosamprenavir, fosphenytoin, H_2 receptor antagonists, proton pump inhibitors (PPIs), rifamycin derivatives, and St. John's wort may decrease the serum concentration of delavirdine.

Efavirenz

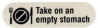

Efavirenz (Sustiva) has a long duration of action relative to other NNRTIs and is dosed only once a day, preferably at bedtime. Patients taking efavirenz should be instructed to take it on an empty stomach. Common side effects include dizziness and headache. The drug may also induce vivid dreams, nightmares, and hallucinations. These side effects typically occur between one and three hours after administration and will usually subside after two to four weeks on the drug.

Contraindications Efavirenz contraindications include concurrent use of bepridil, cisapride, ergot alkaloids, midazolam, pimozide, St. John's wort, and triazolam.

Cautions and Considerations CNS side effects are the most common, and dosing at bedtime can help improve tolerability. Hepatic failure has occurred with use. Patients with moderate-to-severe hepatic dysfunction should avoid efavirenz. Efavirenz may cause false cannabinoid (marijuana) tests. Pregnant women should not take efavirenz.

Drug Interactions Efavirenz is a cytochrome P-450 mixed inhibitor/inducer and has multiple drug interactions. Use of the following drugs should be avoided in patients using efavirenz.

- Efavirenz is a cytochrome P-450 3A4 inducer and may decrease serum concentrations of aripiprazole, axitinib, bedaquiline, bosutinib, enzalutamide, itraconazole, ketoconazole, nisoldipine, olaparib, posaconaozle, and simeprevir.
- Efavirenz may decrease serum concentrations of atovaquone, carbamazepine, elvitegravir, etravirine, palbociclib, and ulipristal.
- Efavirenz may potentiate the toxicities of amodiaquine, dasabuvir, nevirapine, orphenadrine, paraldehyde, paritaprevir, and thalidomide.
- Efavirenz may decrease the serum concentration of boceprevir; boceprevir may increase the serum concentration of efavirenz.
- St. John's wort may decrease the serum concentration of efavirenz.

Etravirine

Etravirine (Intelence) is designed to be given with another HIV drug and should never be given alone. It reduces the HIV level in the blood and increases the levels of WBCs, decreasing the possibility of infections that may occur with a depressed immune system. Commonly reported side effects include rash, nausea, hypersensitivity, and fat redistribution.

Contraindications Etravirine does not have contraindications.

Cautions and Considerations Etravirine should not be used in treatment-naive patients. Etravirine should be taken with food.

Drug Interactions Etravirine has many drug interactions. The following drugs should not be used with etravirine.

- Etravirine may decrease the serum concentrations of axitinib, bedaquiline, bosutinib, carbamazepine, enzalutamide, nisoldipine, olaparib, palbociclib, ritonavir, and simeprevir.
- Etravirine concentrations may be decreased by boceprevir, carbamazepine, efavirenz, fosphenytoin, phenobarbital, phenytoin, primidone, rifamycin derivatives (except rifabutin), St. John's wort, and tipranavir.
- Etravirine may increase serum concentrations of efavirenz, fosamprenavir, and tetrahydrocannabinol.

Nevirapine

Nevirapine (Viramune) is associated with a high incidence of rash, especially during the early phases of treatment. To mitigate this effect, the drug is typically given at a lower dose during the first two weeks of treatment and then increased to the appropriate therapeutic level. Other side effects include liver problems and severe allergic reaction.

TABLE 5.3 Commonly Used Non-Nucleoside Reverse Transcriptase Inhibitors (NNRTIs)

Generic (Brand)	Pronunciation	Dosage Form	Common Dosage	Dispensing Status
delavirdine (Rescriptor)	de-la-VIR-deen	Tablet	400 mg 3 times a day	Rx
efavirenz (Sustiva)	e-FAV-er-enz	Capsule, tablet	600 mg a day	Rx
etravirine (Intelence)	eh-TRAV-er-een	Tablet	200 mg twice a day	Rx
nevirapine (Viramune)	ne-VYE-ra-peen	Oral suspension, tablet	200 mg 1–2 times a day	Rx
rilpivirine (Edurant)	ril-pi-VIR-een	Tablet	25 mg daily	Rx

Contraindications Nevirapine is contraindicated in patients with moderate-to-severe liver impairment and should not be used for postexposure prophylaxis.

Cautions and Precautions Nevirapine has two black box warnings. One warning addresses liver toxicity that may result in liver failure or death. The greatest risk is within the first six weeks of use, and intensive monitoring is required during the first five months of therapy. The second warns of severe and life-threatening skin reactions. As with liver toxicity, the risk is greatest during the first six weeks of therapy.

This drug interferes with the effectiveness of oral contraceptives

Drug Interactions Nevirapine is a cytochrome P-450 inducer. The antibiotic rifampin (a drug used to treat tuberculosis) interferes with the efficacy of nevirapine by reducing its serum concentration in the body. In turn, nevirapine decreases the serum concentration of the protease inhibitor class of antiretrovirals (discussed later in this chapter). As a result, these drugs generally are not prescribed in combination. Nevirapine also decreases the effectiveness of oral contraceptives.

Rilpivirine

Rilpivirine (Edurant) is not for people who have been living with HIV and need antivirals. It is only for first-time users of antiviral medications. It should not be taken with other NNRTIs. It should be taken once daily with a high-fat meal. Depression is the primary side effect. Rash, headache, and insomnia may also occur with use.

Contraindications Rilpivirine contraindications include coadministration with anticonvulsants, antimycobacterials, PPIs, systemic dexamethasone, and St. John's wort.

Cautions and Considerations Because of the lack of data, rilpivirine should be used with caution in patients with a viral load greater than 100,000 copies/mL. A viral load is a measurement taken from a blood sample that determines the level of HIV activity and the effectiveness of antiretroviral therapy.

Drug Interactions Dexamethasone, fosphenytoin, oxcarbazepine, phenobarbital, phenytoin, primidone, PPIs, rifamycin derivatives (except rifabutin), and St. John's wort may decrease rilpivirine concentrations.

- Rilpivirine may increase or decrease serum concentrations of efavirenz and etravirine.
- Ritonavir may increase serum concentrations of rilpivirine.

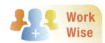

Web

TAKE WITH FOOD

Web

TAKE WITH FOOD

Protease Inhibitors

A **protease inhibitor (PI)** decreases formation of the protease enzyme, which cleaves certain HIV protein precursors that are necessary for the replication of new infectious virions. This mechanism results in the production of immature, noninfectious virions. Figure 5.1 illustrates where PIs work in the HIV life cycle. Most PIs are typically combined with other antiretroviral drugs, and their use has led to marked clinical improvement and prolonged survival among HIV-infected patients. Because PIs are metabolized through cytochrome P-450, drug interactions are common and can be severe. Table 5.4 provides an overview of the most commonly prescribed PIs. Statins should not be given with these drugs.

Side effects associated with all PIs include redistribution of body fat, referred to as "protease paunch" and characterized by a humped back; facial atrophy (a wasting away of facial fat); breast enlargement; hyperglycemia (increased level of glucose in the blood); hyperlipidemia (elevated concentration of lipids in the plasma); and possible increase in bleeding episodes in patients with hemophilia, which is a hemorrhagic condition caused by a deficiency of a coagulation factor.

PIs are notorious for drug interactions. For this reason, only experienced providers should prescribe PIs. Drug interaction data for PIs is regularly updated. The National Institutes of Health (NIH) publishes data on their AIDSinfo website at http://Pharmacology6e.ParadigmCollege.net/AIDSinfo.

Atazanavir

Atazanavir (Reyataz) is dosed once daily and should be given with ritonavir. It does not appear to increase cholesterol or triglyceride levels as most HIV drugs do, but it has other similar side effects. One common side effect is jaundice. Patients using atazanavir may notice yellowing of the skin. Atazanavir should be taken with food.

Contraindications Contraindications to atazanavir include concurrent therapy with alfuzosin, cisapride, ergot derivatives, indinavir, irinotecan, lovastatin, midazolam, nevirapine, pimozide, rifampin, sildenafil, simvastatin, St. John's wort, or triazolam. It should not be coadministered with drugs that strongly induce cytochrome P-450 3A4, which may lead to lower atazanavir exposure and loss of efficacy.

Cautions and Considerations Patients using atazanavir may develop diabetes. Patients should be monitored for signs and symptoms of diabetes. Liver and kidney dysfunction may occur with use.

Drug Interactions PIs have many drug interactions. Please visit the NIH AIDSinfo website at http://Pharmacology6e.ParadigmCollege.net/AIDSinfo to view the most recent interaction information.

Darunavir

Darunavir (Prezista) is a PI that must be administered in combination with ritonavir. The most common side effects are headache, nausea, and diarrhea. Darunavir should be taken with food. It should be stored and dispensed in the original container, tightly closed. This drug received accelerated approval from the US Food and Drug Administration (FDA) so that it could be used in patients resistant to other therapies.

Contraindications Many contraindications to PIs are connected with drug interactions. Contraindications to darunavir include concurrent therapy with alfuzosin, cisapride, ergot derivatives, indinavir, irinotecan, lovastatin, midazolam, nevirapine, pimozide, rifampin, sildenafil, simvastatin, St. John's wort, or triazolam.

TABLE 5.4 Commonly Used Protease Inhibitors (PIs)

Generic (Brand)	Pronunciation	Dosage Form	Common Dosage	Dispensing Status
atazanavir (Reyataz)	at-a-ZAN-a-veer	Capsule, oral packet	300 mg once a day with food (must be taken with ritonavir)	Rx
darunavir (Prezista)	da-ROON-a-veer	Oral suspension, tablet	600–800 mg twice a day with food (must be taken with ritonavir)	Rx
fosamprenavir (Lexiva)	FOS-am-pren-a-veer	Oral suspension, tablet	700–1,400 mg twice a day (must be taken with ritonavir)	Rx
indinavir (Crixivan)	in-DIN-a-veer	Capsule	800 mg every 8–12 hr	Rx
lopinavir-ritonavir (Kaletra)	low-PIN-a-veer rye-TON-a-veer	Oral solution, tablet	400 mg/100 mg twice a day	Rx
nelfinavir (Viracept)	nel-FIN-a-veer	Tablet	1,250 mg 2 times a day with food or 750 mg 3 times a day	Rx
ritonavir (Norvir)	rye-TON-a-veer	Capsule, oral solution, tablet	Up to 600 mg twice daily	Rx
saquinavir (Invirase)	sa-KWIN-a-veer	Capsule, tablet	1,000 mg twice a day (must be taken with ritonavir)	Rx
tipranavir (Aptivus)	tip-RAN-a-veer	Capsule, oral solution	500 mg twice a day (must be taken with ritonavir)	Rx

Coadministration with drugs that strongly induce cytochrome P-450 3A4 may lead to lower darunavir exposure and loss of efficacy.

Cautions and Considerations Darunavir's chemical structure is related to that of sulfa drugs. Patients with sulfa allergies should use darunavir with caution.

- Darunavir use may exacerbate kidney and liver toxicities.
- Darunavir should not be used in children less than three years of age.

Web

Drug Interactions PIs have many drug interactions. Please visit the NIH AIDSinfo website at http://Pharmacology6e.ParadigmCollege.net/AIDSinfo to view the most recent interaction information.

Fosamprenavir

Fosamprenavir (Lexiva) is a prodrug of the PI amprenavir. It is better absorbed and tolerated than amprenavir, with less nausea and diarrhea; therefore, it can be taken without regard for meals. Fosamprenavir has largely replaced the use of amprenavir.

Contraindications Contraindications to fosamprenavir include concurrent therapy with alfuzosin, cisapride, ergot derivatives, irinotecan, lovastatin, midazolam, nevirapine, pimozide, rifampin, sildenafil, simvastatin, St. John's wort, or triazolam.

Cautions and Considerations Fosamprenavir's chemical structure is similar to that of sulfa drugs, and caution must be exercised in patients with a sulfa allergy.

Fosamprenavir is associated with hepatic toxicity. Patients with underlying liver disease should use fosamprenavir with caution.

Drug Interactions PIs have many drug interactions. Please visit the NIH AIDSinfo website at http://Pharmacology6e.ParadigmCollege.net/AIDSinfo.

Indinavir

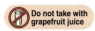

Indinavir (Crixivan) has been shown to be less effective when taken in combination with St. John's wort. Thus, patients who are taking indinavir should be instructed to avoid this herbal remedy. Indinavir is very sensitive to moisture and is therefore always packaged with a **desiccant**. Patients should be instructed to store the drug in its original container. Indinavir should not be taken with high-fat meals or grapefruit juice. It should be taken on an empty stomach or with a low-fat meal. However, if the patient is using indinavir in combination with ritonavir, it may be taken with food. To lower the incidence of kidney stones, the patient should consume 48 ounces of water daily.

Contraindications Contraindications to indinavir include concurrent therapy with alfuzosin, cisapride, ergot derivatives, irinotecan, lovastatin, midazolam, nevirapine, pimozide, rifampin, sildenafil, simvastatin, St. John's wort, or triazolam.

Cautions and Considerations Kidney toxicity is a major concern with indinavir use. Patients using indinavir should be monitored for signs of renal damage.

Drug Interactions PIs have many drug interactions. Please visit the NIH AIDSinfo website at http://Pharmacology6e.ParadigmCollege.net/AIDSinfo to view the most recent interaction information.

Lopinavir-Ritonavir

Lopinavir-ritonavir (Kaletra) is a combination product that shares side effects with ritonavir (discussed later in this section). Because the ritonavir dose is lower when combined with lopinavir, fewer intestinal side effects, such as cramping, are present. Other GI side effects, however, are still present (diarrhea and nausea).

Contraindications Contraindications to lopinavir-ritonavir include concurrent therapy with alfuzosin, cisapride, ergot derivatives, indinavir, irinotecan, lovastatin, midazolam, nevirapine, pimozide, rifampin, sildenafil, simvastatin, St. John's wort, or triazolam. Coadministration with drugs that strongly induce cytochrome P-450 3A4 may lead to lower lopinavir-ritonavir exposure and loss of efficacy. Other side effects include rash, liver dysfunction, and renal dysfunction.

Cautions and Considerations As shown in Table 5.4, lopinavir-ritonavir is available in an oral liquid formula. This formula contains a high percentage of both alcohol and propylene glycol. Patients with cautions or contraindications to alcohol should not use the oral liquid. Patients should not use other medications that contain propylene glycol while using this formulation.

Drug Interactions PIs have many drug interactions. Please visit the NIH AIDSinfo website at http://Pharmacology6e.ParadigmCollege.net/AIDSinfo to view the most recent interaction information.

Nelfinavir

Nelfinavir (Viracept) is well tolerated by patients. Although diarrhea is an initial side effect, it generally resolves itself with continued use. Loperamide and calcium carbonate can help control the diarrhea. Nelfinavir should be taken with food.

Contraindications Nelfinavir should not be used concurrently with alfuzosin, amiodarone, cisapride, ergot derivatives, lovastatin, midazolam, pimozide, quinidine, rifampin, sildenafil, simvastatin, St. John's wort, or triazolam.

Cautions and Considerations Diarrhea occurs frequently with use of nelfinavir. If a patient is unable to swallow nelfinavir tablets, he or she may dissolve a tablet in a small amount of water and consume the solution immediately. The glass used to dissolve the tablet should be rinsed and the contents ingested to ensure the entire dose is taken. Alternatively, the tablets may be crushed and mixed with a small amount of food. Avoid mixing this drug with acidic beverages or acidic food because of its bitter taste.

Drug Interactions PIs have many drug interactions. Please visit the NIH AIDSinfo website at http://Pharmacology6e.ParadigmCollege.net/AIDSinfo to view the most recent interaction information.

Ritonavir

Ritonavir (Norvir) is prescribed primarily for its ability to increase the serum concentrations and decrease the dosage frequency of other PIs (an action known as a **boost**). As such, ritonavir is generally given at a low dose in combination with other drugs. Ritonavir should be taken with food. This drug has many side effects that include an unusual one—an altered sense of taste. Ritonavir, whether in capsule, tablet, or solution form, should be stored in the refrigerator.

Contraindications Ritonavir is contraindicated with the concurrent use of alfuzosin, amiodarone, cisapride, ergot derivatives, flecainide, lovastatin, midazolam, pimozide, propafenone, quinidine, sildenafil, simvastatin, St. John's wort, triazolam, or voriconazole.

Cautions and Considerations Ritonavir has a black box warning for serious and potentially life-threatening drug interactions. Ritonavir should be used cautiously in patients with cardiac arrhythmias due to exacerbations of these conditions.

Drug Interactions Ritonavir is an extremely potent inhibitor of cytochrome P-450 and has many drug interactions. Please visit the NIH AIDSinfo website at http://Pharmacology6e.ParadigmCollege.net/AIDSinfo to view the most recent interaction information.

Saquinavir

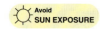

Saquinavir (Invirase) was the first PI to gain FDA approval for HIV treatment. Patients taking this medication should be instructed to avoid sunlight. Saquinavir can also cause diarrhea, nausea, and other abdominal discomfort. Saquinavir must be taken with ritonavir (Norvir). Saquinavir is unique in that it does not cause the lipid abnormalities that other PIs do.

Contraindications Contraindications to saquinavir include congenital or acquired prolongation of the QT interval, refractory hypokalemia or hypomagnesemia, concomitant use of medications that both increase saquinavir plasma concentrations and prolong the QT interval, complete atrioventricular (AV) block, and severe liver impairment. Saquinavir combined with ritonavir is contraindicated with the concurrent use of alfuzosin, amiodarone, bepridil, cisapride, dofetilide, ergot derivatives, flecainide, lidocaine, lovastatin, midazolam, pimozide, propafenone, quinidine, rifampin, sildenafil, simvastatin, trazodone, or triazolam.

Cautions and Considerations Saquinavir may cause QT interval prolongation. It should be used cautiously in patients with a prolonged QT interval or in individuals who are using other medications that have the same effect.

Saquinavir is formulated with lactose. Patients with lactose intolerance should not use saquinavir.

Drug Interactions PIs have many drug interactions. Please visit the NIH AIDSinfo website at http://Pharmacology6e.ParadigmCollege.net/AIDSinfo to view the most recent interaction information.

Tipranavir

Tipranavir (Aptivus) may have some advantages over other PIs. Its structure is more adaptable to protease binding sites than other PIs. It also has a self-emulsifying drug delivery system (SEDDS) in the form of a soft gelatin capsule. This system improves dissolution and the bioavailability of the drug, which increases systemic circulation and reduces the pill burden. Tipranavir is given with ritonavir (Norvir) as a boost and should be taken with food. Common side effects are diarrhea, nausea, vomiting, headache, and fatigue. Capsules should be stored in the refrigerator but are stable for up to 60 days when not refrigerated. The oral solution should be stored at room temperature.

Contraindications Tipranavir is contraindicated in patients with moderate-to-severe liver impairment. Tipranavir in combination with ritonavir should not be used with alfuzosin, amiodarone, bepridil, cisapride, ergot derivatives, flecainide, lovastatin, midazolam, pimozide, propafenone, quinidine, rifampin, sildenafil, simvastatin, St. John's wort, or triazolam.

Cautions and Considerations Tipranavir has a black box warning because intracranial hemorrhages occurred in participants of clinical studies. It has another boxed warning for hepatotoxicity and may cause hepatitis or exacerbate preexisting hepatitis.

Tipranavir capsules contain dehydrated ethanol and should be avoided in patients with cautions or contraindications to ethanol. The oral solution formula contains vitamin E. Those individuals using the oral solution should not take additional vitamin E.

Drug Interactions PIs have many drug interactions. Please visit the NIH AIDSinfo website at http://Pharmacology6e.ParadigmCollege.net/AIDSinfo to view the most recent interaction information.

Fusion Inhibitors

Fusion inhibitors prevent HIV from entering immune cells. This mechanism of action is a major advancement in HIV treatment because older drugs block replication of the virus only after it has entered the cell. Figure 5.1 illustrates where fusion inhibitors work in the HIV life cycle. Table 5.5 lists the only fusion inhibitor available at this time.

Enfuvirtide

Enfuvirtide (Fuzeon) is given subcutaneously. It is administered to HIV patients resistant to older drugs. It is distributed as a powder, and sterile water is the diluent. It takes 30 to 45 minutes to dissolve, and reaction at the injection site is common. Side effects include diarrhea, nausea, and fatigue.

Contraindications Enfuvirtide does not have contraindications.

Cautions and Considerations Enfuvirtide may cause hypersensitivity reactions and pneumonia. Enfuvirtide is not appropriate for treatment-naive patients.

Drug Interactions PIs may increase serum concentrations of enfuvirtide.

Chemokine Coreceptor Antagonists

Chemokine coreceptor (CCR5) antagonists work by preventing HIV from attaching and thereby entering an immune system cell. See Figure 5.1 for an illustration of where CCR5 antagonists work in the HIV life cycle. Currently, there is one drug in this class.

Maraviroc

Maraviroc (Selzentry) is the first drug from the CCR5 class to be approved for the R5 virus, which is a form of HIV. Maraviroc is to be given with other antiretroviral drugs. It is taken without regard to food. The most common side effect is a cough. Other side effects include abdominal pain, dizziness, and fever. Additional information about maraviroc is summarized in Table 5.5.

Contraindications Maraviroc is contraindicated in patients with severe kidney impairment.

Cautions and Considerations Maraviroc has a black box warning for inducing hepatotoxicity with allergic features. While on maraviroc, patients must be monitored closely for infection.

Web

Drug Interactions Maraviroc is a cytochrome P-450 substrate and has many drug interactions. The following list includes drugs that should be avoided when patients are taking maraviroc: conivaptan, fusidic acid, idelalisib, and St. John's wort. Other drug interactions can be found on the NIH AIDSinfo website at http://Pharmacology6e.ParadigmCollege.net/AIDSinfo_2.

TABLE 5.5 Commonly Used HIV Drugs

Generic (Brand)	Pronunciation	Dosage Form	Common Dosage	Dispensing Status
CCR5 Antagonist				
maraviroc (Selzentry)	mah-RAV-er-rock	Tablet	300 mg twice a day	Rx
Fusion Inhibitor				
enfuvirtide (Fuzeon)	en-FOO-vir-tide	Solution for subcutaneous injection	90 mg twice a day	Rx
Integrase Inhibitors				
dolutegravir (Tivicay)	doe-loo-TEG-ra-veer	Tablet	50 mg 1–2 times a day	Rx
elvitegravir (Vitekta)	el-vi-TEG-ra-veer	Tablet	85–150 mg a day	Rx
raltegravir (Isentress)	ral-TEG-ra-veer	Chewable tablet, oral packet, tablet (film coated)	400 mg twice a day	Rx

Integrase Inhibitors

Like reverse transcriptase (blocked by NRTIs, NtRTIs, and NNRTIs) and protease (blocked by PIs), integrase is an enzyme needed for HIV to reproduce. Figure 5.1 illustrates where integrase inhibitors work in the HIV life cycle. Integrase inhibitors are summarized in Table 5.5. Integrase inserts DNA that is produced from viral RNA by reverse transcriptase into the DNA of the host cell. Raltegravir, which blocks the action of integrase, received a priority review and was approved to be used only in combination with other HIV drugs. It reduces the amount of HIV in the blood and increases the WBC count, which helps fight infection. Because HIV patients are immunocompromised, the infection-fighting property of raltegravir is very important.

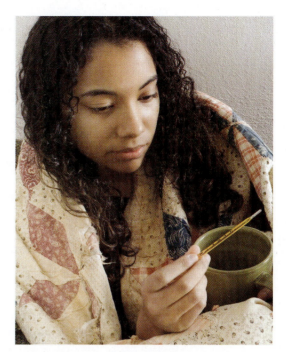

HIV patients are immunocompromised and are vulnerable to illness. Raltegravir increases WBC count and helps fight infections.

Dolutegravir

Dolutegravir (Tivicay) was approved by the FDA in 2013 and is considered to work better than raltegravir or elvitegravir in cases of viral resistance. It may be used in all patients, regardless of their experience with antiviral medications. Compared with other integrase inhibitors, it is well tolerated. Side effects include elevated serum lipase, insomnia, elevated liver enzymes, and hyperglycemia.

Contraindications Dolutegravir should not be used with dofetilide.

Cautions and Considerations Dolutegravir may cause fat redistribution and hypersensitivity reaction.

Drug Interactions Dolutegravir has multiple drug interactions. Drugs that should be avoided when taking dolutegravir include carbamazepine, dofetilide, fosphenytoin, nevirapine, oxcarbazepine, phenobarbital, phenytoin, primidone, and St. John's wort. Multivitamins and zinc salts may decrease dolutegravir concentrations. More information on drug interactions can be found on the NIH AIDSinfo website at http://Pharmacology6e.ParadigmCollege.net/AIDSinfo_3.

Web

Elvitegravir

Elvitegravir (Vitekta) is available alone as a tablet or as a combination product. Common side effects include depression, fatigue, insomnia, headache, diarrhea, and abdominal pain.

Contraindications Elvitegravir does not have contraindications.

Cautions and Considerations Elvitegravir may contribute to lactic acidosis. It should be avoided in patients with severe liver impairment.

Drug Interactions Elvitegravir has many drug interactions. It should be avoided when a patient is using nevirapine, rifabutin, rifampin, or St. John's wort. Elvitegravir may decrease the effectiveness of estrogen-containing contraceptives. Antacids may decrease the serum concentration of elvitegravir. More information on drug interactions can be found on the NIH AIDSinfo website at http://Pharmacology6e. ParadigmCollege.net/AIDSinfo_3.

Web

Work Wise

Raltegravir film-coated tablets, chewable tablets, and oral suspension are not bioequivalent. This means they cannot be substituted on a milligram-to-milligram basis.

Raltegravir

Raltegravir (Isentress) is an integrase inhibitor that is available as a chewable tablet, oral suspension, and film-coated tablet. Side effects include nausea, headache, diarrhea, pyrexia, and creatine kinase elevation.

Contraindications Raltegravir does not have contraindications.

Cautions and Considerations Raltegravir is associated with myopathy and rhabdomyolysis (a condition characterized by muscle breakdown). Caution should be exercised in patients with a history of rhabdomyolysis, myopathy, or creatine kinase elevations.

The chewable tablet formulation contains phenylalanine. Patients with phenylalanine sensitivity should avoid this formulation.

Drug Interactions Aluminum hydroxide and magnesium salts may decrease the serum concentration of raltegravir. Raltegravir may enhance the myopathic effects of fibric acid derivatives and statins (both used for dyslipidemia).

TABLE 5.6 Initial Regimen Recommendations for Adults and Adolescents with HIV

- An antiretroviral regimen for a treatment-naive patient generally consists of two nucleoside reverse transcriptase inhibitors in combination with a third active antiretroviral drug from one of three drug classes: an integrase strand transfer inhibitor, a non-nucleoside reverse transcriptase inhibitor, or a protease inhibitor with a pharmacokinetic enhancer (cobicistat or ritonavir).

- The US Department of Health and Human Services Panel on Antiretroviral Guidelines for Adults and Adolescents classifies the following regimens as recommended therapy for antiretroviral-naive patients:

Regimens Based on Integrase Strand Transfer Inhibitors:
- Dolutegravir-abacavir-lamivudine—only for patients who are HLA-B*5701 negative (AI)
- Dolutegravir plus tenofovir disoproxil fumarate (tenofovir)-emtricitabine (AI)
- Elvitegravir-cobicistat-tenofovir-emtricitabine—only for patients with pre-antiretroviral therapy CrCl >70 mL/min (AI)
- Raltegravir plus tenofovir-emtricitabine (AI)

Regimens Based on Protease Inhibitors:
- Darunavir-ritonavir plus tenofovir-emtricitabine* (AI)

- On the basis of individual patient characteristics and needs, an alternative regimen or, less frequently, another regimen may in some instances be the optimal regimen for a patient.

- Given the large number of excellent options for initial therapy, selection of a regimen for a particular patient should be guided by such factors as virologic efficacy, toxicity, pill burden, dosing frequency, drug-drug interaction potential, resistance testing results, comorbid conditions, and cost.

Rating of Recommendations: *A = Strong; B = Moderate; C = Optional*
Rating of Evidence: *I = Data from randomized controlled trials*
** **Lamivudine:** may substitute for emtricitabine or vice versa*

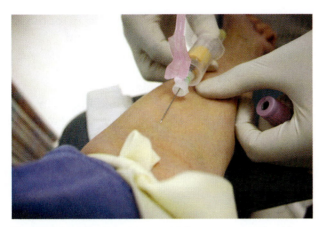

The CDC has developed new guidelines to protect health-care workers. Healthcare workers who are accidentally exposed to blood with a high virus titer should start PEP immediately.

Responding to Exposure to HIV

The **Centers for Disease Control and Prevention (CDC)** have developed guidelines for the management of healthcare worker exposure to HIV. These guidelines include recommendations for the administration of antiretroviral drugs as **postexposure prophylaxis (PEP)**. Healthcare worker risks include exposure to the blood and other body fluids of an HIV-positive patient and needlestick injuries. Following such an exposure, the administration of an appropriate antiretroviral regimen should begin within two hours. Research has shown that prompt treatment can decrease the risk of infection by 80%. Clearly, preventing exposure to HIV through appropriate precautions is the primary means of protection against HIV infection for healthcare workers as well as the public. People accidentally exposed to blood with a high virus titer or to deep needle injury should start PEP immediately (within one to two hours) because they are at a high risk of infection.

Combining Antiretroviral Medications

None of the antiretroviral medications currently available can eradicate HIV, but when used appropriately they can decrease viral replication, improve immunologic status, and prolong life. The standard care for the treatment of HIV is to administer several drugs in combination. The regimens are difficult to follow because the drugs must be taken around the clock. Consequently, patient adherence is frequently poor. Clear written instructions for taking the medications, as well as adequate warnings about the potential for drug interactions, may encourage higher patient adherence. Patients who only have to take a single dose per day show higher adherence to therapy than those individuals on a more complex regimen.

Table 5.6 gives an overview of current recommendations for HIV therapy.

To simplify the drug regimen and decrease pill load, pharmaceutical manufacturers have increasingly moved to drug combinations. There are specific advantages and disadvantages to various combinations. The most obvious advantage is improved patient adherence. A principal disadvantage is that these combination drugs have fixed doses and cannot be used in unstable patients who require frequent dose changes to decrease the viral load.

Atripla (efavirenz-emtricitabine-tenofovir) is a combination of three different classes of antiretrovirals—an NNRTI (efavirenz), an NRTI (emtricitabine), and an NtRTI (tenofovir disoproxil fumarate)—in one pill. The virus can be attacked in three ways simultaneously by the same pill. The side effects are the same as those of the three individual drugs. The big advantage is that Atripla is dosed once a day and improves patient adherence. It is recommended as a first-line therapy unless the patient is in the first trimester of pregnancy. It was approved through an accelerated process. It has a black box warning for lactic acidosis. Atripla must be dispensed in the original unopened container.

Work Wise

The pharmacy technician must display discretion and sensitivity when addressing the needs of patients who have HIV.

Combivir (lamivudine-zidovudine) comes as a capsule and as a syrup for those individuals who have trouble swallowing a capsule. Its ingredients (Epivir and Retrovir) are both NRTIs. The drugs are synergistic, and the pill load is decreased. Because Combivir is a fixed dose, it cannot be used in patients requiring dosage adjustments. It also cannot be used in children under 12 years old.

Epzicom (abacavir-lamivudine) contains two NRTIs (Ziagen and Epivir) in a fixed combination and a single strength. Epzicom can be taken without regard to food, which improves patient adherence. This point is important because partial adherence can lead to resistance. A card packaged with Epzicom states that if the patient has any two of the following symptoms, the prescriber must be contacted immediately and the drug must be discontinued:

- fever

- rash

- nausea and vomiting, or diarrhea and cramping

- extreme tiredness or achiness

- shortness of breath, cough, or sore throat

Pharmacy technicians must ensure that patients receive this card when picking up the medication. Technicians should instruct patients to read the card and to carry the card with them at all times. Providing this patient instruction is *not* considered counseling.

Stribild (elvitegravir-cobicistat-emtricitabine-tenofovir) is a combination product for the treatment of HIV. Stribild may decrease bone mineral density and cause fat redistribution. It may also contribute to lactic acidosis. It should be avoided in patients with severe liver impairment. Stribild is also contraindicated with concurrent use of alfuzosin, cisapride, ergot derivatives, lovastatin, midazolam, pimozide, rifampin, sildenafil, simvastatin, St. John's wort, or triazolam.

Truvada (emtricitabine-tenofovir) has the same drugs as Atripla without Sustiva (efavirenz); that is, this drug is a combination of Emtriva and Viread. It may be an agent to prevent HIV in the future, but not at this time. Currently, it is a drug recommended for occupational exposure to HIV and an option for initial treatment. It is well tolerated and long-acting.

The most commonly used combinations of antiviral drugs are summarized in Table 5.7.

TABLE 5.7 Commonly Used Combination Treatments for HIV

Generic (Brand)	Common Dosage
abacavir-lamivudine (Epzicom)	1 tablet a day
efavirenz-emtricitabine-tenofovir (Atripla)	1 tablet a day
elvitegravir-cobicistat-emtricitabine-tenofovir (Stribild)	1 tablet a day
emtricitabine-tenofovir (Truvada)	1 tablet a day
lamivudine-zidovudine (Combivir)	1 tablet twice a day

Immunization

Immunization is the process whereby a person acquires immunity or resistance to an infectious disease. There are two general ways people acquire immunity: passively and actively. **Passive immunity** occurs when preformed antibodies are transferred to an individual. Examples of passive immunity include a mother transferring antibodies to her fetus during pregnancy (naturally) and injection of immunoglobulins (artificially). Passive immunity provides immediate protection, but the body does not develop immunologic memory.

In contrast to passive immunity, where ready-made antibodies are transferred to an individual, **active immunity** is the process by which a body makes its own antibodies to a pathogen. Active immunity acquired naturally occurs when a person is exposed to certain pathogens; active immunity that is acquired artificially typically results from vaccination. Vaccination is a proven tool for the prevention and elimination of infectious diseases, with an estimated 2 to 3 million deaths prevented worldwide every year by vaccines.

Vaccination may reduce and prevent serious diseases when used universally. For example, vaccination practices have effectively eliminated smallpox worldwide. Vaccination also reduces many other diseases that cause great sickness and disability, especially among children. For instance, vaccines have reduced the impact of measles, polio, and influenza.

Various types of vaccines are available. **Live attenuated vaccines** use live but weakened pathogens to induce an immune response. **Inactivated vaccines** use pathogens that have been killed with chemicals, heat, or radiation.

Immunization Schedule

Several vaccines require multiple doses to produce an adequate immune response and confer full immunity to a disease. The CDC publishes a schedule for childhood and adult vaccines. In Canada, the **Public Health Agency** makes vaccine recommendations. Certain immunizations are recommended for children, whereas others are more appropriate for adults (see Figures 5.2 and 5.3). In most cases, specific vaccines are required for children to enter public school. When the vaccine regimen is complete, most childhood vaccinations lead to lifetime immunity. Others, for example the tetanus and pertussis vaccines, must be readministered periodically as booster shots to continue immunity protection.

Pharmacy technicians should be informed of immunization schedules and be certain they are personally up to date on their immunizations. Working in the healthcare field without being properly vaccinated increases an individual's risk of exposure to diseases and promotes disease transmission. Certain vaccines are recommended for healthcare workers. These immunizations include hepatitis B vaccination and an annual influenza shot. Many healthcare employers require their employees to get these vaccinations and keep all others current as part of employment.

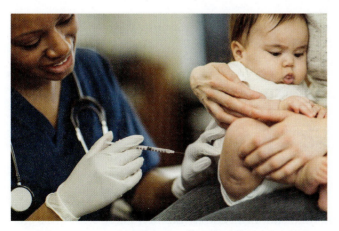

A health care professional administers a vaccine to an infant.

FIGURE 5.2
2016 CDC Immunization Schedule for Adults

The first adult immunization schedule was published by the Centers for Disease Control and Prevention (CDC) in 2002 and is updated annually. The CDC also publishes an adult immunization schedule based on medical and other indications that is designed for use by healthcare professionals.

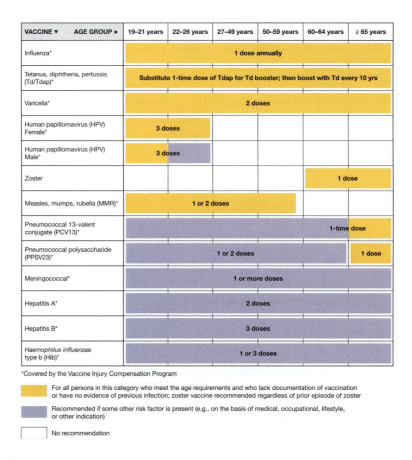

VACCINE ▼ AGE GROUP ►	19–21 years	22–26 years	27–49 years	50–59 years	60–64 years	≥ 65 years
Influenza*	1 dose annually					
Tetanus, diphtheria, pertussis (Td/Tdap)*	Substitute 1-time dose of Tdap for Td booster; then boost with Td every 10 yrs					
Varicella*	2 doses					
Human papillomavirus (HPV) Female*	3 doses					
Human papillomavirus (HPV) Male*	3 doses					
Zoster					1 dose	
Measles, mumps, rubella (MMR)*	1 or 2 doses					
Pneumococcal 13-valent conjugate (PCV13)*						1-time dose
Pneumococcal polysaccharide (PPSV23)*	1 or 2 doses					1 dose
Meningococcal*	1 or more doses					
Hepatitis A*	2 doses					
Hepatitis B*	3 doses					
Haemophilus influenzae type b (Hib)*	1 or 3 doses					

*Covered by the Vaccine Injury Compensation Program

▨ For all persons in this category who meet the age requirements and who lack documentation of vaccination or have no evidence of previous infection; zoster vaccine recommended regardless of prior episode of zoster

▨ Recommended if some other risk factor is present (e.g., on the basis of medical, occupational, lifestyle, or other indication)

☐ No recommendation

Pharm Facts

American physician and researcher Baruch S. Blumberg was a corecipient of the Nobel Prize in Physiology or Medicine in 1976 for his discovery of the hepatitis B virus and the development of a powerful vaccine that fought the virus.

Common Vaccines

Many vaccines are administered in physicians' offices, clinics, or inpatient settings. However, a greater number of vaccines are administered in community pharmacies. For example, many patients now receive their annual influenza vaccine at their local pharmacies. In this setting, it is often the pharmacy technician who screens patients, completes the necessary forms, and stocks and stores the vaccines. Sometimes, the technician may even draw up the vaccine for the pharmacist to administer. Thus, it is important that the pharmacy technician has a working knowledge of this aspect of practice. To learn more about common vaccines, their routes of administration, and their reason for use, see Table 5.8.

Numerous clinics and pharmacies operate **travel immunization clinics**. These clinics can help prepare people for travel and provide immunizations and advice about what vaccines are recommended or necessary for global travel. Examples of **travel vaccines** include those for hepatitis and cholera. These diseases are not common enough to warrant mass vaccination in the United States but are found in other parts of the world. When traveling from an area of low rates of infection to areas with high rates, travel vaccines are recommended or required. Travel vaccines must be given well in advance of a trip to allow the immune system enough time to mount the appropriate response and confer full immunity. Time to level of highest immunity differs among vaccines. Many immunizations should be given two or more weeks before travel.

Side Effects Common side effects of vaccines include fever, headache, upset stomach, local injection-site irritation, mild skin rash, and irritability. These symptoms are related to a systemic immune response, which makes a person feel generally tired and achy. It can feel like the onset of the flu, which is why many patients mistakenly

FIGURE 5.3
2016 CDC Immunization Schedule for Children Ages 0–18

The CDC immunization schedule for children ages 0-18 is published annually.

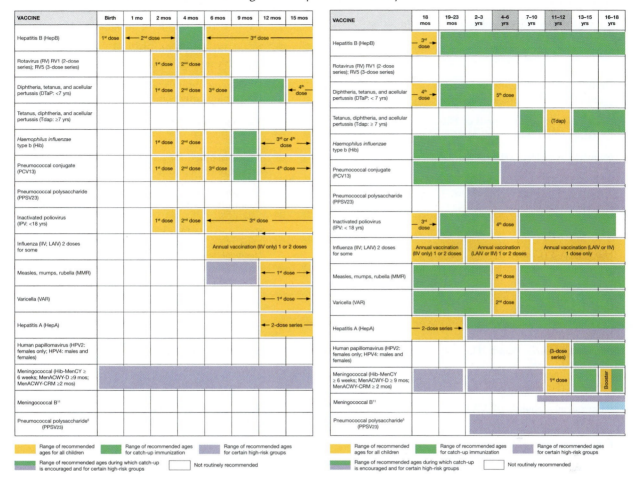

VACCINE	Birth	1 mo	2 mos	4 mos	6 mos	9 mos	12 mos	15 mos
Hepatitis B (HepB)	1st dose	← 2nd dose →			← 3rd dose →			
Rotavirus (RV) RV1 (2-dose series); RV5 (3-dose series)			1st dose	2nd dose				
Diphtheria, tetanus, and acellular pertussis (DTaP: <7 yrs)			1st dose	2nd dose	3rd dose			← 4th dose
Tetanus, diphtheria, and acellular pertussis (Tdap: ≥7 yrs)								
Haemophilus influenzae type b (Hib)			1st dose	2nd dose			3rd or 4th dose →	
Pneumococcal conjugate (PCV13)			1st dose	2nd dose	3rd dose		← 4th dose →	
Pneumococcal polysaccharide (PPSV23)								
Inactivated poliovirus (IPV: <18 yrs)			1st dose	2nd dose	← 3rd dose →			
Influenza (IIV; LAIV) 2 doses for some					Annual vaccination (IIV only) 1 or 2 doses			
Measles, mumps, rubella (MMR)							← 1st dose →	
Varicella (VAR)							← 1st dose →	
Hepatitis A (HepA)							← 2-dose series →	
Human papillomavirus (HPV2: females only; HPV4: males and females)								
Meningococcal (Hib-MenCY ≥ 6 weeks; MenACWY-D ≥9 mos; MenACWY-CRM ≥2 mos)								
Meningococcal B[11]								
Pneumococcal polysaccharide[5] (PPSV23)								

VACCINE	18 mos	19–23 mos	2–3 yrs	4–6 yrs	7–10 yrs	11–12 yrs	13–15 yrs	16–18 yrs
Hepatitis B (HepB)	3rd dose							
Rotavirus (RV) RV1 (2-dose series); RV5 (3-dose series)								
Diphtheria, tetanus, and acellular pertussis (DTaP: < 7 yrs)	4th dose			5th dose				
Tetanus, diphtheria, and acellular pertussis (Tdap: ≥ 7 yrs)						(Tdap)		
Haemophilus influenzae type b (Hib)								
Pneumococcal conjugate (PCV13)								
Pneumococcal polysaccharide (PPSV23)								
Inactivated poliovirus (IPV: < 18 yrs)	3rd dose			4th dose				
Influenza (IIV; LAIV) 2 doses for some	Annual vaccination (IIV only) 1 or 2 doses		Annual vaccination (LAIV or IIV) 1 or 2 doses		Annual vaccination (LAIV or IIV) 1 dose only			
Measles, mumps, rubella (MMR)				2nd dose				
Varicella (VAR)				2nd dose				
Hepatitis A (HepA)	← 2-dose series →							
Human papillomavirus (HPV2: females only; HPV4: males and females)						(3-dose series)		
Meningococcal (Hib-MenCY ≥ 6 weeks; MenACWY-D ≥ 9 mos; MenACWY-CRM ≥ 2 mos)						1st dose	Booster	
Meningococcal B[11]								
Pneumococcal polysaccharide[5] (PPSV23)								

Range of recommended ages for all children
Range of recommended ages for catch-up immunization
Range of recommended ages for certain high-risk groups
Range of recommended ages during which catch-up is encouraged and for certain high-risk groups
Not routinely recommended

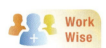
believe that the influenza shot gave them the flu. Such symptoms can also occur after injection of other vaccines. All guidelines state specifically that taking acetaminophen for 24 to 48 hours after immunization usually alleviates these symptoms.

Contraindications The Bacille Calmette-Guerin (BCG) vaccine should not be administered to pregnant women or to patients who are immunocompromised.

The diphtheria, tetanus, and pertussis vaccine is contraindicated in patients with encephalopathy within seven days of administration of a previous dose of vaccine, with or without another identifiable cause. An additional contraindication is progressive neurologic disorder. Certain formulations include latex, and they should not be administered to patients with a latex allergy.

The *Haemophilus influenzae* type b (HIB) vaccine is contraindicated in patients younger than six weeks of age.

The hepatitis A vaccine should not be given to patients with a history of severe reaction to a prior dose of the hepatitis A vaccine or to those patients who are highly sensitive to vaccine additives. The hepatitis B vaccine is contraindicated in individuals with a history of hypersensitivity to yeast.

The vaccine for human papillomavirus (HPV) is contraindicated in patients with yeast hypersensitivity.

TABLE 5.8   Common Vaccines

Generic (Brand)	Route of Administration	Prophylactic Use
Bacille Calmette-Guerin (BCG)	Injection	Recommended for patients at high risk of exposure to tuberculosis Recommended for healthcare workers in high-risk settings only
Diphtheria, tetanus, and pertussis (various combinations available)	Injection	Diphtheria, tetanus, and/or pertussis (whooping cough) in children or adults
Haemophilus influenzae type B or Hib (ActHIB, HibTITER, PedvaxHIB)	Injection	*Haemophilus influenzae* type B in children
Hepatitis A or HAV (Havrix, Vaqta)	Injection	Recommended for patients at high risk of exposure to hepatitis A
Hepatitis B or Hep B (Engerix-B, Recombivax HB)	Injection	Hepatitis B in children Recommended for adults at high risk of exposure to hepatitis B Recommended for healthcare workers
Hib + Hep B (Comvax)	Injection	*Haemophilus influenzae* type B and hepatitis B in children
Human papillomavirus or HPV (Ceravix, Gardasil)	Injection	Gardasil recommended for girls and women 9–26 years old and boys and men 9–26 to prevent genital warts, anal cancer, and in women, cervical cancer.
Influenza (Afluria, Fluarix, FluLaval, Fluvirin, Fluzone)	Injection	Influenza in children and adults
Influenza (FluMist)	Intranasal	Influenza in patients 2–50 years old
Japanese encephalitis (JE-VAX)	Injection	Recommended for patients at high risk of exposure to Japanese encephalitis
Measles, mumps, rubella (MMR II)	Injection	Measles, mumps, and rubella in adults and children
Meningococcal (Menactra, Menomune)	Injection	Recommended for patients at high risk of exposure to *Neisseria meningitidis*
Pneumococcal, conjugate (Prevnar)	Injection	Pneumonia and otitis media (ear infections) in children and certain adults
Pneumococcal, polyvalent (Pneumovax 23)	Injection	Pneumonia in patients <2 years old or >50 years old
Polio, inactivated or IPV (IPOL)	Injection	Poliovirus in children
Rotavirus (Rotarix, RotaTeq)	Oral	Rotavirus in infants and children
Typhoid (Typhim Vi)	Injection	Recommended for patients at high risk of exposure to typhoid fever
Typhoid (Vivotif Berna)	Oral	*Salmonella typhi* in adults and children
Varicella (Varivax)	Injection	Chicken pox in children
Yellow fever (YF-Vax)	Injection	Recommended for patients at high risk of exposure to yellow fever
Zoster (Zostavax)	Injection	Herpes zoster (shingles) in patients 60 years old and older

The influenza vaccine comes in both inactivated and live formulas. The inactivated influenza vaccine is grown in chicken eggs and is contraindicated in patients with egg or chicken allergies. This vaccine should be withheld in children with moderate-to-severe acute febrile illness and administered only after symptoms resolve. However, minor illness with or without fever is not a contraindication.

Some inactivated influenza vaccine formulations contain thimerosal or gelatin; patients with allergies to either of these substances should avoid those formulations. Contraindications to the live influenza vaccine include the following: age younger than two years; history of anaphylactic reaction to gelatin or arginine; long-term aspirin or salicylate therapy; history of Guillain-Barré syndrome; asthma in children younger than five years; recurrent wheezing in children ages two through four years; chronic pulmonary, cardiovascular, renal, hepatic, neurologic, hematologic, or metabolic disorders; pregnancy; known or suspected immunodeficiency; or receipt of other live virus vaccine within the previous four weeks.

The Japanese encephalitis vaccine contains protamine sulfate; therefore, its use should be avoided in patients with protamine hypersensitivity.

Contraindications to the measles, mumps, rubella (MMR) vaccine include anaphylactic reaction to neomycin, pregnancy, and known altered immunodeficiency states. MMR is a live vaccine and use should be withheld in severe febrile illness until the acute illness has subsided.

The rotavirus vaccine is contraindicated in patients with a history of intussusception (a GI disorder) and severe combined immunodeficiency disease.

The oral typhoid vaccine is contraindicated in patients who have immunocompromised states or have an acute febrile illness.

Contraindications to the varicella vaccine include patients in immunocompromised states, for this vaccine contains a live virus.

The yellow fever vaccine should not be given to patients who have a hypersensitivity to egg or chicken protein; children younger than six months; patients who are immunosuppressed (from disorders or use of medications that induce immunosuppression); patients with thymus disorder associated with abnormal immune function; and patients who have undergone organ transplantation.

Contraindications to the herpes zoster vaccine include a history of anaphylactic reaction to gelatin or neomycin; immunosuppression; primary and acquired immunodeficiency states; AIDS or clinical manifestations of HIV; immunosuppressive therapy; or pregnancy.

The meningococcal, pneumococcal, polio (inactivated), and injectable typhoid vaccines do not have contraindications.

Cautions and Considerations Like any drug therapy, immunization is not without risk. Patients must receive written information about risks before getting a vaccination. A **Vaccine Information Statement (VIS)** is available from the CDC for all vaccines on the market. Pharmacy technicians can find samples

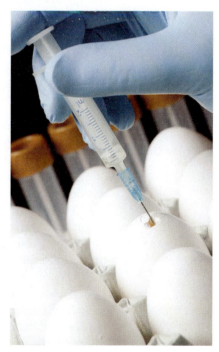

The inactivated form of the influenza vaccine is grown in chicken eggs and should not be administered to patients with egg or chicken allergies.

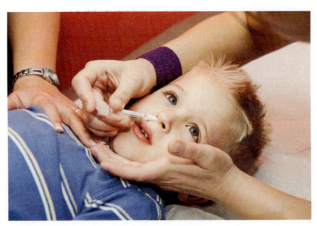

FluMist is a nasal spray option for those who want to get the influenza (flu) vaccine without an injection. This dosage form is only for patients 2 to 50 years of age and contains a live attenuated virus, rather than a deactivated virus. Patients should be aware of the extra precautions and limitations for the use of FluMist.

Web

Practice Tip

The typhoid vaccine is available in an oral dosage form. The oral vaccine is given as four capsules, one capsule every other day. Oral typhoid capsules must be refrigerated and should be taken with cold or lukewarm water about one hour prior to eating a meal. Antibiotics and some malaria medications can decrease the vaccine's effectiveness; consequently, concurrent use should be avoided.

of these sheets on the CDC website (http://Pharmacology6e.ParadigmCollege.net/CDC_Flu). Prior to vaccination, patients must sign a consent form stating that they are making an informed decision to receive a vaccine and verifying they have received a VIS for the appropriate vaccine. Quite often, obtaining these signatures and maintaining documentation records are the responsibilities of technicians when the vaccine is administered in the pharmacy. These responsibilities should not be taken lightly because the patient consent form is required by law.

Healthcare personnel giving immunizations must be trained in administering cardiopulmonary resuscitation (CPR) and other necessary treatments in the event of an anaphylactic reaction.

Most vaccines require storage in either a refrigerator or freezer. The recommended storage temperature range can differ among vaccines and must be strictly followed. Most vaccine products cannot be used if frozen. If allowed to warm to room temperature, most vaccines must be used right away (not refrigerated again). In many cases, daily temperature measurement of refrigerators and freezers is required to ensure that stored vaccines are kept at the appropriate temperature and do not spoil. Vaccines that are supplied as powder for injection usually must be used within minutes to hours after reconstitution. Advance mixing and preparation of multiple doses is not recommended. Vaccines should never be mixed in the same syringe with any other medications. If more than one vaccine is administered at the same time, they should be given at different injection sites.

Complementary and Alternative Therapy

Andrographis (*Andrographis paniculata*) has been widely used in Indian folk medicine and Ayurvedic forms of medicine. In fact, it may colloquially be referred to as "Indian echinacea." There is some information to suggest andrographis may reduce symptom severity and duration of influenza respiratory infections if started quickly (within 36 to 48 hours). Side effects of andrographis include chest discomfort, headache, nausea, and rash. Andrographis may interact with anticoagulants, blood pressure medications, and immunosuppressants.

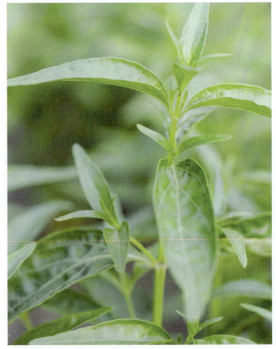

The plant *Andrographis paniculata* may be used to treat influenza respiratory infections.

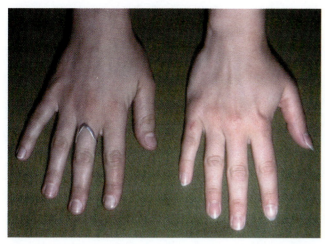

Argyria is an irreversible skin condition that results from silver accumulation.

Colloidal silver is a suspension of submicroscopic silver particles in a colloidal base. Prior to the development of antibiotics, silver-based products were used in the treatment of wounds, and bacterial and viral infections. Colloidal silver is used topically (to treat skin infections) and orally (to treat viral, fungal, or bacterial infections). Some individuals use colloidal silver prophylactically for influenza. Total daily silver intake should not exceed 14 mcg/kg/day. In addition to regular dietary intake of silver, supplemental silver will likely exceed this amount. The risks of silver use are severe. Silver may accumulate in the body and can lead to argyria, an irreversible bluish skin discoloration. Other side effects, such as neurologic deficits and kidney damage, may also occur with use.

Elderberry (*Sambucus nigra*) may be used to treat influenza. Some evidence suggests it may be effective when initiated within 48 hours of influenza symptoms. Elderberry extracts may be well tolerated. However, caution should be exercised when using the raw and unripe fruit, seeds, leaves, and other plant parts because they may contain cyanide-like components. Nausea, vomiting, diarrhea, dizziness, numbness, and stupor have been reported with ingestion of unripened fruit and its juice.

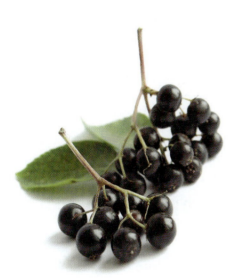

The elderberry has been used to treat influenza.

CHAPTER SUMMARY

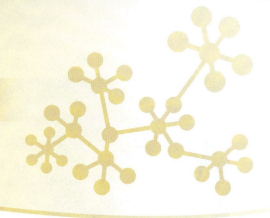

Viruses and Viral Infections

- Viruses are highly specialized infectious agents that replicate within a cell by using the host cell's metabolic processes.

- A virus has a spectrum of cells it can infect, and only in these can it multiply. These host cells can be animal, plant, or bacteria.

- All virus-infected cells have some characteristics that are different from those of uninfected cells. These differences offer ways to block viral replication without affecting normal cells.

- Latency is a problem with viruses. They can lie dormant and then, under certain conditions, reproduce and behave once more like an infectious agent, causing cell damage. Herpesvirus and HIV both have this characteristic.

- Some virus-infected cells produce interferons, which protect neighboring un-infected cells from viral infection.

- Even though the body has defense mechanisms, such as producing interferons, some viruses can cause normal cells to be transformed into cancer cells.

- A major problem in the development of antivirals is the intimate relationship between host and virus. The search for selective inhibitors of viral activity that are not too toxic to the human host is a major area of research. The use of interferons from outside the body is leading the way.

- Antiherpes agents include acyclovir, famciclovir, valacyclovir, and valganciclovir. Valganciclovir has two black box warnings: one for hematologic abnormalities and the other for reproductive toxicity.

- Anti-influenza agents include amantadine, oseltamivir, rimantadine, and zanamivir.

- Ribavirin is another antiviral agent that may be used to treat RSV or hepatitis. Ribavirin has a black box warning for hemolytic anemia and for teratogenic or embryocidal effects.

HIV/AIDS and Antiretroviral Agents

- Human immunodeficiency virus (HIV) is a retrovirus. It converts its RNA into DNA using the reverse transcriptase enzyme and inserts the copy into the DNA of the host cell.

- NRTIs and NtRTIs mimic a DNA building block to inhibit the actions of reverse transcriptase, preventing the multiplication of the virus.

- NNRTIs inhibit the action of reverse transcriptase, preventing the formation of the DNA copy of viral RNA.

- PIs inhibit the protease enzyme, which cleaves certain HIV protein precursors that are necessary for replication of the virus.

- Fusion inhibitors and chemokine coreceptor antagonists prevent HIV from entering the immune cells.

- An integrase inhibitor blocks the enzyme integrase, which inserts DNA produced by reverse transcriptase into the patient's DNA.

- The standard of care for HIV patients involves a combination of antiretroviral drugs. Because these regimens are often complex and difficult to follow, patient adherence is an issue. None of the current drugs can eradicate the disease, but they can improve immunologic status and prolong life.

- An increased number of manufacturers are combining these drugs into one tablet to decrease the pill load and improve patient adherence. This innovation is very important because partial adherence in patients who have HIV can lead to drug resistance.

Immunization

- Immunization can occur naturally, such as in transmission from mother to fetus and through infection exposure.

- Immunization can also occur artificially, through administration of antibodies or through vaccination.

- The administration of vaccines is the most common form of artificial immunization and is estimated to prevent millions of deaths each year.

- Vaccination recommendations and schedules are released by the CDC in the United States and the Public Health Agency in Canada.

- Pharmacies are becoming more popular sites of vaccine administration.

- VIS should be given to patients prior to vaccine administration.

- Special attention should be paid to vaccine storage and administration directions.

acquired immunodeficiency syndrome (AIDS) the advanced and severe form of HIV

active immunity the process by which a person's body makes its own antibodies to a pathogen

acute viral infection an infection that quickly resolves with no latent infection

antiretroviral a drug that limits the progression of HIV or other retrovirus infections

antiviral an agent that prevents virus replication in a host cell without interfering with the host's normal function

boost one drug given to increase the serum concentration of another drug

capsid a protein shell that surrounds and protects the nucleic acid within a virus particle

CD4 cells cells that underlie the immune response in the body

Centers for Disease Control and Prevention (CDC) a US federal agency leading national public health and infection control

chemokine coreceptor antagonist a drug that prevents a strain of HIV from attaching to an immune system cell

chronic viral infection an infection that has a protracted course with long periods of remission interspersed with recurrence

cocktail different drugs used in conjunction as drug therapy

desiccant a substance that maintains dryness

envelope membrane surrounding the capsid in some viruses and carrying surface proteins that attach to cell surface receptors

fusion inhibitor a drug that prevents HIV from entering the immune cells

generalized viral infection an infection that has spread to other tissues by way of the bloodstream or the CNS

genital herpes a sexually transmitted disease caused by the herpes simplex virus; characterized by lesions that cause a burning sensation

hepatitis inflammation of the liver

human immunodeficiency virus (HIV) a retrovirus transmitted in body fluids that causes acquired immunodeficiency syndrome (AIDS) by attacking T lymphocytes

immunization the process whereby a person acquires resistance to an infectious disease

immunocompromised having a deficiency in the immune system response

immunoglobulin an antibody that reacts to a specific foreign substance or organism and may prevent its antigen from attaching to a cell receptor or may destroy the organism

inactivated vaccines vaccines that use pathogens that have been killed with chemicals, heat, or radiation

influenza the flu; a common viral infection

integrase inhibitor a drug that prevents DNA produced by the reverse transcriptase of HIV from becoming incorporated into the patient's DNA

interferon a substance that exerts virus-nonspecific but host-specific antiviral activity by inducing genes coding for antiviral proteins that inhibit the synthesis of viral RNA

latency the ability of a virus to lie dormant and then, under certain conditions, reproduce and again behave like an infectious agent, causing cell damage

live attenuated vaccines vaccines that use live but weakened pathogens to produce an immune response

local viral infection a viral infection affecting tissues of a single system such as the respiratory tract, eye, or skin

naked virus a virus without an envelope covering the capsid

non-nucleoside reverse transcriptase inhibitor (NNRTI) a drug that inhibits HIV reverse transcriptase by preventing the enzyme from working mechanically

nucleoside reverse transcriptase inhibitor (NRTI) a drug that inhibits HIV reverse transcriptase by competing with natural nucleic acid building blocks, causing termination of the DNA chain

nucleotide reverse transcriptase inhibitor (NtRTI) a drug that inhibits HIV reverse transcriptase by competing with natural nucleic acid building blocks, causing termination of chain formulation; is more nearly in the form used by the body than an NRTI

passive immunity immunization when antibodies are transferred to the fetus during pregnancy

postexposure prophylaxis (PEP) the administration of antiretrovirals after exposure to HIV

prodrug a compound that, on administration and chemical conversion by metabolic processes, becomes an active pharmacologic agent

protease inhibitor (PI) a drug that prevents the cleavage of certain HIV protein precursors needed for the replication of new infectious virions

Public Health Agency Canada's agency for public health and emergency preparedness against infections and chronic disease

retrovirus a virus that can copy its RNA genetic information into the host's DNA

reverse transcriptase a retroviral enzyme that makes a DNA copy from an RNA original

slow viral infection an infection that maintains a progressive course over months or years with cumulative damage to body tissues, ultimately ending in the host's death

travel immunization clinics clinical sites that provide immunizations and advice about what vaccines are needed

travel vaccines vaccines given prior to travel to allow the immune system time to confer full immunity

uncoating the removal of the virus capsid proteins to expose the nucleic acid

vaccination the introduction of a vaccine, a component of an infectious agent, into the body to produce immunity to the actual agent

vaccine a substance used to stimulate the production of antibodies and provide immunity

Vaccine Information Statement (VIS) a list of risks associated with a vaccination

virion an individual viral particle capable of infecting a living cell; consists of nucleic acid surrounded by a capsid (protein shell)

virus a minute infectious agent that does not have all the components of a cell and thus can replicate only within a living host cell

DRUG LIST

Antivirals

Systemic Agents
acyclovir (Zovirax)
amantadine (Symmetrel)
famciclovir (Famvir)
oseltamivir (Tamiflu)
ribavirin (Virazole)
rimantadine (Flumadine)
valacyclovir (Valtrex)
valganciclovir (Valcyte)
zanamivir (Relenza)

Antiretrovirals

NRTIs
abacavir (Ziagen)
didanosine (Videx)
emtricitabine (Emtriva)
stavudine (Zerit)
zidovudine (Retrovir)

NNRTIs
delavirdine (Rescriptor)
efavirenz (Sustiva)
etravirine (Intelence)
nevirapine (Viramune)
rilpivirine (Edurant)

PIs
atazanavir (Reyataz)
darunavir (Prezista)
fosamprenavir (Lexiva)
indinavir (Crixivan)
lopinavir-ritonavir (Kaletra)
nelfinavir (Viracept)
ritonavir (Norvir)
saquinavir (Invirase)
tipranavir (Aptivus)

Fusion Inhibitor
enfuvirtide (Fuzeon)

Chemokine Coreceptor Antagonist
maraviroc (Selzentry)

Integrase Inhibitors
dolutegravir (Tivicay)
elvitegravir (Vitekta)
raltegravir (Isentress)

Combinations
abacavir-lamivudine (Epzicom)
efavirenz-emtricitabine-tenofovir
    (Atripla)
elvitegravir-cobicistat-emtricitabine-
    tenofovir (Stribild)
emtricitabine-tenofovir (Truvada)
lamivudine-zidovudine (Combivir)

Black Box Warnings
abacavir-lamivudine (Epzicom)
didanosine (Videx)
efavirenz-emtricitabine-tenofovir (Atripla)
emtricitabine (Emtriva)
ganciclovir (Vitrasert)
lamivudine (Epivir)
lamivudine-zidovudine (Combivir)
maraviroc (Selzentry)
nevirapine (Viramune)
ritonavir (Norvir)
tenofovir (Viread)
tipranavir (Aptivus)
valacyclovir (Valtrex)
zidovudine (Retrovir)

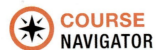

Access interactive chapter review exercises, practice activities, flash cards, and study games.

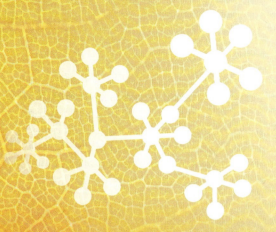

6

Anesthetics and Narcotics

Tina Burke

Learning Objectives

1 Understand the divisions of the nervous system, their functions, and their interactions with drugs.

2 Learn how drugs affect body systems and where they work in the body.

3 Understand the concepts of general and local anesthesia, and know the functions of these agents.

4 Define the action of neuromuscular blocking agents in reducing muscle activity.

5 Understand the different schedules of narcotic and narcotic/nonnarcotic combination drugs and the role of the technician in monitoring use of these drugs.

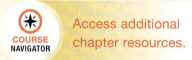

Access additional chapter resources.

The nervous system is the main coordinator and controller for all of the systems in the body. It also acts to interpret, integrate, and respond to the environment around us as well as to our body's internal environment. The nervous system does this through electrical and chemical signals that transmit rapidly through the body. In general, the nervous system works continuously to maintain a state of homeostasis. Most drugs commonly used to anesthetize patients and relieve pain and migraine headache, interact with the body by influencing the electrical and chemical signaling of the nervous system or its target tissues. This chapter will concentrate on these anesthetic agents, narcotic analgesics (pain relievers), and agents for migraine headache relief.

The Nervous System

The nervous system can be divided into anatomical and functional divisions. Understanding these divisions can aid in understanding the site of action, mechanism of action, and effects of a drug in the body.

Anatomical Divisions

The nervous system has two anatomical divisions, the **central nervous system (CNS)** and the **peripheral nervous system (PNS)**. The CNS consists of the brain and spinal cord—the two organs that process and evaluate incoming information and determine responses. The CNS coordinates and controls the activity of the other body systems as well. The PNS consists of nerves and sensory receptors, which are located outside of the CNS. The PNS carries neural signals between the body and the CNS.

Functional Divisions

Functionally, the nervous system consists of sensory and motor divisions, as shown in Figure 6.1. The sensory division carries information from sensory receptors that detect heat, cold, pain, and the presence of chemicals to the CNS. This is called the **afferent system**. The afferent system is further divided into the somatic sensory and visceral sensory systems. The motor division carries information from the CNS to parts of the body to produce a response (e.g., muscles, glands). This is called the **efferent system**. The motor division can be further subdivided into the **autonomic nervous system** and the **somatic nervous system**. The autonomic nervous system regulates motor activity that is involuntary or not consciously controlled (e.g., control of cardiac muscle, smooth muscle, glands). The somatic nervous system regulates motor activity that is voluntary or conscious (e.g., control of skeletal muscles).

FIGURE 6.1   **Functional Organization of the Nervous System**

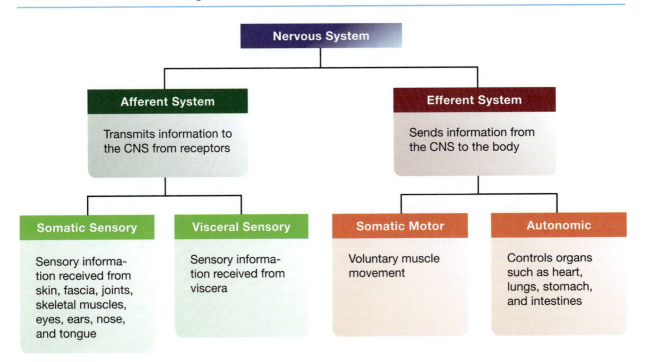

The autonomic nervous system can be further subdivided into the **sympathetic** and **parasympathetic nervous systems** that control specific autonomic functions, as listed in Figure 6.2.

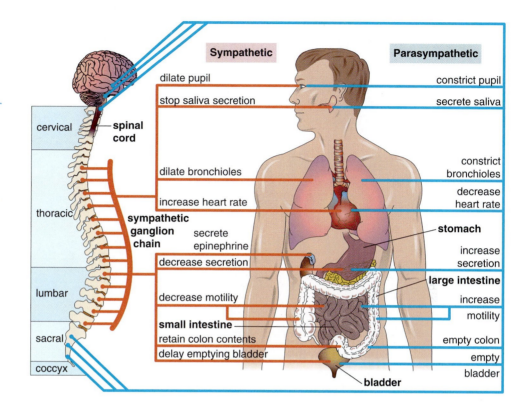

FIGURE 6.2
The Autonomic Nervous System

The autonomic nervous system is divided into the sympathetic and parasympathetic nervous systems. The sympathetic controls the fight/flight functions, and the parasympathetic controls rest, digestion, and homeostasis.

Neurons

The nervous system is responsible for transmitting information over a vast network throughout the body. This network is primarily made up of a specific type of cell, called **neurons**, as well as supporting cells. Neurons transmit information through electrical and chemical signals. Chemical signals, composed of neurotransmitters, are received by receptors on the cell body and **dendrites**, which are branchlike extensions from a neuron's cell body. These chemical signals are converted into an electrical signal, also called an impulse, which travels down the axon of a neuron away from the cell body until it ends at the axon terminal. The axon terminal bulbs of the neuron contain chemical messengers known as neurotransmitters that can then be released onto subsequent cells, as shown in Figure 6.3, to stimulate or inhibit activity of that cell or target tissue.

The process of transmitting signals in the nervous system involves neurotransmitters released at each neuron junction; some are stimulatory and others are inhibitory. The primary CNS transmitters are acetylcholine (ACh), norepinephrine, dopamine, gamma-aminobutyric acid (GABA), glutamate, and serotonin (also known as 5-hydroxytryptamine). Glutamate is the most common neurotransmitter in the brain, and it is always stimulatory. The primary PNS neurotransmitters are ACh and norepinephrine. In the autonomic division, ACh and norepinephrine can be stimulatory or inhibitory; however, ACh is the only neurotransmitter of the somatic division, and it is stimulatory. Neurons voluntarily or involuntarily communicate with a motorneuron in the spinal cord which then stimulates muscle fibers to contract for movement.

FIGURE 6.3 **Neurotransmitters Being Released from a Neuron**

Neurotransmitters are released from one axon and received by another neuron's dendrites.

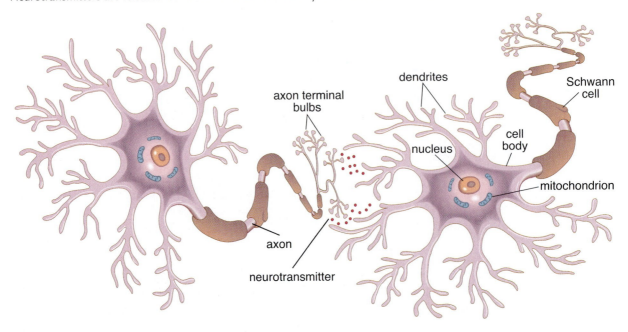

Major Neurotransmitters

- Acetylcholine (ACh)—CNS and PNS; in PNS it stimulates skeletal muscle, inhibits cardiac muscle, and both inhibits and excites smooth muscle and glands
- Gamma-aminobutyric acid (GABA)—CNS; primary inhibitory neurotransmitter in the brain; can impact muscle tone
- Dopamine—CNS; inhibitory neurotransmitter in brain; important roles in cognition (learning, memory), motivation, behavior, and mood
- Epinephrine (adrenaline)—CNS; effects in thalamus, hypothalamus, and spinal cord
- Norepinephrine (noradrenaline)—CNS and PNS; in PNS it modulates the sympathetic nervous system
- Serotonin—CNS; has various functions in the brain related to sleep, appetite, cognition, and mood
- Glutamate—CNS; stimulatory neurotransmitter that increases activity in the nervous system to promote cognitive function in the brain (learning and memory); most common neurotransmitter in the brain

Neurotransmitter Mechanism of Action

When a neurotransmitter binds to a receptor, it causes downstream changes. For many receptors, neurotransmitter binding increases cell membrane permeability to various ions, which then directly stimulates or inhibits an electrical signal in the receiving cell. Other receptors activate enzymatic systems that promote chemical reactions within the cell.

The effect of a neurotransmitter on a cell can depend on the type of receptor it binds to. In the nervous system, adrenergic receptors are sensitive to both epinephrine and norepinephrine. There are three types of adrenergic receptors: alpha, beta-1, and beta-2. Binding of epinephrine and norepinephrine to these receptors facilitates the following responses:

- **Alpha receptors** cause blood vessels to constrict (vasoconstriction, raising blood pressure), but they also cause decongestion.
- **Beta-1 receptors (ß1)** increase the heart rate and contractive force of the heart.
- **Beta-2 receptors (ß2)** influence dilation of both bronchial tubes (bronchodilation) and blood vessels (vasodilation).

In general, the most important action of adrenergic receptors are bronchodilation and heart stimulation. Notice though that alpha and beta-2 receptors have opposite effects on blood vessels. The overall action of adrenergic neurotransmitters depends on the concentration of the neurotransmitter. Beta-2 receptors widen blood vessels in response to moderate neurotransmitter levels, whereas higher levels stimulate the alpha receptors to narrow blood vessels.

The tissue upon which the receptor is found can also affect the cell's response to neurotransmitters. For example, a specific type of acetylcholine receptor called a muscarinic receptor has a very different effect when found on smooth muscle versus cardiac muscle. In smooth muscle, activation of muscarinic receptors will lead to muscle contraction. In cardiac muscle, activation of muscarinic receptors will lead to slowing of the contractions of the heart.

Many drugs facilitate an effect in the body by mimicking or influencing the action of neurotransmitters. The action of a neurotransmitter can be affected by influencing the release of a neurotransmitter, enzyme degradation, and neurotransmitter reabsorption.

Drugs may also act by blocking receptors, thereby preventing the neurotransmitters from binding to them. This can also facilitate a physiologic response that is just the opposite of the normal effect when the neurotransmitter binds to a receptor. For example, anticholinergic drugs block acetylcholine receptors. As described previously, when ACh binds to cardiac muscle, heart rate and force of contractions decrease. When given an anticholinergic drug, heart rate and force of contractions increase.

Anesthetics

Pain is a general sense of the body that detects tissue damage. Pain receptors send impulses through sensory neurons to the central nervous system. Anesthetics work by manipulating the nervous system so that pain or the conscious perception of pain is inhibited.

Before 1846, surgical procedures were uncommon, partly because there were few satisfactory ways to inhibit pain. Although modern anesthetics did not yet exist, some pain relief methods were available. For example, alcohol, hashish, and opium derivatives were taken to relieve pain. Other methods were also sometimes used, such as packing a limb in ice or restricting blood with a tourniquet before an amputation. Unconsciousness was achieved by strangulation or a blow to the head. Most commonly, though, the patient was simply restrained by force during a surgical procedure.

Anesthetic drugs are classified as general or local, according to the type of **anesthesia** (loss of feeling in a person's body or part of the body) they induce. They are provided in a variety of dosage forms and strengths. Choice of anesthetic is determined by clinical needs and, most importantly, patient safety. A physician who oversees administration of anesthesia during surgery is known as an **anesthesiologist**. General anesthetics facilitate a loss of consciousness and overall perception of pain that is reversible, while other vital physiologic functions still occur. The physiologic effects of anesthesia involve many systems, as described in Table 6.1. In contrast, local anesthetics block the transmission of the pain signal to the CNS from a specific anatomic site; however, there are no changes in awareness and sensory perception in other areas.

TABLE 6.1 Physiologic Effects of General Anesthesia

Physiologic System	Effect
Nervous System	All nerve tissue function in the peripheral system is depressed.
Respiratory System	Function is depressed, and the anesthesiologist controls oxygen concentration and ventilation (exchange of air between the lungs and ambient air). Inhaled anesthetics, which are drawn into the lungs, generally irritate the respiratory tract and salivary glands, causing increased mucus secretion, coughing, and spasm.
Endocrine System	Some anesthetics cause pituitary secretion of antidiuretic hormone (ADH), which may cause postoperative urinary retention. The adrenal medulla may release epinephrine and norepinephrine, which can counter depression caused by inhibited nerves.
Cardiovascular System	The activity of cardiac muscle in the myocardium is reduced, and the resultant loss of tone reduces blood pressure. Vagus nerve inhibition increases the heart rate. Some drugs make the heart sensitive, which may cause arrhythmias (variations from the normal rhythm of the heart).
Skeletal Muscular System	Anesthesia depresses systems within the brain and spinal reflexes, causing some muscle relaxation.
GI System	Common GI effects are nausea and vomiting.
Hepatic System	Some medications are suspected of causing liver changes.

General anesthesia is the unique condition of reversible unconsciousness and absence of response to otherwise painful stimuli. It is characterized by four reversible actions:

- unconsciousness (unawareness)
- analgesia (relieving pain)
- skeletal muscle relaxation
- amnesia on recovery

The indicators used to assess the degree of general anesthesia are as follows:

- blood pressure
- hypervolemia (abnormal increase in the volume of circulating fluid—i.e., plasma—in the body) and hypovolemia (abnormal decrease in the plasma volume)

- oxygen level
- pulse
- respiratory rate
- tissue perfusion (the passage of a fluid through the vessels of a specific organ)
- urinary output (reduction in urine volume sends more blood to the brain)

General anesthetics can be administered in different ways, and several factors must be considered before, during, and after their administration. Some of these considerations are briefly discussed in this section.

General Anesthetics: Preanesthetic Medications

Medication is sometimes used preoperatively to control sedation, reduce postoperative pain, cause amnesia, and decrease anxiety. Review of an individual patient's medication history is important in determining which medications to use. Several classes of drugs offer agents to be used before anesthesia:

- Narcotics alleviate pain and depress the respiratory system. Morphine is the standard narcotic analgesic.
- Benzodiazepines are the most commonly used preoperative sedatives. They can cause amnesia, relieve anxiety, as well as act as an anticonvulsant.
- Phenothiazines are often prescribed for their **antiemetic** (prevents vomiting and nausea) properties as well as their sedative effects.

General Anesthetics and Malignant Hyperthermia

Malignant hyperthermia is a rare but serious side effect of anesthesia. It is associated with a sudden and rapid rise in body temperature with accompanying irregularities in heart rhythm and breathing. Body temperature can increase to 110°F or more, and is accompanied by other symptoms that include increased body metabolism and muscle rigidity (inflexibility or stiffness). Malignant

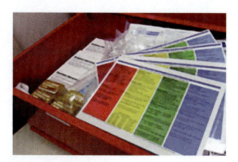

This image is an example of a malignant hyperthermia kit.

hyperthermia is potentially life-threatening and must be treated immediately. If left untreated, death may result from cardiac arrest, brain damage, internal hemorrhaging, or failure of other body systems.

Treatment of malignant hyperthermia involves the intravenous (IV) infusion of the drug **dantrolene (Dantrium, Revonto, Ryanodex)**, a skeletal muscle relaxant also used to treat multiple sclerosis (MS), stroke, cerebral palsy, and spinal cord injury (see Chapter 13 for more information). Dantrolene is thought to reduce muscle tone and metabolism. Hospitals require that a specialized drug kit for the treatment of malignant hyperthermia be immediately accessible wherever anesthesia is administered. It is usually the responsibility of the pharmacy technician to maintain these kits and to make sure that the drugs are up to date because dantrolene has a very short shelf life and must be replenished frequently.

A malignant hyperthermia kit generally contains the following components:

- dantrolene (Ryanodex; older formulations include Dantrium and Revonto)
- sterile water for injection
- sodium bicarbonate, 8.4%
- dextrose, 50%
- calcium chloride, 10%
- regular insulin (refrigerated)
- lidocaine* for injection, 2% (amiodarone or procainamide are also acceptable)
- refrigerated saline solution

*Lidocaine or procainamide should not be given if a wide QRS complex arrhythmia is likely due to hyperkalemia; this may result in asystole.

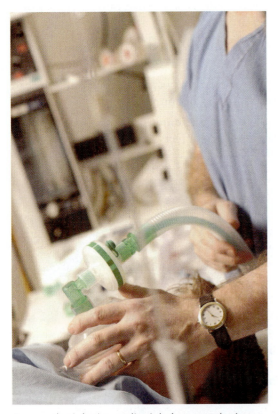
An anesthesiologist applies inhalant anesthetics during surgery.

General Anesthetics: Inhalant Anesthetics

Inhalant anesthetics are stored under high pressure and are provided by the manufacturer in steel cylinders. Though informally referred to as "compressed gas," some of these chemicals are in liquid form in the cylinders and transform into a gas when released. During surgery, anesthesiologists administer inhalant anesthetics through a face mask (at left). Interestingly, the respiratory system will excrete 80%–90% of the inhaled anesthetics. Common side effects associated with inhalant anesthetics include a reduction in blood pressure, **hypervolemia**, reduction in renal function, and nausea and vomiting. The most commonly used inhalant anesthetics are reviewed next and are also listed in Table 6.2.

Nitrous Oxide

Nitrous oxide (N_2O) is not a potent anesthetic, and it usually is used with other agents. Its effects are limited to reducing blood pressure and providing analgesia; it does not induce amnesia or relax skeletal muscle. It may be used alone, as in dental procedures, which is the most common use of this drug. It has the tremendous advantage of being rapidly eliminated; its disadvantage is that it may cause hypoxia, a reduction in the oxygen supplied to a tissue, despite adequate perfusion by blood. In balanced anesthesia, nitrous oxide is supplemented with hypnotics (**barbiturates** or **benzodiazepines**), analgesics (intravenous narcotics), and muscle relaxants. It is administered with more powerful anesthetics to hasten the uptake of the more powerful agent.

Contraindications Nitrous oxide should not be administered with oxygen. No patient should receive more than two hours of continuously inspired nitrous oxide.

TABLE 6.2 Most Commonly Used Inhalant Anesthetics

Generic (Brand)	Pronunciation	Dosage Form	Dispensing Status
desflurane (Suprane)	des-FLOO-rayn	Gas	Rx
enflurane (Ethrane)	EN-floo-rayn	Gas	Rx
isoflurane (Forane)	eye-soe-FLOO-rayn	Gas	Rx
nitrous oxide	NYE-trus OX-ide	Gas	Rx
sevoflurane (Ultane)	see-voe-FLOO-rane	Gas	Rx

Cautions and Considerations Nitrous oxide should not be administered to patients with hypovolemia, shock, or cardiac disease (severe hypotension), as it may cause arrhythmias, cardiac depression, pulmonary hypertension, and systemic hypotension.

Drug Interactions The use of nitrous oxide with other CNS depressants may result in increased or additive CNS depressant effects.

Enflurane

Enflurane (Ethrane) is commonly used in lower doses for labor/delivery, and as a supplement to other general anesthetics during cesarean section because it induces muscle relaxation, specifically in the uterus. Enflurane has the advantages of rapid induction and recovery. A short-acting barbiturate is usually infused first to render the patient unconscious. Enflurane is a mild stimulant of bronchial and salivary secretions. The disadvantages are excessive depression of the respiratory and circulatory systems. High concentrations may stimulate seizures in susceptible patients, and malignant hyperthermia is a possibility.

Contraindications Contraindications include hypersensitivity to enflurane or other halogenated anesthetics (inhaled anesthetics), a history of or suspected genetic susceptibility to malignant hyperthermia, and seizure disorders.

Cautions and Considerations Use with CO_2 absorbents may form carbon monoxide, with potential increases in carboxyhemoglobin levels. Deep anesthesia with enflurane may cause dose-related electroencephalogram (EEG) changes, hypotension, and respiratory depression.

Drug Interactions Concurrent use of nondepolarizing muscle relaxants may result in respiratory depression and apnea. Use of tricyclic antidepressants with enflurane may result in an increased risk of cardiotoxicity and seizure activity. When combined with cisatracurium, enflurane may excessively prolong the neuromuscular blocking effects of cisatracurium. Taking St. John's wort with enflurane may increase the risk of cardiovascular collapse and/or delayed emergence from anesthesia.

Isoflurane

Isoflurane (Forane) produces rapid induction and recovery, with no excessive tracheal or salivary secretions. The disadvantages are progressive respiratory and blood pressure depression, with possible malignant hyperthermia. Isoflurane may cause less renal and hepatic toxicity than any other commonly employed anesthetic.

Contraindications Contraindications include hypersensitivity to isoflurane or other halogenated agents as well as known or suspected genetic susceptibility to malignant hyperthermia.

Cautions and Considerations Use with CO_2 absorbents may form carbon monoxide, with potential increases in carboxyhemoglobin levels. Deep anesthesia with isoflurane may cause dose-related hypotension and respiratory depression, and increases in cerebrospinal fluid pressure. Isoflurane is not recommended for individuals with coronary artery disease as it may increase the risk of myocardial ischemia.

Drug Interactions The use of isoflurane with neuromuscular blocking agents may result in respiratory depression and apnea. Concurrent use of isoflurane and St. John's wort may increase the risk of cardiovascular collapse and/or delayed emergence from anesthesia.

Desflurane

Desflurane (Suprane) is an easily controlled anesthetic with rapid onset and rapid recovery. It is often used in ambulatory surgery. It reduces the required dose of neuromuscular blocking agents. However, it produces a high incidence of moderate-to-severe upper respiratory irritation for children and is therefore not recommended for use in the pediatric population for induction of anesthesia. It can be used for maintenance of general anesthesia.

Contraindications Contraindications include hypersensitivity to desflurane or other halogenated agents as well as known or suspected genetic susceptibility to malignant hyperthermia. Desflurane should not be used with individuals who have a history of moderate to severe hepatic dysfunction after use of halogenated agents. It should not be used to induce anesthesia in pediatric patients.

Cautions and Considerations Desflurane is not recommended as a sole agent for anesthetic induction in individuals with coronary artery disease or other conditions where increases in heart rate or blood pressure are undesirable.

Desflurane dose-related hypotension and respiratory depression, and increases in cerebrospinal fluid pressure may occur.

Drug Interactions The use of desflurane with nitrous oxide may result in a decrease in the minimum alveolar concentration of desflurane. Use with St. John's wort may increase the risk of cardiovascular collapse and/or delayed emergence from anesthesia. When used together, desflurane may excessively prolong the neuromuscular blocking effects of cisatracurium.

Sevoflurane

Sevoflurane (Ultane) is an ether (gas) used for induction and maintenance of general anesthesia. It is usually used with desflurane. It is the preferred agent for mask induction because it is less irritating to mucous membranes.

Contraindications Sevoflurane is contraindicated in patients with hypersensitivity to sevoflurane or other halogenated agents as well as known or suspected genetic susceptibility to malignant hyperthermia.

Cautions and Considerations Dose-related hypotension may occur. Prior exposure to halogenated hydrocarbon anesthetics may increase risk of hepatic injury.

Increased risk of preoperative seizures may occur with administration of sevoflurane, primarily in young adults and children aged two months and older.

Drug Interactions Use with St. John's wort may increase the risk of cardiovascular collapse and/or delayed emergence from anesthesia.

General Anesthetics: Injectable Anesthetics

The injectable anesthetics include the ultrashort-acting barbiturates and benzodiazepines. The IV products are very lipid soluble. They are distributed initially to the brain, liver (where they are metabolized), kidneys, and other organs with high-volume blood flow and later to fat and muscle. Body distribution lowers concentrations that maintain anesthesia. Most of the injectable anesthetics are administered by an IV drip, but some have other dosage forms. Table 6.3 lists the most commonly used injectable anesthesia agents. Almost all of the injectable anesthetics are controlled substances.

Etomidate

Etomidate (Amidate) is used to supplement a weak anesthetic (e.g., nitrous oxide) or for short outpatient procedures, such as gynecologic procedures (e.g., dilation and curettage). It is also used for sedation in rapid sequence intubation. It may cause transient involuntary muscle contractions. Nausea and vomiting are common during the recovery period.

TABLE 6.3 Most Commonly Used Injectable Anesthesia Agents

Generic (Brand)	Pronunciation	Dosage Form	Dispensing Status	Controlled-Substance Schedule
alfentanil (Alfenta)	al-FEN-ta-nil	Injection	Rx	C-II
etomidate (Amidate)	e-TOM-i-date	Injection	Rx	
fentanyl (Sublimaze)	FEN-ta-nil	Injection	Rx	C-II
ketamine (Ketalar)	KET-a-meen	Injection	Rx	C-III
morphine (various brands)	MOR-feen	Injection	Rx	C-II
propofol (Diprivan)	PRO-po-fawl	Injection	Rx	NA
remifentanil (Ultiva)	rem-i-FEN-ta-nil	Injection	Rx	C-II
sufentanil (Sufenta)	soo-FEN-ta-nil	Injection	Rx	C-II
Barbiturates				
methohexital (Brevital)	meth-oh-HEX-i-tal	Injection	Rx	C-IV
Benzodiazepines				
diazepam (Valium)	dye-AZ-e-pam	Injection, oral liquid, tablet	Rx	C-IV
lorazepam (Ativan)	lor-AZ-e-pam	Injection, tablet	Rx	C-IV
midazolam (Versed)	mid-AZ-oh-lam	Injection, syrup	Rx	C-IV

Contraindications Contraindications include hypersensitivity to etomidate.

Cautions and Considerations Etomidate may induce cardiac depression in older patients, especially those with hypertension. Individuals with renal impairment may also be at risk of drug toxicity.

Drug Interactions Taking oxycodone and etomidate may worsen CNS and/or respiratory depression. Use with St. John's wort may increase the risk of cardiovascular collapse and/or delayed submergence from anesthesia.

Fentanyl

Fentanyl (Sublimaze) can be used as a preoperative medication and a narcotic-analgesic. It is used especially for open-heart surgery because it lacks some of the cardiac depressant (diminishing heart function) actions of other anesthetics. It is used as a supplement in balanced anesthesia. Fentanyl is frequently administered intrathecally as part of spinal anesthesia. The lozenge, which is raspberry flavored, is used especially with children and as a preoperative medication. The IV form of this drug is used most often in the operating room. The potency of fentanyl is much greater than that of morphine. It has several analogs that are used exclusively in the operating room. **Alfentanil (Alfenta)** is an ultrashort-acting (5 to 10 minutes) analgesic. **Sufentanil (Sufenta)** is 5 to 10 times more potent than fentanyl. **Remifentani (Ultiva)** is the shortest-acting opioid. It has the benefit of rapid offset, even after prolonged infusions during surgeries. Anesthesiologists prefer anesthetics that promote rapid patient recovery.

Contraindications Contraindications for fentanyl include intolerance to fentanyl products.

Cautions and Considerations There is a high risk of addiction, misuse, and abuse with the use of fentanyl. When fentanyl is taken with strong or moderate cytochrome P-450 3A4 (CYP 3A4) inhibitors, metabolism is decreased, which may result in increased fentanyl plasma concentration, and potentially fatal respiratory depression. Older adults or debilitated patients are at a higher risk of respiratory depression and other adverse events when using fentanyl.

Drug Interactions When fentanyl is taken with CNS depressants (including alcohol), there may be additive respiratory and CNS depressant effects as well as increased sedation and dizziness. Serotonin syndrome may occur when taking fentanyl with monoamine oxidase inhibitors (MAOIs). Taking fentanyl with amphetamines may increase the analgesic effects of fentanyl.

Ketamine

Ketamine (Ketalar) produces a type of anesthesia known as dissociative amnesia, in which the patient appears to be awake but neither responds to pain nor remembers the procedure. This agent enhances muscle tone and increases blood pressure, heart rate, and respiratory secretions. Onset is quick (within 30 seconds), and effects last 5 to 10 minutes.

Contraindications Contraindications for ketamine include conditions where significant elevation in blood pressure would be a serious hazard, and hypersensitivity to ketamine or any other product component.

Cautions and Considerations Ketamine should not be taken with alcohol or given to patients with a history of alcohol abuse. Verbal, tactile, and visual stimulation should be minimized during recovery because postoperative confusion may occur. Rapid administration or overdose of ketamine may increase the risk of respiratory depression, apnea, and enhanced pressor response. Hypertension and cardiac decompensation may occur, so monitoring is recommended.

Drug Interactions Taking St. John's wort and ketamine may increase the risk of cardiovascular collapse and/or delayed emergence from anesthesia. Combined use of ketamine and other CNS depressants may increase the risk of additive CNS depressant effects.

Propofol

Safety Alert

Diprivan and Diflucan might be confused. This could be life-threatening if an ICU patient who needs Diflucan for an infection receives Diprivan instead.

Propofol (Diprivan) is used to maintain anesthesia and sedation or to treat agitation in patients in the intensive care unit (ICU). It has demonstrated antiemetic properties. The side effects are drowsiness, respiratory depression, motor restlessness, and increased blood pressure. Propofol changes urine color to green, pink, or rust. Any unused drug must be discarded after 12 hours. Propofol should be mixed only with 5% dextrose. It is a white emulsion, stable in glass containers, and should be stored at room temperature. Because propofol is the only white emulsion used as an anesthetic, some healthcare workers think it does not need to be labeled, which is incorrect. When drawn up, propofol must be labeled immediately. It is an extremely dangerous drug that should never be used outside the hospital.

Contraindications Contraindications include allergies to eggs, egg products, soybeans, soy products, or peanuts as well as hypersensitivity to propofol or any other product component.

Cautions and Considerations Cardiorespiratory effects, including hypotension and cardiovascular depression, may occur in vulnerable populations. Anaphylactic reactions may occur if the patient is allergic to any of the drug component.

Drug Interactions Taking St. John's wort and ketamine may increase the risk of cardiovascular collapse and/or delayed emergence from anesthesia. Combined use of other anesthetics (e.g., lidocaine and bupivacaine) may increase the hypnotic effect of propofol.

Methohexital

The barbiturate **methohexital (Brevital)** is used primarily for induction in short procedures. Respiratory depression, yawning, coughing, or laryngospasm may occur. In patients who are awake, these agents may cause excitement or delirium in the presence of pain. Methohexital can be used to induce anesthesia prior to administration of another agent or alone for short procedures. The big advantages of the barbiturates are rapid induction, fast recovery, and little post anesthetic excitement or vomiting.

Contraindications Methohexital use is contraindicated in the absence of suitable veins for IV administration, acute intermittent porphyria, or hypersensitivity to barbiturates.

Cautions and Considerations Both of these barbiturate medications should be used with caution in patients with severe cardiovascular disease, hypotension/shock, liver or kidney disease, respiratory impairment or obstruction, and severe anemia.

Drug Interactions Major drug interactions with methohexital include other CNS depressants (e.g., benzodiazepines, opiates), clarithromycin, esomeprazole, and nifedipine.

Benzodiazepines

The benzodiazepines, **diazepam (Valium)**, **lorazepam (Ativan)**, and **midazolam (Versed)**, are used for induction, short procedures, and dental procedures. They are metabolized to active products, so they work longer than barbiturates. Midazolam has the fastest onset of action, greatest potency, and most rapid elimination and is thus the preferred agent. Similar to ketamine, it produces dissociative amnesia and the patient does not remember the procedure even though sometimes the patient can carry on a strange conversation during the procedure. Benzodiazepines are also useful for controlling and preventing seizures.

Contraindications Contraindications for use of benzodiazepines include types of glaucoma, myasthenia gravis, liver disease, or sleep apnea.

Cautions and Considerations Benzodiazepines should be used with caution in psychotic patients, neonates, and older adult patients, and those with anxiety-associated depression, adverse cardiorespiratory events, and a history of alcohol or drug abuse.

Drug Interactions Major drug interactions occur with opioid painkillers, phenytoin, barbiturates, muscle relaxants, mirtazapine, and other CNS depressants.

Antagonist drugs, substances that interfere with or inhibit the physiologic action of another (listed in Table 6.4), are used to reverse the effects of benzodiazepine and narcotic overdoses. All operating rooms and emergency rooms maintain an adequate, quickly accessible supply of these drugs. Wherever narcotics are used, a supply of antagonists must be available.

TABLE 6.4 Most Commonly Used Antagonists to Reverse Overdoses

Generic (Brand)	Pronunciation	Dosage Form	Dispensing Status
flumazenil (Romazicon)	floo-MAZ-eh-nil	Injection	Rx
naloxone (Narcan)	nal-OX-one	Injection	Rx

Flumazenil

Flumazenil (Romazicon) antagonizes benzodiazepines by competing at receptor sites. It blocks sedation, recall, and psychomotor impairment. It is used for complete or partial reversal of sedative effects of the benzodiazepines used as general anesthesia or to reverse the effects of a benzodiazepine overdose. Adverse reactions are headache, nausea, vomiting, dizziness, and agitation.

Contraindications Use of flumazenil is contraindicated with hypersensitivity to flumazenil or benzodiazepines, signs of serious tricyclic antidepressant overdose, and use of a benzodiazepine for control of a life-threatening condition.

Cautions and Considerations Flumazenil carries a black box warning about increased risk of seizures, specifically in association with concurrent major sedative-hypnotic drug withdrawal, recent therapy with repeated doses of parenteral benzodiazepines, myoclonic jerking or seizure activity prior to flumazenil administration in overdose cases, or concurrent serious tricyclic antidepressant overdose. Flumazenil should be used with caution in an ICU setting and with patients who have head injuries, respiratory distress, epilepsy, and drug or alcohol dependence.

Drug Interactions Major drug interactions occur with concurrent use of flumazenil and other benzodiazepines, which may facilitate seizures, and selected benzodiazepine receptor agonists, which can decrease the effectiveness of the receptor agonist.

Naloxone

Naloxone (Narcan) is an antagonist that competes for the opiate receptor sites. Although this drug has a greater affinity for the receptor, its action is much shorter than that of the competing narcotic. Thus, when the naloxone wears off, the opioid will reattach to the receptor. Consequently, naloxone must be given repeatedly until the opioid is cleared from the patient's system. Naloxone must be stored in a dark compartment.

Contraindications Naloxone use is contraindicated in individuals with hypersensitivity to naloxone.

Cautions and Considerations Naloxone should be used with caution in abrupt postoperative reversal of opioids, agitation, during labor, physical dependence of opioids, liver disease, kidney disease, neonates, respiratory depression caused by non-opioid drugs, or septic shock.

Drug Interactions Major drug interactions with naloxone include opioids and clonidine.

Neuromuscular Blocking Agents

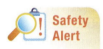

Safety Alert

Most neuromuscular blocking agents must be refrigerated and are expensive. Failure to store them correctly could be very costly.

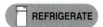

CAUTION PARALYTIC

REFRIGERATE

Neuromuscular blocking agents paralyze the patient's skeletal muscles, which enables a surgeon to operate with greater accuracy and safety. Neuromuscular blocking is often used as an adjunct to general anesthesia to enable **endotracheal intubation**, or the insertion of a tube into the trachea to maintain an open airway and deliver oxygen and general anesthesia directly to the lungs. Neuromuscular blocking agents are some of the most dangerous drugs, because their administration results in immediate skeletal muscle paralysis. When stocking neuromuscular blocking agents, the technician should always flag this type of drug with a label to alert everyone explicitly that the drug will paralyze whoever receives it. Every effort should be made to make sure these agents are not stored close to a look-alike drug. Table 6.5 gives an overview of the most commonly used neuromuscular blocking agents, many of which must be stored in a refrigerator.

There are two mechanisms for achieving neuromuscular blockade. **Succinylcholine (Quelicin)**, often referred to as "sux," is the only agent that works via a depolarizing (neutralizing) mechanism. Succinylcholine works as an agonist of the nicotinic cholinergic receptors. These receptors briefly allow ions to pass through when acetylcholine binds to them, producing a pulse of electrical current that causes the muscle to contract. Succinylcholine holds the ion channels open, causing a persistent depolarization at the motor endplate—in other words, it shorts out the electrical signal.

TABLE 6.5   Most Commonly Used Neuromuscular Blocking Agents

Generic (Brand)	Pronunciation	Dosage Form	Storage	Dispensing Status
Short Duration				
succinylcholine (Quelicin)	sux-in-il-KOE-leen	Injection	Refrigerate	Rx
Intermediate Duration				
atracurium	a-tra-KYOO-ree-um	Injection	Refrigerate	Rx
cisatracurium (Nimbex)	sis-a-tra-KYOO-ree-um	Injection	Refrigerate	Rx
rocuronium (Zemuron)	roe-kyoor-OH-nee-um	Injection	Refrigerate	Rx
vecuronium (Norcuron)	ve-kyoo-ROE-nee-um	Injection	Room temperature	Rx
Extended Duration				
pancuronium (Pavulon)	pan-kyoo-ROE-nee-um	Injection	Refrigerate	Rx

The result is a brief period of skeletal muscle paralysis. Bradyarrhythmias (irregular and slow heartbeats) may occur; if they do, they are reversed with atropine.

Contraindications Succinylcholine use is contraindicated in the acute phase of injury after trauma as it may result in hyperkalemia (high blood potassium levels) and cardiac arrest. It is also contraindicated for patients with a history of malignant hyperthermia, skeletal muscle myopathies, and hypersensitivity to succinylcholine.

Cautions and Considerations Succinylcholine carries a black box warning associated with rare reports of healthy children with previously undiagnosed skeletal muscle myopathy developing acute rhabdomyolysis with hyperkalemia after succinylcholine was administered. This was followed by ventricular dysrhythmias, cardiac arrest, and death. Use of this medication in children is restricted to emergency intubation or situations when the airway must be immediately secured. This medication should also be used with caution in patients with abdominal infections, bradycardia, digoxin toxicity, hyperkalemia and other electrolyte abnormalities, and subarachnoid hemorrhage, or a history of repeated use.

Put Down Roots

Nondepolarizing agents have a longer duration of action than succinylcholine and are categorized accordingly in Table 6.5.

Drug Interactions Major drug interactions with succinylcholine include St. John's wort, systemic lidocaine, digoxin, quinine, aminoglycoside antibiotics (e.g., tobramycin, gentamicin), and donepezil. Concurrent use of these with succinylcholine may result in respiratory depression, cardiovascular distress, or prolongation of the neuromuscular blockade.

The second mechanism for achieving neuromuscular blockade is through nondepolarizing agents that are competitive antagonists to acetylcholine at the nicotinic cholinergic receptors. They prevent acetylcholine from binding to the receptors to start the electrical signal, paralyzing the skeletal muscles. Nondepolarizing agents have a longer duration of action than succinylcholine and are categorized accordingly in Table 6.5.

Contraindications Contraindications include hypersensitivity to nondepolarizing neuromuscular blocking agents. Hypersensitivity to multidose vials containing benzyl alcohol has also been shown in premature infants and contraindicates the use of neuromuscular blocking agents in this patient population.

Cautions and Considerations Patients should be constantly monitored during administration by individuals specifically trained on these medications. Blood pressure, heart rate, peripheral nerve stimulation, blood gases and ventilation should be monitored. Individuals who have a prior history of allergic reactions to nondepolarizing neuromuscular blocking agents should use caution as severe anaphylactic reactions have occurred. Nondepolarizing neuromuscular blocking agents should only be used along with appropriate amounts of anesthesia as these products have not been shown to influence consciousness, thought processes, or pain thresholds.

Both vecuronium and pancuronium have a black box warning and should be administered by trained individuals familiar with its actions, characteristics, and hazards.

Drug Interactions When nondepolarizing neuromuscular blocking agents are given with other anesthetics it can cause prolongation of the neuromuscular blocking effects. The combination of bactericidal antibiotics may also cause prolonged neuromuscular blockade which may lead to respiratory depression and paralysis.

Rocuronium when used with phenytoin may reduce the efficacy of the neuromuscular blockade. Also, when using rocuronium with epinephrine, patients may be at increased risk of postoperative re-paralysis.

Agents to Reverse Neuromuscular Blocking Agents

To reverse the effects of a nondepolarizing neuromuscular blocking drug requires the administration of one of several **anticholinesterase** agents, including **edrophonium (Enlon)**, **neostigmine (Prostigmin)**, and **pyridostigmine (Mestinon)** (see Table 6.6). These drugs potentiate the action of acetylcholine by inhibiting its destruction by the enzyme acetylcholinesterase, thereby restoring the transmission of impulses across the neuromuscular junctions. Many of the anticholinesterase agents are also used in the treatment of myasthenia gravis, a neuromuscular disease that is characterized by weakness of the skeletal muscles of the body.

Contraindications Contraindications for anticholinesterase drugs include hypersensitivity to anticholinesterase drugs, use in patients with intestinal or urinary tract obstruction, and peritonitis.

Cautions and Considerations Anticholinesterase drugs should be used with caution in patients with cardiovascular disease, renal impairment, and hepatic impairment. Vulnerable populations (e.g., infants and small children) may be at an increased risk for complications. Older adult patients should be kept longer to monitor their status during recovery.

TABLE 6.6 Most Commonly Used Anticholinesterase Agents to Reverse Neuromuscular Blocking

Generic (Brand)	Pronunciation	Dosage Form	Dispensing Status
edrophonium (Enlon)	ed-roe-FOE-nee-um	Injection	Rx
neostigmine (Prostigmin)	nee-oh-STIG-meen	Injection, tablet	Rx
pyridostigmine (Mestinon)	peer-id-oh-STIG-meen	Injection, syrup, tablet	Rx

Drug Interactions Taking acetylcholinesterase drugs with succinylcholine may result in increasing the neuromuscular blockade. Also, concurrent use with corticosteroids may decrease the effectiveness of acetylcholinesterase drugs.

Local Anesthetics

Local anesthesia produces a transient and reversible loss of sensation in a defined area of the body without altering alertness or mental function. The introduction of cocaine as a topical ophthalmologic anesthetic in 1884 opened the first era of local anesthesia, and cocaine is still used today for procedures on the eye and nasal passages. Lidocaine, introduced in the 1940s, is now the most widely used local anesthetic. Local anesthetics, especially topical agents, are commonly combined with other drugs. Local anesthetics are available in a variety of dosage forms for use in a range of conditions. These dosage forms and applications are as follows:

- epidural (injection into the space outside the dura mater membrane of the vertebral canal)—to block afferent pain nerve impulses to provide regional anesthesia
- infiltration (superficial injection)—to suture (stitch) cuts, perform dental procedures, and block small nerves
- injection (nerve block)—to prevent transmission of the pain impulse
- IV—for reasons other than anesthesia
- spinal (subarachnoid or intrathecal injection into the innermost space of the spinal cord)—to block afferent pain nerve impulses from the lower part of the body
- topical (drops, sprays, lotions, ointments)—to treat sunburn, insect bites, hemorrhoids

Local anesthetics decrease the neuronal membrane's permeability to ions. This inhibits depolarization with resultant blockade of conduction. Local anesthesia is advantageous because all types of nervous tissue are affected—sensory and motor. The action is reversible, and there is no residual nerve damage. Nerve fibers (cells) determine the degree and speed with which a local anesthetic acts. In response to the activity of the anesthetic, function is lost in the following order:

1. pain perception
2. temperature sensation
3. touch sensation
4. proprioception (recognition of body position/posture and joint positions)
5. skeletal muscle tone

Local anesthetics will depress the small, uninsulated fibers first and larger, insulated nerve fibers last. For these smaller fibers, the onset of action is much shorter. This also means that the concentration of the drug required to depress the sensory signaling is smaller as well. The systemic action that the local anesthetic has on the nervous tissue depends on the time that the drug is in contact with that nerve tissue. The action of a local anesthetic can also depend on other factors. For example, inflammation in the tissue and dilation of the blood vessels in the area has the potential to reduce drug activity and duration of action. On the other hand, adding a vasoconstrictor (e.g., epinephrine) will slow the absorption of a drug into the bloodstream allowing for a longer duration of action. Dentists commonly employ the use of epinephrine to keep the local anesthetic drug at the injection site so that the numbness from the local anesthetic will last longer.

Local anesthetics are classified by their chemical structures into esters and amides. An **ester** is relatively easily broken down, so local anesthetics that are esters are short-acting and are metabolized in the plasma and tissue fluids. An **amide** is more difficult to break down, so amide-containing local anesthetics are longer-acting and are metabolized by liver enzymes. Metabolites of both classes are excreted in urine. Table 6.7 lists the most commonly used local anesthetics in these two classes.

All local anesthetics, except cocaine (used for eye and nose surgery), cause relaxation of vascular smooth muscles and can lead to vascular collapse. Hypersensitivity or an allergy to a particular local agent can cause histamine release at the injection site. The most common reactions to the ester class of local anesthetics are skin rashes, edema (an abnormal accumulation of fluid in interstitial spaces of the body), and asthma. This hypersensitivity usually develops when the agent is used frequently or for prolonged periods. An amide can generally be substituted for an ester to prevent these hypersensitivity reactions.

Although local anesthetics are given to produce a pharmacologic response in a well-defined area of the body, occasionally, the anesthetic is absorbed into the blood from the administration site. It can then affect organs along the way, with the most serious effects on the blood vessels, heart, and brain.

TABLE 6.7 Most Commonly Used Local Anesthetics

Generic (Brand)	Pronunciation	Dosage Form	Dispensing Status
Esters			
benzocaine (Americaine)	BEN-zoe-kayn	Cream, ear drops, gel, lozenge, ointment, oral liquid, oral paste, spray	OTC
chloroprocaine (Nesacaine)	klor-oh-PROE-kayn	Injection	Rx
dyclonine (Cepacol Maximum Strength Sore Throat Spray, Sucrets, Dyclone)	DYE-kloe-neen	Liquid spray, lozenge/troche, solution	OTC, Rx
tetracaine (Cepacol Viractin, Pontocaine)	TET-ra-kayn	Gel, injection, ophthalmic solution, oral liquid	OTC, Rx
Amides			
bupivacaine (Marcaine)	byoo-PIV-a-kayn	Injection	Rx
lidocaine (L-M-X, Lidoderm, Solarcaine Aloe Extra Burn Relief, Xylocaine)	LYE-doe-kayn	Cream, gel, injection, lotion, ointment, oral, patch, solution (external and mouth/throat), topical	OTC
lidocaine-epinephrine (Xylocaine with Epinephrine)	LYE-doe-kayn ep-i-NEF-rin	Injection	Rx
lidocaine-prilocaine (EMLA)	LYE-doe-kayn PRIL-oh-kayn	Cream	Rx
mepivacaine (Carbocaine)	me-PIV-a-kayn	Injection	Rx

Lidocaine

Lidocaine (L-M-X, Lidoderm, Solarcaine Aloe Extra Burn Relief, Xylocaine) can be administered with a patch, an adhesive strip that should be placed directly onto dry, clean skin at the site of pain. The patch should be applied only to intact skin and may be cut with scissors to fit a smaller area. As many as three patches may be applied in one area if the patch is too small to cover the painful area. The patch is worn for 12 hours and then removed for 12 hours. Hands should be washed immediately after applying the patch. Patches are especially useful to treat pain caused by shingles.

Contraindications Lidocaine use is contraindicated in patients with a history of hypersensitivity to local amide anesthetics.

Cautions and Considerations Lidocaine (topical solution) carries a black box warning for risk of seizures, cardiopulmonary arrest, and death when not administered according to dosing and administration instructions. Lidocaine should be used with caution in patients with severe shock, bradycardia, impaired cardiovascular function, acute porphyria, severe liver disease, and epilepsy, and with geriatric and pediatric patients.

Drug Interactions Major drug interactions with lidocaine include antiarrhythmic drugs, metoprolol, St. John's wort, phenytoin, propofol, and propranolol because potentially toxic side effects may lead to cardiovascular collapse, seizures, and respiratory depression.

Pain Management

As described earlier, **pain** is a general sense of the body. Pain receptors are activated when a stimulus is sufficient to damage tissue. Pain perception arises from the transmission of nerve impulses from these receptors. Pain is primarily a protective signal to warn of damage or the presence of disease—it is also a normal part of healing. This process involves inflammation, in which protective cells move into the injured area and release chemical mediators that cause fluids and plasma proteins to leak into the surrounding tissue.

Because the perception of pain can be subjective, thorough patient assessment and selection of the most successful and cost-effective therapy in pain management is challenging. Goals of management include enhancing functionality and productivity to improve the patient's quality of life. Studies have demonstrated that pain is often undertreated, and this deficiency can, in some cases, delay recovery from the condition causing the pain. To adequately control pain, the appropriate medication must sometimes be administered around the clock.

In January 2001, the Joint Commission on the Accreditation of Healthcare Organizations—now known as the Joint Commission—issued its pain management standards, which are used to evaluate the performance of healthcare providers. The standards emphasize the right of patients to receive appropriate pain management and education. The standards define pain as the "fifth" vital sign, along with temperature, pulse, respiration, and blood pressure. Healthcare providers must make regular pain intensity assessments. Pain is classified as acute, chronic nonmalignant, and chronic malignant:

- **Acute** pain is associated with trauma or surgery. Acute pain is usually easier to manage by identifying and treating the cause, and it usually disappears when the body heals.

- **Chronic Nonmalignant** pain may have a diagnosed or an undiagnosed cause, such as a nonmalignant disease. The pain lasts for more than three months and may respond poorly to treatment. Chronic nonmalignant pain may have signs and symptoms of depression in patients with a high tolerance of pain. The neurotransmitters involved in pain transmission are the same as those involved with depression (norepinephrine, dopamine, serotonin). Chronic pain syndrome is a form of this type of pain. In this syndrome, pain lasts longer than three months, may or may not have an identifiable physical or chemical basis, creates an overwhelming lifestyle burden for the patient, and does not respond to medication.
- **Chronic Malignant** pain accompanies malignant disease and often increases in severity as the disease progresses.

Acute and chronic pain differ in one important way. Whereas acute pain has a beginning and an end and warns of a problem, chronic pain does not cease when an illness or injury is cured or healed. With chronic pain, the suffering includes a sense of helplessness and hopelessness. Chronic pain has physical, psychological, social, and spiritual components. Adequate sleep, mood elevation, diversion, sympathy, and understanding all can raise an individual's pain threshold. Alternatively, fatigue, anxiety, fear, anger, sadness, depression, and isolation can lower the pain threshold.

Physiologic responses to pain vary and include the following:

- catabolism (tissues such as muscle are broken down)
- delayed stomach and bowel function
- impaired immune response
- increased autonomic activity (heart rate and blood pressure)
- increased metabolism
- muscle rigidity
- negative emotional response (depression)
- shallow breathing
- water retention

Inadequate treatment of pain can have adverse physiological, psychological, and immunological effects. Good clinical care must be based on the optimization of risk-benefit considerations. The major sources of pain, its characteristics, and their treatment are listed in Table 6.8.

TABLE 6.8 Major Sources of Pain

Source	Areas Involved	Characteristics	Treatment
Somatic	Body framework (bones, muscles, ligaments)	Throbbing, stabbing, well localized	Narcotics, NSAIDs, nerve blockers
Visceral	Kidneys, intestines, liver	Aching, throbbing, sharp, gnawing, cramping, deep squeezing; associated with sweating, nausea, vomiting	Narcotics, NSAIDs, nerve blockers, antiemetics
Neuropathic	Nerves (destruction)	Burning, aching, numbing, tingling, viselike, knifelike, constant	Antidepressants, anticonvulsants
Sympathetically mediated	Overactivity in sympathetic nervous system	Occurring when no pain should be felt	Nerve blockers

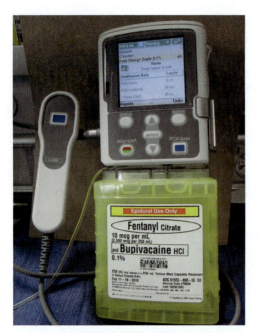

A patient-controlled analgesia pump allows the patient to regulate the amount of pain medication he or she receives. This results in better pain control with less drug used.

Sympathetically mediated pain occurs when nerve fibers are overactive and send pain signals when no pain should be felt. Sympathetically mediated pain is often associated with nerve damage, which usually occurs as a result of trauma to the area.

Narcotics

A **narcotic** is a pain-modulating chemical that tends to cause insensibility or stupor. Generally, a narcotic is an **opiate**, which is a substance that is either derived from opium (juice from the unripe seed capsule of the opium poppy, *Papaver somniferum*) or chemically resembles the opium derivatives. Morphine and codeine are examples of opiate narcotics.

Opiates are agonists of **opioid** receptors that affect the CNS, GI tract, and to a lesser extent, peripheral tissues. The body (specifically, the brain) produces three types of natural opioids—endorphins, enkephalins, and dynorphins—in response to pain stimuli. As pain increases, the levels of these chemicals also increase. When opioid receptors are activated, nerve transmission to CNS centers for pain processing is decreased, so the sensation of pain is diminished. Narcotics bind to the same receptors as these natural substances, causing activation. The pain receptors in the CNS are in the limbic system, thalamus, hypothalamus, midbrain, and spinal cord. Additional receptors are found in the adrenal medulla and nerve plexus. The primary opioid receptors associated with analgesia are denoted as mu, delta, and kappa.

Narcotics have the following effects:

- **Analgesia** Narcotics reduce pain from most sources (organs, trauma, myocardial infarction, terminal illness, and surgical wounds). Some pain is unresponsive to opiates.

- **Sedation** Narcotics allay anxiety and cause drowsiness.

- **Euphoria and Dysphoria** Narcotics produce feelings of well-being or feelings of disquiet, restlessness, or malaise. In addition, all narcotics have the potential to induce tolerance and dependence.

Narcotics also reduce the cough reflex and respiratory drive; increase mental clouding; and can cause nausea, vomiting, and constipation.

Patients can develop tolerance to pain therapy within days or weeks. As a result, dosages may need to be titrated (adjusted) every day or two. A good rule of thumb is to increase the current dose by 50% when needed, based on evaluation of pain control. After long-term treatment and disease regression, dosage may often be reduced without signs of withdrawal or recurrence of pain. Patients in pain have activated endorphin systems and are pharmacologically, physiologically, and biochemically different from drug abusers. Patients with medical reasons for their pain who are treated with appropriate opiates rarely become addicted.

Although opioids frequently impair judgment and psychomotor function for a period following the onset or acceleration of therapy, after a few days these adverse effects usually diminish markedly.

Opioids are associated with a high incidence of constipation. Thus, an opioid regimen often requires a clinically prescribed bowel program, such as stimulant laxatives, to produce an adequate response if constipation develops. Nausea is also a side effect of narcotics. An antiemetic will likely be prescribed for these patients.

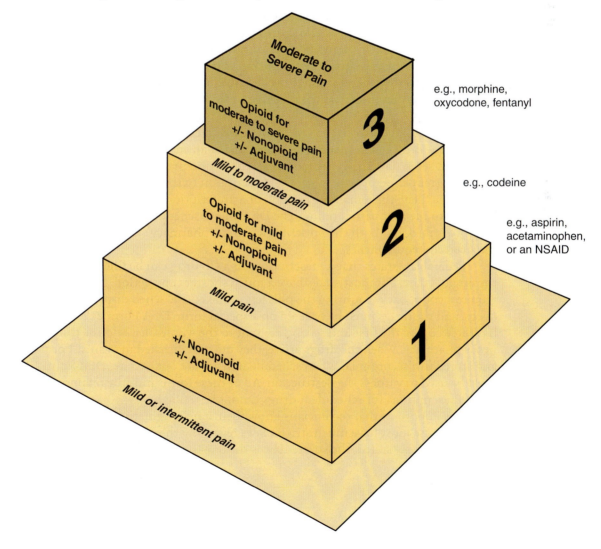

This PCA pump button should be pushed only BY THE PATIENT

An effective means of controlling pain in hospitalized patients is the **patient-controlled analgesia (PCA) pump**. The patient regulates, within certain limits, the amount of drug received by pushing a button controlled only by the patient. Better pain control can be achieved with lower doses when patients administer the drug at the onset of pain. Once pain has been ongoing for a long time, it is much more difficult to control. Another remarkable development in pain control is the transdermal patch. By providing stable blood levels of drug, the patch seems to control pain more effectively than other forms of delivery while allowing the patient to remain more alert.

Persistent pain should be treated in a stepwise fashion: first acetaminophen, then **nonsteroidal anti-inflammatory drugs (NSAIDs)**, and then the opioids. A simple scheme for analgesic selection is known as the **analgesic ladder**, which is illustrated in Figure 6.4.

FIGURE 6.4 Analgesic Ladder

The World Health Organization analgesic ladder for pain relief. Source: World Health Organization

1. Mild to moderate pain is treated with acetaminophen or an NSAID (prototype: aspirin) and an adjuvant (enhancement) analgesic.
2. If adequate relief is not achieved, a nonnarcotic analgesic (e.g., an NSAID) is given with a "weak" opioid (prototype: codeine).
3. If this fails, the patient is given a strong opioid (e.g., morphine), with an adjuvant analgesic if indicated.

Symptoms of narcotic overdose are respiratory depression, decreased body temperature, decreased blood pressure, tachycardia (abnormally rapid heart rate), and coma. The treatment is assisted ventilation and a narcotic antagonist.

Schedule II Drugs

Most narcotics are schedule II drugs. Schedule II drugs (C-II) have their own rules about where they are stored, how prescriptions must be written, how they are dispensed, and how they are ordered. They have the highest potential for abuse and addiction. They are not more likely to be involved in medication errors, but if they are, there is a greater likelihood that the patient will be harmed. They are kept in highly secure storage areas. If the pharmacist has to get a key to get to the drug, it is likely that it is a schedule II drug.

The US Drug Enforcement Administration (DEA) stipulates the federal requirements for laws regarding schedule II drugs, but each state determines its own regulations, which are usually stricter. The stricter rule is the one that must be followed; therefore, it is imperative that the technician is aware of the state laws regarding these drugs, as well as the federal regulations described next in this section.

Federal law requires that the pharmacist filling the drug must have the original, signed hard copy of the prescription with a DEA number. There are a few exceptions, however, including hospice and emergency care. In these situations, only a few days worth of the drug will be dispensed. In the case of an emergency, the prescriber has no more than seven days to get the hard copy to the pharmacy. Most state laws require a much shorter period of time to get the prescription to the pharmacy. If a partial prescription is filled, the remaining portion of a prescription must be filled within 72 hours of the first partial filling. The DEA allows schedule II drugs to be electronically prescribed, but both the prescriber's and the pharmacy's computer systems must meet certain requirements.

Federal law states that a prescription for a CII drug can be filled within a year of the original date, but most states have a much shorter time period. Some pharmacies require a count back (counting the pills left in the bottle) when dispensing these drugs, and the drugs must be ordered on a special form, DEA Form 222. This form has three copies: the first and second are sent to the wholesaler, and the third is kept in the pharmacy. When the drugs arrive, they must be checked in against Form 222 and stored in a secure area. When schedule II drugs are out of date, DEA Form 106 must be used to witness the destruction. All of these forms must be retained for two years. Prescriptions for schedule II drugs cannot be refilled.

It is important that technicians know their state's regulations for schedule II drugs, because most have much stricter laws regarding the dispensing of these drugs, and, as previously stated, the stricter law is the one that must be followed.

Pharm Facts

In March of 2016, the CDC released a new guideline for prescribing opioids for chronic pain. The guideline provides recommendations for primary care clinicians and addresses

1) when to initiate or continue opioids for chronic pain,

2) opioid selection, and

3) assessing risk and addressing harms of opioids.

Addiction and Dependence

Underprescribing opioids for nonmalignant pain is not uncommon. These are controlled substances that may cause addiction, and physicians are concerned with regulatory authorities as well as the risk that the patient may become addicted. Now, however, healthcare providers are increasingly aware that chronic pain is not being adequately treated and that opioids are appropriate when other treatments fail or are not tolerated. Chronic opioid therapy has a low risk of addiction when used appropriately for pain.

Although patients undergoing chronic opioid therapy do become physically dependent, addiction must not be confused with dependence. Recall from Chapter 2 that dependence is a physical and emotional reliance on a drug. Patients who are dependent will experience an abstinence syndrome (withdrawal) when drug therapy is discontinued or when the dose is reduced substantially.

In contrast, addiction is a compulsive disorder that leads to continued use of the drug despite harm to the user. Symptoms of addiction include preoccupation with drugs, refusal to taper off medication, a strong preference for a specific opioid (usually for short-acting over long-acting drugs), and a general decrease in ability to function. An addicted patient generally does not take the medication as prescribed. Opioid addicts have a tendency to rely on multiple prescribers and pharmacies to conceal their behavior. Pharmacy technicians must be alert to these signs of addiction when dispensing opioids, because it is their legal and moral responsibility to notify the pharmacist and/or prescribing physician if drug-seeking behavior is suspected. The technician should always watch for signs of abuse of these drugs, without prejudging patients.

The pharmacy technician should be alert to the following signs of addiction:

- Forged prescriptions
- Frequent prescription loss
- Changes made to the prescription; for example, adding a zero to the number 10
- Unsanctioned dose escalation
- Patient repeatedly saying he or she was shorted when medication was dispensed

One of the most difficult tasks for the pharmacy team is to assess narcotic use in patients. The pharmacy team commonly does not know what illness is being treated. Never hesitate to call the prescribing physician to verify and clarify a prescription for pain. Although the intention is certainly not to cause patients to feel uncomfortable or embarrassed, the pharmacy team must always be on the alert for those who abuse these medications, because addiction itself is an illness.

A patient will be more successful at overcoming addiction if the symptoms of withdrawal are handled appropriately, which means administering drugs that bind tightly to the opioid receptors. An agent with a stronger attraction for a receptor will replace another agent with a weaker attraction. The opioid antagonists work in this manner because they have a stronger attraction for receptors than analgesic agents do. Blocking the opioid action may prevent withdrawal symptoms. Table 6.9 lists drugs commonly used to treat addiction.

It is highly important that the pharmacy team acknowledge the value of opioids in the treatment of pain as well as the potential for drug diversion. The federal regulation pertinent to controlled substances states that prescriptions can be "issued for a legitimate medical purpose by an individual practitioner acting in the usual course of his or her professional practice." It is imperative that documentation be in the medical records. The pharmacy team must serve as both gatekeeper and advocate for patients who are in pain.

TABLE 6.9 Most Commonly Used Drugs to Treat Addiction

Generic (Brand)	Pronunciation	Dosage Form	Dispensing Status	Controlled Substance Schedule
buprenorphine (Buprenex, Subutex)	byoo-pre-NOR-feen	Injection, sublingual tablet	Rx	C-III
buprenorphine-naloxone (Suboxone, Butrans)	byoo-pre-NOR-feen nal-OX-oan	Sublingual tablet	Rx	C-III
methadone (Dolophine)	METH-a-doan	Injection, oral liquid, tablet	Rx	C-II

Buprenorphine

Buprenorphine (Buprenex, Subutex) is used to manage moderate-to-severe pain and to prevent opioid withdrawal. This drug attaches to the opioid receptors and acts as both agonist and antagonist.

Contraindications Buprenorphine use is contraindicated in patients with a history of hypersensitivity to buprenorphine.

Cautions and Considerations These medications should be used with caution in geriatric or debilitated patients and those with adrenal insufficiency, acute alcoholism, compromised pulmonary function, CNS depression, delirium, head injury, and hypothyroidism. Buprenorphine should not be swallowed.

Drug Interactions Major drug interactions with buprenorphine include naltrexone, phenobarbital, opioids, and carbamazepine and other CNS depressants, which may increase toxicity and result in CNS depression or respiratory depression.

Buprenorphine-Naloxone

Buprenorphine-naloxone (Suboxone, Butrans) is given after the patient has completed a course of buprenorphine, which takes three to four days. The patient is then maintained on this drug. It is only approved to treat opioid dependence. Prescribers must have two DEA numbers to write for this drug, and the second number is issued when the prescriber has met the appropriate requirements. The pharmacy technician must always check for this second DEA number on all prescriptions for Suboxone. It is a schedule III drug and is limited to qualifying prescribers. Like buprenorphine, it too is administered sublingually. Butrans is a transdermal patch that is applied to the upper arm, upper chest, upper back, or side of the chest, in rotation. Patients must wait at least three weeks before reusing a patch site. Nausea, headaches, dizziness, and vomiting may occur; overdose is possible.

Methadone

Methadone (Dolophine) is used as a pain reliever and to prevent withdrawal symptoms in patients addicted to opiate drugs who are enrolled in a treatment program. Alcohol, when added to methadone, can slow breathing and cause death. The concentrated form of methadone is packaged as a dispersible tablet and as a concentrated solution. Both must be mixed with four ounces of liquid. Patients should ingest the prepared solution immediately after it is mixed. Methadone is a schedule II controlled substance.

Contraindications Methadone use is contraindicated in patients with acute asthma, significant respiratory depression, or hypersensitivity to methadone.

Cautions and Considerations Methadone has black box warnings based upon the dosage form of the drug. In methadone injectable solution, QT interval prolongation and serious arrhythmias have been observed during treatment, with most cases occurring in individuals receiving higher doses. Use of oral tablet and solution methadone increases the risk of opioid addiction, abuse, or misuse, and death. Methadone oral tablets in suspension have been associated with deaths caused by titration that is too rapid, drug interactions, or cardiac and respiratory side effects.

In general methadone should be used with caution in patients with a history of substance abuse, respiratory depression, cardiovascular disease, hypotension, adrenal insufficiency, hypothyroidism, severe obesity, gastrointestinal obstruction, liver disease, kidney disease, and preexisting chronic obstructive pulmonary disease (COPD). Methadone should also be used cautiously in older adults and pregnant patients.

Drug Interactions Major drug interactions with methadone include antifungals (e.g., fluconazole), ziprasidone, dronedarone, linezolid, hydroxychloroquine, additional opioids, donepezil, selective serotonin reuptake inhibitor (SSRI) antidepressants, and ciprofloxacin.

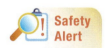

Safety Alert

The words *codeine* and *Lodine* (an NSAID) can look alike if written with poor handwriting.

Narcotic Analgesics

A drug that alleviates pain is known as an **analgesic**. An analgesic medication that consists of or is derived from an opioid is a **narcotic analgesic**. Table 6.10 describes the most commonly used single narcotic analgesics. Table 6.11 gives an overview of pharmacotherapeutic options for moderate to severe pain.

Narcotics have no set or optimal dose. Dose requirements vary with the severity of pain, the individual's response to pain, the patient's age and weight, and the presence of concomitant disease. Morphine is the standard against which all other narcotics are measured. Some drugs are more potent than morphine, but none are more effective when given in equianalgesic doses (a dose which would offer an equal amount of analgesia). Table 6.12 lists common narcotic analgesics and provides dosage equivalents to 10 mg of morphine.

Narcotics can be delivered by several routes. Oral doses of most drugs are essentially equivalent to rectal suppository doses, and intramuscular doses are essentially equivalent to subcutaneous doses. A subcutaneous dose of morphine is two to three times as potent as an oral dose. When patients cannot tolerate oral medications (e.g., because they suffer from nausea or vomiting), the rectal suppository route should be considered. Another alternative is subcutaneous or IV infusion. Intravenous doses are usually more potent than intramuscular or subcutaneous doses. The route and administration affect both the onset and duration of action. Long-acting opioids are usually better choices because there is less euphoria, lower potential for addiction, and fewer sleep disturbances. Even though the patient still needs to take pills, quality of life is improved because fewer pills are required.

Doses should be titrated, and the dose should be repeated at a time *before* the pain recurs (adjusted to each individual). The right dose is the dose that controls pain without excessive or intolerable adverse effects.

Narcotics may produce a range of side effects in individual patients. Side effects should be anticipated and minimized so that pain relief is not offset by creating other distressing symptoms. Some common effects are mental confusion, reduced alertness, nausea, vomiting, dry mouth, constipation, urinary retention, histamine release (flush, wheal, and flare), vessel dilation, inflammatory process, and bronchial constriction (especially in persons with asthma).

Narcotics inhibit normal peristalsis in the GI system (waves of contractions that pass along tubular organs to propel their contents), causing local spasms and reduced linear movement. All patients taking regular doses of a narcotic become constipated and should be maintained on some form of stimulant laxative from the outset of narcotic therapy. Stool softeners and increased fluid intake may be of benefit. Urinary retention can result because of spasmodic activity of the urethra (the tubular organ through which urine passes from the bladder) and major sphincter (ringlike muscle that closes a natural orifice) of the bladder. This can last from 24 to 48 hours and is most pronounced in patients over 55 years of age. Patients can also experience postural hypotension.

Respiratory depression is dose related. Appropriately prescribed narcotics rarely cause clinically significant respiratory depression. Any narcotic should be used with caution in patients with COPD or asthma; for these patients, reduction of the dosage is necessary.

TABLE 6.10 Most Commonly Used Narcotic Analgesics

Generic (Brand)	Pronunciation	Dosage Form	Dispensing Status	Controlled Substance Schedule
butorphanol (Stadol, Stadol NS)	byoo-TOR-fa-nawl	Injection, nasal spray	Rx	C-IV
codeine (various brands)	KOE-deen	Tablet	Rx	C-II
fentanyl (Abstra, Abstral, Actiq, Duragesic, Fentora, Ionsys, Lazanda, Onsolis, Subsys)	FEN-ta-nil	Injection, sublingual liquid, oral lozenge, intranasal solution, buccal tablet, sublingual tablet, buccal film	Rx	C-II
hydromorphone (Dilaudid, Exalgo)	hye-droe-MOR-foan	Injection, oral liquid, tablet, suppository	Rx	C-II
meperidine (Demerol)	me-PER-i-deen	Injection, syrup, tablet	Rx	C-II
morphine (Astramorph/PF, Avinza, DepoDur, Duramorph, Kadian, MS Contin, MSIR)	MOR-feen	Capsule, injection, oral solution, suppository, tablet	Rx	C-II
nalbuphine (Nubain)	NAL-byoo-feen	Injection	Rx	Varies
oxycodone (Oxecta, OxyContin, OxyIR, Roxicodone)	ok-see-KOE-doan	Capsule, oral liquid, tablet	Rx	C-II
oxymorphone (Numorphan, Opana, Opana ER)	ok-see-MOR-foan	Injection, suppository, tablet	Rx	C-II
pentazocine (Talwin)	pen-TAZ-oh-seen	Injection	Rx	C-IV
tapentadol (Nucynta)	ta-PEN-ta-dol	Tablet	Rx	C-II

TABLE 6.11 Pharmacotherapeutic Options for Moderate-to-Severe Pain

Indication	Pharmacotherapeutic Options for Treatment
Bone pain	NSAIDs, calcitonin, dexamethasone, prednisone
Cancer pain	Opioids
Fibromyalgia	Antidepressants, opioids
Lower back pain	Muscle relaxants, opioids
Neuropathic pain	Antidepressants, anticonvulsants
Osteoarthritis	NSAIDs, glucocorticoid injections

TABLE 6.12 Comparative Doses of Narcotic Analgesics

Generic (Brand)	Dose Equivalent to 10 mg IM Morphine
codeine (various brands)	130 mg, injection
fentanyl (Sublimaze)	0.1 mg, IV
hydromorphone (Dilaudid)	1.5 mg, injection
meperidine (Demerol)	300 mg, oral
methadone (Dolophine)	10–20 mg, oral
oxycodone-acetaminophen (Percocet)	30 mg, oral
oxycodone-aspirin (Endodan, Percodan)	30 mg, oral
oxymorphone (Numorphan)	1.5 mg, IV

Note: These equivalents will vary slightly, depending on reference.

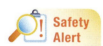

Safety Alert

Percocet is packaged in different strengths. Technicians must be careful to fill the prescription in the correct strength.

Narcotics act on an area identified as the chemoreceptor trigger zone (CTZ), which in turn acts on the vomiting center to produce emesis (the act of vomiting). This can be very dangerous in a patient heavily sedated with narcotics, because it can result in vomit blocking the airway. Morphine is especially likely to cause nausea because of the drug's stimulatory effect on the CTZ and inhibitory effect on GI motility. Antiemetics may be given to prevent or offset this reaction.

Narcotics can also stimulate seizures in patients with convulsive disorders. Most narcotics are metabolized by the liver; thus, serious liver disease may cause the patient to become comatose (a state of profound unconsciousness). Reduced doses must be used in these patients.

Consumption of alcohol with any of these drugs is very dangerous. It can result in the absorption and rapid release of the opioid, which leads to breathing depression and potentially death.

When these drugs are dispensed, *they must always be counted twice*. The number is then circled on either the label of the bottle or the label attached to the back of the prescription. It is not unusual for abusers to call back and say they were shorted. These circles will show that whoever dispensed the drug did count it twice, and it is not likely to be short.

Butorphanol

Butorphanol (Stadol, Stadol NS) is an analgesic that is more potent than morphine, yet it has fewer cardiovascular effects and lower respiratory sensitivity. It is a synthetic opiate that is a partial agonist. It binds to opiate receptors in the CNS. It is often used to manage pain during early labor, and it may be administered intranasally for migraine headaches.

Contraindications Butorphanol use is contraindicated in patients with a history of hypersensitivity to butorphanol or benzethonium chloride.

Cautions and Considerations Butorphanol should be used with caution in patients with a history of drug abuse, opioid dependence, cardiovascular disease, head injury, liver and kidney disease, hypertension, and respiratory insufficiency.

Drug Interactions Major drug interactions with butorphanol include naltrexone, other opioids and CNS depressants, propofol, and donepezil.

Codeine

Codeine is an opioid analgesic primarily used as an antitussive (coughing) or anti-diarrheal medicine, but it can also be used as an analgesic. It is an alkaloid derived from opium. Codeine is converted to morphine in the liver, is not approved for IV administration, and is most frequently marketed with acetaminophen. Combinations of codeine with another drug used for mild-to-moderate pain or diarrhea are schedule III, schedule IV, or schedule V controlled substances. Even in those locales where diluted codeine preparations are available OTC, very few pharmacists will sell them without a prescription. To do so, they must maintain a log. Many states have their own laws regarding these products. Codeine is considered less addictive than other opiates.

Contraindications Codeine use is contraindicated in patients with acute asthma or hypersensitivity to codeine, and pediatric patients undergoing tonsillectomy and/or adenoidectomy.

Cautions and Considerations Codeine should be used with caution in patients who are older adults or have a history of substance abuse or dependence, acute pancreatitis, constipation, head injury, liver and kidney disease, hypotension, hypothyroidism, respiratory insufficiency, and seizures.

Drug Interactions Major drug interactions include concurrent use with other opioid analgesics and CNS depressants, which may result in additive respiratory and cardiovascular depression.

Fentanyl

Fentanyl can be administered as a patch **(Duragesic)** or as a lozenge **(Actiq)**. Before these dosage forms were available, fentanyl was rarely prescribed outside of the operating room (OR) or ICU. The transdermal patches are used for chronic pain management. They should not be used for acute pain, such as that experienced immediately after surgery. Prescribers are not always aware of this limitation; if the prescriber is unaware, it is the pharmacy technician who has to catch this inappropriate use of fentanyl. The patch is applied to a dry area on the body and left in place for 72 hours. The patch works by releasing fentanyl into body fats. The fatty tissue stores the drug and slowly releases it into the bloodstream. These patches must not be cut. Body temperature, skin type, and placement of the patch all determine how effective the pain control is.

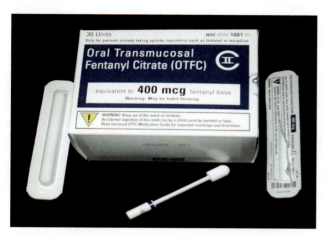

This image shows an example of an oral transmucosal fentanyl lozenge.

Ionsys is a transdermal system that transports the drug into the body through a three-volt lithium battery.

Fentanyl lozenges are berry flavored and should be swabbed on the mucosal surfaces inside the mouth and under the tongue. They are most effective when consumed over a period of 10 to 15 minutes. The lozenge is less effective if swallowed. A disadvantage of this dosage form is that it is very hard for nurses to document how much of the lozenge has been consumed.

Fentora, the buccal pellet, is effervescent and absorbed through the buccal mucosa. An advantage of this dosage form is quicker absorption into the bloodstream at lower dosage levels.

Abstral is a sublingual form of fentanyl. It is not equivalent to other dosage forms. It comes in a blister pack that must be peeled back. The pill must not be pushed through, as this could damage the pill and alter the dosing. **Subsys** is a sublingual spray. It is not comparable to other fentanyl dosage forms because there are differences in the pharmacologic profile. It is available only through a Risk Evaluation Mitigation Strategy (REMS). Healthcare professionals who want to prescribe or dispense the drug must enroll in the program. **Lazanda** is a nasal spray to be used for breakthrough pain. Like Subsys, it is not equivalent to other products. **Onsolis** is a buccal-soluble film used for breakthrough pain. Onsolis is restricted in its distribution and requires enrollment in the FOCUS Program by the prescriber, pharmacy, and patient. None of these durgs can be substituted for another formulation of fentanyl.

Contraindications Fentanyl use is contraindicated in acute or postoperative pain including headache/migraine or dental pain, intolerance or hypersensitivity to fentanyl, or opioid naïve patients. Transmucosal use is contraindicated in the emergency room.

Cautions and Considerations Different fentanyl products should not be converted on a mcg per mcg basis. Fentanyl should be used with caution in patients with bradycardia, COPD or other respiratory disorders, liver or kidney disease, or head injury. Caution is also required if the patient is taking other opioids or CNS depressants, consumes alcohol, or is an older adult. Hypoventilation may occur at any dose with transmucosal administration.

Drug Interactions Major drug interactions with fentanyl include naltrexone, antivirals, nifedipine, amiodarone, citalopram, MAOI antidepressants, other opioids, barbiturates, carbamazepine, and donepezil.

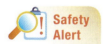
Safety Alert

Lortab and Lorabid (a cephalosporin antibiotic; see Chapter 4) can be confused. The dosing should help identify the prescribed drug.

Hydrocodone

Hydrocodone (Lorcet, Lortab, Norco, Vicodin) was the top-selling drug in the United States in 2006. It is sold only in combination with other drugs, such as acetaminophen or aspirin. It is very popular as an antitussive in cough syrups, many of which were removed from the market by the FDA in 2008. (See information in Table 6.13, which lists combinations of opioids and analgesics used for pain control.) Hydrocodone is a semisynthetic opioid derived from either codeine or thebaine, two naturally occurring opiates. It relieves pain by binding to opioid receptors in the

TABLE 6.13 Most Commonly Used Combination Drugs for Control of Pain

Generic (Brand)	Pronunciation	Dosage Form	Dispensing Statu	Controlled Substance Schedule
acetaminophen-codeine (Phenaphen with Codeine, Tylenol with Codeine)	a-seat-a-MIN-oh-fen KOE-deen	Capsule, elixir, tablet	Rx	C-III, C-V
hydrocodone-acetaminophen (Lorcet, Lortab, Norco, Vicodin)	hye-droe-KOE-done a-seat-a-MIN-oh-fen	Capsule, elixir, tablet	Rx	C-II
meperidine-promethazine (Mepergan)	me-PER-i-deen proe-METH-a-zeen	Capsule	Rx	C-II
oxycodone-acetaminophen (Endocet, Percocet, Tylox)	ox-i-KOE-done a-seat-a-MIN-oh-fen	Capsule, oral solution, tablet	Rx	C-II
oxycodone-aspirin (Endodan, Percodan)	ox-i-KOE-done AS-pir-in	Tablet	Rx	C-II
oxycodone-ibuprofen (Combunox)	ox-i-KOE-done eye-byoo-PROE-fen	Tablet	Rx	C-II
pentazocine-naloxone (Talwin NX)	pen-TAZ-oh-seen nal-OX-one	Tablet	Rx	C-IV

brain and spinal cord. Because hydrocodone is frequently abused, in 2014 the FDA changed the regulatory status from schedule III to the more regulated schedule II.

Contraindications Hydrocodone use is contraindicated in patients with acute asthma, significant respiratory depression, or hypersensitivity reactions to opioids.

Cautions and Considerations These medications should be used with caution in patients who are pregnant or those who have respiratory depression, history of substance or alcohol abuse, hypotension, decreased bowel motility, liver or kidney disease, head injury, and other CNS depressants.

Drug Interactions Drugs that have major interactions with hydrocodone include naltrexone, which may result in withdrawal symptoms; MAOI antidepressants; other opioids; and CNS depressants, which may result in additive respiratory and cardiovascular depression.

Safety Alert

To help reduce medication error, verify both the total dose in mg and the total volume in mL between HYDROmorphone and HYDROmorphone HP, because confusion between the two may result in accidental overdose and death.

Hydromorphone

Hydromorphone (Dilaudid) is becoming more popular in the treatment of chronic pain. It is preferred over morphine in many cases because of its superior solubility and speed of onset. Hydromorphone has a less troublesome side effect profile. Furthermore, patients experience less nausea and vomiting with hydromorphone than with alternatives, and it has no troublesome metabolites. The brand name for the extended release form is **Exalgo**. It is for patients who need around-the-clock medication.

Contraindications Hydromorphone use is contraindicated in acute asthma, opioid naïve patients, significant respiratory depression, or hypersensitivity reactions.

Cautions and Considerations Hydromorphone should be used with caution in patients with a history of substance abuse or addiction, respiratory insufficiency, alcoholism, hypotension, adrenal insufficiency, GI obstruction, and seizure disorders. It should also be used with care in the geriatric patients.

Drug Interactions Drugs that have major interactions with hydromorphone include naltrexone, other opioids, muscle relaxants, barbiturates, MAOI antidepressants, and antipsychotics.

Meperidine

Meperidine (Demerol) changes the way the body senses pain. It is used to control mild-to-moderate pain. Meperidine produces less nausea than most of the other opioids. However, it produces a metabolite that can cause serious problems when used over long periods. For that reason, it should never be used long term. The syrup should be diluted to prevent numbing of the mouth. It can be used as an adjunct to anesthesia.

Morphine

Morphine (Kadian, MS Contin, MSIR) is the principal alkaloid obtained from opium. It is an extremely versatile drug used in many different settings. Morphine is a strong analgesic used for the relief of severe and chronic pain, for preoperative sedation, and as a supplement to anesthesia. It is the drug of choice for the pain of myocardial infarction (heart attack). As with other opiate agonists, clinical effects other than pain relief include cough suppression, hypotension, nausea, and vomiting. Morphine is also very dangerous. An overdose causes the patient to stop breathing.

Morphine is administered orally, parenterally, intrathecally, epidurally, and rectally. When administered via the intravenous route, it is three to six times more potent than when it is administered orally. Morphine has significant first-pass metabolism and is readily absorbed from the gut and is absorbed even faster rectally. Kadian is also a slow-release form of this drug.

Some confusion arises with the morphine sulfate forms of morphine. There are two types of morphine sulfate: MSIR and MS Contin. MSIR (morphine sulfate immediate release) is immediately available and is used for breakthrough pain. The other sulfate form of morphine, MS Contin, is used for pain control over a longer period (continuous release). When a prescriber writes a prescription for morphine, he or she usually means the sustained release form, but it is always best to call to make sure if the prescriber does not indicate which form is being prescribed. MS Contin is usually dosed for 12 hours, whereas MSIR is usually dosed for 4 hours. The minimum effective plasma concentration varies widely from patient to patient. Many factors affect the minimum concentration, including age, prior opiate therapy, medical condition, and emotional state. Yet another morphine sulfate product, **DepoDur**, is an extended-release epidural injection that works for up to 48 hours.

Contraindications Morphine use is contraindicated with acute alcoholism, brain tumors, cardiac arrhythmias, severe CNS or respiratory depression, head injury, heart failure, and hypersensitivity reactions.

Cautions and Considerations Morphine carries multiple black box warnings associated with misuse, abuse, and concentration confusion that may result in an increased risk for overdose, seizures, respiratory depression, and death. These medications should be used with caution in neonatal and older adult patients and those with a history of substance abuse, respiratory depression, reduced cardiac output, hypotension, tachycardias, adrenal insufficiency, GI obstruction, liver or kidney disease, seizure disorders, and MAOI antidepressants.

Drug Interactions Drugs that have major interactions with morphine include naltrexone, muscle relaxants, other opioids, CNS depressants, cyclosporine, barbiturates, MAOI antidepressants, and donepezil.

Nalbuphine

Nalbuphine (Nubain) is injected into a large muscle, and it inhibits pain pathways by changing the perception of pain. It is used to control pain primarily during labor. CNS depression is a side effect.

Contraindications Contraindications to this medication include patients with hypersensitivity to nalbuphine or to any component of the product.

Cautions and Considerations Precautions for nalbuphine include use in patients who have a potential for drug abuse, concomitant use of CNS depressants including alcohol, or hepatic impairment.

Drug Interactions Drug interactions include concurrent use with opioid analgesics, as this may precipitate withdrawal symptoms or additive CNS and respiratory depression.

Oxycodone

Oxycodone (OxyContin, OxyIR, Roxicodone) is used to relieve mild-to-severe pain. It is provided in either liquid or tablet form. The most commonly used forms of this drug are combined with other analgesics such as acetaminophen or aspirin. Oxycodone causes CNS depression, which impedes mental abilities. It is a much abused drug and has a high street value. Oxycodone has high potential for abuse in patients as well as by pharmacy staff. When a prescriber writes an order for OxyContin, the extended release (ER) form must be used.

The pharmaceutical industry has started making abuse-deterrent formulations of medications recognized for high abuse potential. These unique compounds serve to take opioid formulations that will deter tampering. A recent formulation of OxyContin forms a viscous hydrogel when mixed with aqueous liquid for dissolution.

Contraindications Contraindications for oxycodone include use in patients with significant respiratory depression.

Cautions and Considerations Oxycodone should be used with caution in patients who have a potential for abuse, severe hypotension, or severe hepatic impairment.

Drug Interactions Drug interactions include concurrent use with sertraline, as this may result in an increased risk of serotonin syndrome; or other CNS depressing medications, as this may increase the risk for CNS or respiratory depression.

Oxymorphone

Oxymorphone (Numorphan, Opana, Opana ER) is a morphinelike opioid agonist. It is a semisynthetic compound that stimulates opioid receptors in the CNS, producing analgesia. Oxymorphone is approximately three times as potent as oral morphine. It is indicated for the management of moderate-to-severe pain when an opioid analgesic is needed around the clock for an extended period. Oxymorphone doses must not be broken, chewed, or dissolved, because doing so would lead to rapid release and a fatal overdose. Unlike other opioids, oxymorphone should be taken on an empty stomach, because taking it with food can lead to excessive peak levels.

Contraindications Contraindications to oxymorphone include use in patients with moderate or severe hepatic impairment, or significant respiratory depression.

Cautions and Considerations Oxymorphone should be used with caution in patients who have a potential for abuse, upper airway obstruction, or cardiovascular disease.

Drug Interactions Drug interactions include concurrent use with benzodiazepines, as this may result in additive respiratory depression.

Pentazocine

Pentazocine (Talwin) is a synthetically prepared narcotic used to treat mild-to-moderate pain. It is sold only in combination with other drugs. It is more likely to cause hallucinations than other opioids.

Contraindications The contraindications to this medication include hypersensitivity to pentazocine.

Cautions and Considerations Pentazocine should be used with caution in patients with acute myocardial infarction, asthma, head injury, or history of drug abuse.

Drug Interactions Drug interactions include concurrent use with opioid analgesics, as this may result in an increased risk for CNS and respiratory depression.

Tapentadol

Tapentadol (Nucynta) is a centrally acting opioid analgesic to be used for chronic, malignant pain. It should not be used as needed, such as to control pain after surgery. It is a more potent version of tramadol. The mechanism of action is unknown. It is only to be used in patients 18 years or older. The most common side effects are nausea, dizziness, vomiting, and drowsiness. It is associated with improved mental/physical abilities. Patients must be monitored closely for abuse and addiction, so it is a schedule II drug. The analgesic potency is somewhere between morphine and tramadol. It also may be very useful in patients who cannot tolerate the gastric distress (nausea) of other opioids. It is as successful as low-dose oxycodone in many people. There is also an extended release form of this drug.

Contraindications Contraindications to this medication include patients with gastrointestinal obstruction or significant respiratory depression.

Cautions and Considerations Tapentadol carries a black box warning for the potential for abuse, addiction, or misuse, which may lead to overdose and death. Tapentadol should be used with caution in patients with severe hepatic impairment, respiratory depression, or concurrent use of CNS depressants, including alcohol.

Drug Interactions Drug interactions include concurrent use of opioid analgesics, because this may result in additive CNS and respiratory depression.

Combination Drugs for Managing Pain

The combination of a narcotic and a nonnarcotic oral analgesic often results in analgesia superior to that produced by either agent alone. Relieving pain on two fronts (peripherally and centrally) enhances relief and facilitates use of lower doses of each agent. This produces a more favorable side effect profile. For example, combining meperidine and promethazine causes less nausea than other similar agents because the promethazine helps to control it. This combination is useful for patients who develop nausea from taking opioids. This combination also has strong sedative properties.

The purpose of combining drugs is twofold: (1) increasing pain relief through drug synergy, and (2) limiting the intake of addictive substances. Many combination drugs come in varying strengths. Oxycodone and hydrocodone both come in several combinations of doses of both the analgesic and the narcotic. It is important to make sure that both strengths agree with the prescription. The most commonly used combinations of drugs for controlling pain are listed in Table 6.13.

Because of the serious risk of aspirin and acetaminophen toxicity associated with combination drugs, they now contain less aspirin and acetaminophen. When a prescription is filled, the pharmacy technician should check to make sure the patient is not getting more than four grams of aspirin or acetaminophen per day. Often, prescribers are more concerned with the addiction potential of the narcotic component and overlook the potential for toxicity.

Acetaminophen is the leading cause of liver failure due to unintentional overdoses of combination analgesics. To decrease the probability of accidental overdose, most combination analgesics now contain a maximum of 325 mg of acetaminophen per tablet or capsule.

Pharmacy technicians must also be on alert regarding schedule III, schedule IV, and schedule V drugs. Prescriptions for these substances may be refilled no more than five times and are good for no more than six months. After this time, the patient must get a new prescription. Schedule II substances have absolutely no refills.

Migraine Headaches

A **migraine headache** is a severe, throbbing, unilateral headache accompanied by neurologic and GI disturbances that can severely affect quality of life and daily function. The headache is caused by dilation of cerebral surface vessels. Vomiting and anorexia are common, and approximately 90% of all migraine sufferers report nausea. Photophobia (sensitivity to light), phonophobia (sensitivity to sound), and hyperesthesia (increased sensitivity to stimulation) are also common.

A classic migraine has five components: prodrome (a symptom indicating the onset), aura, headache, headache relief, and postdrome (knowing it is gone). About 30% of migraine attacks are preceded by a subjective sensation or motor phenomenon known as an **aura**, which entails visual or sensory disturbances, or both: flashing lights; shimmering heat waves; bright lights; dark holes in the visual field; blurred, cloudy vision; or transient loss of vision. The headache generally dissipates in six hours, but sometimes lasts one to two days.

The pathogenesis of the migraine is not completely understood. One well-known theory, referred to as the **vascular theory**, proposes that migraines are caused by vasodilation and the concomitant mechanical stimulation of sensory nerve endings. Researchers suspect that the mechanism is more complicated than this.

The neurotransmitter serotonin (also known as 5-hydroxytryptamine or 5-HT) appears to be involved in the pathogenesis of a migraine. Serotonin is a potent vasoconstrictor, and its concentration in platelets increases just before migraine attacks and decreases afterward. Thus, changes in serotonin level parallel the migraine symptoms. It has been theorized that stimulating certain subclasses of serotonin receptors in the cerebral and temporal arteries will cause vasoconstriction, which inhibits neural transmission, thereby alleviating migraine caused by excessive dilation of cranial arteries. As a result of this theory, several serotonin receptor agonists are now being used to treat migraine headaches.

Diet, stress, sleep habits, certain medications, hormonal fluctuations, depression, atmospheric changes, and environmental irritants have all been implicated as causative factors that lower the threshold for neural transmission in the trigeminal nerve system, which is implicated in migraines. Oral contraceptives can exacerbate migraine, partly because of their estrogen component.

The initial treatment for a migraine should focus primarily on nondrug interventions. Identifying and eliminating trigger factors may be effective for many patients. For example, a quiet environment and sleep may help as many as 25% of patients during an acute attack. Lying down in a dark room often helps. When symptoms are severe or debilitating and attacks are frequent, drug therapy may be indicated. Sedative, antiemetic, and narcotic agents are helpful.

The medications used in migraine therapy can be divided into two classes: prophylactic therapy and abortive therapy, each of which is discussed briefly in the following paragraphs.

Prophylactic therapy is aimed at preventing or reducing recurrence. Prophylaxis is indicated if migraines occur more than twice a month, occur in predictable patterns, or become refractory (stop responding) to acute therapy. **Propranolol (Inderal)** is the drug of choice for prophylaxis for migraines. Prophylactic therapies for migraines include the following classes of drugs:

- anticonvulsants
- beta blockers
- calcium channel blockers
- estrogen (can also be a causative factor)
- feverfew (an herb frequently used but without scientific data to support its use)
- NSAIDs
- SSRIs
- tricyclic antidepressants

Abortive therapy for migraine headaches treats acute migraine headaches after they occur. The abortive drugs should be taken at the first sign of a headache. Patients must be educated about the importance of treating the attack as soon as possible—long before it develops into a full migraine, when treatments are much less effective. Abortive therapy is most effective when it begins at the first sign of aura or headache. The traditional therapies for acute migraine include simple analgesics, NSAIDs, serotonin receptor agonists, and ergotamine-containing medications.

Research has shown that combination regimens are more effective at treating migraine headaches and have lower recurrence rates than monotherapy. These advantages are especially true for combinations of a triptan and an NSAID.

Table 6.14 gives an overview of the most commonly used agents for migraine headaches. Several groups of drugs used to treat migraine headaches are discussed in the sections that follow.

TABLE 6.14 Most Commonly Used Agents for Migraine Headaches

Generic (Brand)	Pronunciation	Dosage Form	Dispensing Status	Controlled-Substance Schedule
Triptans—Selective 5-HT Receptor Agonists				
almotriptan (Axert)	al-moe-TRIP-tan	Tablet	Rx	
eletriptan (Relpax)	el-ih-TRIP-tan	Tablet	Rx	
frovatriptan (Frova)	froe-va-TRIP-tan	Tablet	Rx	
naratriptan (Amerge)	NAR-a-trip-tan	Tablet	Rx	
rizatriptan (Maxalt, Maxalt-MLT)	rye-za-TRIP-tan	Sublingual tablet, tablet	Rx	
sumatriptan (Imitrex)	soo-ma-TRIP-tan	Injection, nasal spray, patch, tablet	Rx	
sumatriptan-naproxen (Treximet)	soo-ma-TRIP-tan na-PROX-en	Tablet	Rx	
zolmitriptan (Zomig, Zomig ZMT)	zohl-mi-TRIP-tan	Nasal spray, sublingual tablet, tablet	Rx	
Ergot Derivatives				
dihydroergotamine (Migranal)	dye-hye-droe-er-GOT-a-meen	Injection, nasal spray	Rx	
ergotamine (Ergomar)	er-GOT-a-meen	Sublingual tablet	Rx	
Antiemetic Agents				
chlorpromazine (Thorazine)	klor-PROE-ma-zeen	Injection, tablet	Rx	
metoclopramide (Reglan)	met-oh-KLOE-pra-mide	Injection, oral liquid, tablet	Rx	
Opioid Analgesic				
butorphanol (Stadol, Stadol NS)	byoo-TOR-fa-nawl	Injection, nasal spray	Rx	C-IV
Beta Blocker				
propranolol (Inderal)	proe-PRAN-oh-lawl	Capsule, injection, oral liquid, tablet	Rx	
Other				
butalbital-acetaminophen-caffeine (Fioricet)	byoo-TAL-bi-tal a-seet-a-MIN-oh-fen KAF-een	Capsule, oral liquid, tablet	Rx	
butalbital-aspirin-caffeine (Fiorinal)	byoo-TAL-bi-tal AS-pir-in KAF-een	Capsule, tablet	Rx	C-III
tramadol (Ultram)	TRA-ma-dawl	Capsule, cream, oral suspension, tablet	Rx	C-IV

Triptans—Selective Serotonin Receptor Agonists

Migraine-specific products called **triptans** offer good efficacy and rapid onset of action. They bind to serotonin receptors, causing dilated blood vessels in the dura mater to constrict. They are available in various dosage forms. If a patient does not respond to one, he or she may respond well to another.

Almotriptan

Almotriptan (Axert) has one of the highest oral bioavailabilities. It is also better tolerated than some of the other migraine medications.

Eletriptan

Eletriptan (Relpax) has quite a few drug interactions, so the technician should check the computer system before dispensing. The maximum is two doses in 24 hours, but the effects seems to last longer than most migraine treatments.

Frovatriptan

Frovatriptan (Frova) has a slow onset but a relatively long half-life.

Naratriptan

Naratriptan (Amerge) is the gentlest triptan because it has slow onset and a favorable safety profile. It has a long half-life, which is generally associated with a low likelihood of migraine recurrence.

Rizatriptan

Rizatriptan (Maxalt, Maxalt-MLT) oral tablets are quickly absorbed and have the most rapid onset of action of all the oral migraine therapies. Many patients experience relief as soon as 30 minutes after taking this drug. The tablet is dissolved under the tongue. Maxalt is not absorbed as rapidly as Maxalt-MLT.

Sumatriptan

Sumatriptan (Imitrex) first entered the market as a subcutaneous injection and now is also available in tablet form and as a nasal spray. When injected, sumatriptan is effective in approximately 15 minutes. Sumatriptan may cause tingling, warm sensation, chest discomfort, dizziness, vertigo, and discomfort at the injection site. It has little or no activity on dopamine, beta-adrenergic, and alpha-adrenergic receptors. Side effects, including nausea, vomiting, and peripheral vasoconstriction, are relatively uncommon. The use of alcohol should be avoided because alcohol is a major contributor to migraines. The maximum recommended adult dose (subcutaneous route) is two 6-mg doses in 24 hours. A second dose may be administered at least one hour after the first dose if some improvement occurs but the migraine is still not relieved. The subcutaneous administration route is especially beneficial to patients with diminished gastric absorption or nausea and vomiting. The autoinjector is very easy to use. The patient should receive an injection at the first sign of a headache.

Sumatriptan-Naproxen

Sumatriptan-naproxen (Treximet) is used for the acute treatment of migraine. If there is no response to the first dose, then a second dose may be taken within two hours. Only these two doses should be taken in 24 hours. The first dose should be taken as soon as symptoms appear.

Zolmitriptan

Zolmitriptan (Zomig, Zomig ZMT) is similar to sumatriptan. It constricts cerebral blood vessels and reduces inflammation of sensory nerves. The dose can be repeated in two hours, but the patient should never take more than 10 mg in 24 hours.

Contraindications Contraindications to triptans include patients with cerebro-vascular syndromes, ischemic cardiac syndromes, uncontrolled hypertension, and hepatic impairment.

Cautions and Considerations Precautions for triptan drug use include risk factors for coronary artery disease or patients with hepatic impairment. Patients with concurrent use of SSRIs, serotonin-norepinephrine reuptake inhibitors (SNRIs), tricyclic antidepressants, or MAOIs may be at risk for serotonin syndrome.

Drug Interactions Drug interactions include concurrent use of amphetamines and SSRIs, which may increase the risk of serotonin syndrome. Concurrent use of ketoconazole, itraconazole, and amiodarone may increase toxicity.

Ergot Derivatives

Ergotamine, an alkaloid derived from the **ergot** group of fungi, which live parasitically on grasses such as rye, is used in the treatment of migraine headaches. The ergotamine molecule is similar to several neurotransmitters; its effectiveness with migraines is due to its activity as a vasoconstrictor. To be effective, ergotamine therapy should be initiated early in the attack.

Ergotamine has significant adverse effects that limit its usefulness. The most common, regardless of the administration route, are nausea and vomiting. These effects may be exacerbated if a rectal suppository is used, because absorption is enhanced. Ergotism (a syndrome of progressive vasoconstriction and ischemia of vital organs) and ergot headache (a medication-headache cycle occurring with daily use of ergotamine) have been reported. To avoid these adverse effects, patients should be told the maximum daily and weekly dosages and the importance of avoiding ergotamine use on consecutive days or more than twice a week.

Dihydroergotamine

Dihydroergotamine (Migranal) is a nasal spray that constricts peripheral and cranial blood vessels. This drug does not work as quickly as sumatriptan, but the effect lasts longer. Patients should administer one spray in each nostril, repeating every 15 minutes for a total of four sprays. The head should be held upright while spraying so that the drug remains in the nostril for absorption. Any drug not used within 24 hours should be discarded. Once the vial is opened, the drug loses its potency.

Ergotamine

Ergotamine (Ergomar) is a direct vasoconstrictor of smooth muscle in cranial blood vessels and is used to treat migraines. The dose should be titrated to each patient. The patient should be told to initiate treatment at the first sign of an attack and not to exceed the recommended dose.

Contraindications Ergot derivative contraindications include patients who have myocardial infarction and those who are pregnant or lactating.

Cautions and Considerations Ergot derivatives carry a risk for serious and/or life-threatening peripheral ischemia with the concurrent use of CYP 3A4 inhibitors. Derivatives should also be used with caution in patients at risk for cardiovascular or cerebrovascular events.

Drug Interactions Concurrent use of ergot derivative drugs with ketoconazole, voriconazole, or macrolide antibiotics may increase the risk of nausea/vomiting.

Antiemetic Agents

As described previously in this chapter, antiemetics are commonly prescribed to treat nausea and vomiting, as well as dizziness. There are a number of agents that can be used as an antiemetic treatment. Most of these agents work by blocking specific neurotransmitters. These can include serotonin, dopamine, acetylcholine, and histamine antagonists. Antimetic agents can alleviate nausea and vomiting associated with migraine headaches.

Chlorpromazine

Chlorpromazine (Thorazine) is effective in some migraines unresponsive to ergotamines. It has antiemetic properties. The side effects include drowsiness, extrapyramidal side effects, and orthostatic hypotension. This drug is also used to treat hiccups.

Contraindications Antiemetic agents are contraindicated in patients with epilepsy or gastrointestinal hemorrhage, concurrent use with large doses of CNS depressants, or hypersensitivity to antiemetic medications.

Cautions and Considerations Precautions for antiemetic agent use include patients with liver disease, congestive heart failure, or concomitant use with alcohol. The antiemetic drugs described previously both carry black box warnings. Metoclopramide treatment is associated with an increased risk of tardive dyskinesia, a serious movement disorder. Chlorpromazine treatment is not approved for patients with dementia-related psychosis, because it is associated with an increased risk of death.

Drug Interactions Drugs that may interact with chlorpromazine include tricyclic antidepressants or trazodone, because they may increase the risk for extrapyramidal reactions or neuroleptic malignant syndrome. Amitriptyline should not be used with chlorpromazine because it may increase the risk of fatal heart arrhythmia.

Metoclopramide

Metoclopramide (Reglan) can be used to reduce nausea and vomiting and enhance the absorption of other antimigraine products by reducing gastritis (inflammation of the stomach). Currently, many physicians are prescribing 1,000 mg of aspirin with 10 mg of metoclopramide in place of oral sumatriptan. This combination seems to have fewer side effects. Metoclopramide tends to cause drowsiness, but sumatriptan is more likely to cause nausea, fatigue, and weakness.

Opioid Analgesic

Butorphanol (Stadol, Stadol NS) is a mixed narcotic agonist-antagonist. The nasal spray form has central analgesic actions. It is used to manage moderate-to-severe pain. It can be addictive and is a schedule IV drug. Each bottle of the nasal spray delivers only 14 doses—fewer if it is primed before each use. The nasal spray is most commonly used, but the drug also comes as an injection that can be given either by IV or intramuscularly.

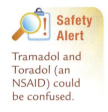

Safety Alert

Tramadol and Toradol (an NSAID) could be confused.

Other Antimigraine Agents

Other antimigraine agents include tramadol and butalbital combinations, as described below.

Tramadol

Tramadol (Ultram) is a synthetic agent that acts centrally. It binds to opiate receptors and inhibits reuptake of norepinephrine and serotonin. It is used for moderate-to-severe pain. The most common side effects include dizziness, vertigo, nausea, constipation, and headache. When given in combination with Tylenol, it has a high success rate in treating pain. Because the drug has a slow onset, it was originally promoted as a nonaddictive substance. However, with evidence for potential addiction to this drug, it was classified as a Schedule IV controlled substance in 2014.

Contraindications Contraindications to this medication include acute intoxication with alcohol, narcotics, or opioids because they may worsen CNS response and increase respiratory depression.

Cautions and Considerations Precautions for tramadol include concurrent alcohol use, misuse/abuse potential, and cirrhosis.

Drug Interactions Drug interactions include concurrent use with trazodone, as it may increase the risk of serotonin syndrome; or other CNS depressants because it may increase the risk of CNS depression.

Butalbital Combinations

Butalbital-acetaminophen-caffeine (Fiorcet) and **butalbital-aspirin-caffeine (Fiorinal)** are combination drugs often used to treat migraine, tension, or muscle contraction headaches. The butalbital-aspirin combination is regulated as a controlled substance, whereas the acetaminophen combination is not.

Contraindications Contraindications to butalbital combination drugs include hemorrhagic medical conditions, peptic ulcer (or other serious gastrointestinal lesions), porphyria, or hypersensitivity to any component of the medication.

Cautions and Considerations Butalbital combination drugs should be used with precaution in pediatric patients or those with severe hepatic impairment. Fioricet carries a black box warning for liver failure associated with acetaminophen use greater than 4 g a day.

Drug Interactions Drug interactions include the concurrent use of SSRIs as they may result in an increased risk for bleeding. Concurrent use with benzodiazepines or opioid analgesics may result in additive respiratory depression.

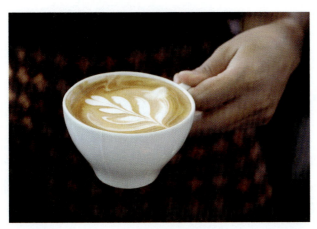

The caffeine in coffee can sometimes be used to treat headaches, fatigue, and drowsiness.

Complementary and Alternative Therapies

Caffeine is a CNS stimulant used in combination with other analgesics to treat headache. It is sometimes used to treat fatigue and drowsiness in doses of 100–200 mg. It should not be used more than every three to four hours. Caffeine is available in tablets, capsules, gum, and lozenges. Side effects include rapid heartbeat, palpitations, insomnia, restlessness, ringing in the ears, tremors, light-headedness, nausea, vomiting, stomach pain, and an itchy skin rash. Taking caffeine with food can help with these effects, and typically doses should be decreased if such effects occur.

Capsaicin is a chemical derived from cayenne peppers that is used as a topical treatment for pain. It has been found to be effective in diabetic neuropathy, arthritis, and headache pain. It works by exhausting the supply of substance P, a substrate in pain nerve endings in the skin. At first, burning, itching, and tingling occur, and then analgesic effects take hold once substance P is depleted. It should not be taken orally, inhaled, or applied to the eye because severe burning can occur. Patients should wear gloves during application and wash their hands thoroughly afterward to avoid these effects.

Feverfew is a plant product used orally for migraine pain. It is occasionally used to treat other pain conditions, including menstrual cramps and arthritis. It has been found to improve nausea, vomiting, and light sensitivity experienced during a migraine. Feverfew is generally well tolerated, but side effects include heartburn, nausea, diarrhea, constipation, abdominal pain, and gas. Chewing on feverfew leaves has caused mouth ulceration. Feverfew is dosed as 50–100 mg a day to prevent a migraine, rather than treating a migraine once it has already started.

Cannabis sativa, commonly known as *marijuana*, is a plant that is used for medical and recreational purposes. Synthetic and natural extracts may be used to provide relief of chronic or neuropathic pain. Medical marijuana can be administered via oral, sublingual, intramuscular, and inhalation routes, and its side effects include dizziness, weight gain, and heart disease. Inhaled marijuana may increase the risk of lung cancer.

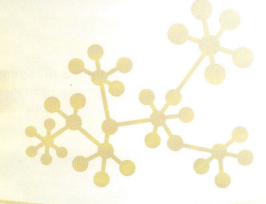

CHAPTER SUMMARY

The Nervous System

- The primary CNS neurotransmitters are acetylcholine, norepinephrine, dopamine, GABA, glutamate, and serotonin.

- The primary PNS neurotransmitters are acetylcholine and norepinephrine.

- The major neurotransmitters of the sympathetic nervous system are acetylcholine, norepinephrine, dopamine, and epinephrine.

- The only neurotransmitter of the parasympathetic nervous system is acetylcholine.

- If a drug is classified as an anticholinergic, the following side effects may occur: decreased GI motility, decreased urination, pupil dilation, decreased sweating, dry eyes, and dry mouth.

Anesthetics

- Drugs that allow painless, controlled surgical, obstetric, and diagnostic procedures constitute the cornerstone of modern pharmacologic therapy.

- One anesthetic may be superior to another, depending on the clinical circumstances. Final selection is based on those drugs and anesthetic techniques judged to be safest for the patient.

- General anesthesia is the unique condition of reversible unconsciousness and absence of response to stimulation. It is characterized by four actions: unconsciousness, analgesia, skeletal muscle relaxation, and amnesia on recovery.

- The purposes of premedication are sedation, reduction of postoperative pain, and relief of anxiety.

- Dantrolene is a skeletal muscle relaxant; it is the drug of choice to treat malignant hyperthermia.

- The advantage of nitrous oxide is that it is rapidly eliminated.

- Fentanyl is used extensively for open-heart procedures because it lacks some of the cardiac depressant actions of other anesthetics.

- Naloxone (Narcan) and flumazenil (Romazicon) are given to reverse overdoses of specific drugs.

- Neuromuscular blocking is important as an adjunct to general anesthesia to facilitate endotracheal intubation and to ensure that the patient does not move during surgery.

- Neuromuscular blocking agents act via a depolarizing mechanism or as antagonists to acetylcholine at receptors on the muscle cell.

- Anticholinesterase agents reverse neuromuscular blockers.

- Local anesthetics are advantageous because they affect all types of nervous tissue. They relieve pain without decreasing the level of alertness or mental function.

Pain Management

- Pain itself can be a disease; it is classified as acute, chronic nonmalignant, or chronic malignant.

- Pain is now considered to be the "fifth" vital sign.

- All narcotics have the potential to induce tolerance and dependence.

- The effects of narcotics are different for each individual.

- The patient-controlled analgesia (PCA) pump is an effective means of controlling pain; the pump allows the patient to regulate, within certain limits, the amount of drug received. Better pain control is achieved with less drug.

- The transdermal patch controls pain and allows the patient to remain more alert than with most other methods.

- Methadone (Dolophine), buprenorphine (Buprenex, Subutex), and buprenorphine-naloxone (Suboxone) are used to treat opioid addiction.

- Morphine is the standard against which all other narcotic analgesics are measured.

- Fentanyl is manufactured as a lozenge, spray, buccal film sublingual, and a patch. The patch is approved for chronic use, not acute pain following surgery.

- Narcotics act on the chemoreceptor trigger zone (CTZ) of the brain, which in turn stimulates the vomiting center.

- It is as important to monitor the aspirin or acetaminophen dose in narcotic combination analgesics as it is to monitor the narcotic dose.

- The pharmacy team must serve as the advocate and gatekeeper when dispensing narcotics.

- There are special laws regarding the ordering, dispensing, prescribing, and wasting of Schedule II drugs. Know your state's laws.

Migraine Headaches

- Patients with migraine headaches should initiate therapy at the first hint of an episode.

- Treatments for migraine headaches are divided into two groups: abortive and prophylactic therapies.

- Prophylactic drugs include anticonvulsants, beta blockers, calcium channel blockers, estrogen, feverfew, NSAIDs, SSRIs, and tricyclic antidepressants.

- Sumatriptan (Imitrex) is used for the relief of migraine headaches. It should be used at the first sign of headache. If it brings partial, but not total, relief, the patient may receive a second dose at least one hour after the first dose.

- Butalbital is combined with other drugs to treat headaches.

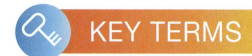

KEY TERMS

acute short, severe course

afferent system the nerves and sense organs that bring information to the CNS; part of the peripheral nervous system

alpha receptors nerve receptors that control vasoconstriction, pupil dilation, and relaxation of the GI smooth muscle in response to epinephrine

amide a longer-acting local anesthetic that is metabolized by liver enzymes

analgesic a drug that alleviates pain

analgesic ladder a guideline for selecting pain-relieving medications according to the severity of the pain and whether agents lower on the ladder have been able to control the pain

anesthesia loss of feeling in a person's body or part of the body

anesthesiologist a physician who oversees administration of anesthesia during surgery

anticholinesterase a drug that potentiates the action of acetylcholine by inhibiting the enzyme acetylcholinesterase, which breaks down acetylcholine

antiemetic agent prevents vomiting and nausea

aura a subjective sensation or motor phenomenon that precedes and marks the onset of a migraine headache

autonomic nervous system the part of the efferent system of the PNS that regulates activities of body structures not under voluntary control

barbiturates a depressant for the central nervous system that also acts as an antianxiety, hypnotic, and anticonvulsant

benzodiazepines a class of drugs that acts as a sedative, hypnotic, antianxiety, and anticonvulsant

beta-1 receptors (ß1) nerve receptors on the heart that control the rate and strength of the heartbeat in response to epinephrine

beta-2 receptors (ß2) nerve receptors that control vasodilation and relaxation of the smooth muscle of the airways in response to epinephrine

central nervous system (CNS) the brain and spinal cord

chronic malignant pain that accompanies malignant disease and often increases in severity as the disease progresses

chronic nonmalignant pain that lasts for more than three months and may respond poorly to treatment

dendrites branchlike extensions from a neuron's cell body

efferent system the nerves that dispatch information out from the CNS; part of the peripheral nervous system

endotracheal intubation insertion of a tube into the trachea to keep it open

ergot derivatives drugs derived from ergotamine, an alkaloid derived from the ergot group of fungi

ester a short-acting local anesthetic, metabolized by pseudocholinesterase of the plasma and tissue fluids

euphoria and dysphoria feelings of well-being or feelings of disquiet, restlessness, or malaise; common in narcotics

general anesthesia a condition characterized by reversible unconsciousness, analgesia, skeletal muscle relaxation, and amnesia on recovery

hypervolemia an excess of circulating fluid resulting in an increase in blood volume

local anesthesia the production of transient and reversible loss of sensation in a defined area of the body

malignant hyperthermia a rare but serious side effect of anesthesia associated with an increase in intracellular calcium and a rapid rise in body temperature

migraine headache a severe, throbbing, unilateral headache, usually accompanied by nausea, photophobia, phonophobia, and hyperesthesia

narcotic a pain-modulating chemical that tends to cause insensibility or stupor

narcotic analgesic pain medication containing an opioid

neuromuscular blocking skeletal muscle paralysis

neuron the type of cell making up the nervous system

nonsteroidal anti-inflammatory drug (NSAID) a drug such as aspirin or ibuprofen that reduces pain and inflammation

opiate a narcotic that is either derived from opium or synthetically produced to resemble opium derivatives chemically

opioid a substance, whether a drug or a chemical naturally produced by the body, that acts on opioid receptors to reduce the sensation of pain

pain the activation of electrical activity in afferent neurons with sensory endings in peripheral tissue with a higher firing threshold than those of temperature or touch; a protective signal to warn of damage or presence of disease; the fifth vital sign; classified as acute, chronic nonmalignant, and chronic malignant

parasympathetic nervous systems the rest and digest system; slows heart rate, increases intestinal and gland activity, and relaxes gastrointestinal tract sphincters

patient-controlled analgesia (PCA) pump a means of pain control whereby the patient can regulate, within certain limits, the administration of pain medication

peripheral nervous system (PNS) the nerves and sense organs outside the CNS

sedation state of calm of sleep typically induced by narcotics

somatic nervous system the part of the efferent system of the PNS that regulates the skeletal muscles

sympathetic nervous system activates the fight or flight response

triptans drugs that offer good efficacy and rapid onset of action for migraines

vascular theory a theory that proposes that migraine headaches are caused by vasodilation and the concomitant mechanical stimulation of sensory nerve endings

DRUG LIST

Inhalant Anesthetics

desflurane (Suprane)
enflurane (Ethrane)
isoflurane (Forane)
nitrous oxide, N_2O
sevoflurane (Ultane)

Injectable Anesthetics

alfentanil (Alfenta)
etomidate (Amidate)
fentanyl (Sublimaze)
ketamine (Ketalar)
morphine (Astramorph/PF, Duramorph, Kadian, MS Contin, MSIR)
propofol (Diprivan)
remifentanyl (Ultiva)
sufentanil (Sufenta)

Barbiturates

methohexital (Brevital)

Benzodiazepines

diazepam (Valium)
lorazepam (Ativan)
midazolam (Versed)

Antagonist to Reverse Malignant Hyperthermia

dantrolene (Dantrium, Revonto, Ryanodex)

Antagonists to Reverse Overdoses

flumazenil (Romazicon)
naloxone (Narcan)

Neuromuscular Blocking Agents

atracurium (Tracrium)
cisatracurium (Nimbex)
pancuronium (Pavulon)
rocuronium (Zemuron)
succinylcholine (Quelicin)
vecuronium (Norcuron)

Agents to Reverse Neuromuscular Blocking

edrophonium (Enlon)
neostigmine (Prostigmin)
pyridostigmine (Mestinon)

Local Anesthetics

Esters

benzocaine (Americaine)
chloroprocaine (Nesacaine)
dyclonine (Cepacol Maximum Strength, Sucrets)
tetracaine (Cepacol Viractin, Pontocaine)

Amides

bupivacaine (Marcaine)
lidocaine (L-M-X, Lidoderm, Solarcaine Aloe Extra Burn Relief, Xylocaine)
lidocaine-epinephrine (Xylocaine with Epinephrine)
lidocaine-prilocaine (EMLA)
mepivacaine (Carbocaine)

Drugs Used to Treat Addiction

buprenorphine (Buprenex, Subutex)
buprenorphine-naloxone (Butrans, Suboxone)
methadone (Dolophine)

Narcotic Analgesics

butorphanol (Stadol, Stadol NS)
codeine
fentanyl (Abstral, Actiq, Duragesic, Fentora, Ionsys, Lazanda, Onsolis, Subsys)
hydrocodone (Lorcet, Lortab, Norco, Vicodin)
hydromorphone (Dilaudid, Exalgo)
meperidine (Demerol)
morphine (DepoDur, Duramorph, Kadian, MS Contin, MSIR)
nalbuphine (Nubain)

oxycodone (Oxecta, OxyContin, OxyIR, Roxicodone)
oxymorphone (Numorphan, Opana, Opana ER)
pentazocine (Talwin)
tapentadol (Nucynta)

Combination Drugs

acetaminophen-codeine (Phenaphen with Codeine, Tylenol with Codeine)
hydrocodone-acetaminophen (Lorcet, Lortab, Norco, Vicodin)
meperidine-promethazine (Mepergan)
oxycodone-acetaminophen (Endocet, Percocet, Tylox)
oxycodone-aspirin (Endodan, Percodan)
oxycodone-ibuprofen (Combunox)
pentazocine-naloxone (Talwin NX)

Migraine Headaches

Triptans—Selective 5-HT Receptor Agonists

almotriptan (Axert)
eletriptan (Relpax)
frovatriptan (Frova)
naratriptan (Amerge)
rizatriptan (Maxalt, Maxalt-MLT)
sumatriptan (Imitrex)
sumatriptan-naproxen (Treximet)
zolmitriptan (Zomig, Zomig ZMT)

Ergot Derivatives

dihydroergotamine (Migranal)
ergotamine (Ergomar)

Antiemetic Agents

chlorpromazine (Thorazine)
metoclopramide (Reglan)

Opioid Analgesic

butorphanol (Stadol, Stadol NS)

Beta Blocker

propranolol (Inderal)

Other

butalbital-acetaminophen-caffeine (Fioricet)
butalbital-aspirin-caffeine (Fiorinal)
tramadol (Ultram)

Black Box Warnings

(Note that only certain forms and not all the drugs have this warning.)
bupivacaine (Marcaine)
buprenorphine (Buprenex, Subutex)
buprenorphine-naloxone (Suboxone)
dantrium (Dantrolene)
fentanyl (Abstral, Actiq, Duragesic, Fentora, Ionsys, Lazanda, Onsolis, Subsys)
flumazenil (Romazicon)
hydromorphone (Dilaudid, Exalgo)
ketamine (Ketalar)
methadone (Dolophine)
midazolam (Versed)
morphine (DepoDur, Duramorph, Kadian, MS Contin, MSIR)
oxycodone (Oxycontin)
oxymorphone (Opana ER)
pentazocine-naloxone (Talwin NX)
rocuronium (Zemuron)
succinylcholine (Quelicin)
vecuronium (Norcuron)

Medication Guides

buprenorphine (Buprenex, Subutex)
buprenorphine-naloxone (Suboxone)
fentanyl (Abstral, Actiq, Duragesic, Fentora, Ionsys, Lazanda, Onsolis, Subsys)
methadone (Dolophine)
morphine (Avinza, MS Contin)
oxycodone (Oxycontin)
oxycodone-ibuprofen (Combunox)
oxymorphone (Opana)
sumatriptin-naproxen (Treximet)

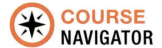

Access interactive chapter review exercises, practice activities, flash cards, and study games.

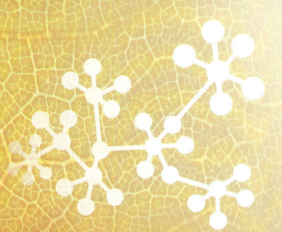

7

Psychiatric and Related Drugs

Learning Objectives

1. Differentiate antidepressant, antipsychotic, and antianxiety agents.

2. Discuss the antidepressant classes, their uses, and their side effects.

3. Describe the mechanism of lithium and other drugs used in treating bipolar disorders.

4. List the antipsychotics and the drugs that prevent their side effects.

5. Define anxiety, state its symptoms, and describe the drugs used in its treatment.

6. Recognize the course and treatment of panic disorder, insomnia, and alcoholism.

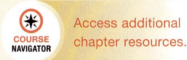

COURSE NAVIGATOR

Access additional chapter resources.

Psychiatric disorders are among the most disabling conditions that healthcare professionals encounter. Many of these disorders have their cause in the interaction of central nervous system (CNS) chemicals. Often, control of symptoms is the only treatment that can be offered. Psychiatric disorders include depression, posttraumatic stress disorder, seasonal affective disorder, bipolar disorder, psychotic disorders, anxiety, panic attacks, sleep disorders, and alcohol abuse.

Depression and Mood Disorders

Depression is the most common severe psychiatric disorder. Depression is characterized by feelings of pessimism, worry, intense sadness, loss of concentration, slowing of mental processes, and problems with eating and sleeping. Its symptoms may include dysphoric mood or loss of interest in almost all usual activities, low self-esteem, pessimism, self-pity, weight loss or gain, insomnia or hypersomnia, extreme restlessness, loss of energy, feelings of worthlessness, diminished ability to think, feelings of guilt, recurrent thoughts of death, and suicide attempts. Women are more likely than men to have depression, with the peak years usually from ages 35 to 45. Depression usually occurs later in life in men.

In addition to depression, there are several recognized types of mood disorders. **Mania** is a mood of extreme excitement, excessive elation, hyperactivity, agitation, and increased psychomotor activity.

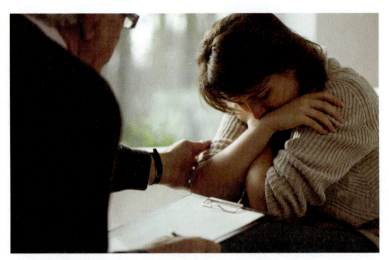

According to the World Health Organization, more than 350 million individuals worldwide have depression—the majority of whom are women.

Patients with **bipolar disorder** have mood swings that alternate between periods of major depression and periods of mild-to-severe chronic agitation (mania). Major depressive disorder (MDD) is depression with no previous occurrence of mania. **Posttraumatic stress disorder (PTSD)**, a mental health condition triggered by a terrifying event, is now the fourth most common psychiatric illness. Most people involved in a traumatic event have a brief period of difficulty, but if persistent anxiety or recurrent fear lasts more than a month after the end of the traumatic event or disturbs work or personal life, the disorder should be treated.

Finally, **seasonal affective disorder (SAD)** is a form of major depression that occurs in the fall and winter and remits in the spring and summer.

A **neurotransmitter** is a chemical produced by a nerve cell and is involved in transmitting information in the body. Neurotransmitters are important in mood disorders and other mental disorders. Drug therapy for depression is aimed at changing the levels of neurotransmitters, specifically serotonin, norepinephrine, and dopamine. Antidepressants are classified based on which neurotransmitter they affect and how.

Unlike most other drugs, antidepressants generally have a delay of onset of 10 to 21 days. These medications should never be used on an "as needed" basis to treat depression. As a pharmacy technician, you will be required by the US Food and Drug Administration (FDA) to include a medication guide for all antidepressants. These guides address concerns regarding the drug class and must be given to all patients with every dispensing of an antidepressant. Medication guides are "required for drug products that present a serious and significant" concern. Technicians should make sure that every antidepressant has this medication guide attached to promote the safe use of the drug. It is also important to remember that antidepressants are *not* controlled substances.

Selective Serotonin Reuptake Inhibitors

A **selective serotonin reuptake inhibitor (SSRI)** blocks the reuptake (i.e., reabsorption) of serotonin, thus increasing the concentration of that neurotransmitter with little effect on another important neurotransmitter, norepinephrine. SSRIs have the benefit of producing fewer side effects than historically older antidepressants.

Common side effects of SSRIs include nausea, vomiting, dry mouth, drowsiness, insomnia, headache, and diarrhea. These side effects can subside over time, but if bothersome, a different agent may be prescribed. Most of these medications can also cause sexual dysfunction, including decreased libido, inability to achieve orgasm, or impaired ejaculation. In fact, sexual dysfunction is a frequent reason that patients stop SSRI therapy. You can learn more about drug safety and side effects at http://Pharmacology6e.ParadigmCollege.net/DrugSafety.

SSRIs and **serotonin-norepinephrine reuptake inhibitors (SNRIs)** are generally safer than tricyclic antidepressants or TCAs (discussed later). However, if combined with

Practice Tip

Patients who have been prescribed antidepressants should be aware that it may take four weeks for these drugs to achieve full effect. However, antidepressants should help with sleep problems within a week or so.

Pharm Facts

PTSD was first recognized in World War I combat veterans. At that time, this disorder was called "shell shock." PTSD emerged as a major civilian illness after the Iraq War and Hurricane Katrina.

Web

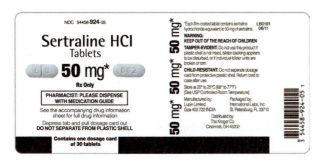

Sertraline is a commonly used SSRI.

certain other drugs, they can be fatal. This effect is known as **serotonin syndrome**, and it occurs when drugs that increase serotonin levels are combined with drugs that themselves stimulate the serotonin receptors, causing the receptors to be overstimulated. Although serotonin syndrome is rare, it can be fatal, partly because it is difficult to diagnose. It causes mental state changes and neuromuscular abnormalities, as well as other symptoms. Many prescribers are unaware of these dangerous interactions, but pharmacy technicians should know about them; they will see warnings on their computer screen (from pharmacy database information) and from insurance companies. If a patient is prescribed drugs that could cause such interactions, the pharmacy technician should notify both the pharmacist and the prescriber.

The most commonly used SSRIs for the treatment of depression are listed in Table 7.1.

Fluoxetine

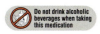

Fluoxetine (Prozac) is indicated for major depression and **obsessive-compulsive disorder (OCD)**, which is characterized by recurrent, persistent urges to perform repetitive acts such as handwashing. Adverse effects include nervousness, insomnia, drowsiness, **anorexia** (loss of appetite), nausea, and diarrhea. Most patients lose weight with fluoxetine use, but some may gain weight. Patients should avoid alcohol. Patients should take the drug in the morning to prevent insomnia. Fluoxetine plus light therapy (exposure to white light for a specific time period early in the morning, upon awakening) may be effective to treat SAD. Sarafem is a brand of fluoxetine specifically targeted for women suffering from **premenstrual dysphoric disorder (PMDD)**, which is a severe form of premenstrual syndrome (PMS). Serotonin levels are thought to influence the hormonal fluctuation that occurs just prior to the onset of menstruation. Although some women will benefit by taking the drug only during the week before menses, most women will need to take it daily to achieve the desired effect. It comes in a seven-day pack containing 10 mg or 20 mg capsules.

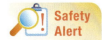

Safety Alert

Prozac and Proscar (finasteride, used to treat prostate enlargement), can look almost exactly alike.

TABLE 7.1 Most Commonly Used SSRIs and Related Drugs for Depression

Generic (Brand)	Pronunciation	Dosage Form	Common Dosage	Dispensing Status
citalopram (Celexa)	sye-TAL-oh-pram	Oral solution, tablet	10–40 mg a day	Rx
escitalopram (Lexapro)	es-sye-TAL-oh-pram	Oral liquid, tablet	5–20 mg a day	Rx
fluoxetine (Prozac, Sarafem)	floo-OX-e-teen	Capsule, oral liquid, tablet	10–80 mg a day	Rx
fluvoxamine (Luvox)	floo-VOX-a-meen	Capsule, tablet	25–150 mg a day	Rx
paroxetine (Paxil)	pa-ROX-e-teen	Oral liquid, tablet	10–60 mg a day	Rx
sertraline (Zoloft)	SER-tra-leen	Oral liquid, tablet	50–200 mg a day	Rx

Contraindications SSRIs are contraindicated with the use of monoamine oxidase inhibitors (MAOIs) intended to treat psychiatric disorders. SSRIs should not be started in patients who are receiving linezolid or intravenous (IV) methylene blue. Pimozide use is contraindicated with SSRIs. Fluoxetine should not be used with thioridazine.

Cautions and Considerations SSRIs have been associated with an increased risk of suicide in the first few weeks of therapy, especially in pediatric and adolescent patients. Because of this potentially fatal hazard, there is a black box warning for children, adolescents, and young adults. Patients should be monitored closely, particularly until the drug's full effects are experienced. Patients should be offered counseling and psychotherapy in addition to medication. The FDA has a warning that discusses the dangers of combining triptans (serotonin receptor agonists used to treat migraines, discussed in Chapter 6) with antidepressants, a combination that can occur frequently because many people who suffer from migraine headaches are also depressed.

Drug Interactions Fluoxetine may increase the effects of metoprolol and propranolol. It may increase the levels of the antiepileptics carbamazepine and phenytoin and the antipsychotics clozapine, haloperidol, and risperidone. Fluoxetine and paroxetine may increase each other's concentrations.

The sedating side effects of alcohol, benzodiazepines, and sibutramine may be increased by SSRIs. The anticoagulant effect of warfarin may be enhanced with SSRI use. SSRIs may lower the seizure threshold and should be used cautiously in patients taking antiepileptic drugs. The risk of gastrointestinal (GI) bleeding increases when nonsteroidal anti-inflammatory drugs (NSAIDs) are used with SSRIs. MAOIs when combined with SSRIs may lead to an increased risk of hypertensive crisis. SSRIs can increase the risk of serotonin syndrome when combined with other serotonergic drugs (such as triptans, TCAs, lithium, tramadol, tryptophan, and buspirone). Fluoxetine may enhance the effects of other medications that prolong the QT interval. Examples include haloperidol, ivabradine, mifepristone, ondansetron, pimozide, propafenone, thioridazine, and ziprasidone. Fluoxetine may increase the serum concentration of mequitazine. Pharmacists and technicians should be alert for possible inter-action with phenytoin (Dilantin). This interaction can raise the serum phenytoin to toxic levels.

Citalopram

Citalopram (Celexa) is considered to be an SSRI, although it is structurally different from the other drugs in this class. Citalopram has relatively few drug interactions because it is metabolized through an alternative pathway. It is ideal for patients who are required to take a number of different prescriptions concurrently. In addition to depression, citalopram is approved to treat OCD. Some of the most common adverse effects include insomnia, headache, drowsiness, anxiety, nervousness, and yawning.

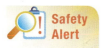

Safety Alert

Celexa is often confused with Cerebyx (fosphenytoin, an anticonvulsant) and Celebrex (celecoxib, for treating arthritis pain); be careful in dispensing.

Contraindications SSRIs are contraindicated with the use of MAOIs intended to treat psychiatric disorders. SSRIs should not be started in patients who are receiving linezolid or IV methylene blue. Pimozide use is contraindicated with SSRIs.

Cautions and Considerations SSRIs have been associated with an increased risk of suicide in the first few weeks of therapy, especially in pediatric and adolescent patients. Because of this potentially fatal hazard, there is a black box warning for children, adolescents, and young adults. Patients should be monitored closely, particularly until the drug's full effects are experienced. Patients should be offered counseling and psychotherapy in addition to medication.

Drug Interactions The sedating side effects of alcohol, benzodiazepines, and sibutramine may be increased by SSRIs. The anticoagulant effect of warfarin may be enhanced with SSRI use. SSRIs may lower the seizure threshold and should be used cautiously in patients on antiepileptic drugs. The risk of GI bleeding increases when NSAIDs are used with SSRIs. MAOIs when combined with SSRIs may lead to an increased risk of hypertensive crisis. SSRIs can increase the risk of serotonin syndrome when combined with other serotonergic drugs (such as triptans, TCAs, lithium, tramadol, tryptophan, and buspirone).

Escitalopram

Escitalopram (Lexapro) is the *S*-isomer of citalopram. An isomer is a chemical compound of identical composition but with a different arrangement of atoms. It is more potent, and patients generally experience fewer side effects. Escitalopram is used to treat both depression and generalized anxiety disorder.

Contraindications SSRIs are contraindicated with the use of MAOIs intended to treat psychiatric disorders. SSRIs should not be started in patients who are receiving linezolid or IV methylene blue. Pimozide use is contraindicated with SSRIs.

Cautions and Considerations SSRIs have been associated with an increased risk of suicide in the first few weeks of therapy, especially in pediatric and adolescent patients. Because of this potentially fatal hazard, there is a black box warning for children, adolescents, and young adults. Patients should be monitored closely, particularly until the drug's full effects are experienced. Patients should be offered counseling and psychotherapy in addition to medication.

Drug Interactions The sedating side effects of alcohol, benzodiazepines, and sibutramine may be increased by SSRIs. The anticoagulant effect of warfarin may be enhanced with SSRI use. SSRIs may lower the seizure threshold and should be used cautiously in patients taking antiepileptic drugs. The risk of GI bleeding increases when NSAIDs are used with SSRIs. MAOIs when combined with SSRIs may lead to an increased risk of hypertensive crisis. SSRIs can increase the risk of serotonin syndrome when combined with other serotonergic drugs (such as triptans, TCAs, lithium, tramadol, tryptophan, and buspirone). Conivaptan, fusidic acid, and idelalisib may increase concentrations of escitalopram.

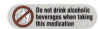

Name Exchange

Fluvox, the first brand name of fluvoxamine, has been voluntarily removed from the market. Yet many prescribers still write Fluvox on prescriptions and medication orders. In those situations, Luvox should be dispensed instead.

Fluvoxamine

Fluvoxamine (Luvox) is effective for the treatment of major depression and may be useful in managing anxiety; it is also approved for treatment of OCD. The primary side effect is nausea. Alcohol should be avoided, as should administration of phenytoin (Dilantin). Hard candy can relieve the side effect of dry mouth.

Contraindications Fluvoxamine should not be used with thioridazine, alosetron, ramelteon, and tizanidine. SSRIs are contraindicated with the use of MAOIs intended to treat psychiatric disorders. SSRIs should not be started in patients who are receiving linezolid or IV methylene blue. Pimozide use is contraindicated with SSRIs.

Cautions and Considerations SSRIs have been associated with an increased risk of suicide in the first few weeks of therapy, especially in pediatric and adolescent patients. Because of this potentially fatal hazard, there is a black box warning for children, adolescents, and young adults. Patients should be monitored closely, particularly until the drug's full effects are experienced. Patients should be offered counseling and psychotherapy in addition to medication.

Drug Interactions The sedating side effects of alcohol, benzodiazepines, and sibutramine may be increased by SSRIs. The anticoagulant effect of warfarin may be enhanced with SSRI use. SSRIs may lower the seizure threshold and should be used cautiously in patients taking antiepileptic drugs. The risk of GI bleeding increases when NSAIDs are used with SSRIs. MAOIs when combined with SSRIs may lead to an increased risk of hypertensive crisis. SSRIs can increase the risk of serotonin syndrome when combined with other serotonergic drugs (such as triptans, TCAs, lithium, tramadol, tryptophan, and buspirone). Fluvoxamine has many drug interactions. Fluvoxamine may decrease the metabolism of ramelteon and increase the serum concentration of pirfenidone, pomalidomide, and thioridazine. Avoid combining fluvoxamine with these medications.

Paroxetine

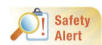

The indications for **paroxetine (Paxil)** are depression, OCD, and panic disorder. Side effects include nausea, headache, ejaculatory disturbances, and sweating.

Contraindications SSRIs are contraindicated with the use of MAOIs intended to treat psychiatric disorders. SSRIs should not be started in patients who are receiving linezolid or IV methylene blue. Pimozide use is contraindicated with SSRIs.

Cautions and Considerations SSRIs have been associated with an increased risk of suicide in the first few weeks of therapy, especially in pediatric and adolescent patients. Because of this potentially fatal hazard, there is a black box warning for children, adolescents, and young adults. Patients should be monitored closely, particularly until the drug's full effects are experienced. Patients should be offered counseling and psychotherapy in addition to medication.

Drug Interactions The sedating side effects of alcohol, benzodiazepines, and sibutramine may be increased by SSRIs. The anticoagulant effect of warfarin may be enhanced with SSRI use. SSRIs may lower the seizure threshold and should be used cautiously in patients taking antiepileptic drugs. The risk of GI bleeding increases when NSAIDs are used with SSRIs. MAOIs when combined with SSRIs may lead to an increased risk of hypertensive crisis. SSRIs can increase the risk of serotonin syndrome when combined with other serotonergic drugs (such as triptans, TCAs, lithium, tramadol, tryptophan, and buspirone).

Paroxetine may increase the effects of metoprolol, propranolol, and rivaroxaban. Paroxetine may increase the levels of the antiepileptics carbamazepine and phenytoin and the antipsychotics clozapine, haloperidol, and risperidone. Fluoxetine and paroxetine may increase each other's concentrations. It may decrease the effects of tamoxifen.

SSRIs increase the concentration of dosulepin and IV methylene blue. SSRIs may decrease the effects of tamoxifen. SSRIs decrease the metabolism of mexiletine. Tryptophan may enhance the serotonergic effects of SSRIs.

Sertraline

May Cause DROWSINESS

Sertraline (Zoloft) is indicated for depression and OCD. The primary side effect reported by patients is nausea when they first begin to take the drug; it may also cause drowsiness. It should be taken once daily without regard for food. Patients should show improvement in the first eight weeks of therapy.

Contraindications SSRIs are contraindicated with the use of MAOIs intended to treat psychiatric disorders. SSRIs should not be started in patients who are receiving linezolid or IV methylene blue.

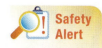
Cautions and Considerations SSRIs have been associated with an increased risk of suicide in the first few weeks of therapy, especially in pediatric and adolescent patients. Because of this potentially fatal hazard, there is a black box warning for children, adolescents, and young adults. Patients should be monitored closely, particularly until the drug's full effects are experienced. Patients should be offered counseling and psychotherapy in addition to medication.

Drug Interactions The sedating side effects of alcohol, benzodiazepines, and sibutramine may be increased by SSRIs. The anticoagulant effect of warfarin may be enhanced with SSRI use. SSRIs may lower the seizure threshold and should be used cautiously in patients taking antiepileptic drugs. The risk of GI bleeding increases when NSAIDs are used with SSRIs. MAOIs when combined with SSRIs may lead to an increased risk of hypertensive crisis. SSRIs can increase the risk of serotonin syndrome when combined with other serotonergic drugs (such as triptans, TCAs, lithium, tramadol, tryptophan, and buspirone).

Serotonin-Norepinephrine Reuptake Inhibitors

When SSRIs are not effective, SNRIs offer potential relief. SNRIs affect both serotonin and norepinephrine reuptake, which may make them more effective for treating pain than drugs that affect only one neurotransmitter. These drugs may be prescribed for pain alone. The most commonly used SNRIs in the treatment of depression are listed in Table 7.2. SNRIs are commonly associated with nausea, vomiting, insomnia, agitation, and drowsiness. SNRIs, like SSRIs, may cause sexual dysfunction.

Desvenlafaxine

Desvenlafaxine (Pristiq), the major metabolite of venlafaxine, is approved to treat depression and hot flashes. Pharmacokinetically, it works in the same way as venlafaxine, but it does not produce all of the unpleasant side effects. Additionally, desvenlafaxine is currently the only nonestrogenic drug available for hot flashes. This distinction is significant because many of the estrogens previously used for hot flashes have been taken off the market. It is anticipated that many women who cannot tolerate estrogen will be prescribed desvenlafaxine. Desvenlafaxine is also used for fibromyalgia and neuropathic pain.

TABLE 7.2 Most Commonly Used Serotonin and Norepinephrine Reuptake Inhibitors

Generic (Brand)	Pronunciation	Dosage Form	Common Dosage	Dispensing Status
desvenlafaxine (Pristiq)	des-ven-la-FAX-een	Tablet	50 mg a day	Rx
duloxetine (Cymbalta)	doo-LOX-a-teen	Capsule	20–60 mg a day	Rx
levomilnacipran (Fetzima)	lee-voe-mil-NAY-ci-pran	Capsule	20–120 mg a day	Rx
venlafaxine (Effexor)	ven-la-FAX-een	Capsule, tablet	75–375 mg a day	Rx

Contraindications Desvenlafaxine is contraindicated in patients with a hypersensitivity to venlafaxine.

SNRIs are contraindicated with the use of MAOIs intended to treat psychiatric disorders. SNRIs should not be started in patients who are receiving linezolid or IV methylene blue.

Cautions and Considerations Desvenlafaxine should not be used in pediatric patients.

SNRIs have a black box warning for an increased risk of suicidal thoughts and behavior in children, adolescents, and young adults. Patients, however, of all ages should be closely monitored for the emergence of suicidal thoughts and behaviors.

Drug Interactions Dapoxetine may increase the adverse effects of SNRIs. SNRIs may diminish the therapeutic effects of iobenguane I-123. Linezolid, MAOIs, and IV methylene blue may enhance the serotonergic effects of SNRIs. SNRIs may enhance the anticoagulant effects of urokinase.

Duloxetine

Duloxetine (Cymbalta) is approved for the treatment of major depression and the management of pain associated with diabetic neuropathy. It is a potent inhibitor of serotonin and norepinephrine and a weak inhibitor of dopamine reuptake, providing a more balanced reuptake inhibition. Duloxetine cannot be discontinued abruptly; instead, its dosage must be tapered. It has more interactions than the other drugs in this class.

NDC 0002-3270-30
Oral capsules • 60 mg

Cymbalta®

duloxetine HCl

60 mg • 30 capsules

Rx only

Cymbalta (duloxetine), a an SNRI, has recently been approved by the FDA for the treatment of major depression.

Contraindications SNRIs are contraindicated with the use of MAOIs intended to treat psychiatric disorders. SNRIs should not be started in patients who are receiving linezolid or IV methylene blue.

Cautions and Considerations SNRIs have a black box warning warning for an increased risk of suicidal thoughts and behavior in children, adolescents, and young adults. However, patients of all ages should be closely monitored for the emergence of suicidal thoughts and behaviors.

Drug Interactions Duloxetine inhibits cytochrome P-450 2D6 and, therefore, may increase levels of drugs metabolized by this enzyme (such as TCAs, carvedilol, diphenhydramine, fluoxetine, metoclopramide, metoprolol, tamoxifen, and venlafaxine). Concurrent use of anticoagulant drugs should be avoided when possible.

SNRIs should not be used with MAOIs due to an increased risk of serotonin syndrome. SNRIs should be used cautiously with other serotonergic drugs such as SSRIs, triptans, TCAs, lithium, tramadol, tryptophan, and buspirone.

Levomilnacipran

Levomilnacipran (Fetzima) is an SNRI for the treatment of MDD. It is a more potent inhibitor of norepinephrine reuptake than the other SNRIs. Food may improve the ability to tolerate this medication. The drug must be titrated. If the drug is discontinued, the dosage must be tapered.

Contraindications Levomilnacipran is contraindicated in patients with a hypersensitivity to milnacipran and in individuals with narrow-angle glaucoma.

SNRIs are contraindicated with the use of MAOIs intended to treat psychiatric disorders. SNRIs should not be started in patients who are receiving linezolid or IV methylene blue.

Cautions and Considerations Use with caution in older adults and in those individuals with kidney dysfunction.

SNRIs have a black box warning for an increased risk of suicidal thoughts and behavior in children, adolescents, and young adults. However, patients of all ages should be closely monitored for the emergence of suicidal thoughts and behaviors.

Drug Interactions SNRIs should not be used with MAOIs due to an increased risk of serotonin syndrome. SNRIs should be used cautiously with other serotonergic drugs such as SSRIs, triptans, TCAs, lithium, tramadol, tryptophan, and buspirone.

Venlafaxine

Venlafaxine (Effexor) blocks reuptake of both serotonin and norepinephrine and is prescribed for depression. A sustained increase in blood pressure may result from its use, and it may produce manic episodes. Side effects include sweating, headache, drowsiness, nausea, vomiting, dry mouth, blurred vision, and abnormal ejaculation or orgasm. At lower doses, venlafaxine primarily affects serotonin, whereas at higher doses, it also affects norepinephrine.

Contraindications SNRIs are contraindicated with the use of MAOIs intended to treat psychiatric disorders. SNRIs should not be started in patients who are receiving linezolid or IV methylene blue.

TABLE 7.3 Most Commonly Used Cyclic Antidepressants

Generic (Brand)	Pronunciation	Dosage Form	Common Dosage	Dispensing Status
Tricyclic Antidepressants (TCAs)				
amitriptyline (Elavil)	a-mee-TRIP-ti-leen	Tablet	30–300 mg a day	Rx
clomipramine (Anafranil)	cloe-MIP-ra-meen	Capsule	25–75 mg a day	Rx
desipramine (Norpramin)	des-IP-ra-meen	Tablet	75–200 mg a day	Rx
doxepin (Sinequan, Zonalon)	DOX-e-pin	Capsule, cream, oral liquid	25–150 mg a day	Rx
imipramine (Tofranil)	im-IP-ra-meen	Capsule, tablet	75–200 mg a day	Rx
nortriptyline (Aventyl, Pamelor)	nor-TRIP-ti-leen	Capsule, oral liquid	25–100 mg a day	Rx
Tetracyclic Antidepressants				
mirtazapine (Remeron)	meer-TAZ-a-peen	Tablet	15–45 mg a day	Rx

Cautions and Considerations SNRIs have a black box warning for an increased risk of suicidal thoughts and behavior in children, adolescents, and young adults. However, patients of all ages should be closely monitored for the emergence of suicidal thoughts and behaviors.

Drug Interactions SNRIs should not be used with MAOIs due to an increased risk of serotonin syndrome. SNRIs should be used cautiously with other serotonergic drugs such as SSRIs, triptans, TCAs, lithium, tramadol, tryptophan, and buspirone. Avoid the concurrent use of QT-prolonging agents.

Cyclic Antidepressants

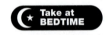

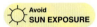

The cyclic antidepressants include varieties that contain three fused rings (tricyclic) and four fused rings (tetracyclic) of carbon atoms. Tricyclic antidepressants (TCAs) produce a response in greater than 50% of patients. Usually, a therapeutic course of 10 to 20 days is needed before improvements are apparent. Once the acute phase has subsided, the patient should continue to take the drug for 6 to 12 months to reduce the risk of relapse. TCAs have anticholinergic effects (blocking the neurotransmitter acetylcholine), which can decrease urinary urgency; therefore, TCAs may be used in children with bed-wetting problems. Table 7.3 lists the most commonly used cyclic antidepressants. Table 7.4 lists the anticholinergic and sedative properties of antidepressants.

TCAs can be cardiotoxic in high doses, and this primary side effect should be monitored. Patients, particularly older adults, may experience postural hypotension (a blood pressure decrease of at least 20 mm Hg). An overdose of TCAs may result in CNS toxicity and potentially fatal cardiac arrhythmias. Treatment should begin with a low dose and should be increased as needed to attain a response. Sedation is a common side effect, especially in the first few days of treatment. This effect may last several weeks; however, most patients become tolerant to this effect. It is usually prudent to advise the patient to take these drugs at bedtime. Dry mouth, blurred vision, constipation, and urinary retention (an anticholinergic effect) may all resolve within a few weeks. Patients also need to avoid prolonged sun exposure.

TABLE 7.4   Anticholinergic and Sedative Properties of Common Antidepressants

Generic Name	Properties	
	Anticholinergic	Sedative
amitriptyline	+ + + + +	+ + + +
bupropion	–	–
citalopram	–	–
clomipramine	+ + + +	+ + + +
desipramine	+ +	+ +
doxepin	+ + +	+ + + +
duloxetine	+	+
escitalopram	–	–

Note: The greater the number of + signs, the stronger the property. The – sign means there is no property.

Tricyclic Antidepressants

Amitriptyline, clomipramine, desipramine, doxepin, imipramine, and nortriptyline are all TCAs. As a class, they behave similarly. There are, however, some differences. **Doxepin (Sinequan, Zonalon)** has some unusual dosage forms. As a cream (Zonalon), it is used for pruritus (itching) in adults and older adults. Zonalon is applied three or four times a day. The topical form should not be used for more than eight days. The oral liquid is used by dentists as a topical for "burning mouth syndrome." The oral form is best taken at bedtime because it does cause drowsiness. It should not be taken with carbonated beverages or grape juice because these drinks can reduce its effectiveness. Overall, doxepin is a very versatile drug. **Imipramine (Tofranil)** is used primarily for nocturnal enuresis (bed-wetting) in children.

Contraindications TCAs should not be used with MAOIs because serotonin syndrome could develop. If a TCA is not working and an MAOI must be tried, the TCA must be discontinued for two weeks prior to initiation of an MAOI. This time in between therapies is called a **washout period**.

Amitriptyline, clomipramine, desipramine, and imipramine are contraindicated in the phase immediately after a heart attack. Clomipramine, desipramine, and imipramine are contraindicated in patients using linezolid or IV methylene blue.

Cautions and Considerations TCAs have a black box warning for an increased risk of suicidal thoughts and behavior in children, adolescents, and young adults. However, patients of all ages should be closely monitored for the emergence of suicidal thoughts and behaviors.

TCAs can cause cardiotoxicity and heart arrhythmias. Patients with preexisting heart conditions or who have recently had a heart attack should not take TCAs. These drugs can also cause **orthostatic hypotension** (a drop in blood pressure on sitting or standing up). Patients should change positions slowly—that is, from a supine position to a seated position, or from a seated position to a standing position.

TCAs can lower the seizure threshold, so most patients with seizure disorders should not take these drugs. Because these agents can also cause liver toxicity, patients with liver problems should not take TCAs. Periodic blood tests are required to monitor liver function.

An overdose of TCAs can be fatal, so prescriptions written for a large supply of medication all at once can be dangerous. Pharmacists may be resistant to filling such prescriptions for patients at risk for suicide. Be aware that many prescribers are also wary of warning patients that an overdose could be lethal because that message could suggest a pathway to suicide. It is important for healthcare prescribers to assess a patient's risk for suicide when prescribing these TCAs.

Drug Interactions Aclidinium, ipratropium, and umeclidinium may enhance the anticholinergic effects of TCAs. TCAs may enhance the CNS depressant effects of azelastine, paraldehyde, thalidomide, and tiotropium. TCAs may increase the adverse effects of glucagon.

Linezolid, MAOIs, and IV methylene blue may enhance the serotonergic effects of TCAs.

Amitriptyline may enhance the arrhythmogenic effect of cisapride.

Despiramine may increase the concentrations of bosutinib, ibrutinib, ivabradine, lomitapide, naloxegol, olaparib, simeprevir, thioridazine, tolvaptan, trabectedin, and ulipristal.

Clomipramine and imipramine may increase concentration of thioridazine.

Tetracyclic Antidepressants

Mirtazapine (Remeron) is a tetracyclic antidepressant used to treat mild-to-severe depression. It may be useful for patients who suffer from nausea. It is an alpha-2 adrenergic agonist. Like other antidepressants, mirtazapine increases active levels of serotonin and norepinephrine in the synapse. But rather than blocking the reuptake of these neurotransmitters, it is thought to work by blocking receptors that normally inhibit the release of the neurotransmitters. Mirtazapine seems to have some anti-anxiety effects and should be taken at bedtime.

Contraindications Mirtazapine is contraindicated in patients using MAOIs intended to treat psychiatric conditions. Mirtazapine should not be initiated in patients receiving linezolid or IV methylene blue.

Cautions and Considerations Mirtazapine has a black box warning for an increased risk of suicidal thoughts and behavior in children, adolescents, and young adults. However, patients of all ages should be closely monitored for the emergence of suicidal thoughts and behaviors.

Drug Interactions Alcohol, azelastine, orphenadrine, paraldehyde, and thalidomide may enhance the CNS side effects of mirtazapine.

Linezolid, MAOIs, and IV methylene blue may enhance the serotonergic effects of mirtazapine.

Pimozide concentrations may be increased by mirtazapine.

Conivaptan, fusidic acid, and idelalisib may increase the concentration of mirtazapine.

Monoamine Oxidase Inhibitors

Monoamine oxidase inhibitors (MAOIs) inhibit the activity of the enzymes that break down catecholamines (a group of neurotransmitters used by the sympathetic nervous system, including epinephrine, dopamine, and norepinephrine), thus allowing these transmitters to build up in the synapse. MAOIs are not first-line treatments for depression because of their many interactions with foods and other drugs, but they may be effective for certain patients. These drugs may be beneficial in atypical depression. They are similar in efficacy and adverse effects to TCAs, but they are not as cardiotoxic and may offer some advantages to patients with angina and cardiac conduction defects. At present, they are primarily used to treat conditions other than depression. Table 7.5 lists the most commonly used MAOIs.

When dispensing any of these drugs, the pharmacist should check the patient profile for interactions with other drugs. If a patient is taking an MAOI and the physician changes to another class of antidepressant, the patient must wait at least two weeks for the MAOI to clear his or her system (sometimes referred to as a washout period) before starting the second drug. MAOIs generally cause weight gain and edema. Severe interactions may also occur when someone taking an MAOI takes amphetamine, ephedrine, levodopa, meperidine, or methylphenidate. MAOIs impact serotonin and may increase the risk of serotonin syndrome, especially when used with other drugs that effect serotonin.

Severe hypertensive reactions have occurred when an MAOI is taken with food containing a high level of tyramine, a compound that occurs in aged cheese and many meats and vegetables. The clinical result is a sudden onset of a painful, throbbing, occipital headache; if severe, the condition may progress to severe hypertension; profuse sweating; pallor; palpitations; and, occasionally, death. Patients taking these drugs

TABLE 7.5 Most Commonly Used Monoamine Oxidase Inhibitors (MAOIs)

Generic (Brand)	Pronunciation	Dosage Form	Common Dosage	Dispensing Status
phenelzine (Nardil)	FEN-el-zeen	Tablet	45–90 mg a day	Rx
selegiline (Eldepryl, Emsam)	seh-LEDGE-i-leen	Capsule, patch, tablet	6–12 mg a day	Rx
tranylcypromine (Parnate)	tran-il-SIP-roe-meen	Tablet	30–60 mg a day	Rx

should never ingest aged cheeses, concentrated yeast extracts, pickled fish, sauerkraut, or broad bean pods because of the high levels of tyramine in these foods.

Selegiline

Selegiline (Eldepryl, Emsam) may be used to treat depression but is primarily used in Parkinson's disease as an adjunct in the management of patients in whom levodopa-carbidopa therapy is becoming ineffective. Selegiline may also be used in the management of Alzheimer's disease. Selegiline can be administered either orally or via a patch. The patch has some distinct advantages over the oral form. For one, the patch allows selegiline to bypass the first-pass effect, which allows it to reach higher levels in the CNS than can be achieved with oral administration. Patch administration also carries less potential for food interactions, although patients still need to be mindful of their diets. A patch should be used immediately upon removal from the sealed packet; applied to dry, intact skin on the upper body; and worn for 24 hours. The patch should increase patient adherence. Because of the potential of serotonin syndrome, this drug should not be taken with other antidepressants.

Contraindications MAOIs should not be used in patients with cardiovascular disease, cerebrovascular defect, a history of headache or liver disease, pheochromocytoma, or severe kidney impairment. MAOIs are also contraindicated with the use of antihistamines, blood pressure medications, bupropion, buspirone, caffeine (excessive use), depressants (such as alcohol), dextromethorphan, diuretics, general anesthetics, meperidine, other MAOIs or TCAs, carbamazepine, SNRIs, SSRIs, spinal anesthesia, sympathomimetics, and foods high in tyramine content.

Cautions and Considerations MAOIs interact with tyramine, a substance found in aged and pickled foods. This interaction causes serotonin syndrome, a life-threatening condition involving a rapid heart rate, high blood pressure, headache, and fever. Patients who take MAOIs should avoid consuming foods and beverages containing tyramine, such as aged cheeses, beer, wine, sauerkraut, and other pickled foods.

Drug Interactions These agents interact with numerous other drugs. When patients are taking an MAOI, they should work closely with their physicians and pharmacists to manage any additional prescription or over-the-counter (OTC) medications they want to take.

Other Antidepressant Drugs

Table 7.6 presents the most commonly used antidepressant medications that do not fit into the previously discussed drug classifications.

Bupropion

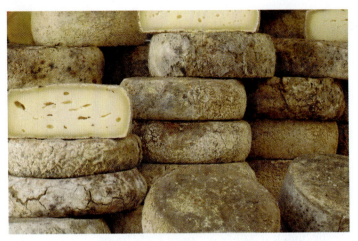

Tyramine-rich foods—such as aged cheese, concentrated yeast extracts, pickled fish, sauerkraut, or broad beans—should be avoided in patients taking MAOIs.

Bupropion (Aplenzin, Buproban, Forfivo, Wellbutrin, Zyban) is a dopamine-norepinephrine reuptake inhibitor with no direct effect on serotonin or monoamine oxidases, and it does not present anticholinergic, antihistaminic, or adrenergic effects. Bupropion has also been approved to treat SAD and as an aid to smoking cessation. The maximum daily dose of bupropion should not exceed 450 mg. It may take three to four weeks for the full effects to be realized. Bupropion should not be discontinued abruptly.

Bupropion is manufactured in several forms, which can cause confusion for the pharmacy technician. At times it is difficult to determine which dosage form the prescriber intended. Forms of bupropion, together with daily dosing rates, include the following:

- Wellbutrin, three times a day
- Wellbutrin SR, twice a day
- Wellbutrin XL, once per day

Prescriptions for bupropion may be written in any of these forms. The dosing indicates which drug you will need to dispense. When in doubt, always clarify the form and dosage with the prescriber. Zyban for smoking cessation is initiated at once a day for 3 days, then twice a day for 7 to 12 weeks. Aplenzin is a once-daily dose that allows the patient to take one dose of 300 mg or greater.

Bupropion has negligible anticholinergic and adrenergic effects. It does not cause sedation, blood pressure effects, or electrocardiographic changes. Effects that may occur are headache, impairment of cognitive skills, nausea and vomiting, dry mouth, constipation, seizures, and impotence. Bupropion may cause less erectile dysfunction than other antidepressants.

Contraindications Contraindications to bupropion include seizure disorder; history of anorexia/bulimia; abrupt discontinuation of ethanol or sedatives, including benzodiazepines, barbiturates, or antiepileptic drugs; use of MAOIs concurrently or within 14 days of discontinuing either bupropion or the MAOI; initiation of bupropion in a patient receiving linezolid or IV methylene blue; and the concurrent use of other dosage forms of bupropion.

Aplenzin and Wellbutrin XL should not be used in patients with other conditions that increase seizure risk, including arteriovenous malformation, severe head injury, severe stroke, CNS tumor, and CNS infection.

Cautions and Considerations Bupropion has two black box warnings. The first warning is for a risk of suicidal thoughts and behavior in children, adolescents, and young adults. However, patients of all ages should be closely monitored for the emergence of suicidal thoughts and behaviors. The second warning describes serious neuropsychiatric events that can occur in patients taking bupropion for smoking cessation.

TABLE 7.6 Most Commonly Used Miscellaneous Antidepressant Drugs

Generic (Brand)	Pronunciation	Dosage Form	Common Dosage	Dispensing Status
bupropion (Aplenzin, Buproban, Forfivo XL, Wellbutrin, Wellbutrin SR, Wellbutrin XL, Zyban)	byoo-PROE-pee-on	Tablet	100–450 mg daily	Rx
trazodone (Desyrel)	TRAZ-oh-done	Tablet	150–600 mg a day	Rx

Drug Interactions MAOIs may enhance the hypertensive effects of bupropion. Bupropion may increase concentrations of pimozide and thioridazine. Bupropion may decrease concentrations of tamoxifen.

Trazodone

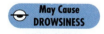

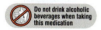

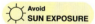

Trazodone (Desyrel) exerts its effect by preventing the reuptake of serotonin and norepinephrine. It is a serotonin inhibitor/antagonist, which means its mechanism of action is slightly different from that of the SNRIs. It has fewer side effects than the TCAs. It has no anticholinergic effects and no effects on cardiac conduction. It may cause orthostatic hypotension, which can be offset by changing positions gradually. There is much concern that it might have a serious interaction with ginkgo biloba. The drug should be given at bedtime because it can cause drowsiness. Patients should avoid alcohol and sun exposure.

Contraindications Trazodone is contraindicated in patients using MAOIs. In addition, trazodone should not be given to a patient receiving linezolid or IV methylene blue.

Cautions and Considerations Trazodone has a black box warning for risk of suicidal thoughts and behavior in children, adolescents, and young adults. However, patients of all ages should be closely monitored for the emergence of suicidal thoughts and behaviors.

If trazodone is to be used in combination with other antidepressants, such as SNRIs, SSRIs, TCAs, or MAOIs, the patient should be monitored closely for symptoms of serotonin syndrome. Therapy should be stopped immediately if any of the following symptoms occur, especially if in combination: fever, agitation, hallucinations, racing heart rate, flushing, tremors, diarrhea, or nausea and vomiting.

Trazodone has been associated with a serious and potentially fatal cardiac arrhythmia called *torsades de pointes*. Patients with a history of heart disease should not take trazodone. Trazodone has also been associated with lowering blood pressure and subsequent fainting. Therefore, it should be used with caution in combination with anti-hypertensive medications.

Cases of abnormal penile erection (**priapism**) have been reported with trazodone use; some patients have even required surgical intervention. This drug should not be prescribed for young males but can provide very effective relief of depression in older men.

Drug Interactions Trazodone may increase the CNS side effects of CNS depressants. Serotonergic drugs may increase the risk of serotonin syndrome.

Trazodone may increase digoxin blood levels and the risk of bleeding with anticoagulants.

Drugs Used to Treat Bipolar Disorder

Bipolar disorder is related to the dysfunction of neurotransmitters such as gamma-aminobutyric acid (GABA), serotonin, and norepinephrine. This disorder is characterized by periods of depression alternating with periods of mania, during which the patient exhibits irritability, elevated mood, excessive involvement in work or other activities, grandiose ideas, racing thoughts, and a decreased need for sleep. Patients vary in how much they experience mania versus depression.

Patients with bipolar disorder can struggle with psychotic features, such as thought disorders, hallucinations, or delusions. Half of patients with bipolar disorder will have at least one psychotic episode at least once in their lifetime. Frequently, other psychiatric disorders coexist with bipolar disorder. If a patient is experiencing signs of increased mood or activity or three or more of the following symptoms, the diagnosis could be mania:

- decreased need for sleep
- increased distractibility
- elevated or irritable mood
- excessive involvement in pleasurable activities with a large potential for painful consequences (e.g., financial irresponsibility, sexual indiscretions, alcohol or drug abuse, or reckless driving)
- grandiose ideas
- increase in activity (socially, at work, or sexually)
- emotional lability
- racing thoughts

Depressive episodes are characterized by the following symptoms:

- sadness or excessive crying
- low energy
- loss of pleasure
- difficulty concentrating
- irritability
- thoughts of death or suicide

The first episode of bipolar disorder typically occurs at about age 30 years, may last several months, and usually remits spontaneously. Without treatment, however, many patients experience one or more subsequent episodes. The objective of therapy is to treat acute episodes and prevent subsequent attacks.

Lithium is a commonly prescribed drug in the treatment of bipolar disorder. It works best when combined with psychotherapy, counseling, or cognitive behavioral therapy. An antipsychotic agent may be added initially to the regimen to control the hostility and agitation that sometimes accompany mania. Valproic acid and lamotrigine, traditionally thought of as anticonvulsants, are also commonly used (see Chapter 8 for more details on these medications). Antidepressants and some antipsychotic medications can also be used in the treatment of bipolar disorder, but close monitoring is required. Antidepressants are used very carefully when a patient is in the depressive pole because they can trigger a manic episode. Table 7.7 presents the drugs most often used to treat bipolar disorder.

Lithium

Lithium (Lithobid) compounds are the most commonly prescribed drugs for bipolar mood disorders; these compounds are generally referred to simply as "lithium."

The specific mechanism underlying the effectiveness of lithium is unknown, but it is believed to alter levels of specific brain chemicals (neurotransmitters) or cause changes in brain receptor sensitivity.

Lithium may indirectly interfere with sodium transport in nerve and muscle cells. It also affects the synthesis and storage of CNS neurotransmitters. Lithium promotes norepinephrine reuptake and increases the sensitivity of serotonin receptors. A common dosage of lithium is 300 mg, two to three times daily. Therapeutic blood levels are usually attained within 5 to 10 days after the start of therapy. Levels of 0.6 to 0.8 mEq/L are effective for most patients. To prevent toxicity, the patient must have regular blood tests and take the medication at a specific time. Even if the patient is taking a therapeutic dosage, slight tremors, especially of the hands, may occur. Lithium may also cause liver damage. Salt intake should remain constant during treatment because it can affect lithium blood levels. Alcohol intake increases the potential for toxicity.

Lithium is a common choice for treating bipolar (manic-depressive) disorder and acute mania, and for prophylaxis of unipolar and bipolar disorders. When the blood level of lithium reaches therapeutic levels, the antipsychotic can be discontinued. Lithium is the only mood stabilizer that has consistently been shown to decrease the risk of suicide for bipolar patients.

Common side effects that can occur when initiating lithium therapy include dry mouth, thirst, fine hand tremors, and mild nausea. These effects usually subside with continued treatment. Patients taking lithium sometimes complain of fatigue, mental dullness, somnolence, and impotence. These side effects may be chronic; therefore, patients should discuss these effects with their prescribers before stopping therapy on their own. Symptoms associated with elevated levels of lithium in the blood include diarrhea, vomiting, muscular weakness, slowed heart rate, low blood pressure (which can result in fainting), blackouts, incontinence, frequent urination, confusion, and hallucinations. If any of these effects occur, patients should seek medical attention right away.

Contraindications Contraindications to lithium include severe cardiovascular or kidney disease, dehydration, and sodium depletion.

Cautions and Considerations Lithium can become toxic, even in doses at the upper end of the normal dosing range; so regular laboratory tests to check blood concentration are needed to appropriately dose and monitor therapy. Lithium should be used with caution in patients with kidney disease, cardiovascular disease, or dehydration, as these conditions could increase the risk of lithium toxicity.

Drug Interactions Patients taking diuretics or angiotensin-converting enzyme (ACE) inhibitors should not take lithium, as these medications could also increase the risk of lithium toxicity. Patients taking NSAIDs or thyroid hormone with lithium should be monitored closely.

TABLE 7.7   Most Commonly Used Drugs to Treat Bipolar Disorder

Generic (Brand)	Pronunciation	Dosage Form	Dispensing Status
carbamazepine (Epitol, Tegretol)	kar-ba-MAZ-e-peen	Capsule, oral liquid, tablet	Rx
divalproex (Depakote)	dye-VAL-pro-ex	Capsule, tablet	Rx
lithium (Lithobid)	LITH-ee-um	Capsule, oral liquid, tablet	Rx
valproic acid (Depakene)	val-PRO-ik AS-id	Capsule, injection, oral liquid	Rx

Carbamazepine

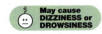

Carbamazepine (Epitol, Tegretol) affects the sodium channels that regulate nerve cells. This drug is indicated in bipolar disorder and is also used as an anticonvulsant. It is considered a second-line treatment to lithium and is used for patients who do not respond to lithium or cannot tolerate its side effects. Carbamazepine produces a response in many manic patients within 10 days. Side effects, which may be alleviated by briefly decreasing the dose to slow the rate of accumulation in the blood, include dizziness, ataxia (irregularity of muscular action), clumsiness, slurred speech, double vision, and drowsiness. More information on carbamazepine can be found in Chapter 8.

Divalproex and Valproic Acid

Divalproex (Depakote) and **valproic acid (Depakene)**, referred to as *valproates*, are particularly effective in older adults and in those patients with rapid changes of mood (rapid cyclers). These medications also work well as an adjunct to lithium and may replace lithium for some patients. They should be taken with food or milk but not with carbonated beverages. Bleeding or bruising symptoms of thrombocytopenia (a decrease in the number of platelets), should be reported to the physician. Valproates may also cause drowsiness and impair judgment or coordination. Please see Chapter 8 for more information on these medications.

Schizophrenia and Psychosis

The primary indication for using **antipsychotic drugs** (or **neuroleptic drugs**, as they are sometimes called) is schizophrenia. **Schizophrenia** is a chronic psychotic disorder manifested by retreat from reality, delusions, hallucinations, ambivalence, withdrawal, and bizarre or regressive behavior. In general, schizophrenia comprises positive symptoms (including hallucinations and delusions) and negative symptoms (including withdrawal, ambivalence, behavior changes, memory loss, and confusion). Negative symptoms are associated with thought disorders in which the patient displays language and communication that is illogical, contradictory, irregular, distracting, and tangential. Onset of symptoms usually occurs in the teenage or early adult years.

Dopamine and, to a lesser degree, serotonin are the major neurotransmitters implicated in schizophrenia. Dopamine receptors are present in four pathways: the limbic system (nerve fibers surrounding the upper brain stem), which controls emotions; the frontal cortex, which controls thought, learning, and memory; the basal ganglia, which affect control of voluntary muscle movement; and the pathway for the release of the hormone prolactin, which can cause sexual dysfunction. The first of these four pathways, involving the limbic system, is the one responsible for psychotic experiences when dopamine levels are excessive. The "older" or "typical" antipsychotic drugs antagonize dopamine receptors in all four of the dopamine pathways, leading to unfavorable side effects. In particular, drug action in the pathway involving the basal ganglia causes muscle control problems, referred to as **extrapyramidal symptoms (EPS)** or **EPS effects**.

At the beginning of the 21st century, antipsychotic agents were developed that had improved efficacy and fewer negative side effects. The "new" or "atypical" antipsychotic medications are designed to limit dopamine-blocking ability to the limbic system pathway rather than all four pathways. The atypical agents are now considered first-line agents in the treatment of schizophrenia.

Antipsychotic drugs are chosen on the basis of cost, degree of adverse effects, and a patient's response history. Drugs do not alter the natural course of schizophrenia. They do reduce symptoms such as thought disorders, hallucinations, and delusions, but medications rarely eliminate them. Symptoms such as emotional and social withdrawal, ambivalence (conflicting emotional attitudes), and poor self-care usually do not respond to drug treatment. Most therapeutic gains occur in the first 6 weeks, but maximum response may take up to 12 to 18 weeks. Discontinuation of these drugs leads to relapse of symptoms. Evidence shows that drug therapy does not reverse memory impairment, confusion, or intellectual deterioration.

Typical Antipsychotic Medications

"Typical" or "first generation" antipsychotics may be effective, but serious long-term side effects limit their use. Table 7.8 lists the typical antipsychotic medications that are most commonly prescribed; however, prescribers are moving toward the newer "atypical" antipsychotics, described in a later section.

Side effects of antipsychotic drugs run the gamut from minor annoyances to serious irreversible problems. Sedation that lasts as long as two weeks is a common side effect, which is minimized by administering the total daily dose at bedtime. The patient may also experience the following side effects:

- **Anticholinergic** Dryness of the mouth, eyes, and throat; blurred vision; and constipation. Problems occur at the beginning of treatment, but the patient develops tolerance.
- **Cardiovascular** Postural hypotension and an increase in pulse rate of about 20 beats per minute (bpm) with a change in position. These events may cause fainting or falling, most often in older adults.
- **Dermatologic** Excessive tanning or burning and a steely gray appearance to the skin after years of therapy, due to drug accumulation in melanocytes. With increased usage of the newer drugs, this effect is becoming rare.
- **Endocrine** Hyperglycemia (high blood glucose), lack of menses, lactation in nonpregnant females, breast enlargement in males, change in sexual function and drive (increased in females; decreased in males). Patients taking antipsychotics should be monitored closely for weight gain, development of diabetes, and an increase in cholesterol levels.
- **Hematologic** Reversible or irreversible bone marrow depression.
- **Ophthalmologic** Deposit of melanin–drug complex in lens and retina, resulting in blindness.
- **Withdrawal** Relapse.

Practice Tip

In low doses, **prochlorperazine (Compazine)** is commonly used as an antiemetic. In high doses, however, it can be used as an antipsychotic. It is rarely prescribed this way, but it may be used under unusual circumstances. Pharmacy technicians should be aware of this usage.

Safety Alert

The only antipsychotic drug that has a ceiling dose is **thioridazine (Mellaril)**, which should not exceed 800 mg per day because abnormal pigment deposits in the retina may result in blindness.

- **Neurologic** EPS effects due to an imbalance of cholinergic and dopaminergic transmitters. Dopaminergic blockade results in excessive cholinergic effects. Coadministration of anticholinergic drugs can balance some of these effects. Side effects develop in 40%–60% of patients, with early-onset symptoms developing within the first four weeks.

The following muscle coordination conditions develop as early-onset symptoms from the cholinergic and dopaminergic imbalance:

- **Dystonia** Involuntary tonic contraction of skeletal muscles, mostly of the head, face, and shoulders. The tongue may protrude, and the patient experiences difficulty talking and swallowing.

- **Akathisia** Motor restlessness. Patients complain that they are unable to sit or stand still and that they feel a compulsion to pace. Feelings of apprehension, irritability, and uneasiness may also appear. While standing, the patient may rock to and fro or shift weight from one leg to the other. This symptom occurs most frequently in middle-aged patients, especially women.

- **Pseudoparkinsonism** Tremors, rigidity, and slow movement; apathy with little facial expression; difficulty in walking or a shuffling gait; and drooling. The treatment is reducing the dose, changing to an agent less likely to produce EPS effects, or prescribing anticholinergics.

TABLE 7.8 Most Commonly Used Typical Antipsychotic Drugs

Generic (Brand)	Pronunciation	Dosage Form	Common Dosage	Dispensing Status
fluphenazine (Prolixin)	floo-FEN-a-zeen	Injection, oral liquid, tablet	IM: 12.5–25 mg every 2–4 weeks PO: 2.5–20 mg a day	Rx
haloperidol (Haldol)	hal-oe-PAIR-i-dawl	Injection, oral liquid, tablet	IM: 50–200 mg every 4 weeks PO: 0.5–30 mg a day	Rx
perphenazine (Trilafon)	per-FEN-a-zeen	Tablet	4–64 mg a day	Rx
prochlorperazine (Compazine)	proe-klor-PAIR-a-zeen	Injection, suppository, tablet	IM: 10–40 mg a day IV: 2.5–10 mg a day PO: 15–40 mg a day	Rx
thioridazine (Mellaril)	thye-oh-RID-a-zeen	Tablet	100–800 mg a day	Rx
trifluoperazine (Stelazine)	trye-floo-oh-PAIR-a-zeen	Tablet	2–20 mg a day	Rx

TABLE 7.9 Most Commonly Used Drugs to Minimize the Side Effects of Antipsychotic Drugs

Generic (Brand)	Pronunciation	Dosage Form	Common Dosage	Dispensing Status
benztropine (Cogentin)	BENZ-troe-peen	Injection, tablet	1–6 mg a day	Rx
diphenhydramine (Benadryl)	dye-fen-HYE-dra-meen	Capsule, injection, oral liquid, tablet	25–50 mg a day	OTC, Rx

Late-onset neurologic side effects occur after six months of treatment. **Tardive dyskinesia** involves involuntary movements of the mouth, lips, and tongue that are sometimes accompanied by involuntary movements of the limbs or trunk. These actions are worsened by emotional distress and disappear during sleep. Onset can be insidious and often occurs while the patient is taking the drug. The condition is potentially irreversible, even if the drug is discontinued. Drug withdrawal reveals the presence and severity of tardive dyskinesia. Once tardive dyskinesia appears, it is rarely progressive and usually either becomes static or slows, improving gradually over weeks or months. Currently, there is no satisfactory treatment for this condition. Anticholinergics make the condition worse.

Table 7.9 lists drugs that are commonly used to minimize the side effects of antipsychotic medications. **Benztropine (Cogentin)** is an anticholinergic that may produce an immediate but not necessarily complete response to excessive muscle activity resulting from antipsychotic administration. **Diphenhydramine (Benadryl)** is an antihistamine.

Atypical Antipsychotic Medications

The mechanisms of action for **atypical antipsychotics** are not fully understood and vary among agents. Some block dopamine and others enhance it. Atypical antipsychotics are first-line therapy for schizophrenia and other psychoses. Each agent varies in its effectiveness for individual patients. If one agent does not work, others are tried until a medication and dose are found that control symptoms (see Table 7.10). Unlike typical antipsychotics, atypical antipsychotics may be effective for the negative symptoms of schizophrenia.

Although atypical antipsychotic agents are much better tolerated than the older agents, they are associated with metabolic side effects, such as weight gain, hyperglycemia, new-onset diabetes, and dyslipidemia. The most commonly prescribed atypical antipsychotic medications are listed in Table 7.10 and briefly discussed here.

Side effects are similar to those of typical antipsychotics, but their incidence is lower. Common side effects of atypical antipsychotics include drowsiness, headache, constipation, dry mouth, urinary incontinence or retention, rash, excitation, and, occasionally, frequent hiccups. Taking these medications at bedtime can help with drowsiness, an effect that decreases with time. Atypical antipsychotic agents can cause EPS effects, but to a much lesser extent than do typical antipsychotic agents. Quetiapine can increase a patient's risk for cataracts, so regular eye examinations are necessary. Decreases in blood pressure can also occur, especially when changing to a standing or seated position. Patients should rise slowly after sitting or lying down.

Older patients should be especially careful until they know how these medications will affect them. Significant weight gain occurs for many patients on these medications. This weight gain is often associated with high cholesterol levels and new-onset diabetes. Many patients taking atypical antipsychotic agents will need medication for type 2 diabetes. Some atypical antipsychotics can cause arrhythmias and QT-interval prolongation. These effects can be problematic in patients with heart disease. Close cardiac monitoring is necessary.

Aripiprazole

Aripiprazole (Abilify) is a dopamine system stabilizer. Unlike typical antipsychotic agents, its actions may vary throughout the brain, depending on endogenous dopamine activity. Also, unlike some atypical antipsychotics, aripiprazole does not prolong the **QT interval**, and it may cause less weight gain than a typical antipsychotic drugs. These drug characteristics could make aripiprazole a favorable option for treatment of schizophrenia. It is thought that this drug improves dopamine activity and modulates motor function and prolactin secretion. Aripiprazole has a low risk of motor and other side effects. This drug is used primarily for bipolar disorder but has also received approval for major depressive disorder.

Clozapine

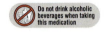

Clozaril and Clinoril (sulindac, a medication for rheumatoid arthritis pain) can be confused.

Clozapine (Clozaril), a blocker of D_2 dopamine receptors and serotonin type 2A receptors, is indicated for managing patients who have schizophrenia. It also blocks other dopaminergic, alpha-adrenergic, and histamine CNS receptors. Its most serious side effect is a reduction in white blood cells (WBCs), and leukocyte counts should be obtained weekly for the duration of therapy. Frequent blood samples *must* be taken, and the results documented by the pharmacy. Before the drug is dispensed, the pharmacy must receive blood work reports, and the technician must document that the WBC count is greater than $3,500/mm^3$ and that the absolute neutrophil count (ANC) is greater than $2,000/mm^3$. The patient should report any lethargy, fever, sore throat, flulike symptoms, or symptoms of infection. However, the medication should not be stopped abruptly.

Cautions and Considerations Atypical antipsychotics have black box warnings. The first warning is for an increased mortality in older adults with dementia-related psychosis. Another warning is for a risk of suicidal thoughts and behavior in children, adolescents, and young adults. However, patients of all ages should be closely monitored for the emergence of suicidal thoughts and behaviors. Clozapine's most serious side effect is a reduction in WBCs (**agranulocytosis**), for which it carries a black box warning. Patients showing hematologic changes should be monitored. Another black box warning is for orthostatic hypotension, bradycardia, and cardiac arrest. Seizure risk, which is thought to be dose-related, carries another warning. Clozapine carries a warning for potentially fatal myocarditis and cardiomyopathy.

Clozapine may cause QT-prolongation, which can lead to serious and life-threatening arrhythmias.

Patients with liver or kidney problems should avoid taking atypical antipsychotics, if possible.

TABLE 7.10 Most Commonly Used Atypical Antipsychotic Drugs

Generic (Brand)	Pronunciation	Dosage Form	Common Dosage	Dispensing Status
aripiprazole (Abilify)	air-i-PIP-ra-zole	Injection, oral disintegrating tablet, oral solution, tablet	IM: 5.25–15 mg every 2 hrs (daily maximum = 30 mg) PO: 10–30 mg a day	Rx
clozapine (Clozaril)	KLOE-za-peen	Oral disintegrating tablet, oral suspension, tablet	25–500 mg a day	Rx
olanzapine (Zydis, Zyprexa)	oh-LAN-za-peen	Injection, oral disintegrating tablet, tablet	IM: 150–300 mg every 2 weeks or 300–405 mg every 4 weeks PO: 5–20 mg a day	Rx
paliperidone (Invega)	pal-ee-PAIR-i-doan	Injection, tablet	IM: 39–234 mg every 4 weeks PO: 6–12 mg a day	Rx
quetiapine (Seroquel)	kwe-TYE-a-peen	Tablet	300–800 mg a day	Rx
risperidone (Risperdal)	ris-PAIR-i-doan	Injection, oral disintegrating tablet, oral solution, tablet	IM: 25–50 mg every 2 weeks PO: 1–8 mg a day	Rx
ziprasidone (Geodon)	zi-PRAS-i-doan	Capsule, injection	IM: 10 mg every 2 hrs or 20 mg every 4 hrs (daily maximum = 40 mg) PO: 40–160 mg a day	Rx

Atypical antipsychotics should be used with caution in older adults because excessive dizziness, drops in blood pressure, and sedation can cause falls. Patients must be monitored closely. Because kidney and liver functions are often reduced in older adult patients, they cannot effectively eliminate these medications. Therefore, reduced doses are necessary.

Because patients at any age who have schizophrenia or psychosis can have thought disorders, it is important for patients to be monitored closely and offered counseling or psychotherapy in addition to drug treatment.

Patients should not drink alcohol while taking atypical antipsychotic medications because excessive sedation and hallucinations can occur. The pharmacy technician should affix an auxiliary warning label about alcohol use when dispensing these medications.

Drug Interactions Clozapine may enhance the effects of other medications that prolong the QT interval (such as quinolones and ivabradine). Clozapine may enhance anticholinergic side effects of other drugs (such as ipratropium and umeclidinium) and the CNS depressant effects of other drugs (such as alcohol, azelastine, and thalidomide). Carbamazepine and other myelosuppressive drugs may increase the hematologic adverse effects of clozapine. Metoclopramide may increase the adverse effects of antipsychotics.

Olanzapine

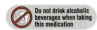

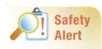

Olanzapine (Zyprexa) is used to treat schizophrenia. Like clozapine and risperidone, olanzapine blocks dopamine and serotonin receptors, but it causes fewer movement disorders. It does not affect WBCs as clozapine does, so frequent blood monitoring is not necessary. Side effects are dizziness, drowsiness, constipation, dry mouth, and weight gain. Patients *must* avoid alcohol. This drug appears to help patients by decreasing distorted thinking or obsessive-compulsive behavior concerning food. It helps patients respond better to behavioral therapy. It can be used for either anorexia nervosa or weight gain.

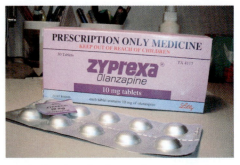

Atypical antipsychotics, such as olanzapine (Zyprexa), can be used to treat schizophrenia.

Olanzapine has a once monthly injectable dosage form, which may improve patient adherence.

Contraindications Olanzapine does not have any contraindications.

Cautions and Considerations Atypical antipsychotics have black box warnings. The first warning is for an increased mortality in older adults with dementia-related psychosis. Another warning is for a risk of suicidal thoughts and behavior in children, adolescents, and young adults. However, patients of all ages should be closely monitored for the emergence of suicidal thoughts and behaviors.

Atypical antipsychotics can lower the seizure threshold, so patients with seizure disorders must be monitored closely when taking these medications. Patients with liver or kidney problems should avoid taking atypical antipsychotics, if possible. Some atypical antipsychotics can cause bone marrow suppression, a rare but serious side effect. Regular laboratory tests are necessary to check for this condition.

Atypical antipsychotics should be used with caution in older adults because excessive dizziness, drops in blood pressure, and sedation can cause falls. Patients must be monitored closely. Because kidney and liver functions are often reduced in older adult patients, they cannot effectively eliminate these medications. Therefore, reduced doses are necessary.

Because patients at any age who have schizophrenia or psychosis can have thought disorders, it is important for patients to be monitored closely and offered counseling or psychotherapy in addition to drug treatment.

Patients should not drink alcohol while taking atypical antipsychotic medications because excessive sedation and hallucinations can occur. The pharmacy technician should affix an auxiliary warning label about alcohol use when dispensing these medications.

Drug Interactions Olanzapine may enhance the adverse effects of benzodiazepines. It may also increase the anticholinergic side effects of other anticholinergic drugs (such as diphenhydramine and umeclidinium).

Antipsychotics may increase the adverse effects of CNS depressants. Metoclopramide may increase the adverse effects of antipsychotics.

Quetiapine

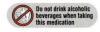

Quetiapine (Seroquel) is structurally related to clozapine but has a lower incidence of the hematologic toxicities associated with clozapine.

Contraindications Quetiapine does not have contraindications.

Cautions and Considerations Atypical antipsychotics have black box warnings. The first warning is for an increased mortality in older adults with dementia-related psychosis. Another warning is for a risk of suicidal thoughts and behavior in children, adolescents, and young adults. However, patients of all ages should be closely monitored for the emergence of suicidal thoughts and behaviors.

Atypical antipsychotics can lower the seizure threshold, so patients with seizure disorders must be monitored closely when taking these medications. Patients with liver or kidney problems should avoid taking atypical antipsychotics, if possible. Some atypical antipsychotics can cause bone marrow suppression, a rare but serious side effect. Regular laboratory tests are necessary to check for this condition.

Atypical antipsychotics should be used with caution in older adults because excessive dizziness, drops in blood pressure, and sedation can cause falls. Patients must be monitored closely. Because kidney and liver functions are often reduced in older adult patients, they cannot effectively eliminate these medications. Therefore, reduced doses are necessary.

Patients should not drink alcohol while taking atypical antipsychotic medications because excessive sedation and hallucinations can occur. The pharmacy technician should affix an auxiliary warning label about alcohol use when dispensing these medications.

Drug Interactions Antipsychotics may increase the CNS effects of azelastine and thalidomide. Metoclopramide may increase the adverse effects of antipsychotics.

Risperidone and Paliperidone

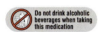

Risperidone (Risperdal) is a mixed serotonin-dopamine antagonist. It binds to serotonin receptors in the CNS and the peripheral nervous system with a very high affinity, and it binds to dopamine receptors with less affinity. The binding of serotonin receptors and dopamine receptors is thought to improve negative symptoms of psychosis and reduce the incidence of EPS effects. Risperidone is indicated for the management of psychotic disorders (e.g., schizophrenia) and dementia in older adults. The primary side effects of risperidone are hypotension, sedation, and anxiety.

Paliperidone (Invega) is an active metabolite of risperidone. It is used in the treatment of schizophrenia. Paliperidone works as well as risperidone, but it causes fewer side effects. It is a sustained-release tablet and is dosed once a day. There are few interactions with other drugs because it is not extensively metabolized in the liver. Advantages of paliperidone include low weight gain, fewer EPS effects, and significant efficacy in the treatment of schizophrenia. Invega uses an extended-release technology called osmotic controlled-release oral delivery system (OROS), in which the drug dissolves through pores in the tablet shell. When the tablet is empty, the tablet shell, known as a **ghost tablet**, is excreted in the stool. These tablets must not be crushed or broken. It is recommended that the drug be taken in the morning. One potential side effect of paliperidone that should be monitored is orthostatic hypotension.

Contraindications Risperidone does not have contraindications. Paliperidone is contraindicated in patients with risperidone hypersensitivity.

Cautions and Considerations Risperidone and paliperidone have black box warnings for an increased mortality in older adults with dementia-related psychosis. Paliperidone comes in extended-release tablets only. Consequently, these tablets should not be chewed or crushed.

Atypical antipsychotics can lower the seizure threshold, so patients with seizure disorders must be monitored closely when taking these medications. Patients with liver or kidney problems should avoid taking atypical antipsychotics, if possible. Some atypical antipsychotics can cause bone marrow suppression, a rare but serious side effect. Regular laboratory tests are necessary to check for this condition.

Atypical antipsychotics should be used with caution in older adults because excessive dizziness, drops in blood pressure, and sedation can cause falls. Patients must be monitored closely. Because their kidney and liver functions are often reduced in older adult patients, they cannot effectively eliminate these medications. Therefore, reduced doses are necessary.

Because patients at any age who have schizophrenia or psychosis can have thought disorders, it is important for patients to be monitored closely and offered counseling or psychotherapy in addition to drug treatment.

Patients should not drink alcohol while taking atypical antipsychotic medications, because excessive sedation and hallucinations can occur. The pharmacy technician should affix an auxiliary warning label about alcohol use when dispensing these medications.

Drug Interactions Risperidone has a significant drug interaction with the SSRI paroxetine. Risperidone levels may be increased with concurrent use.

The effects of agents that prolong the QT interval may be enhanced when used with risperidone or paliperidone.

Antipsychotics may increase the adverse CNS effects of azelastine and thalidomide. Metoclopramide may increase the adverse effects of antipsychotics.

Ziprasidone

Ziprasidone (Geodon), which is used to treat schizophrenia, may cause less weight gain than other antipsychotic agents. This drug characteristic is an important advantage because weight gain is often the reason that patients quit taking their antipsychotic medication. The major problem with ziprasidone is that it prolongs the QT interval, which may lead to arrhythmia and death. Ziprasidone can be given intramuscularly.

Contraindications Contraindications to ziprasidone include a known history of QT prolongation, recent acute myocardial infarction, uncompensated heart failure, and concurrent use of other drugs that prolong the QT interval (including arsenic trioxide, chlorpromazine, dofetilide, dolasetron, droperidol, gatifloxacin, mefloquine, moxifloxacin, other Class Ia and III antiarrhythmics, pentamidine, pimozide, quinidine, sotalol, tacrolimus, or thioridazine).

Cautions and Considerations Atypical antipsychotics have black box warnings. The first warning is for an increased mortality in older adults with dementia-related psychosis. Another warning is for a risk of suicidal thoughts and behavior in children, adolescents, and young adults. However, patients of all ages should be closely monitored for the emergence of suicidal thoughts and behaviors.

Atypical antipsychotics can lower the seizure threshold, so patients with seizure disorders must be monitored closely when taking these medications. Patients with liver or kidney problems should avoid taking atypical antipsychotics, if possible. Some atypical antipsychotics can cause bone marrow suppression, a rare but serious side effect. Regular laboratory tests are necessary to check for this condition.

Atypical antipsychotics should be used with caution in older adults because excessive dizziness, drops in blood pressure, and sedation can cause falls. Patients must be monitored closely. Because their kidney and liver functions are often reduced in older adult patients, they cannot effectively eliminate these medications. Therefore, reduced doses are necessary.

Because patients at any age who have schizophrenia or psychosis can have thought disorders, it is important for patients to be monitored closely and offered counseling or psychotherapy in addition to drug treatment.

Patients should not drink alcohol while taking atypical antipsychotic medications because excessive sedation and hallucinations can occur. The pharmacy technician should affix an auxiliary warning label about alcohol use when dispensing these medications.

Drug Interactions Antipsychotics may increase the CNS side effects of azelastine and thalidomide. Metoclopramide may increase the adverse effects of antipsychotics.

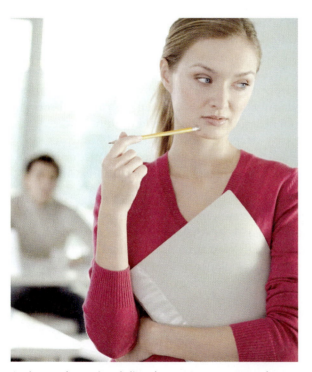

Anxiety and emotional disorders can separate people from their friends and loved ones. Medications can relieve the symptoms so that patients may lead productive, positive lives.

Anxiety

Anxiety is a state of uneasiness characterized by apprehension and worry about possible events. Anxiety is a common complaint made to physicians. It is a collection of unpleasant feelings identical to the fearful feelings experienced under conditions of actual danger. The patient feels generalized tension and apprehension and startles easily. Other symptoms include uneasiness and nervousness at work or with people, or vague, nagging uncertainty about the future. These feelings may lead to chronic fatigue, headaches, and insomnia.

Exogenous anxiety (anxiety caused by factors outside the organism) develops in response to external stresses. The response may be appropriate if conditions warrant apprehension and fear.

Endogenous anxiety (anxiety caused by factors within the organism) is not related to any identifiable external factors but occurs spontaneously as a result of a defined abnormality in cellular function in the CNS. The most common way that people deal with anxiety is by consuming excessive alcohol.

Antianxiety Agents

Antianxiety agents include both noncontrolled and controlled substances (see Table 7.11). SSRIs and SNRIs are key therapies used to treat anxiety. Benzodiazepines, which are also effective in the treatment of insomnia, panic disorders, alcohol withdrawal syndrome, convulsive disorders, and muscle spasms, are also used to treat anxiety. When used short term, they can be effective in controlling anxiety. They are used in the lowest possible doses that control the symptoms while minimizing side effects.

Patients taking antianxiety drugs should be monitored closely for the onset of depression, which occurs in about one-third of cases. Patients who discontinue medication have a high rate of relapse. The drug must be tapered to avoid withdrawal reactions.

Benzodiazepines

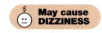

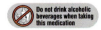

Benzodiazepines are used to treat anxiety, panic disorder, and PTSD. They are regularly used as preanesthetic medications to calm patients prior to procedures such as a colonoscopy or surgery. Benzodiazepines are also part of the standard treatment for alcohol withdrawal symptoms and status epilepticus.

Benzodiazepines work by stimulating GABA receptors in the CNS, thereby causing drowsiness and relaxation. When used to treat anxiety, benzodiazepines have a calming and sometimes euphoric effect. When used for sleep, they reduce the time it takes to fall asleep, decrease early morning wakening, and generally improve sleep quality.

Safety Alert

Patients who consistently request refills of benzodiazepines a few days early could be exhibiting physical or psychological dependence. Alert the prescriber if you receive frequent refill authorization requests from the pharmacy as this could be a sign that dependence is developing. Some patients may need help to stop taking these drugs and may benefit from intervention.

Common side effects of benzodiazepines include muscle weakness, impaired reflexes, and constipation. Patients may also experience difficulty waking up in the morning and residual drowsiness the following day. Pharmacy technicians should affix an auxiliary warning label about drowsiness to each benzodiazepine prescription. Other concerning effects include drowsiness, oversedation, and respiratory depression (slowed breathing). Patients should be informed of these effects and notify their physicians if they occur. In settings where patients taking benzodiazepines can be observed, such as in inpatient or long-term care facilities, caregivers should monitor these patients for slowed breathing and excessive sleepiness. Patients should not drink alcohol or take other medications that cause sedation (e.g., opiate pain medications) because excessive sedation and drastically slowed breathing can occur. Breathing can slow to the point of causing death.

Contraindications Alprazolam is contraindicated in patients with narrow-angle glaucoma and in individuals taking ketoconazole or itraconazole. Clonazepam should not be used in patients with acute narrow-angle glaucoma or liver disease. Clorazepate is contraindicated in patients with narrow-angle glaucoma. Contraindications to diazepam include myasthenia gravis, respiratory insufficiency, liver disease, sleep apnea, and acute narrow-angle glaucoma. Lorazepam is contraindicated in patients with acute narrow-angle glaucoma, sleep apnea, and respiratory insufficiency. Chlordiazepoxide and oxazepam do not have contraindications.

Cautions and Considerations All benzodiazepines have dependence and abuse potential. Consequently, they are considered Schedule IV controlled substances. Patients can become both physically and psychologically dependent on benzodiazepines, making it difficult to stop therapy. Patients should be aware of this potential and should understand that benzodiazepines should be used only for a short time. If used for longer than a couple of weeks, doses must be slowly tapered to avoid withdrawal symptoms.

Because they are controlled substances, benzodiazepine prescriptions have a limited number of refills and may have specific storage requirements. You should be familiar with regulations and follow your facility's policies and procedures for dispensing benzodiazepines at your practice site. Patients with heart conditions may not be able to take benzodiazepines and should be monitored closely. These medications can increase heart rate.

TABLE 7.11   Most Commonly Used Antianxiety Agents

Generic (Brand)	Pronunciation	Dosage Form	Dispensing Status	Control Schedule
SSRIs/SNRIs				
citalopram (Celexa)	sye-TAL-oh-pram	Oral solution, tablet	Rx	
duloxetine (Cymbalta)	doo-LOX-a-teen	Capsule	Rx	
escitalopram (Lexapro)	es-sye-TAL-oh-pram	Oral liquid, tablet	Rx	
paroxetine (Paxil)	pa-ROX-e-teen	Oral liquid, tablet	Rx	
sertraline (Zoloft)	SER-tra-leen	Oral liquid, tablet	Rx	
venlafaxine (Effexor)	ven-la-FAX-een	Capsule, tablet	Rx	
Benzodiazepines				
alprazolam (Xanax)	al-PRAZ-oh-lam	Oral disintigrating tablet, oral liquid, tablet	Rx	C-IV
chlordiazepoxide (Librium)	klor-dye-az-e-POX-ide	Capsule	Rx	C-IV
clorazepate (Tranxene)	klor-AZ-e-pate	Tablet	Rx	C-IV
clonazepam (Klonopin)	kloe-NA-ze-pam	Oral disintegrating tablet, tablet	Rx	C-IV
diazepam (Valium)	dye-AZ-e-pam	Injection, oral liquid, tablet	Rx	C-IV
lorazepam (Ativan)	lor-AZ-e-pam	Injection, oral liquid, tablet	Rx	C-IV
oxazepam (Serax)	ox-AZ-e-pam	Capsule	Rx	C-IV
Other Antianxiety Agents				
buspirone (BuSpar)	byoo-SPYE-rone	Tablet	Rx	
hydroxyzine (Atarax, Vistaril)	hye-DROX-i-zeen	Capsule, injection, oral solution, syrup, tablet	Rx	

Drug Interactions The effects of CNS depressants may be enhanced by benzodiazepines. Azole antifungals may decrease the metabolism of benzodiazepines. Digoxin and phenytoin concentrations may be increased by benzodiazepines. TCA levels may increase when used with benzodiazepines. Benzodiazepines may cause physical or psychological dependence, or both.

Other Antianxiety Agents

Buspirone (BuSpar) acts by selectively antagonizing serotonin receptors without affecting the receptors for benzodiazepine and GABA. Buspirone is not a controlled substance. Buspirone should be taken with food, and the patient should report any changes in the senses (hearing, smell, or taste). It takes about two weeks to see the full effect of this drug. It has few side effects; nausea and headache are the most common. Buspirone has shown little potential for abuse. It is also used for depression.

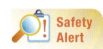
Contraindications Buspirone does not have contraindications.

Cautions and Considerations Buspirone has been associated with depression and increased suicidal tendencies. Patients taking this medication should be monitored closely. Counseling should accompany buspirone therapy when warranted.

Drug Interactions Buspirone, when combined with MAOIs, may elevate blood pressure. Do not use with sedative hypnotic drugs because it may increase CNS depression. Buspirone may worsen OCD in patients using fluoxetine.

Hydroxyzine Pamoate (Vistaril), used for some anxious patients, is a sedative and is widely used as a preoperative sedative and sleeping pill. This drug is thought to depress subcortical areas of the CNS. (Hydroxyzine chloride [Atarax] is used for itching.)

Panic Disorder

Panic disorder is a form of intense, overwhelming, and uncontrollable anxiety. It is neither a voluntary, controllable emotion nor a condition that can be avoided by ignoring it or wishing it away.

Panic attacks have a definite onset and end spontaneously. They occur in public or at home, sometimes interrupting sleep. They are characterized by a sense of fear, apprehension, a premonition of serious illness, and fear of a life-threatening attack. The criteria for diagnosis are three attacks in a three-week period, not stimulated by physical exertion, life-threatening situations, or exposure to phobic stimulus; and at least four of the following symptoms: dyspnea (labored breathing), palpitations, chest pain or discomfort, choking sensation, dizziness, feelings of unreality, tingling in the hands or feet, hot or cold flashes, sweating, numbness, and trembling.

Panic disorder appears to result from a neurochemical defect in part of the brain. In some persons, the brain stem functions abnormally. This abnormality, often characterized by progressive oversensitivity, can develop at any age and occurs in the *locus coeruleus*, a group of synapses in the brain stem at the level of the pons and medulla. The locus coeruleus determines the organism's level of arousal. Sensory information that arrives from all parts of the body passes through this major neurologic junction before being distributed to other parts of the brain. If an abnormality occurs in the locus coeruleus, incoming signals are affected, depending on both the current state of the organism and the nature of the arriving messages. If incoming messages are inappropriately amplified to signal a life-threatening stress, the organism is aroused to defense or flight. Excessive amplification of incoming messages gives rise to a state of excessive arousal, excessive autonomic discharges, and increased respiratory drive. If the incoming message is calm and nonthreatening, the stimuli are subdued, and the locus coeruleus does not overreact.

Patients who have panic disorder are unusually sensitive to the stimulant effects of low doses of caffeine and sodium lactate that, when infused, alter intracellular pH and increase impulse transmission through the brain, causing panic symptoms.

Treatment of Panic Disorder

A panic attack is postulated to be of neurochemical origin and has both emotional and physical components. The most successful treatment combines medication and behavioral therapy.

Psychotherapy is the preferred treatment in panic disorders for patients whose symptoms cause significant discomfort or impairment. Panic disorders have a true biochemical basis and can be effectively treated. These disorders should be viewed with the same objectivity as other chronic, incurable diseases that can be controlled with medications.

Short-term administration of an antianxiety agent may be indicated. Drug therapy blocks the autonomic expression of the panic. SSRIs, benzodiazepines, buspirone, and, to a lesser extent, the beta-adrenergic blocking agents are the most appropriate pharmacologic alternatives. Diphenhydramine, hydroxyzine, and other antihistamines are sometimes prescribed, especially for older adults. TCAs have also proven to be effective.

Sleep and Sleep Disorders

Sleep is fundamental to human health (as well as the health of all mammals and many other vertebrates). Sleep research has recognized four stages of sleep:

- Stage I involves nonrapid eye movements (NREM). The subject is somewhat aware of his or her surroundings and is relaxed (4 %–5% of sleep time).
- Stage II also involves NREM. The subject is unaware of surroundings but can be easily awakened (50% of sleep time).
- Stages III and IV involve rapid eye movements (REMs). The subject's sleep is characterized by increased autonomic activity and by episodes of REM sleep with dreaming, if possible. This deep sleep (20%–25% of sleep time), which occurs four to five times per night (for a total of >90 minutes), is important for physical rest.

Insomnia

Many adults have trouble sleeping. Approximately 6% of these individuals seek a physician's help. **Insomnia** is characterized by difficulty falling or staying asleep and by not feeling refreshed on awakening. The symptoms of insomnia are indications for using a **hypnotic** (a drug that induces sleep).

Insomnia may be a chronic condition or an occasional or short-term problem. Transient insomnia is not really a sleep disorder. It is usually a response to an acute stressful event and can typically be expected to improve with time as the person adapts to the stress. Chronic insomnia most often has multifaceted origins. The first evaluation of patients should include sleep, drug, medical, and psychiatric histories.

Some types of sleep disorders can be caused by various events or conditions. The causes can be:

- situational: job stress, hospitalization, or travel;
- medical: pain, respiratory problems, or GI problems;
- psychiatric: schizophrenia, depression, or mania;
- drug induced: alcohol, caffeine, or sympathomimetic agents.

In these cases, diagnosis and effective treatment of the cause can usually eliminate the need for using hypnotic drugs. Treating only the symptoms of insomnia can make it difficult to recognize and treat the underlying illness. Furthermore, it can subject patients to psychological or physical dependence on the drugs.

Narcolepsy

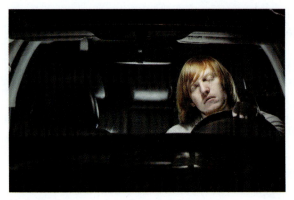

Narcolepsy occurs more frequently in men.

Narcolepsy is a sleep disorder involving recurring inappropriate episodes of sleep during the daytime hours. There is no known cause. Onset usually occurs in adolescents or young adults, and this disorder continues throughout life. It occurs four times more frequently in men than women. Narcolepsy exhibits four characteristic symptoms. First, the patient feels sleepy during the daytime, proceeding almost immediately into REM sleep without first entering NREM. The patient can only briefly resist the desire to sleep. Second, the patient experiences **cataplexy**, or short periods of muscle weakness or loss of muscle tone, associated with sudden emotions such as joy, fear, or anger. Third, sleep paralysis occurs as the patient falls asleep or immediately upon awakening. The patient wishes to move but finds that, for a brief period, he or she cannot. Fourth, the patient has vivid hallucinations at the onset of sleep.

Treatment of Narcolepsy

Therapeutic approaches include drug and nondrug therapy. Nondrug therapy includes lifestyle changes to establish a consistent sleep schedule, avoidance of shift work, and avoidance of alcohol. Stimulants such as methylphenidate and dextroamphetamine have been the drug therapy mainstay for sleepiness. (These drugs will be discussed in Chapter 8.) TCAs and SSRIs work well in the treatment of cataplexy. Two drugs specifically approved for narcolepsy are listed in Table 7.12.

One drug approved for narcolepsy is **modafinil (Provigil)**. It is a nonamphetamine stimulant, but it is a Schedule IV controlled substance. Modafinil is also approved for shift-work sleep disorder, which is a disturbance in the circadian rhythm (body cycles that occur within a 24-hour period at about the same time each day) and is a response to changes in exposure to light and dark. This problem affects people who work at night. The mechanism of action is unclear, but modafinil does increase mental alertness.

Contraindications Hypersensitivity to armodafinil contraindicates the use of modafinil.

Cautions and Considerations Modafinil may impair the ability to engage in hazardous activities, and patients should be warned about performing activities that require mental alertness, such as driving.

TABLE 7.12 **Drugs Used to Treat Narcolepsy**

Generic (Brand)	Pronunciation	Dosage Form	Common Dosage	Dispensing Status	Control Schedule
armodafinil (Nuvigil)	ar-moe-DAF-i-nil	Tablet	150 to 250 mg once daily	Rx	C-IV
modafinil (Provigil)	moe-DAF-i-nil	Tablet	200 mg once daily	Rx	C-IV

Modafinil may increase blood pressure and heart rate. Use with caution in patients with cardiac issues.

Patients should avoid alcohol when using modafinil.

Drug Interactions Modafinil may decrease concentrations of axitinib, bosutinib, enzalutamide, nisoldipine, olaparib, simeprevir, and sofosbuvir. Conivaptan may increase modafinil levels. Idelalisib and pimozide concentrations may increase with modafinil use.

Armodafinil (Nuvigil) is structurally related to modafinil. It is approved for excessive sleepiness caused by sleep apnea, narcolepsy, or shift-work sleep disorder. The mechanism of action is unknown. Armodafinil should be taken in the morning or one hour before going to work if taken for shift-work sleep disorder. It will not cure sleep apnea, but it will help diminish the symptoms. Armodafinil should not be taken close to the time of sleep and should not be taken for longer than 12 weeks. When prescribed to treat sleep apnea, armodafinil is commonly combined with a continuous positive airway pressure (CPAP) machine. The CPAP machine consists of an air pump, connected to a mask, that blows pressurized air into the nose while sleeping. It does not interrupt normal sleep patterns. The most serious side effect of armodafinil is a skin rash. If a rash appears, the patient should immediately stop taking armodafinil.

Contraindications Hypersensitivity to modafinil contraindicates its use.

Cautions and Considerations Armodafinil may impair the ability to engage in hazardous activities, and patients should be warned about performing activities that require mental alertness, such as driving. Because the drug works on the CNS, alcohol should be avoided while taking this drug.

Armodafinil should never be used in place of getting enough sleep, and it may decrease the effectiveness of oral contraceptives.

Drug Interactions Conivaptan and fusidic acid may increase armodafinil levels. Idelalisib concentrations may increase with armodafinil use.

Treatment of Sleep Disorders

Effective treatment of sleep disorders necessitates both pharmacologic and nonpharmacologic measures. For patients with clearly defined insomnia, pharmacologic treatment consists primarily of the adjunctive use of hypnotics. Table 7.13 lists the most commonly used agents for sleep disorders, several of which are among the antianxiety medications listed in Table 7.11. Nonpharmacologic treatment includes supportive counseling and behavioral treatment. The components of this therapy include:

- normalizing the sleep schedule for bedtime and waking time
- increasing physical exercise during the daytime
- discontinuing use of alcohol as a sedative
- sleeping a total of only 7–8 hours in a 24-hour period
- reducing caffeine and nicotine intake
- eliminating any drug (e.g., decongestant) that could lead to insomnia

A person facing a clearly identified external stress (i.e., grief reaction) may become anxious and have difficulty sleeping. A one- to three-week course of treatment with a hypnotic agent may be justified in such instances. Hypnotic drugs should be used only as an adjunct to medical therapeutic measures.

TABLE 7.13 Most Commonly Used Sleep Agents

Generic (Brand)	Pronunciation	Dosage Form	Common Dosage	Dispensing Status	Controlled-Substance Schedule
Benzodiazepines					
estazolam (ProSom)	es-TAZ-oe-lam	Tablet	1–2 mg	Rx	C-IV
flurazepam (Dalmane)	floo-RAZ-e-pam	Capsule	15–30 mg	Rx	C-IV
quazepam (Doral)	KWA-ze-pam	Tablet	7.5–15 mg	Rx	C-IV
temazepam (Restoril)	tem-AZ-e-pam	Capsule	7.5–30 mg	Rx	C-IV
triazolam (Halcion)	trye-AY-zoe-lam	Tablet	0.25–0.5 mg	Rx	C-IV
Hypnotics					
ramelteon (Rozerem)	ra-MEL-tee-on	Tablet	8 mg within 30 minutes of bedtime	Rx	
Z-Drugs					
eszopiclone (Lunesta)	es-zo-PIK-lone	Tablet	1–3 mg immediately before bedtime	Rx	C-IV
zaleplon (Sonata)	ZAL-e-plon	Capsule	5–20 mg immediately before bedtime	Rx	C-IV
zolpidem (Ambien, Zolpimist)	ZOLE-pi-dem	Spray, tablet	5–12.5 mg immediately before bedtime	Rx	C-IV

Therapy with hypnotic agents decreases the time it takes to fall asleep, reduces early-morning awakenings, increases total sleep, and improves quality of sleep. Three specific criteria guide the choice when prescribing a hypnotic drug:

- The agent must have low addiction and suicide potential.
- The agent must minimally alter electroencephalographic patterns (brain activity) and not depress REM sleep.
- The agent must have minimal interaction with other drugs.

Patients should be informed of the limitations of drugs used to induce sleep. To reduce the risk of habituation and increase the duration of effectiveness, they should be taken as needed, rather than every night. It is easy to slip into the habit of taking these drugs every day, and the patient may not be able to sleep without them. Therapy should be started with a small dose, to be increased only if the initial dose is ineffective. Sleep agents are best administered one hour before bedtime.

The primary side effect of sleep medications (seen more often with high doses) is CNS depression, which results in dizziness, confusion, next-day drowsiness, and impaired reflexes. Some patients, particularly older adults, may exhibit paradoxical reactions (excitation, irritability, and, occasionally, aggressive behavior). Anterograde amnesia (impaired memory of the event) may also occur after taking a hypnotic.

Benzodiazepines

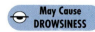

Benzodiazepines, discussed earlier with antianxiety agents, are also used for insomnia. The FDA has specifically approved five benzodiazepines for hypnotic use: estazolam,

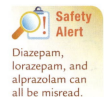
flurazepam, quazepam, temazepam, and triazolam. Common side effects of benzodiazepines include muscle weakness, impaired reflexes, and constipation. Patients may also experience difficulty waking up in the morning and residual drowsiness the following day. Pharmacy technicians should affix an auxiliary warning label about drowsiness to each benzodiazepine prescription.

Contraindications Benzodiazepines are contraindicated in pregnant women. They may cause fetal damage when administered during pregnancy. Allergy to one benzodiazepine contraindicates use of others.

Quazepam is contraindicated in patients with established or suspected sleep apnea and pulmonary insufficiency.

Triazolam is contraindicated in patients using cytochrome P-450 3A4 inhibitors (such as itraconazole, ketoconazole, and several HIV protease inhibitors).

Cautions and Considerations All benzodiazepines have dependence and abuse potential. Consequently, they are considered Schedule IV controlled substances. Patients can become both physically and psychologically dependent on benzodiazepines, making it difficult to stop therapy. Patients should be aware of this potential and should understand that benzodiazepines should be used only for a short time. If used for longer than a couple of weeks, doses must be slowly tapered to prevent withdrawal symptoms. Because they are controlled substances, benzodiazepine prescriptions have a limited number of refills and may have specific storage requirements. You should be familiar with regulations and follow your facility's policies and procedures for dispensing benzodiazepines at your practice site. Patients with heart conditions may not be able to take benzodiazepines and should be monitored closely. These medications can increase heart rate.

Drug Interactions The effects of CNS depressants may be enhanced by benzodiazepines. Azole antifungals may decrease the metabolism of benzodiazepines. Digoxin and phenytoin concentrations may be increased by benzodiazepines. TCA levels may increase when used with benzodiazepines.

Ramelteon

Ramelteon (Rozerem) is approved for sleep-onset insomnia. It is a melatonin receptor agonist, so there is no potential for abuse, and it is not a controlled substance. It is more potent than melatonin. It has not been shown to be effective in sleep maintenance disorders, just for initiating sleep. It has a rapid onset and no next-day morning grogginess.

Contraindications Contraindications include a history of angioedema with previous ramelteon therapy and concurrent use with fluvoxamine.

Cautions and Considerations CNS depression may result from the use of ramelteon, including impaired physical and mental capabilities. Patients should be warned about performing tasks that require mental alertness.

Hypnotics are associated with behavior changes and abnormal thinking. Aggression, bizarre behavior, agitation, and hallucinations have all occurred in patients using hypnotics.

Ramelteon should not be taken with or immediately following a high-fat meal. Patients with liver problems should discuss use of ramelteon with their healthcare practitioners before taking it.

Drug Interactions Ramelteon is a CNS depressant and may enhance the effects of other CNS depressants (such as azelastine, orphenadrine, paraldehyde, sodium oxybate, and thalidomide). Fluvoxamine may decrease the metabolism of ramelteon.

Z-Drugs

A newer class of drugs called the Z-drugs has emerged for the treatment of sleep disorders. Z-drugs have relatively short half-lives and, unlike other hypnotics, do not significantly impact REM sleep.

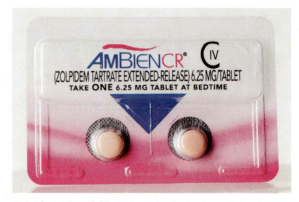

Zolpidem is available in a controlled-release formulation under the brand name Ambien CR.

Side effects of the Z-drugs may include sleepwalking or eating, with no recall of the events. There have also been reports of people driving (sleepdriving) with no recall of the event. The FDA is investigating these reports and encouraging manufacturers to include these side effects in their labeling. Patients using a hypnotic should use it only a limited number of times each week, and that use should be restricted to a four- to six-week period.

Eszopiclone (Lunesta) is similar to zolpidem; however, the FDA has approved it for chronic insomnia. It may cause an unpleasant taste, which usually disappears after a couple of weeks. The medication should be taken immediately before bedtime.

Zaleplon (Sonata), the shortest-acting hypnotic, has a four-hour duration of action. It can be taken in the middle of the night. Depending on when the drug is taken, there should be little leftover morning grogginess. Use should be limited to 7–10 days. Zaleplon has the advantage of having the lowest risk of next-day impairment of cognitive function. Patients should be warned to take this drug right before going to bed and allow enough time to sleep before the drug wears off.

Zolpidem (Ambien, Zolpimist) has the hypnotic (and many of the anxiolytic) properties of the benzodiazepines, but it is structurally dissimilar. It has a high affinity for the benzodiazepine receptors, especially the omega$_1$ receptors, but it has reduced effects on skeletal muscle and seizure threshold. Rarely is mechanical ventilation required for an overdose. Zolpidem is used for short-term treatment of insomnia. The side effects are dizziness, headache, nausea, diarrhea, and next-day drowsiness. Like zaleplon, this drug also should not be taken for more than 10 days. The pharmacy technician should monitor the prescriptions and alert the pharmacist if it is prescribed for a longer period. Of course, there may be exceptions. Ambien CR is approved for long-term use. It is a controlled-release form that contains 12.5 mg, of which 10 mg is released immediately, then 2.5 mg later in the night to help maintain sleep. It prevents early awakening. Zolpimist is the spray form.

Contraindications The Z-drugs do not have contraindications.

Cautions and Considerations Eszopiclone, zaleplon, and zolpidem are controlled substances. Pharmacy technicians should be aware of laws regarding controlled substances in the state in which they practice.

CNS depression may result with Z-drug use, including impaired physical and mental capabilities. Patients should be warned about performing tasks that require mental alertness.

Hypnotics are associated with behavior changes and abnormal thinking. Aggression, bizarre behavior, agitation, and hallucinations have all occurred in patients using hypnotics.

Drug Interactions The Z-drugs cause CNS depression and enhance the adverse effects of other CNS depressants (such as opioids, orphenadrine, paraldehyde, and thalidomide).

Conivaptan and fusidic acid may increase levels of Z-drugs.

Alcohol Dependence

Alcohol dependence, sometimes referred to as alcoholism, is a pattern of alcohol use that involves problems controlling drinking, preoccupation with alcohol, use of alcohol even when it causes problems, drinking more to get the same effect, or having withdrawal symptoms with rapidly decreasing or stopping drinking. The World Health Organization estimates that 75 million people suffer from alcohol dependence globally. Genetic, psychological, social, and environmental factors all contribute to alcohol dependence. Theories suggest that, for certain people, drinking has a different and stronger impact that can lead to alcohol use disorder.

Alcohol abuse can impact health. Liver disease, digestive problems, cardiac complications, diabetes, sexual dysfunction, immune system weakening, and neurologic complications can all result. Furthermore, alcohol abuse can impact safety and increase the risk of motor vehicle accidents, drowning, and legal problems.

Alcoholism is a complex genetic disease. The abuser has different levels of brain chemicals, different levels of enzymes, or altogether different enzymes that metabolize the alcohol at different rates and quantities than in nonalcoholics. Thus, genetic makeup may affect a person's likelihood of becoming an alcohol abuser.

Ethanol (alcohol) is an anesthetic. As with any anesthetic, intake of a large quantity of ethanol causes loss of consciousness. However, the margin between loss of consciousness and medullary paralysis is smaller than with general anesthetics. The **emetic (vomit-inducing)** action usually prevents death by reducing absorption of lethal concentrations. Many deaths from alcohol are due to cirrhosis (irreversible damage) of the liver or aspiration of vomitus during unconsciousness.

The habitual drinker has an increased ability to metabolize ethanol rapidly, which increases tolerance. Neurons in the CNS adapt to the presence of ethanol, and the drinker learns to compensate to some extent for the depressant action.

Abuse of alcohol takes a heavy toll on many aspects of health. Heavy drinking may lead to the serious complication of obesity coupled with vitamin deficiency. In the later stages of alcoholism, gastritis and loss of appetite, organic brain damage, alcoholic psychosis, and dementia occur. Cirrhosis of the liver results from fatty synthesis and excessive buildup of lipid compounds.

Dependence and Withdrawal from Alcohol

Chemical dependence is the inability to control the use of some physical substance; the person is unable to stop the use or limit the amount taken. Dependence is often a physical condition that cannot be cured by willpower. A person can be chemically dependent without showing obvious signs. Table 7.14 lists symptoms of dependence. To resolve their problem, alcohol abusers must take four steps toward recovery:

1. Acknowledge the problem.
2. Limit the time spent with substance users.
3. Seek professional help.
4. Seek support from recovering alcoholics.

TABLE 7.14   Alcohol Dependence Symptoms

Blackouts or lapses of memory
Concerns of family, friends, and employers about drinking
Doing things while under the influence of alcohol that cause regret afterward
Financial or legal problems from drinking
Loss of pleasure without alcohol
Neglecting responsibilities
Trying to cut down or quit drinking but failing
Drinking alone; hiding evidence
Drinking to forget about problems
Willingness to do almost anything to get alcohol

TABLE 7.15   Alcohol Withdrawal Symptoms

Agitation	Mental disturbances
Circulatory disturbances	Nausea and vomiting
Convulsions	Restlessness
Delirium tremens (DTs)	Sweating
Digestive disorders	Temporary suppression of REM sleep
Disorientation	Tremors
Extreme fear	Weakness
Hallucinations	

Abrupt withdrawal of alcohol can precipitate a variety of symptoms, some of which are serious and even life-threatening. Table 7.15 lists withdrawal symptoms. The first signs of withdrawal appear within a few hours. In mild withdrawal, symptoms may disappear in one to two days; in severe withdrawal, symptoms may last one to two weeks.

Benzodiazepines are frequently used for detoxification. Their dosage must be adjusted to the needs of individual patients. Benzodiazepines will also prevent detoxification-related seizures and **delirium tremens (DTs)**, a condition caused by cessation of alcohol consumption, in which coarse, irregular tremors are accompanied by vivid hallucinations.

Therapy may also necessitate administering a sedative, anticonvulsant, beta blocker, antipsychotic drug, or a combination of these drugs. In addition, when an alcoholic enters a treatment program, comes to an emergency room, or is admitted into the hospital, the patient is usually given folic acid (Folvite), thiamine (vitamin B_1), and a multipurpose vitamin. This treatment is given because liver damage, imbalanced fluid intake, and imbalanced nutrition cause alcoholics to be deficient in vitamins, particularly the water-soluble ones.

Alcohol Antagonists

There are three drugs approved for treating alcohol dependence (see Table 7.16). Any drug regimen must be accompanied by psychosocial support.

Acamprosate

Acamprosate (Campral) is thought to work by restoring balance between neuronal excitation and neuronal inhibition. This reestablishment of balance reduces the negative effects of abstinence from alcohol and ideally diminishes the chances of a relapse. A combination of disulfiram and acamprosate may work better than either drug alone. The most common adverse effects include headache, diarrhea, flatulence, and nausea. Drug therapy should be combined with a comprehensive management program that includes psychosocial support. Acamprosate is taken three times a day, with meals—because food increases absorption. This regimen may also improve patient adherence and may help prevent alcohol cravings and relapses. Acamprosate, however, is not an effective treatment for delirium tremens.

Contraindications Acamprosate is contraindicated in patients with severe renal failure.

Cautions and Considerations Acamprosate use may cause CNS depression. Patients using acamprosate have attempted suicide. Patients should be monitored for depression and suicidal thinking. Dose adjustment is needed in patients with renal insufficiency.

Drug Interactions There are no known drug interactions.

Disulfiram

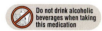

Disulfiram (Antabuse) stops the metabolism of alcohol at the acetaldehyde stage, allowing the latter to accumulate in body tissues. When a patient taking disulfiram consumes alcohol, the acetaldehyde causes violent side effects almost instantaneously. These side effects include:

- blurred vision
- confusion
- difficulty breathing
- hot, flushed face
- intense throbbing in head and neck
- chest pain

- nausea
- severe headache
- severe vomiting
- thirst
- uneasiness

These side effects are known as disulfiram-like reactions. The patient usually becomes exhausted and sleeps for several hours after symptoms have worn off. Patients who are taking disulfiram must examine food labels to be sure they do not inadvertently ingest alcohol in an everyday product (e.g., cough medicines, mouthwashes, salad dressings, and wine vinegars). Several other prescription drugs can produce a disulfiram-like reaction when combined with alcohol. These medications

TABLE 7.16 Most Commonly Used Alcohol Antagonists

Generic (Brand)	Pronunciation	Dosage Form	Common Dosage	Dispensing Status
acamprosate (Campral)	a-kam-PROE-sate	Tablet	666 mg three times daily	Rx
disulfiram (Antabuse)	dye-SUL-fi-ram	Tablet	125–500 mg daily	Rx
naltrexone (ReVia, Vivitrol)	nal-TREX-one	Tablet, injectable	oral 50 mg a day; IM 380 mg every 4 weeks	Rx

include metronidazole, some cephalosporins, and certain oral hypoglycemic drugs. Pharmacy technicians should place an auxiliary warning label about alcohol use to these medication containers during the dispensing process.

Contraindications Contraindications to disulfiram include severe myocardial disease and/or coronary occlusion, psychosis, or known hypersensitivity to the medication or other thiuram derivatives. Disulfiram is generally avoided in pregnant and nursing women.

Cautions and Considerations Disulfiram has a black box warning. It should never be administered to a patient during a state of ethanol intoxication or without the patient's knowledge.

Liver dysfunction is associated with disulfiram use. Consequently, liver function should be monitored in patients.

Drug Interactions The adverse effects of alcohol and products that contain alcohol (such as lopinavir-ritonavir and ritonavir oral solution) are potentiated with disulfiram use. Disulfiram may enhance the adverse effects of metronidazole. The body levels of paraldehyde and phenytoin may be increased by disulfiram. Tinidazole may enhance the adverse effects of disulfiram.

Naltrexone

Naltrexone (ReVia) is a pure opiate antagonist that blocks the effects of endogenous opioids released as a result of alcohol consumption, making alcohol consumption less pleasurable. It is used to treat alcohol dependence. Naltrexone can cause an acute withdrawal syndrome, including nausea, dizziness, headache, and weight loss, in opiate-dependent patients. The patient should be stable after alcohol withdrawal before starting this drug. To prevent withdrawal symptoms, those individuals with a history of opiate intake must be opiate-free before starting the drug. Vivitrol is the injectable extended-release form of this drug. It decreases the effectiveness of opiates for pain, cough, and diarrhea. Patients taking this drug should wear a medical alert pendant or bracelet so that, if they end up in the emergency room, the staff will know not to provide opiates. The drug must be refrigerated, except for the week just before injection. It is packaged in a single-use carton that contains the drug in powdered form, diluent, and syringe. It is administered intramuscularly, monthly, in alternating buttocks.

Contraindications Contraindications include opioid dependence or current use of opioid analgesics (including partial opioid agonists), acute opioid withdrawal, and failure to pass the naloxone challenge or positive urine screen for opioids.

Cautions and Considerations Accidental opioid overdose may occur with naltrexone use. Patients using naltrexone may respond to lower opioid doses than previously used, leading to life-threatening opioid intoxication.

Use naltrexone with caution in patients with hepatic dysfunction.

Drug Interactions Naltrexone may enhance the adverse effects of methylnaltrexone and naloxegol.

Complementary and Alternative Therapies

Melatonin is used for sleep and insomnia disorders as well as for benzodiazepine and nicotine withdrawal. It is used occasionally for a variety of other disorders including headache.

Melatonin is a naturally produced hormone that helps regulate circadian rhythms (the sleep-wake cycle). People generally take 0.3 to 5 mg before bedtime to induce sleep. Common side effects include drowsiness, headache, and dizziness. Melatonin can also cause mild tremors, anxiety, abdominal cramps, irritability, confusion, nausea, and low blood pressure. Melatonin interacts with other medications; it should never be taken with CNS depressants because excessive sedation could occur.

Kava is used to treat anxiety and insomnia. It has been found to be effective but dangerous. Kava can induce hepatotoxicity and liver failure, so patient self-treatment is not recommended. Kava lactone is the active ingredient and is thought to work by affecting GABA and dopamine in the brain. Other side effects include stomach upset, headache, dizziness, drowsiness, dry mouth, and EPS effects. Patients should also realize that herbal, dietary, and other supplements are not subject to the standardization among manufacturers that are required for prescription and OTC drugs.

St. John's wort is taken orally for mild depression with some success. It has also been used to relieve the psychological symptoms of menopause when used with black cohosh (Remifemin). Patients should discuss St. John's wort with their healthcare practitioners before taking it and make sure it is documented in their medication history.

The active ingredient in St. John's wort is hypericin, which has activity similar to that of SSRIs. Common starting doses range from 300 to 400 mg three times daily. Maintenance doses are often lower and may range from 300 to 900 mg daily. Side effects include insomnia, vivid dreams, restlessness, anxiety, irritability, upset stomach, diarrhea, fatigue, dry mouth, dizziness, and headache. Usually these effects are mild. St. John's wort can cause photosensitivity, so proper skin protection should be used.

St. John's wort should not be taken with other antidepressants because serotonin syndrome could develop. In addition, it should not be taken with CNS depressants, such as digoxin, phenytoin, or phenobarbital. St. John's wort can alter the effectiveness of these and other drugs, including warfarin and some drugs for HIV and acquired immune deficiency syndrome (AIDS).

Patients taking natural products for mood disorders or insomnia should discuss this therapy with their healthcare practitioners. Herbal and dietary supplements may not adequately treat symptoms of depression or insomnia. Patients who display symptoms of mental illness should be evaluated by a physician and should not be self-treated. Encourage patients to communicate with their healthcare practitioners.

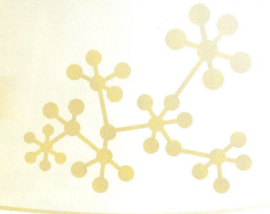

CHAPTER SUMMARY

Depression and Mood Disorders

- Antidepressants are not controlled substances.

- Antidepressants are classified as SSRIs, tricyclic and tetracyclic antidepressants, SNRIs, and MAOIs.

- SSRIs block the reuptake of serotonin, with little effect on norepinephrine. They have fewer side effects than the older antidepressant medications.

- TCAs can be cardiotoxic in high doses.

- MAOIs are not first-line therapy for depression because of their many interactions with drugs and foods.

- It may take at least two weeks for some of the antidepressants to be effective.

- Lithium is commonly used to treat bipolar (manic-depressive) disorder and acute mania and for prophylaxis of unipolar and bipolar disorders.

- A patient taking lithium must have frequent blood tests to assess lithium levels and maintain a therapeutic range.

- Carbamazepine (Tegretol) or divalproex (Depakote) may be used to treat bipolar disorder.

Psychosis

- The older agents are identified as "typical" or first-generation antipsychotics and are effective, but serious long-term side effects limit their use. Prescribers are moving away from these drugs and toward the newer "atypical" antipsychotics, such as aripiprazole (Abilify), clozapine (Clozaril), olanzapine (Zyprexa), paliperidone (Invega), quetiapine (Seroquel), risperidone (Risperdal), and ziprasidone (Geodon).

- Anticholinergics can minimize some of the side effects of typical antipsychotic drugs.

Anxiety

- Anxiety is a state of uneasiness characterized by apprehension and worry about possible events.

- SSRIs, SNRIs, benzodiazepines, buspirone, and hydroxyzine are used to treat anxiety.

Sleep and Sleep Disorders

- Benzodiazepines that are FDA-approved for hypnotic use are estazolam (ProSom), flurazepam (Dalmane), quazepam (Doral), temazepam (Restoril), and triazolam (Halcion).

- Hypnotic medications should be administered one hour before bedtime.

- Rozerem is not a controlled substance because it works in a different way from other hypnotics.

- The Z-drugs are the preferred treatment for sleep disorders.

- Zaleplon (Sonata) is the shortest-acting hypnotic, with a duration of action of four hours. Therefore, it may be taken in the middle of the night.

- Zolpidem (Ambien), a Schedule IV drug, has many of the same properties as the benzodiazepines, but it is structurally dissimilar.

- Eszopiclone (Lunesta) is approved for long-term use.

Alcohol Abuse

- Alcohol abuse is a serious disorder.

- Alcohol abusers have an increased ability to metabolize ethanol rapidly, and neurons in the CNS adapt to the presence of ethanol.

- Three drugs have been approved for treatment of alcoholism; they are disulfiram (Antabuse), acamprosate (Campral), and naltrexone (ReVia).

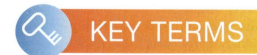 KEY TERMS

agranulocytosis a reduction in white blood cells

alcohol dependence a pattern of alcohol use that involves problems controlling drinking and preoccupation with alcohol; also known as *alcoholism*

anorexia loss of appetite for food

antipsychotic drugs drugs that are used to treat schizophrenia; reduce symptoms of hallucinations, delusions, and thought disorders; also called *neuroleptics*

anxiety a state of uneasiness characterized by apprehension and worry about possible events

atypical antipsychotic drugs first-line therapy for schizophrenia and other psychoses that address specific neurotransmitters

bipolar disorder a condition in which a patient presents with mood swings that alternate between periods of major depression and periods of mild-to-severe chronic agitation

cataplexy short periods of muscle weakness and loss of muscle tone associated with sudden emotions such as joy, fear, or anger; a symptom of narcolepsy

chemical dependence the inability to control the use of some physical substance

delirium tremens (DTs) a condition caused by cessation of alcohol consumption in which coarse, irregular tremors are accompanied by vivid hallucinations

depression a condition characterized by anxiety, hopelessness, irritability, intense sadness, loss of concentration, pessimism, and problems with eating and sleeping

emetic a substance that induces vomiting

endogenous anxiety anxiety caused by factors within the organism

exogenous anxiety anxiety caused by factors outside the organism

extrapyramidal side (EPS) effects disorders of muscle movement control caused by blocking dopamine receptors in the basal ganglia

ghost tablet empty shell of an OROS tablet; excreted in the stool after the drug has dissolved

hypnotic a drug that induces sleep

insomnia difficulty falling asleep or staying asleep, or not feeling refreshed on awakening

mania a state of overly high energy, excitement, hyperactivity, optimism, and increased psychomotor activity

monoamine oxidase inhibitor (MAOI) an antidepressant drug that inhibits the activity of the enzymes that break down catecholamines (such as norepinephrine) and serotonin

narcolepsy a sleep disorder in which inappropriate attacks of sleep occur during the daytime hours

neuroleptic drugs see *antipsychotic drugs*

neurotransmitter a chemical substance emitted by a neuron to communicate, such as serotonin, dopamine, or norepinephrine

orthostatic hypotension a drop in blood pressure on sitting or standing up

osmotic controlled-release oral delivery system (OROS) a drug delivery system that allows the drug to dissolve through pores in the tablet shell; the empty shell, called a *ghost tablet*, is passed in the stool

panic intense, overwhelming, and uncontrollable anxiety

posttraumatic stress disorder (PTSD) a disorder characterized by persistent agitation or persistent, recurrent fear after the end of a traumatic event and lasting for over a month or impairing work or relationships

premenstrual dysphoric disorder (PMDD) a severe form of premenstrual syndrome (PMS)

priapism a prolonged penile erection

QT interval the time between depolarization and repolarization of the ventricles of the heart during a heartbeat, as shown on an electrocardiogram

schizophrenia a chronic mental-health disorder with mental and emotional fragmentation and retreat from reality, hallucinations, ambivalence, and bizarre or regressive behavior

seasonal affective disorder (SAD) a form of depression that recurs in the fall and winter and remits in the spring and summer

selective serotonin reuptake inhibitor (SSRI) an antidepressant drug that blocks the reabsorption of serotonin, with little effect on norepinephrine and fewer side effects than other antidepressant drugs

serotonin-norepinephrine reuptake inhibitor (SNRI) an antidepressant drug that blocks the reabsorption of both serotonin and norepinephrine, increasing the levels of both neurotransmitters

serotonin syndrome a possibly fatal condition caused by combining antidepressants that increase serotonin levels with other medications that also stimulate serotonin receptors

tardive dyskinesia involuntary movements of the mouth, lips, and tongue

tricyclic antidepressant (TCA) one of a class of antidepressant drugs, developed earlier than the SSRIs and SNRIs, that also prevent neuron reuptake of norepinephrine and/or serotonin

washout period the time period one must wait before changing drug therapies so the first drug is out of the patient's system before the new drug takes effect

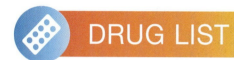

DRUG LIST

Antidepressants

amitriptyline (Elavil)
citalopram (Celexa)
clomipramine (Anafranil)
desipramine (Norpramin)
desvenlafaxine (Pristiq)
doxepin (Sinequan, Zonalon)
duloxetine (Cymbalta)
escitalopram (Lexapro)
fluoxetine (Prozac, Sarafem)
fluvoxamine (Luvox)
imipramine (Tofranil)
mirtazapine (Remeron)
nortriptyline (Aventyl, Pamelor)
paroxetine (Paxil)
phenelzine (Nardil)
selegiline (Eldepryl)
sertraline (Zoloft)
tranylcypromine (Parnate)
venlafaxine (Effexor)

Miscellaneous Antidepressants

bupropion (Aplenzin, Wellbutrin, Zyban)
trazodone (Desyrel)

Drugs to Treat Bipolar Disorders

carbamazepine (Epitol, Tegretol)
divalproex (Depakote)
lithium (Eskalith, Lithobid)
valproic acid (Depakene)

Antipsychotics

aripiprazole (Abilify)
clozapine (Clozaril)
fluphenazine (Prolixin)
haloperidol (Haldol)
olanzapine (Zyprexa)
paliperidone (Invega)
perphenazine (Trilafon)
prochlorperazine (Compazine)
quetiapine (Seroquel)
risperidone (Risperdal)
thioridazine (Mellaril)
trifluoperazine (Stelazine)
ziprasidone (Geodon)

Drugs Used to Minimize the Effects of Antipsychotics

benztropine (Cogentin)
diphenhydramine (Benadryl)

Antianxiety Agents

buspirone (BuSpar)
citalopram (Celexa)
duloxetine (Cymbalta)
escitalopram (Lexapro)
hydroxyzine (Atarax, Vistaril)
paroxetine (Paxil)
sertraline (Zoloft)
venlafaxine (Effexor)

Benzodiazepines

alprazolam (Xanax)
chlordiazepoxide (Librium)
clonazepam (Klonopin)
clorazepate (Tranxene)
diazepam (Valium)
estazolam (ProSom)
flurazepam (Dalmane)
lorazepam (Ativan)
oxazepam (Serax)
quazepam (Doral)
temazepam (Restoril)
triazolam (Halcion)

Stimulants

armodafinil (Nuvigil)
modafinil (Provigil)

Sleep Agents

diphenhydramine (Benadryl)
eszopiclone (Lunesta)
hydroxyzine (Atarax, Vistaril)
ramelteon (Rozerem)
zaleplon (Sonata)
zolpidem (Ambien, Zolpimist)

Alcohol Antagonists

acamprosate (Campral)
disulfiram (Antabuse)
naltrexone (ReVia)

Black Box Warnings

aripiprazole (Abilify)
armodafinil (Nuvigil)
bupropion (Aplenzin, Wellbutrin, Zyban)
citalopram (Celexa)
clomipramine (Anafranil)
clozapine (Clozaril)
desipramine (Norpramin)
desvanlafaxine (Pristiq)
doxepin (Sinequan, Zonalon)
duloxetine (Cymbalta)

escitalopram (Lexapro)
fluoxetine (Prozac, Sarafem)
fluvoxamine (Luvox)
imipramine (Tofranil)
lithium (Eskalith, Lithobid)
mirtazapine (Remeron)
modafinil (Provigil)
naltrexone (ReVia)
nortriptyline (Aventyl, Pamelor)
olanzapine (Zyprexa)
paliperidone (Invega)
paroxetine (Paxil)
phenelzine (Nardil)
propranolol (Inderal)
quetiapine (Seroquel)
risperidone (Risperdal)
selegiline (Eldepryl)
sertraline (Zoloft)
tranylcypromine (Parnate)
trazodone (Desyrel)
venlafaxine (Effexor)
ziprasidone (Geodon)

Medication Guides

Note that bipolar drugs (except for Lithobid)
all get a medication guide.

aripiprazole (Abilify)
armodafinil (Nuvigil)
clorazepate (Tranxene)
estazolam (ProSom)
eszopiclone (Lunesta)
flurazepam (Dalmane)
levomilnacipran (Fetzima)
modafinil (Provigil)
olanzapine (Zyprexa)
paroxetine (Paxil)
quazepam (Doral)
quetiapine (Seroquel)
ramelteon (Rozerem)
triazolam (Halcion)
zaleplon (Sonata)
zolpidem (Ambien, Zolpimist)

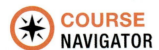

Access interactive chapter review exercises, practice activities, flash cards, and study games.

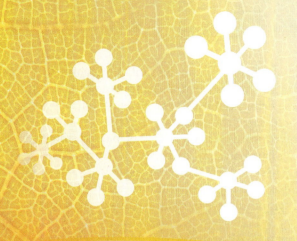

8

Drugs for Central Nervous System Disorders

Learning Objectives

1. Describe the physiologic processes that occur in epilepsy.

2. Classify seizures and the goals of antiseizure therapy.

3. Describe the specific drugs used in the treatment of different classes of seizures.

4. Describe the pathophysiology and manifestations of Parkinson's disease.

5. Explain drug treatments for Parkinson's disease.

6. Identify drugs used to treat attention-deficit disorders.

7. Recognize drugs used to manage Alzheimer's disease.

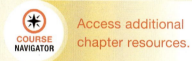

Access additional chapter resources.

Central nervous system (CNS) disorders cause a range of complex, distressing, and life-threatening symptoms, some of which are nonresponsive to treatment. These disorders often leave a patient unable to function normally. The chemicals involved in the thought process and motor activity cause some of these diseases and provide rationales for their treatments. These diseases include epilepsy in its various forms, Parkinson's disease, myasthenia gravis, attention-deficit disorders, amyotrophic lateral sclerosis, multiple sclerosis, Alzheimer's disease, restless leg syndrome, fibromyalgia, and Huntington's disease. For some of these diseases, medical research is still searching for definitive treatments.

Seizure Disorders

A **seizure** is caused by abnormal electrical discharges in the cerebral cortex (the main portion of the brain), resulting in a change in behavior. Conscious periods may or may not be accompanied by loss of control over movements or distortion of the senses. When body movement is lost, it may be in only one area of the body or in the entire body.

Seizures result from the sudden, excessive firing of a small number of neurons, often without an exogenous (outside the organism) trigger, and the spread of the electrical activity to adjacent neurons. These firings can result in a **convulsion**, an involuntary contraction or series of contractions, of the voluntary muscles.

Epilepsy is a fairly common neurologic disorder characterized by **paroxysmal** (sudden and recurring) seizures. It involves disturbances of neuronal electrical activity that interfere with normal brain function. These abnormal discharges may occur only in a specific area of the brain or may spread extensively throughout the brain. Though seizures may not provoke obvious clinical symptoms, seriously imbalanced chemical discharges may still occur.

Epilepsy is a symptom of brain dysfunction. All epilepsy patients have seizures, but not all patients with seizures have epilepsy. Some have a single unprovoked seizure in their lifetime; 1%–2% have chronic epilepsy.

Seizures

Every neuron is in one of three states: resting, firing, or returning to rest. The balance between excitatory and inhibitory impulses determines whether a neuron fires. Neurons operate through the movement of ions across the cell membrane. When negatively charged ions, such as chloride, enter a neuron, they inhibit firing; conversely, when positively charged ions, such as sodium and calcium, enter the cell, they excite it and make it more likely to fire.

The flow of ions is controlled ion channels, or molecules in the cell membrane. These channels are controlled by **neurotransmitters**. Some neurotransmitters bind to receptors that let positive ions in and excite the cell, whereas others bind to receptors that let negative ions in and inhibit firing. Healthy individuals have a balance between excitation and inhibition, but in individuals diagnosed with epilepsy, there is an imbalance. When excitation is excessive relative to inhibition, neurons can fire uncontrollably, leading to a seizure. Glutamate, an excitatory amino acid neurotransmitter, and gamma-aminobutyric acid (GABA), an inhibitory neurotransmitter, play the greatest role in seizures. Other contributors are CNS chemicals involved in thought process and motor activity, such as the following:

- acetylcholine (ACh)
- aspartate
- dopamine
- glutamate
- glycine
- norepinephrine
- serotonin

The levels of neurotransmitters are determined in part by the levels of the **enzymes** (biological molecules that catalyze chemical reactions in the body) that produce them. Upsetting the enzymes disrupts the balance and leads to seizures, especially if the disruption results in a high ratio of glutamate to GABA. The majority of seizures are caused by the following events or conditions:

- alcohol or drug withdrawal
- epilepsy
- high fever

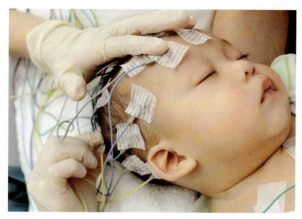

An electroencephalogram can provide vital information on the cause of seizures, helping the physician to select the best option for treatment.

- hypoglycemia (low blood glucose) or hyperglycemia (high blood glucose)
- infection (meningitis)
- neoplasm (brain tumor)
- trauma or injury (head, hematoma)

The two major types of seizures are partial and generalized (see Figure 8.1). Each type is further subdivided according to their manifestations.

Partial Seizures

A **partial seizure** is localized in a specific hemisphere or area of the brain. Partial seizures generally result from injury to the cerebral cortex. They occur in two distinct types, each of which can progress to generalized seizures.

In a **simple partial seizure**, the patient does not lose consciousness and may have:

- some muscular activity manifested as twitching
- sensory hallucinations (visual or auditory phenomena)

In a **complex partial seizure**, the patient experiences:

- impaired consciousness, often with confusion
- a blank stare
- postseizure amnesia

FIGURE 8.1
Partial and Generalized Seizure Activity

A partial seizure and a generalized seizure affect brain activity differently, as shown on the simulated electro-encephalogram (EEG).

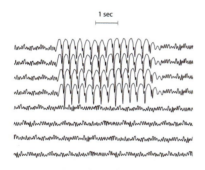

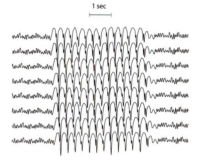

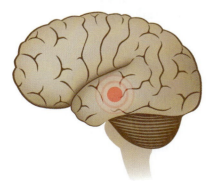

Partial seizure

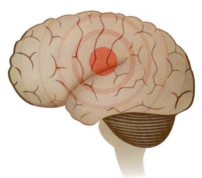

Generalized seizure

Generalized Seizures

A **generalized seizure** involves simultaneous malfunction in both hemispheres of the brain and has no local origin. This type of seizure sometimes occurs in the absence of injury or known structural abnormality. Generalized seizures are classified by type and include tonic-clonic, absence, myoclonic, and atonic seizures.

- A **tonic-clonic seizure** (formerly called a **grand mal seizure**) occurs in two general phases. The tonic portion of the seizure begins with the patient's body becoming rigid, which may result in a fall. This phase lasts for a minute or less. The clonic portion usually is initiated with muscle jerks and may be accompanied by shallow breathing, loss of bladder control, and excess salivation (foaming at the mouth). Jerking continues for a few minutes. After the attack, the patient is drowsy and confused for moments or hours.

- **Status epilepticus** is a serious disorder involving continuous tonic-clonic convulsions, with or without a return to consciousness, that last at least 30 minutes. It is characterized by a high fever and lack of oxygen severe enough to cause brain damage or death. Of the patients who have convulsive status epilepticus, 10% die regardless of treatment, often as a complication of sudden drug withdrawal.

- An **absence seizure** (formerly called a **petit mal seizure**) begins with interruption of the patient's activities by some or all of the following signs: blank stare, rotating eyes, uncontrolled facial movements, chewing, rapid eye blinking, and twitching or jerking of an arm or a leg, but no generalized convulsions. Absence seizures can last from 10 seconds to 2 minutes but are rarely longer than 30 seconds. The patient may experience up to 100 attacks a day. Often, the person has a premonition of the attack through unusual sensations of light, sound, and taste, known as an **aura**. After the attack, the patient continues normal activities. Seizures are most prevalent during the first 10 years of life; 50% of children with absence seizures have tonic-clonic activity as they grow older.

- A **myoclonic seizure** occurs with a sudden, massive, brief muscle jerks, which may throw the patient down, or nonmassive, quick jerks of the arms, hands, legs, or feet. Consciousness is not lost, and this seizure type can occur during sleep.

- An **atonic seizure** begins with sudden loss of both muscle tone and consciousness. The patient may collapse, the head may drop, and the jaw may slacken. An arm or a leg may go limp. The seizure lasts a few seconds to a minute, and then the patient can stand and walk again.

Antiepileptic Drug Therapy

Epilepsy can have profound effects on an individual's health, quality of life, and ability to function. The optimum antiepileptic therapy would be complete seizure control without compromising the patient's quality of life. Thus, therapy with anticonvulsant drugs has two goals: (1) to control seizures or reduce their frequency so that the patient can live an essentially normal life, and (2) to prevent emotional and behavioral changes that may result from the seizures.

As described previously, seizures occur when the effect of excitatory neurotransmitters is excessive relative to the effect of inhibitory neurotransmitters. Drugs to

Safety Alert

There is risk of fetal malformation with the use of certain anticonvulsants. *Valproate, phenytoin, carbamazepine, phenobarbital,* and *topiramate* are all associated with higher than usual fetal malformations. However, having seizures also presents significant risk to a developing fetus. Patients and providers must complete risk-benefit evaluations to manage epilepsy during pregnancy.

control seizures work by reducing the excitation or increasing the inhibition so that neurons do not fire out of control. Not surprisingly, many drugs used to control seizures are used, or have been used, to treat other conditions characterized by excessive excitation, such as mania, anxiety, or panic.

Monotherapy is tried first, and other agents may be added to control seizures. Except in life-threatening situations, single-drug therapy should be initiated at one-fourth to one-third of the usual daily dosage. The dosage is then increased gradually over three to four weeks until seizures are controlled or adverse side effects occur. Once an optimal dosage has been determined, it is essential that the plasma concentration of the drug remain stable to ensure seizure control and minimize the risk of side effects. **Combination therapy** or polytherapy, is using two or more drugs from different classes. Polytherapy is common among patients with severe forms of epilepsy. It can take up to a month to see the full benefit from these drugs. Monotherapy is preferred to polytherapy because it costs less and patients may have fewer adverse effects, drug interactions, and compliance problems.

One possible reason for nonresponsiveness to antiepileptic drug therapy is that the agent is inappropriate for the seizure type. In the past, most patients with epilepsy were treated with phenytoin, phenobarbital, or both drugs. Clinicians now recognize that different seizure types respond better to specific antiepileptic agents. A drug that controls one seizure type may exacerbate another type. The newer drugs are seizure-specific; that is, their pharmacologic action is directed toward controlling a certain type of seizure activity.

The need for therapy should be evaluated periodically. Some patients can discontinue therapy if they have been seizure-free for several years. To discontinue an antiepileptic drug, the dosage should be decreased gradually over two to six months. Abrupt discontinuation should be avoided because of the risk of triggering status epilepticus or other withdrawal seizures.

The potential for drug interactions during antiepileptic therapy is high. Antiepileptic drugs interact with each other and with other drugs through two major mechanisms. They can induce or inhibit the liver enzymes responsible for drug metabolism. They can also displace drugs from their binding sites on plasma proteins.

Table 8.1 presents the most commonly used **anticonvulsant drugs** (drugs used to control seizures). These drugs have relatively narrow therapeutic ranges. In some patients, even minor changes in bioavailability can compromise control or result in toxicity. Factors that affect bioavailability include storage conditions, the drug's physical and chemical characteristics, the dosage form, and the patient's physical condition.

Anticonvulsants have many drug interactions, which can also impact therapeutic ranges (see Table 8.2). Because of the narrow therapeutic ranges of this class of drugs, even the very small allowable differences in manufacturing can affect the ability of the drug to control episodes. For this reason, prescribers may not allow generic drugs to be used, so pharmacy technicians should watch for these drugs to be written DAW (dispense as written), or "brand only." If the computer automatically changes the drug's brand name to its generic name, the technician may have to change it back to the brand name. Medication guides are required when dispensing all antiepileptics.

Sodium Channel Blockers

Sodium channel blockers work on fast sodium channels. Blocking sodium (a positive ion) makes neurons less likely to fire. Alteration of sodium currents is the most common mechanism of action of existing anticonvulsants.

TABLE 8.1 Commonly Used Anticonvulsants

Generic (Brand)	Pronunciation	Dosage Form	Dispensing Status	Control Schedule
Sodium Channel Blockers				
carbamazepine (Carbatrol, Epitol, Tegretol, Teril)	kar-ba-MAZ-e-peen	Capsule, suspension, tablet	Rx	
fosphenytoin (Cerebyx)	fos-FEN-i-toyn	Injection	Rx	
lacosamide (Vimpat)	la-KOE-sa-mide	Injection, solution, tablet	Rx	C-V
oxcarbazepine (Trileptal)	ox-kar-BAZ-e-peen	Suspension, tablet	Rx	
phenytoin (Dilantin)	FEN-i-toyn	Capsule, injection, suspension, tablet	Rx	
vigabatrin (Sabril)	vye-GA-ba-trin	Oral powder, tablet	Rx	
Calcium Channel Blockers				
ethosuximide (Zarontin)	eth-oh-SUX-i-mide	Capsule, syrup	Rx	
valproic acid (Depakene, Depakote)	val-PRO-ik AS-id	Capsule, injection, syrup, tablet	Rx	
zonisamide (Zonegran)	zoh-NIS-a-mide	Capsule	Rx	
GABA Enhancers				
gabapentin (Neurontin)	gab-a-PEN-tin	Capsule, oral solution, tablet	Rx	
phenobarbital (Luminal)	fee-noe-BAR-bi-tal	Elixir, injection, tablet	Rx	C-IV
pregabalin (Lyrica)	pree-GAB-a-lin	Capsule, oral solution	Rx	C-V
primidone (Mysoline)	PRYE-mih-done	Tablet	Rx	
tiagabine (Gabitril)	te-AG-a-been	Tablet	Rx	
Glutamate Inhibitors				
felbamate (Felbatol)	FEL-ba-mate	Suspension, tablet	Rx	
lamotrigine (Lamictal)	la-MOE-tri-jeen	Tablet	Rx	
topiramate (Topamax)	toe-PYRE-a-mate	Capsule, tablet	Rx	
Unknown Mechanism				
levetiracetam (Keppra)	lev-a-tur-AS-a-tam	Injection, oral solution, tablet	Rx	

TABLE 8.2 Common Uses, Side Effects, and Drug Interactions for Anticonvulsants

Generic (Brand)	Common Use(s)	Side Effects	Selected Drug Interactions
Sodium Channel Blockers			
carbamazepine (Carbatrol, Epitol, Tegretol, Teril)	Tonic-clonic, partial seizure (no effect on absence seizure)	Dizziness, drowsiness, nausea, unsteadiness, vomiting, abnormal vision, hyponatremia, hepatotoxicity, arrhythmias, increased suicide risk	Cimetidine, diltiazem, erythromycin, isoniazid, itraconazole, nefazodone, theophylline, and troleandomycin increase concentrations. Phenobarbital, phenytoin, theophylline, and valproic acid decrease concentrations.
fosphenytoin (Cerebyx)	Status epilepticus (short-term use until phenytoin can be given)	Dizziness, itching, numbness, headache, tiredness, decreased movement, hypotension, cardiovascular collapse (rare but serious)	Anticoagulants, chloramphenicol, cimetidine, diltiazem, disulfiram, isoniazid, phenylbutazone, sulfonamides, and trimethoprim may increase phenytoin concentrations. Phenytoin may increase anticoagulant effects and chloramphenicol concentrations. Antineoplastic drugs, diazoxide, folic acid, and rifampin may decrease the effect of phenytoin.
lacosamide (Vimpat)	Partial seizure	Dizziness, fatigue, headache, nausea, tremors, slurred speech, blurred or double vision	Delavirdine and nicardipine may increase concentrations. Carbamazepine, fosphenytoin, phenobarbital, and phenytoin may decrease concentrations.
oxcarbazepine (Trileptal)	Partial seizure (alternative uses: bipolar disorder, diabetic neuropathy, neuralgia)	Abdominal pain, headache, trouble walking, abnormal or double vision, difficulty moving, dizziness, fatigue, nausea, tremors, vomiting, hyponatremia	Carbamazepine, phenobarbital, phenytoin, valproic acid, and verapamil may decrease levels. Oxcarbazepine may decrease the effects of oral contraceptives, felodipine, and lamotrigine. Oxcarbazepine may increase levels of phenobarbital and phenytoin.
phenytoin (Dilantin)	Tonic-clonic, partial seizure, status epilepticus	Decreased coordination/movement, mental confusion, slurred speech, dizziness, headache, insomnia, twitches, nervousness, hepatotoxicity, gingival hyperplasia, hair growth	Anticoagulants, chloramphenicol, cimetidine, diltiazem, disulfiram, isoniazid, phenylbutazone, sulfonamides, and trimethoprim may increase phenytoin concentrations. Phenytoin may increase anticoagulant effects and chloramphenicol concentrations. Antineoplastic drugs, diazoxide, folic acid, and rifampin may decrease the effect of phenytoin.
vigabatrin (Sabril)	Partial seizure	Fatigue, headache, confusion, poor coordination, memory loss, tremors, weight gain, blurred vision, depression	Vigabatrin may decrease fosphenytoin and phenytoin levels. Vigabatrin enhances the effects of other CNS depressants.

Calcium Channel Blockers

ethosuximide (Zarontin)	Absence seizure	Drowsiness, headache, dizziness, hiccups, aggression, fatigue, difficulty moving, loss of appetite, stomach upset, diarrhea, nightmares	Carbamazepine, nevirapine, phenytoin, phenobarbital, primidone, ritonavir, and valproic acid decrease levels.
valproic acid (Depakene, Depakote)	Partial, absence seizures, and tonic-clonic seizures	Dizziness, headache, nausea, vomiting, tremors, diarrhea, tiredness, hair loss, hepatotoxicity	Estrogen-containing oral contraceptives, meropenem, and rifampin concentrations. Salicylates increase effects.
zonisamide (Zonegran)	Partial seizure (alternative uses: binge-eating disorder, obesity)	Tiredness, dizziness, loss of appetite, headache, nausea, irritability, difficulty thinking, sulfa allergy, kidney stones	Carbamazepine, phenobarbital, and phenytoin may decrease levels.

GABA Enhancers

gabapentin (Neurontin)	Partial seizure (alternative uses: diabetic neuropathy, neuralgia, shingles, fibromyalgia, hot flashes, hiccups, restless legs syndrome, others)	Dizziness, drowsiness, tiredness, nausea, vomiting, diarrhea, dry mouth, swelling in legs/arms, abnormal thinking, difficulty moving, weight gain	Gabapentin enhances the effects of other CNS depressants.
phenobarbital (Luminal)	Tonic-clonic, status epilepticus (alternative use: sedative for anxiety and insomnia)	Tiredness, drowsiness, hepatotoxicity, aggression or mood changes, hypotension	Oxycarbazepine, phenytoin, rufinamide, and valproic acid increase levels. Alcohol ingestion may enhance CNS depression.
pregabalin (Lyrica)	Partial seizure, neuropathic pain, fibromyalgia	Dizziness, drowsiness, dry mouth, blurred vision, fluid retention, weight gain	Pregabalin enhances the effects of other CNS depressants.
primidone (Mysoline)	Tonic-clonic seizure (alternative use: tremors)	Difficulty moving, dizziness, nausea, loss of appetite, vomiting, fatigue, mood changes, impotence, double vision	Carbamazepine and phenytoin decrease levels of primidone and its metabolite, phenobarbital. Primodone deceases levels of carbamazepine, dronedarone, protease inhibitors, ticagrelor, and tolvaptan. Levels and the effects of estrogen-based oral contraceptives are decreased. Alcohol ingestion may enhance CNS depression.
tiagabine (Gabitril)	Partial seizure (alternative use: bipolar disorder)	Dizziness, tiredness, nausea, nervousness, tremors, abdominal pain, abnormal thinking, depression	Barbiturates, carbamazepine, and phenytoin decrease levels. Tiagabine enhances the effects of other CNS depressants.

Glutamate Inhibitors

felbamate (Felbatol)	Tonic-clonic, partial seizure	Insomnia, loss of appetite, weight loss, nausea, vomiting, headache, dizziness, tiredness, acne, rash, constipation, diarrhea	Carbamazepine and phenytoin decrease levels. Felbamate enhances the effects of drugs that increase the QT interval.
lamotrigine (Lamictal)	Tonic-clonic, partial seizure (alternative use: bipolar disorder)	Rash, decreased coordination/movement, dizziness, headache, insomnia, tiredness, rash, nausea, vomiting, blurred or double vision	Acetaminophen, carbamazepine, estrogen-containing oral contraceptives, phenobarbital, phenytoin, and rifampin decrease concentrations. Valproic acid increases levels.
topiramate (Topamax)	Tonic-clonic, partial seizure (alternative use: migraine)	Dizziness, numbness, memory problems, depression, kidney stones, insomnia, nausea, tiredness, loss of appetite, weight loss	Carbamazepine, phenytoin, and valproic acid decrease levels. Hydrochlorothiazide increases concentrations. Topiramate may decrease the effectiveness of digoxin, oral contraceptives, and valproic acid.

Unknown Mechanism

levetiracetam (Keppra)	Partial seizure	Dizziness, tiredness, lack of energy, depression, behavioral changes and/or psychosis	Levetiracetam enhances the effects of other CNS depressants.

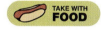

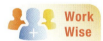

Work Wise

Carbamazepine has a narrow therapeutic window, and maintaining therapeutic drug concentrations is important. Patients may need to use carbamazepine produced by only one manufacturer, which may require the pharmacy to dispense the brand-name drug, not a generic drug.

Carbamazepine (Carbatrol, Epitol, Tegretol, Teril) is a sodium channel blocker used in the prophylaxis of generalized tonic-clonic, partial, and mixed or generalized seizure disorders. It is also used to treat bipolar disorders, as described in Chapter 7. The antiepileptic effect may be related to its effects on sodium channels to limit sustained, repetitive firing and alter synaptic transmission. Blood monitoring is important because carbamazepine induces its own metabolism. Carbamazepine has two black box warnings. One warning is for potentially fatal dermatologic reactions that certain patient populations are more likely to experience. For this reason, genotype testing is recommended for Asian patients who are at a higher risk than other ethnicities. The other boxed warning is for aplastic anemia and agranulocytosis. The most common side effect is a rash that occurs after several weeks of use. The patient should report bleeding, bruising, jaundice, abdominal pain, pale stools, mental disturbances, fever, chills, sore throat, or mouth ulcers. Carbamazepine may also cause drowsiness. As with all anticonvulsant medications, carbamazepine has many drug interactions. The drug should be taken with food to offset gastrointestinal (GI) disturbances.

Lacosamide (Vimpat) has few interactions and is a Schedule V drug because it promotes a sensation of euphoria. Common side effects of lacosamide include dizziness, fatigue, ataxia, tremors, headache, and blurred vision.

Oxcarbazepine (Trileptal) blocks voltage-sensitive sodium channels and thereby stabilizes hyperexcited neurons. This drug is most frequently used as an adjunct to other therapies, but it can be used as monotherapy for partial seizures.

Female patients taking oxcarbazepine must be warned that this drug decreases the effectiveness of oral contraceptives. Patients should also be warned about the potentially debilitating drowsiness associated with oxcarbazepine therapy.

Phenytoin (Dilantin) is used to manage generalized tonic-clonic, simple-partial, and complex-partial seizures and to prevent seizures after head trauma and neurosurgery. It works in the motor cortex by promoting sodium ion outflow from cells, thus stabilizing the membrane threshold. In some patients, small changes in dosage result in large changes in serum concentration. Side effects may or may not be related to dosage and may be reversible when the dosage is reduced. Table 8.3 lists phenytoin's dose-related and non-dose-related side effects.

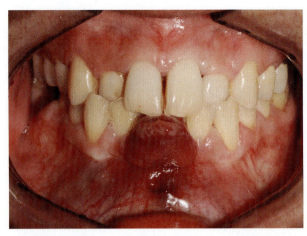

Gingival hyperplasia, or overgrowth of the gingiva, is a side effect of phenytoin use.

Phenytoin should be discontinued if a rash appears. A phenytoin rash, even a mild one, can progress to life-threatening Stevens-Johnson syndrome and should prompt concern. Due to absorption problems, phenytoin and antacids should be administered several hours apart. Phenytoin is unique in that it has many drug interactions; it is important for technicians to obtain accurate drug lists for patients using phenytoin.

Intravenous (IV) phenytoin is considered a "high alert" drug due to safety concerns with use. This drug is considered a vesicant, and injection can cause **phlebitis** (inflammation of the vein). Extravasation should be avoided. Additionally, IV phenytoin may cause hypotension and should be infused no faster than 50 mg/min.

TABLE 8.3   Phenytoin's Side Effects

Dose-Related	Ataxia (irregularity of muscular action)
	Diplopia (the perception of two images of a single object)
	Dizziness
	Drowsiness
	Encephalopathy (degenerative brain disease)
	Involuntary movements (when concentration is greater than 30 mcg/mL)
Non-Dose-Related	Gingival hyperplasia (abnormal tissue growth that increases the volume of the tissue covering the tooth-bearing border of the jaw)
	Peripheral neuropathy (noninflammatory pathologic disturbance or pathologic change in peripheral nerves, commonly in the arms or legs; pain in the extremities)
	Vitamin deficiencies

Phenytoin is a drug for which pharmacy technicians may receive requests to dispense the brand-name product. Requests to use the same manufacturer for all phenytoin dispenses for a particular patient may also occur. The rationale behind these requests is based on the drug's narrow therapeutic index, which is so small that legally allowable differences in drug formulations may pose problems for patients. For most drugs, changes this small are negligible, but for antiepileptic drugs, these changes can result in significant variations in efficacy.

NDC 49349-099-02
30 mg

Dilantin®

Oral capsules

30 mg · 100 capsules

Phenytoin (Dilantin) is most often administered orally. For intravenous administration, fosphenytoin is more frequently used.

Fosphenytoin (Cerebyx) can be used instead of IV phenytoin. It is a prodrug (precursor or inactive form) that is rapidly converted to phenytoin after administration. It has the advantage of being water-soluble and, therefore, better tolerated. This drug characteristic means fewer infusion reactions (pain, burning, or tissue damage) and more reliable treatment. It does have an unusual side effect of brief, intense itching, usually in the groin, which might be a reaction to the phosphate in the injection, but this reaction is not an allergic response. Fosphenytoin has a black box warning regarding the rate of infusion. It should not exceed 150 mg phenytoin equivalents per minute due to the risk of severe hypotension and cardiac arrhythmias.

Vigabatrin (Sabril) is used only as an add-on drug for seizures that do not respond to other drugs because it can cause permanent loss of vision. Only qualified prescribers (those who have undergone required training) can order this drug, and it is shipped directly to the patient. Patients using the drug receive baseline vision testing as well as follow-up visits every three months. These visits continue for up to six months after the patient has stopped taking the drug.

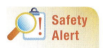
Safety Alert

When diluting phenytoin for a safe infusion, normal saline is the only suitable vehicle. Phenytoin is one of the few drugs that might be mixed by a nurse outside the pharmacy because it precipitates so quickly.

Contraindications The sodium channel blockers have multiple contraindications. Carbamazepine use is contraindicated in bone marrow depression, with or within 14 days of monoamine oxidase inhibitor (MAOI) use, and with concurrent use of nefazodone. Use of delavirdine or other nonnucleoside reverse transcriptase inhibitors is contraindicated with carbamazepine, phenytoin, and fosphenytoin drug therapy. Fosphenytoin and phenytoin should be avoided in patients who have a variety of cardiac issues (including sinus bradycardia, sinoatrial block, second- and third-degree atrioventricular [AV] block, and Adams-Stokes syndrome), an occurrence of rash during treatment, and treatment of absence seizures. Fosphenytoin and phenytoin should be avoided in patients with a hypersensitivity to hydantoins. Use of lacosamide is contraindicated in patients with liver abnormalities and blood disorders. Oxcarbazepine and vigabatrin do not have contraindications.

Cautions and Considerations Carbamazepine has a black box warning for potentially fatal dermatologic reactions; for that reason, genotype testing is recommended for Asian patients (high risk). Another boxed warning is for aplastic anemia and agranulocytosis. Hyponatremia is a concern with carbamazepine and oxcarbazepine. However, oxcarbazepine more commonly causes hyponatremia. Sodium levels should be monitored in patients using either drug.

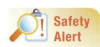

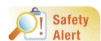

Lacosamide has cardiac side effects. Cardiac function should be monitored in patients using it.

Phenytoin is highly bound to protein in the bloodstream, and it interacts with many other medications that are also bound to protein. All alerts for drug interactions should be taken seriously, and the pharmacist must evaluate each one carefully. Phenytoin can adhere to nasogastric tubing. If it is given through a tube into the stomach, it must be mixed well with normal saline and separated by two hours from feedings given through the same tube. IV phenytoin should be mixed or prepared using only normal saline. Suspensions of phenytoin must be shaken well—as should any medication in suspension form.

Serious vision problems may occur in patients who take vigabatrin, so frequent eye examinations are necessary.

Drug Interactions Selected drug interactions are listed in Table 8.2.

Calcium Channel Blockers

Calcium channel blockers are anticonvulsants that work to stabilize the neuronal membrane. Calcium is a positively charged ion, which excites neuronal cells and makes them more likely to fire. Blocking calcium channels makes neurons less likely to inappropriately fire.

Ethosuximide (Zarontin) is used for absence seizures and increases the seizure threshold. Because of its long half-life, it can usually be given once daily to achieve therapeutic plasma concentrations, but it is often divided between two daily doses to reduce GI side effects. The patient should be told to take the dose with food and not to discontinue it abruptly. Patients should have a complete blood count (CBC) every four months during therapy. The drug may cause drowsiness and impair judgment. Other side effects include headache, dizziness, nausea, and vomiting.

Valproate is a drug available as **valproic acid (Depakene)** and **divalproex sodium (Depakote)**. Valproate blocks calcium and sodium channels and also increases GABA levels. It is also indicated for treating manic episodes in bipolar disorder (Chapter 7) and for managing simple and complex absence seizures, mixed seizure types, and generalized tonic-clonic seizures. Valproic acid may also be effective for partial seizures and infantile (early childhood) spasms. Patients should take oral valproic acid with water (not with a carbonated beverage) and should not chew, break, or crush the tablets or capsules. Patients should be warned not to use aspirin or aspirin products because these products could lead to serious valproic acid toxicity. Routine hepatic and hematologic tests are indicated during therapy. Patients should report severe or persistent sore throat, fever, fatigue, bleeding, or bruising. Side effects include drowsiness and impaired judgment or coordination.

Zonisamide (Zonegran) is a sulfonamide with anticonvulsant activity. Patients must be warned about potentially serious sulfonamide reactions, and the pharmacy technician should check for sulfa allergies when dispensing this drug. Patients should also be instructed to report any skin rashes and to drink six to eight glasses of water a day to reduce the risk of developing kidney stones.

Contraindications Ethosuximide is contraindicated in patients with a history of sensitivity to succinimides. Valproate and valproic acid should not be used in patients who have a hypersensitivity to divalproex or divalproex derivatives, liver disease, urea cycle disorders, and mitochondrial disorders. Zonisamide use should be avoided in patients with a sulfonamide hypersensitivity.

Cautions and Considerations Valproic acid has several black box warnings. One warning is for liver failure, which usually occurs within the first six months of therapy. The risk is increased in patients with inherited deoxyribonucleic acid (DNA) mutations. Liver function tests should be performed in patients using valproic acid. Other boxed warnings are for pancreatitis and for the risk of fetal malformations when used during pregnancy. Valproic acid tablets should be swallowed whole, not crushed or chewed. (Chewing can interfere with the extended-release properties of some dosage forms.) These tablets should not be taken with aspirin or carbonated beverages. Aspirin competes with valproic acid for protein-binding sites, and carbonated beverages can break down valproic acid before absorption can occur. Ethosuximide, however, works best when taken with food.

Abrupt withdrawal of antiepileptic drugs should always be avoided because sudden discontinuation may trigger seizures. The dosage should be slowly tapered if a patient needs to stop taking an anticonvulsant.

Drug Interactions Selected drug interactions are listed in Table 8.2.

GABA Enhancers

GABA is a neurotransmitter that is present throughout the CNS. GABA is capable of inhibiting neuron firing. Reducing GABA can be proconvulsant; increasing GABA can be anticonvulsant.

Gabapentin (Neurontin) is used as an adjunct (a drug added to existing therapy) for drug-refractory (not responsive to treatment) partial seizures. It is not effective for absence seizures. Gabapentin was designed to mimic the neurotransmitter GABA, but studies have shown that it must have another mechanism of action.

Unlike other anticonvulsant drugs, it does not modify plasma concentrations of standard anticonvulsant medications. Side effects are somnolence (sleepiness or unnatural drowsiness), dizziness, ataxia (irregular muscle movements), fatigue, nystagmus (involuntary, rapid movement of the eyeballs), tremors, and double vision. Renal function should be monitored. Gabapentin is a well-accepted treatment option for patients with neuropathic pain, a stinging and burning pain that results from nerve damage due to conditions such as diabetes or herpes. Other uses not as well documented include bipolar disorder, migraine prevention, hot flashes, multiple sclerosis, attention-deficit disorders, and alcohol withdrawal. Because it is generally well tolerated and easy to use, gabapentin is a very popular drug.

Phenobarbital (Luminal) is used for generalized tonic-clonic and partial seizures because it interferes with the transmission of impulses from the thalamus to the cortex of the brain. Use of alcohol and other CNS depressants should be avoided. The drug should not be stopped abruptly. Phenobarbital is a Schedule IV agent because it has abuse potential. It can cause drowsiness and paradoxical hyperexcitability in children and older adults. Periodic blood tests are required. When filling a prescription for phenobarbital, the pharmacy technician should always check the patient's profile in the computer for other drugs being prescribed because phenobarbital has several interactions. If the patient has a rash or exhibits excessive drowsiness, ataxia, dysphagia (difficulty swallowing), slurred speech, or confusion while taking this drug, the prescriber should be notified immediately.

Pregabalin (Lyrica) reduces the release of several neurotransmitters, including glutamate, norepinephrine, and substance P (a sensory neurotransmitter mediating pain, touch, and temperature; a potent vasoactive substance). Pregabalin is thought to bind to calcium channels and modulate calcium influx. Pregabalin is structurally similar to gabapentin. Pregabalin produces fewer side effects than gabapentin and other anticonvulsant drugs, probably because it is efficacious at lower doses.

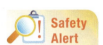

Safety Alert

Neurontin and Noroxin can be confused, but they can be differentiated by dose. Neurontin is usually 100 mg, and Noroxin is 400 mg.

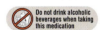

Do not drink alcoholic beverages when taking this medication

Pregabalin can be titrated more readily and may have a faster onset. It is approved as an adjunct only (added onto another drug) for partial seizures. It is important to remember that pregabalin is classified as a controlled substance (Schedule V) because it can cause euphoria and withdrawal. It is also approved to treat diabetic neuropathy and nerve pain that continues after shingles. It must not be stopped abruptly.

Primidone (Mysoline) is indicated in generalized tonic-clonic and complex partial seizures. Metabolic reactions in the liver transform primidone into phenobarbital, so the therapeutic and side effect profiles are similar to those of phenobarbital. Because megaloblastic anemia is a rare and serious side effect of primidone, annual CBCs are recommended.

Tiagabine (Gabitril) blocks the reabsorption of GABA, which allows it to bind to nerve cells that may enhance normal brain activity. Tiagabine should be taken with food and must be tapered if stopped. Tiagabine can cause seizures, which has occurred in patients who do not have epilepsy but take tiagabine for other uses. The US Food and Drug Administration (FDA) has issued a black box warning about taking tiagabine for off-label uses because prescribers would not expect a drug used to treat seizures to cause them instead.

Contraindications Gabapentin and pregabalin do not have contraindications. Phenobarbital should not be used in patients with liver impairment, shortness of breath or airway obstruction, porphyria, or sedative addiction. Primidone use is contraindicated in porphyria. Tiagabine has no contraindications.

Cautions and Considerations Tiagabine has a boxed warning for an increased risk of seizures when used to treat conditions other than epilepsy. Phenobarbital and primidone are controlled substances. With the use of these drugs, patients can develop tolerance. Consequently, special storage and handling requirements are needed. Some pharmacies require double and triple counting of controlled substances. In addition, refills are limited on controlled substances.

Drug Interactions Selected drug interactions are listed in Table 8.2.

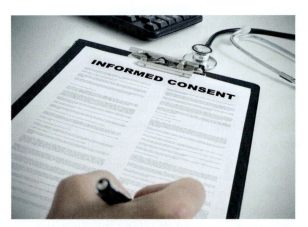
Due to serious adverse effects, felbamate requires patient or guardian signature consent to use.

Glutamate Inhibitors

Glutamate is an excitatory neurotransmitter. Increasing glutamate levels is proconvulsant. Blocking glutamate decreases neuron activity and is anticonvulsant.

Felbamate (Felbatol) is used for tonic-clonic and partial seizures. Felbamate poses the risk of developing aplastic anemia and/or liver failure (both black box warnings). For these reasons, patients must be fully advised of these risks and sign a waiver consenting to the use of the drug.

Lamotrigine (Lamictal) provides add-on therapy for adults with partial seizures, with or without generalized secondary seizures. It can also be used to treat bipolar disorder. Lamotrigine works by blocking sodium channels, thereby reducing neuron excitation. Lamotrigine does not affect serum concentrations of phenobarbital, phenytoin, or primidone, but it may affect the pharmacokinetics or pharmacodynamics of carbamazepine and valproic acid. The drug has a black box warning about fatal rashes in the FDA-approved product information. The patient should be advised to call his or her physician immediately if a rash appears, but the drug should not be discontinued abruptly. Life-threatening rashes with this drug are much more common in children, and lamotrigine is not to be used in patients less than 16 years old.

Topiramate (Topamax) is prescribed for treating partial-onset seizures in adults. Although its mechanism of action is not well understood, the most common theories propose that topiramate blocks sodium channels, subsequently enhancing the activity of GABA and antagonizing glutamine receptors. It is used as an add-on therapy to carbamazepine or phenytoin. It works well but causes significant cognitive effects (e.g., slowed thinking, slowed speech, and difficulty concentrating). Therapy should start with a low dose and be titrated slowly over eight weeks. Topiramate can increase phenytoin levels. It is a weak carbonic anhydrase inhibitor, so it increases the risk of kidney stones. Patients should drink plenty of water during use.

Contraindications Felbamate use should be avoided in patients with carbamate sensitivity, a history of blood dyscrasia, or liver impairment. Topiramate in the extended-release formula is contraindicated in patients with recent alcohol use and in those with metabolic acidosis who are also taking metformin. Lamotrigine and immediate-release topiramate have no contraindications.

Cautions and Considerations Felbamate has black boxed warnings for aplastic anemia and liver failure. Felbamate should not be used in patients with liver dysfunction or hematologic problems. Both conditions may be exacerbated by felbamate.

Lamotrigine has a boxed warning for potentially fatal rashes. In fact, lamotrigine doses must be titrated slowly because of the risk of rash. Slow titration decreases the incidence of rash.

Topiramate may cause metabolic acidosis. Blood chemistries should be monitored in patients using topiramate.

Drug Interactions Selected drug interactions are listed in Table 8.2.

Other Anticonvulsants

Levetiracetam (Keppra) is an adjunctive therapy for partial seizures. Its mechanism of action is unknown, and it is structurally unrelated to other anticonvulsants. It was initially developed to improve cognition (the ability to perceive, think, and remember). The pharmacokinetics of this drug are predictable. There is little potential for drug interactions and no serum monitoring is required, so dispensing this drug is fairly easy. However, there is no evidence that dosages greater than 3,000 mg per day are effective, so the pharmacy technician should watch the dosage and alert the pharmacist if a prescriber orders a higher dosage. Levetiracetam causes drowsiness.

Contraindications Levetiracetam has no contraindications.

Cautions and Considerations Levetiracetam may cause CNS depression. It should be used with caution in patients using other CNS depressants.

Psychiatric symptoms such as psychosis, paranoia, and hallucinations may occur with use. Suicidal ideation may also occur. Patients should be monitored for changes in behavior that suggest suicidal thoughts and depression.

Drug Interactions Selected drug interactions are listed in Table 8.2.

Parkinson's Disease

Parkinson's disease (PD) is characterized by muscular difficulties and postural abnormalities. It usually affects individuals over age 60. Three characteristic signs of PD are tremors while resting, rigidity, and akinesia (absence of movement). These signs may manifest as poor posture control, shuffling gait, and loss of overall muscle control (e.g., flexed stance, difficulty in turning, and hurried gait). With the population of older adults increasing in number, this debilitating disease may become more prevalent in the coming years.

Pathophysiology of Parkinson's Disease

PD occurs as a result of pathologic alterations in the extrapyramidal system, a complex functional unit of the CNS involved in controlling motor activities. The extrapyramidal system is composed of the **basal nuclei** (also called the basal ganglia); these are symmetric, subcortical masses of gray matter embedded in the lower portions of the cerebral hemisphere. PD is the most common of the extrapyramidal diseases. No definitive test exists for this disease, so it is diagnosed almost exclusively by its symptoms.

Voluntary movement requires complex neurochemical messaging in the brain. Electrical currents and neurotransmitters carry nerve impulses from the cerebral cortex to the basal nuclei and back to the cerebral cortex via the thalamus (see Figure 8.2 for the features of the brain). Transmission of information about the initiation of movement, muscle tone, and posture is affected by the balance of neurotransmitters in the basal nuclei. Normal movement requires that the two primary neurotransmitters—dopamine, an inhibitor, and ACh, a stimulator—be in balance.

FIGURE 8.2
Cutaway View of the Brain

The features of the brain.

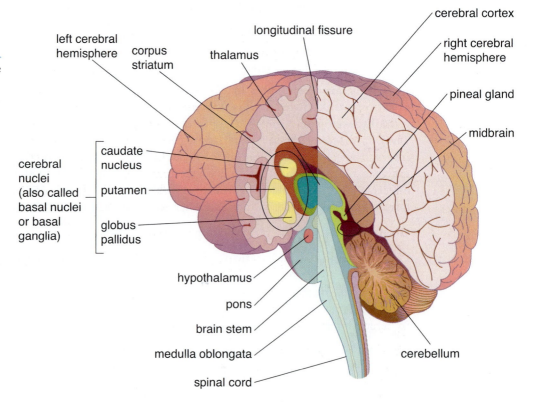

FIGURE 8.3
Substantia Nigra

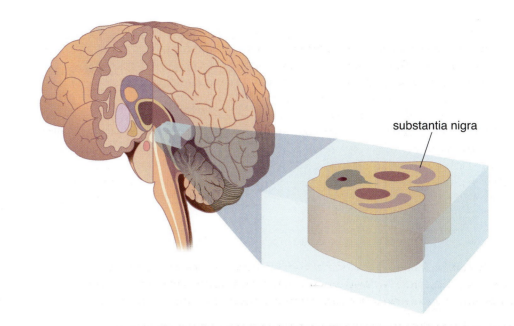

substantia nigra

In a healthy person, dopaminergic neurons (neurons that release dopamine when they fire) in the **substantia nigra** (a collection of dark gray substance, found deep within the midbrain and illustrated in Figure 8.3) release an amount of dopamine sufficient to control the stimulating effect of ACh on large-motor and fine-muscle movements. In PD, however, there is progressive destruction of dopaminergic neurons in the nigrostriatal pathway, so an insufficient amount of dopamine is produced to counterbalance ACh production. This dopamine deficiency results in a predominance of cholinergic neuronal activity, which produces excessive motor-nerve stimulation.

Drug Therapy for Parkinson's Disease

Currently, there is no cure for PD, so the goals of treatment are to minimize disability and help patients maintain the highest possible quality of life. Drug therapy for PD has greatly improved the functional ability and clinical status of patients, and temporary remission from the disease can allow patients to live productive lives. Nevertheless, drug therapy is aimed only at symptomatic relief; it cannot alter the underlying disease process. Levodopa is the most commonly used drug therapy for PD, but the search continues for new agents to prolong the length of effective treatment or reverse the disease. Table 8.4 presents the most commonly used agents for patients who have PD.

The side effects of the drugs can be a problem in the treatment of PD, which may necessitate constant changes in medication. Often, the patient will need emotional and psychological support as well.

Levodopa-Carbidopa and Dopamine Agonists

Dopamine agonists are the mainstay of treatment for PD. This group of drugs either replaces dopamine or mimics its action in the brain. In effect, these agents either raise the level of dopamine in the brain or provide a drug that has the same action. Levodopa is widely recognized as the most effective treatment for PD because it significantly improves movement and restores normal function. Unfortunately, the effects of this drug (i.e., its ability to restore control of movement, or "on" time to patients) wear off over time. Dopamine agonists offer another alternative without

TABLE 8.4 Commonly Used Agents for Parkinson's Disease

Generic (Brand)	Pronunciation	Dosage Form	Dispensing Status
amantadine (Symmetrel)	a-MAN-ta-deen	Capsule, oral liquid, tablet	Rx
benztropine (Cogentin)	BENZ-troe-peen	Injection, tablet	Rx
bromocriptine (Parlodel)	broe-moe-KRIP-teen	Capsule, tablet	Rx
entacapone (Comtan)	en-TAK-a-pone	Tablet	Rx
levodopa-carbidopa (Sinemet)	lee-voe-DOE-pa kar-bi-DOE-pa	Tablet	Rx
levodopa-carbidopa-entacapone (Stalevo)	lee-voe-DOE-pa kar-bi-DOE-pa en-TAK-a-pone	Tablet	Rx
pramipexole (Mirapex)	pra-mi-PEX-ole	Tablet	Rx
rasagiline (Azilect)	ra-SAJ-i-leen	Tablet	Rx
ropinirole (Requip)	ro-PIN-a-role	Tablet	Rx
selegiline (Eldepryl, Zelapar)	seh-LEDGE-ah-leen	Capsule	Rx
tolcapone (Tasmar)	TOLE-ka-pone	Tablet	Rx
trihexyphenidyl (Trihexy)	trye-hex-ee-FEN-i-dill	Oral liquid, tablet	Rx

some of the movement effects that levodopa causes, but they are not always as effective as levodopa. The average period for which a dopaminergic drug will work without significant side effects is about five years.

Levodopa-carbidopa (Sinemet) is probably the most commonly used drug for patients who have PD. Levodopa crosses the blood-brain barrier and is metabolized in the brain into dopamine, which does not itself cross the blood-brain barrier. Levodopa is also converted into dopamine by the peripheral tissues, so the brain does not receive the full dose. On its own, this drug has very undesirable effects.

The dosage of levodopa-carbidopa must be limited because of the potential for nausea, vomiting, and cardiac arrhythmia. However, the addition of carbidopa prevents loss of levodopa from the CNS by conversion to dopamine in the peripheral nervous system, resulting in fewer dopaminergic side effects. Carbidopa does not affect the CNS metabolism of levodopa, and lower doses of levodopa can be used as brain concentrations of dopamine increase. There is a smoother, more rapid induction into therapy with this drug.

Another problem with levodopa is the **on-off phenomenon**, which occurs in as many as two-thirds of patients after about five years of therapy. This phenomenon is a wide fluctuation of functional states, ranging from hyperkinetic to hypokinetic, potentially occurring several times a day. The hyperkinetic (abnormally increased motor function) state is characterized by **dyskinesia** (impairment of the power of voluntary movement) and good functional status; the hypokinetic (abnormally diminished motor activity) state is characterized by akinesia or "freezing" episodes and painful dystonic spasms. These fluctuations are associated primarily with the availability of levodopa at postsynaptic dopamine receptors in the CNS.

Patients may be well controlled on levodopa for several years and then suddenly assume a state of akinesia, masked facies (a relentless, unblinking stare without emotional expressiveness), and stooped posture. The drug may just as suddenly start working again. It also causes neuropsychiatric disorders, dementia (organic loss of intellectual function), loss of memory, hallucinations, and orthostatic hypotension (reduced blood pressure in certain positions, due to inhibition of neurons responsible for vasoconstriction). Levodopa should be carefully titrated to provide optimal control at minimal doses so that the on-off phenomenon is delayed as long as possible.

Apomorphine is a self-injected agent used for acute treatment of intermittent "off" time (the inability to move). Despite its name, apomorphine is not an opioid drug. It should not be used regularly; instead, it is saved for when levodopa wears off more quickly than anticipated. Apomorphine boosts the effects of levodopa until the next dose can be taken. If repeated doses of apomorphine are needed, adjustments in other therapies should be made to prevent frequent off times. Apomorphine is only available through specialty pharmacies.

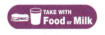

Bromocriptine (Parlodel) is an ergot alkaloid with dopaminergic properties. It improves symptoms of PD by directly stimulating dopamine receptors in the corpus striatum. It is usually used with levodopa or levodopa-carbidopa. The drug should be taken with food or milk. The patient should limit use of alcohol and avoid exposure to cold. Blood pressure should be closely monitored. Drowsiness, nausea, and hypotension are the most common side effects. It also inhibits prolactin secretion and has been used to stop milk production in breast-feeding mothers.

Pramipexole (Mirapex), a dopamine agonist, is more selective for dopamine D_2 receptors but has also been shown to bind to D_3 and D_4 receptors. This drug works as well as other antiparkinsonian drugs but has fewer side effects. Unlike bromocriptine, pramipexole is not an ergot derivative. Pramipexole should be prescribed early in the disease, either as a monotherapy or in combination with levodopa-carbidopa. It should be taken with food to reduce nausea. Pramipexole is approved for restless leg syndrome (see the section on restless leg syndrome later in this chapter). It may help with the pain of fibromyalgia and bipolar disorder but is not yet approved for these uses.

Ropinirole (Requip), like pramipexole, is a dopamine agonist, binding with higher affinity at the D_3 receptors. The precise mechanism of action is unknown. It can be taken without regard to food. Hypotension, especially at the beginning of therapy or dose escalation, can cause severe dizziness, especially with a change in position. Ropinirole is also approved for restless leg syndrome.

Pharm Facts

Michael J. Fox, a popular television and film actor, announced he had PD in his thirties. Since then, Fox has raised awareness of the disease through his speaking engagements and fund-raising efforts.

Contraindications Use of levodopa-carbidopa is contraindicated in patients with narrow-angle glaucoma, recent MAOI use, and melanoma or undiagnosed skin lesions. Apomorphine should not be administered intravenously, and its use is contraindicated in patients taking a serotonin (5-HT) antagonist. Bromocriptine should be avoided in patients with a hypersensitivity to ergot alkaloids. Pramipexole and ropinirole do not have contraindications.

Cautions and Considerations Apomorphine should not be taken along with antiemetic agents such as ondansetron, granisetron, or alosetron. If a patient complains of nausea and drug treatment is needed, other antiemetic medications should be used.

Apomorphine comes in a self-injector pen. The pharmacist should teach the patient how to use the pen if he or she has not been instructed already. Ampules and cartridges for the injector can be stored at room temperature. If syringes are prefilled with apomorphine, they can be stored in the refrigerator for one day.

Drug Interactions Antipsychotics and anticholinergics may diminish the antiparkinsonian effects of these drugs. The adverse effects of bupropion may be enhanced by levodopa and dopamine agonists. These agents may enhance the hypotensive effects of MAOIs.

Apomorphine's hypotensive effects may be enhanced by serotonin antiemetics. Apomorphine may enhance the effects of agents that prolong the QT interval. Apomorphine may also increase the serum concentration of pimozide.

Pramipexole and ropinirole may diminish the therapeutic effect of sulpiride. Sulpiride may diminish the therapeutic effect of pramipexole and ropinirole.

Amantadine and Anticholinergics

These agents are used early in PD to treat mild symptoms (primarily tremors). They are used later in the disease progression as adjunct therapy for the movement side effects caused by levodopa. By blocking muscarinic receptors in the brain, anticholinergics help balance cholinergic activity and reduce tremors. Amantadine, an antiviral drug used for influenza, inhibits the reuptake of dopamine into presynaptic nerve endings. This inhibition allows dopamine to accumulate in the synaptic cleft and stimulate more dopamine receptors. (See Table 8.4 for information on these drugs.)

Amantadine (Symmetrel), an antiviral discussed in Chapter 4 as a prophylactic agent and treatment for influenza, is also used to treat PD. It works by blocking the reuptake of dopamine into presynaptic neurons and causing direct stimulation of postsynaptic dopamine receptors. It is taken once or twice daily, and the second dose of the day should be taken in the early afternoon to decrease the incidence of insomnia. Abrupt discontinuation of therapy should be avoided.

Benztropine (Cogentin) blocks central cholinergic receptors, helping to balance cholinergic activity in the basal ganglia. Indications for the use of this drug are acute dystonic reactions, PD, and drug-induced extrapyramidal reactions (such as those caused by antipsychotics). Benztropine may also prolong dopamine's effects by blocking dopamine reuptake and storage at central receptor sites. This drug should be administered after meals to prevent GI irritation. Constipation is the primary side effect. The drug should not be discontinued abruptly.

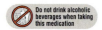

Trihexyphenidyl (Trihexy) is a centrally acting anticholinergic. It appears to be useful for relieving tremors in PD. Trihexyphenidyl is a widely used anticholinergic agent. The starting dosage of trihexyphenidyl is 0.5 to 1 mg twice daily, with a gradual increase to 2 mg three times daily.

Contraindications Benztropine should not be prescribed for children younger than three years old. Amantadine and trihexyphenidyl do not have contraindications.

Cautions and Considerations Because these agents can cause drowsiness and confusion, patients should avoid alcohol, which can intensify these effects. Patients may also be advised to drink plenty of fluids and eat foods high in fiber to counteract the constipation these agents can cause.

Drug Interactions These agents increase the anticholinergic effects of other anticholinergics.

Catechol-O-Methyltransferase Inhibitors

Catechol-O-methyltransferase (COMT) inhibitors are drugs that inhibit the action of catechol-O-methyl transferase. As an adjunct therapy, COMT inhibitors, such as entacapone and tolcapone, help when levodopa starts to wear off at the end of each dosing interval. Typically, one of these agents (see Table 8.4) is given with each dose of levodopa to increase the amount of "on" time by one to two hours each day. Usually, the levodopa dosage is decreased by approximately 100 mg a day when one of these drugs is added. This class of drug works by blocking an enzyme that metabolizes dopamine. COMT inhibitors boost the effects of levodopa and dopamine by allowing dopamine to remain active longer.

Tolcapone (Tasmar) was the first COMT inhibitor to be discovered. The inhibition of COMT allows greater amounts of levodopa to reach the brain, thereby extending the drug's beneficial life. The COMT inhibitors have no clinical effect unless they are combined with levodopa. Tolcapone was approved by the FDA in 1998, but it has since been linked to three fatal liver injuries. As a result, the medication now carries a warning label recommending that its use be limited to people who do not respond to or are not appropriate candidates for other available treatments. Tolcapone has been shown to increase patient "on time" by an average of two to three hours per day. The drug should be discontinued if the patient does not demonstrate any improvement within three weeks.

Entacapone (Comtan) is the second COMT inhibitor to be approved by the FDA. Whereas tolcapone penetrates the CNS, entacapone acts peripherally. Thus, entacapone is expected to be less toxic than tolcapone. Entacapone is indicated for patients who are experiencing a deteriorating response to levodopa in the earlier stages of motor fluctuations. This drug can be taken without regard to food.

Contraindications Entacapone does not have contraindications. Tolcapone is contraindicated in patients with liver disease.

Cautions and Considerations Entacapone can cause urine discoloration (urine may appear red, brown, or black), so patients should be warned about this sometimes alarming but harmless effect. Tolcapone has a black box warning for liver damage, so this medication should be used only when other drug therapies for PD fail.

Drug Interactions COMT inhibitors can enhance the side effects of CNS depressants.

Monoamine Oxidase Inhibitors

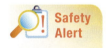

Mild dopamine-boosting drugs that are used early on in disease progression or as adjunct therapy in advanced PD are MAOIs. Rasagiline is often used for mild PD symptoms. Selegiline is usually used as an adjunct therapy when levodopa begins wearing off. (See Table 8.4 for information on these drugs.) These agents block monoamine oxidase (MAO), an enzyme that breaks down dopamine in neurons.

Rasagiline (Azilect) is an MAOI, so it blocks the breakdown of dopamine. It is similar to selegiline. Rasagiline is used as initial therapy in early stages of PD to improve symptoms. It can also be added to levodopa to prolong the effects of levodopa. Rasagiline should not be taken for two weeks prior to surgery. Like other MAOIs, rasagiline can cause a hypertensive crisis, as described in Chapter 7, if the patient ingests foods that contain tyramine. Examples of tyramine-containing foods include aged cheese, concentrated yeast extracts, pickled fish, sauerkraut, soy sauce, beer, and broad beans.

Selegiline (Eldepryl, Emsam, Zelapar) is a potent MAOI that affects MAO type B, found primarily in the brain. Selegiline plays a major role in the metabolism of dopamine and may increase dopaminergic activity by interfering with dopamine breakdown. The daily dose should not exceed 10 mg. Zelapar is a form that dissolves in the mouth. Because absorption is higher with Zelapar, doses are lower than with related drugs. Emsam is the transdermal form of selegiline and is approved only for depression, not for the treatment of PD; therefore, Emsam was discussed in Chapter 7.

Contraindications Rasagiline should be avoided with concurrent use of other MAOIs, meperidine, methadone, tramadol, cyclobenzaprine, dextromethorphan, or St. John's wort. Selegiline should not be used with meperidine. Patients using the oral disintegrating tablet form of selegiline should not concurrently use dextromethorphan,

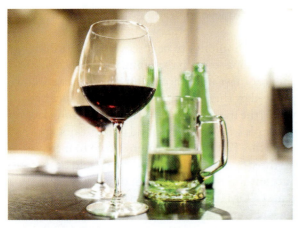

Red wine and beer are among beverages that contain tyramine. Tyramine-containing foods and beverages should be avoided in patients using MAOIs.

methadone, tramadol, or other MAOIs. The transdermal form of selegiline is contraindicated in pheochromocytoma; concomitant use of bupropion, serotonin reuptake inhibitors, tricyclic antidepressants, tramadol, propoxyphene, methadone, dextromethorphan, St. John's wort, mirtazapine, cyclobenzaprine, oral selegiline and other MAOIs, carbamazepine, and oxcarbazepine; elective surgery requiring general anesthesia; use of sympathomimetics; foods high in tyramine (see Cautions and Considerations section below); and supplements containing tyrosine, phenylalanine, tryptophan, or caffeine.

Cautions and Considerations MAOIs block the metabolism of tyramine, a substance in many aged and pickled foods. If tyramine concentrations rise high enough in the blood, blood pressure may increase to dangerous levels. Therefore, patients should be instructed to limit their intake of the following tyramine-rich foods and beverages:

- aged cheese
- beef
- beer
- peppers
- red wine
- sauerkraut
- sausage

Drug Interactions MAOIs have many serious drug interactions. In particular, they should never be administered with tramadol, methadone, dextromethorphan, sympathomimetics, fluoxetine, or fluvoxamine.

Other Central Nervous System Disorders

Several other neurologic disorders share signs and symptoms with the convulsive disorders and PD. They include myasthenia gravis, amyotrophic lateral sclerosis (ALS), multiple sclerosis (MS), Huntington's disease, Alzheimer's disease, and attention-deficit/hyperactivity disorder (ADHD). Restless leg syndrome and fibromyalgia are treated with many of the same drugs, so they will be discussed in this section of the text.

Myasthenia Gravis

Myasthenia gravis is a disorder of the interface between nerves and muscles, resulting from autoimmune damage to ACh receptors at the **motor end plate** (connection between a nerve and a muscle; see Figure 8.4). As a result, the muscles cannot respond to the nerve signal to contract. The disorder is characterized by weakness and increased fatigability, especially of the skeletal muscles. For some individuals, weakness is relatively constant; for others, weakness is typically caused by exercise and diminishes with rest. The first symptoms may be **ptosis** (paralytic drooping of the upper eyelid), **diplopia** (double vision), or blurred vision; these symptoms may be

FIGURE 8.4
Neuro-muscular junction

The interface between the nervous system and the muscular system is the neuromuscular junction.

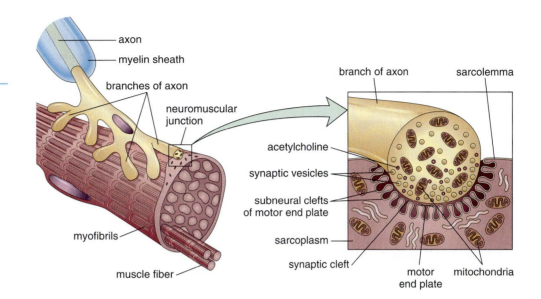

accompanied or followed by **dysarthria** (imperfect articulation of speech), **dysphagia** (difficulty in swallowing), extremity weakness, and respiratory difficulty. The clinical course is variable and includes spontaneous remissions and exacerbations.

Treatments for Myasthenia Gravis

Symptomatic treatment of myasthenia gravis includes several different agents. Acetylcholinesterase inhibitors (commonly pyridostigmine) can be used to treat symptoms. Acetylcholinesterase inhibitors can produce clinical improvement in all forms of myasthenia gravis. They allow ACh to remain longer in the neuromuscular junction and may be used with corticosteroids. Although drug therapy does not inhibit or reverse the basic immunologic flaw, it does enable the ACh remaining in the junctions to interact with ACh receptors for longer periods. In addition, many patients require the use of immunotherapy (such as azathioprine and cyclophosphamide). Table 8.5 lists the most commonly used drugs for the treatment of myasthenia gravis.

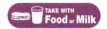

Pyridostigmine (Mestinon) is used to treat myasthenia gravis or to reverse the effects of nondepolarizing muscle relaxants. Pyridostigmine blocks ACh hydrolysis by cholinesterase, resulting in ACh accumulation at cholinergic synapses and thereby increasing stimulation of cholinergic receptors at the neuromuscular junction. Pyridostigmine interacts with procainamide, quinidine, corticosteroids, succinylcholine, and magnesium. It should be taken with food or milk. It is equally important to take it exactly as directed and at the same time each day. When pyridostigmine is delivered by oral, intramuscular, or IV routes, it facilitates transmission of impulses across the neuromuscular junction. Side effects are generally due to exaggerated

TABLE 8.5 Commonly Used Agents for Myasthenia Gravis

Generic (Brand)	Pronunciation	Dosage Form	Dispensing Status
azathioprine (Imuran)	ay-za-THYE-oh-preen	Injection, tablet	Rx
cyclophosphamide (Cytoxin)	sye-kloe-FOS-fa-mide	Capsule, injection, tablet	Rx
pyridostigmine (Mestinon)	peer-id-oh-STIG-meen	Injection, oral liquid, tablet	Rx

pharmacologic effects. The most common side effects are salivation and **muscle fasciculation** (a small, local, involuntary muscular contraction visible under the skin). The prescriber should be notified of any nausea, vomiting, muscle weakness, severe abdominal pain, or difficulty in breathing.

Azathioprine (Imuran) suppresses cell-mediated hypersensitivity and alters antibody production. It is taken with food to prevent nausea. The side effects of immunosuppressive drugs are leukopenia (reduction of leukocytes), pancytopenia (abnormal depression of blood cell levels), infection, GI irritation, and abnormal liver function tests.

Cyclophosphamide (Cytoxan), an alkylating agent, prevents cell division by cross-linking DNA strands. Cyclophosphamide is covered in-depth in Chapter 16. Guidelines for preparing and disposing of chemotherapeutic agents should be followed. Fluids should be taken liberally (3 L per day). Cystitis is a frequent side effect, even months after therapy has been discontinued. Other urinary tract effects may include urinary bladder fibrosis, hematuria, and renal tubular necrosis. Uric acid, CBCs, and renal and hepatic functions should be monitored. Alopecia (hair loss) is a side effect, as are nausea, vomiting, and bone marrow depression.

Pharm Facts

ALS is also known as Lou Gehrig's disease after the New York Yankees star who died of the disease in 1941.

Amyotrophic Lateral Sclerosis

Amyotrophic lateral sclerosis (ALS) is a progressive, degenerative disease of the nerves that leads to muscle weakness, paralysis, and, eventually, death. It is thought to be caused by excessive levels of glutamate, an excitatory neurotransmitter that causes nerve damage.

Riluzole

Riluzole (Rilutek) inhibits the release of glutamate, inactivates sodium channels, and interferes with intracellular events following neurotransmitter binding at excitatory receptors. Riluzole is the only drug that prolongs ALS patient survival. Riluzole is generally well tolerated. Weakness, dizziness, GI effects, and liver enzyme elevation are the most common side effects.

Multiple Sclerosis

Multiple sclerosis (MS) is an autoimmune disease in which the myelin sheaths around nerves, which serve as electrical insulation, degenerate. The patient loses use of the muscles, and eyesight is also often affected. In the later stages of the disease, there is severe trembling. Some drugs can slow the progression of the disease, but there is no cure. Table 8.6 lists the agents most commonly used to treat MS.

Interferon Betas

Interferons are used for a variety of conditions affecting the immune system, including MS. Interferon betas closely resemble interferons (cytokines) naturally produced by the body. The exact way that interferon betas help in the treatment of MS is not fully understood. However, they can prevent CNS inflammation and demyelination. Interferon therapy is costly (tens of thousands of dollars a year) and often dispensed only in specialty pharmacies or hospitals. Interferon betas have many side effects, which are described in Table 8.6. Injection-site reactions are common and can include skin necrosis.

Interferon beta-1a (Avonex, Rebif) is used for ambulatory patients with relapsing-remitting MS. It reduces the frequency of attacks in patients with this form of MS and delays disability. It is dosed every other day. Most patients report flu-like symptoms; to avoid these symptoms, prophylaxis with acetaminophen is indicated. It is also recommended that the drug be taken in the evening. A photosensitivity reaction may occur. The drug should not be exposed to high temperatures or freezing.

Interferon beta-1b (Betaseron, Extavia) is approved to reduce the frequency of episodes and for patients with a single episode plus consistent magnetic resonance imaging (MRI) findings. It is injected subcutaneously every other day.

Interferon beta-1b differs from naturally occurring protein by a single amino acid and the lack of carbohydrate side chains. Its mechanism of action in MS is unknown, but it does suppress T-cell activity, thereby reducing MRI lesions, decreasing relapses, and lessening the severity of these relapses.

Contraindications Interferons are contraindicated in patients with a hypersensitivity to human albumin.

Cautions and Considerations Hypersensitivity reactions are a concern with interferon betas. Anaphylaxis is associated with interferon use and may occur immediately after initiation of therapy or after prolonged use.

The interferon betas are associated with asymptomatic liver dysfunction. Caution should be exercised in patients using other potentially hepatotoxic drugs.

Hematologic abnormalities including leukemia and anemia have been reported with use of interferon betas. Routine monitoring of CBCs is recommended.

Other Disease-Modifying Therapies

There are several disease-modifying therapies for MS in addition to the interferon betas (see Table 8.6). Unlike interferon betas, which are injectable products, these medications are available in various dosage forms. Side effects of disease-modifying therapies for MS are detailed in Table 8.6.

Dimethyl fumarate (Tecfidera) is an oral drug used to reduce relapse rates and the development of new brain lesions in patients who have MS. Side effects include flushing and GI symptoms. The starting dose is titrated after approximately a week.

Fingolimod (Gilenya) is an immune modulator that prevents lymphocyte cells from migrating to the CNS. It reduces the frequency of exacerbations and delays disability. Patients should be tested for immunity to chicken pox and varicella zoster, and these immunizations should not be administered until at least one month after the patient has completed treatment with this drug. The primary side effects are cardiac. The once daily dosage is a positive attribute because patients are more likely to be adherent to therapy.

REFRIGERATE

Glatiramer acetate (Copaxone) seems to block the autoimmune reaction against myelin that leads to nerve damage. It decreases the frequency of relapses, but it has not been shown to slow disease progression. Glatiramer acetate is given every day by subcutaneous injection. The injection must be refrigerated when stored but brought to room temperature before injection. It may cause local injection-site reactions and brief flushing, chest pain, and shortness of breath; these side effects are bothersome but benign.

Mitoxantrone (Novatrone) is a chemotherapeutic agent. It has been shown to slow the progression of MS and to reduce relapses. It is given intravenously every three months. Because of the serious risk of leukemia, it is reserved for patients with worsening conditions.

Natalizumab (Tysabri) is used for relapsing forms of MS. Its use is associated with progressive multifocal leukoencephalopathy (black box warning), which can be fatal. For this reason, natalizumab is part of a Risk Evaluation and Mitigation Strategy (REMS) program. REMS programs are risk management plans that use risk minimization strategies beyond the professional labeling to ensure that the benefits of certain drugs outweigh the risks. Patients must be enrolled in a REMS program to receive natalizumab. Natalizumab is given as an IV infusion every four weeks.

Teriflunomide (Aubagio) is used for relapsing forms of MS. Oral dosing is a main advantage of teriflunomide. Hepatotoxicity may occur with use. A unique side effect is hair thinning. More information on side effects can be found in Table 8.6.

TABLE 8.6 Commonly Used Agents for Multiple Sclerosis

Generic (Brand)	Pronunciation	Dosage Form	Common Dosage	Dispensing Status	Side Effects
Beta Interferons					
interferon beta-1a (Avonex)	in-ter-FEER-on BAY-ta won-aye	Injection	30 mcg once a week	Rx	Flulike symptoms, anemia, injection-site reactions
interferon beta-1a (Rebif)	in-ter-FEER-on BAY-ta won-aye	Injection	22–44 mcg 3 times a week	Rx	Flulike symptoms, injection-site reactions, leukopenia, increased liver enzymes
interferon beta-1b (Betaseron, Extavia)	in-ter-FEER-on BAY-ta won-bee	Injection	0.25 mg every other day	Rx	Flulike symptoms, injection-site reactions, asthenia, menstrual disorders
Other Disease-Modifying Therapies (Noninterferons)					
dimethyl fumarate (Tecfidera)	dye-METH-il FUE-ma-rate	Capsule	240 mg twice a day	Rx	Flushing, abdominal pain, diarrhea
fingolimod (Gilenya)	fin-GO-li-mod	Capsule	0.5 mg once a day	Rx	Increased liver enzymes, infections, diarrhea
glatiramer acetate (Copaxone)	gla-TIR-a-mer	Injection	20 mg once a day	Rx	Injection-site reactions, chest pain, flushing, dyspnea
mitoxantrone (Novatrone)	mye-toe-ZAN-trone	Injection	12 mg/m^2 every 3 months up to a lifetime dose of 140 mg/m^2	Rx	Nausea, alopecia, menstrual disorders
natalizumab (Tysabri)	na-ta-LI-zoo-mab	Injection	300 mg every 4 weeks	Rx	Headache, fatigue, arthralgia
teriflunomide (Aubagio)	ter-i-FLOO-noe-mide	Tablet	7–14 mg once a day	Rx	Diarrhea, nausea, hair thinning

Contraindications Fingolimod is contraindicated in heart disease, stroke, heart failure, AV block, and sick sinus syndrome. It should also not be used concurrently with Class Ia antiarrhythmics (disopyramide, procainamide, quinidine) or Class III antiarrhythmics. Contraindications to glatiramer include mannitol hypersensitivity. Natalizumab should not be used by patients with a history of progressive multifocal leukoencephalopathy. Teriflunomide is contraindicated in patients with severe liver impairment, women of childbearing age who do not use contraception reliably, and women who are pregnant. Dimethyl fumarate and mitoxantrone do not have contra-indications.

Cautions and Considerations Dimethyl fumarate may decrease lymphocyte counts; consequently, these counts should be monitored while patients are undergoing therapy. Fingolimod is associated with the risk of varicella-zoster virus infections and tumor development. Mitoxantrone therapy may lead to bone marrow suppression and typically should not be used in patients with neutropenia. Myocardial toxicity may occur with mitoxantrone use, and the risk increases with cumulative dosing. Severe local tissue damage can occur with mitoxantrone extravasation. Natalizumab may increase the risk of developing fatal or disabling progressive multifocal leuko-encephalopathy. Routine monitoring of signs and symptoms of this condition is required. Teriflunomide use is associated with a risk of liver toxicity; therefore, patients with liver disease should be cautious when taking this drug. This agent is not recommended during pregnancy, so women of childbearing age should also be cautious.

Drug Interactions These drugs increase the adverse effects of live vaccines:

- Fingolimod has an additive effect with other drugs that prolong the QT interval. It may enhance the arrhythmogenic effects of antiarrhythmic agents.
- Glatiramer acetate may enhance the adverse effects of immunosuppressants.
- Mitoxantrone may decrease levels of digoxin and hydantoins.
- Natalizumab may enhance the adverse effects of other immunosuppressants.
- Teriflunomide may enhance the adverse effects of other immunosuppressants.

Huntington's Disease

Huntington's disease (also known as Huntington's chorea) is a neurodegenerative disorder characterized by brief, repetitive, jerky, involuntary movements (known as chorea). It is also characterized by emotional disturbances and other problems with brain function, such as memory and reasoning skills.

Tetrabenazine (Xenazine) is approved to treat this condition. This drug works by reducing the activity of chemicals (especially dopamine) in the brain, thereby reducing the involuntary movements associated with the disease. Tetrabenazine must be dose-titrated to the optimal dose. It also has serious side effects, including neurologic side effects, which should be carefully monitored. The drug is dispensed from a specialty pharmacy.

Restless Leg Syndrome and Fibromyalgia

Restless leg syndrome (RLS) causes pain or unpleasant sensations in the legs, especially between the knees and ankles. These sensations can be so uncomfortable and overwhelming that they force an individual to move his or her legs to find relief. The cause is generally unknown, although stress can worsen the condition. This syndrome occurs most often in middle-aged or older adults, usually at bedtime, which can create serious sleep disturbances. RLS may be linked to kidney disease, diabetes, PD, peripheral neuropathy, and iron deficiency. Pregnancy or withdrawal from sedatives may also cause these symptoms, as well as the use of lithium, calcium channel blockers, or caffeine. The cause of RLS is thought to be genetic, although the responsible abnormality has not yet been identified.

A person with **fibromyalgia** suffers from long-term pain across the entire body, as well as tenderness in the joints, muscles, and tendons. This syndrome has been linked to sleep problems, fatigue, headaches, anxiety, and depression. There is no known cause, but the disorder may be triggered by trauma, sleep disturbances, or infection. Fibromyalgia is most common in women age 20 through 50 years old.

There is no cure for RLS or fibromyalgia, so treatment is focused on relieving pain and stress. For RLS, a healthcare practitioner may recommend stretching exercises, massage, or warm baths. **Gabapentin (Horizant, Neurontin)** is approved to treat RLS. Antiparkinsonian medications, such as **pramipexole (Mirapex)** and **ropinirole (Requip)**, are also used to treat this ailment.

In treating fibromyalgia, a physician may start by recommending physical therapy, an exercise and fitness regimen, light massage, and relaxation techniques. Again, there is no consensus on proper treatment, but prescribers may try an antidepressant such as duloxetine (Cymbalta) or an anticonvulsant such as pregabalin (Lyrica). Both medications are discussed in Chapter 7.

Alzheimer's Disease

Alzheimer's disease was first described by Alois Alzheimer, a German psychiatrist, in 1907. It is a degenerative disorder of the brain that leads to progressive dementia (loss of memory, intellect, judgment, orientation, and speech) and changes in personality and behavior. In the early stages of the disease, the patient complains of memory deficit, forgetfulness, and/or misplacement of ordinary items. Depression is a part of the disease profile. As the disease progresses, complex tasks become impossible (for example, managing personal finances), and concentration becomes poor. In the final stages, the patient suffers complete incapacitation, disorientation, and failure to thrive.

Two neurochemical mechanisms for cognitive impairment have been identified. One underlying cause is that not enough of the neurotransmitter ACh is produced to transmit reliable signals through cholinergic pathways. The other underlying cause is that some of the receptors for the neurotransmitter glutamate are hyperactive and cause the neuron to fire even when there is no glutamate present.

Table 8.7 lists drugs most commonly used to manage Alzheimer's disease. These drugs slow the disease but do not cure or reverse it. There are no agents that will reverse the cognitive abnormalities. The depression associated with the disease is often treated with antidepressants, as determined by existing symptoms and adverse drug reaction profiles. Amitriptyline should be avoided in these patients because it blocks ACh receptors. Agitation and sleep disturbances should be treated with short-acting benzodiazepines.

TABLE 8.7 **Most Commonly Used Agents for Alzheimer's Disease**

Generic (Brand)	Pronunciation	Dosage Form	Common Dosage	Dispensing Status
donepezil (Aricept)	don-EP-a-zil	Tablet	5–23 mg a day	Rx
galantamine (Razadyne)	ga-LAN-ta-meen	Capsule, oral liquid, tablet	8–24 mg a day	Rx
memantine (Namenda)	MEM-an-teen	Capsule, oral solution, tablet	5–20 mg a day	Rx
rivastigmine (Exelon)	riv-a-STIG-meen	Capsule, oral liquid, patch	3–12 mg a day	Rx

Cholinesterase Inhibitors and Memantine

Cholinesterase inhibitors and memantine are used to treat mild symptoms early in disease progression and will not work once severe memory and functional loss have occurred. These agents work by inhibiting enzymes that break down ACh, a neurotransmitter thought to be deficient in the early stages of Alzheimer's disease. Common side effects of cholinesterase inhibitors include nausea, vomiting, agitation, rash, loss of appetite, weight loss, and confusion. These effects can be significant, so doses must be started low and increased slowly. If these effects do not ease with time or are particularly bothersome, the drug should be discontinued.

Donepezil (Aricept) is a cholinesterase inhibitor that improves memory and alertness, but donepezil is more selective for the cholinesterase that is in the CNS. Donepezil is taken orally, only once a day at bedtime.

Galantamine (Razadyne) is a cholinesterase inhibitor derived from daffodil bulbs. It may be better tolerated than rivastigmine, but not as well tolerated as donepezil. The oral forms of the drug should be taken with meals. This drug is rarely used because of deaths reported in some of the clinical trials.

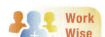
Memantine (Namenda) works by blocking the glutamate receptors known as NMDA receptors (named as such because they also respond to the chemical *N*-methyl-D-aspartate). These receptors are excessively excitable in Alzheimer's disease and can cause neurons to fire even without the neurotransmitter. Memantine may have less severe side effects and may be better tolerated than other drugs used to treat this disease. Some common side effects of memantine include dizziness, headache, sleepiness, constipation, vomiting, confusion, high blood pressure, and rash. If a patient experiences difficulty breathing, he or she should seek medical care immediately. The prescriber will provide starter doses to titrate the patient to the optimal dose. After the patient is stabilized and the optimal dose is established, the pharmacy will get a prescription. The results of clinical trials suggest that memantine slows advancement of Alzheimer's disease.

Rivastigmine (Exelon) is similar to donepezil, but it may be more difficult to dose and administer. The patch form was specifically designed for patients with Alzheimer's disease. It is a matrix formulation. This drug is thought to increase brain ACh levels through inhibition of acetylcholinesterase. It is approved to treat mild-to-moderate dementia associated with PD or Alzheimer's disease.

Contraindications Donepezil is contraindicated in patients with piperidine hypersensitivity. Contraindications to rivastigmine include a hypersensitivity to related compounds and a history of an application-site reaction to a rivastigmine patch. Memantine and galantamine do not have contraindications.

Cautions and Considerations Patients with cardiac disease, liver problems, or PD should not take donepezil.

Memantine should be used with caution in patients with the following conditions: seizure disorder, heart disease, kidney disease, or liver disease.

Drug Interactions Donepezil can interact with nonsteroidal anti-inflammatory drugs (NSAIDs), theophylline, and nicotine (through smoking). These substances should be avoided while taking donepezil. Galantamine may increase the adverse effects of other agents that prolong the QT interval. Trimethoprim may enhance the adverse effects of memantine. Rivastigmine may decrease the effects of anticholinergic agents.

Attention-Deficit/Hyperactivity Disorder

Attention-deficit/hyperactivity disorder (ADHD) has received a lot of media attention and carries with it many misconceptions about diagnosis and treatment. The condition is characterized by inattention, impulsivity, and hyperactivity. To be diagnosed with ADHD, an individual must exhibit six or more symptoms of inattention and six or more symptoms of hyperactivity/impulsivity that impair daily life in at least two settings for at least six months. Although many people think environment and stressors cause an individual to have ADHD, research has shown that these factors merely exacerbate the condition rather than cause it.

Some estimate that 3%–10% of school-aged children have some aspect of the disorder, whereas 5% of adults have ADHD. Onset occurs by age three years and is more prevalent in boys. Although hyperactivity symptoms decline with age, the inattention and impulsivity can persist into adulthood for half of those individuals who have this condition. Usually, symptoms improve after puberty when the frontal lobe of the brain fully matures. Several other disorders can coexist with ADHD. Most often these disorders include learning disabilities and, sometimes, depression or anxiety. Proper diagnosis and assistance with all learning disabilities are important steps in helping children with ADHD perform well in school. Counseling and behavioral strategies can help develop good coping mechanisms. Without adequate treatment and effective coping mechanisms, adults with ADHD can sometimes have problems with substance abuse. Therefore, ADHD and its coexisting conditions can be a difficult mix to treat effectively.

Central Nervous System Stimulants

Common therapy for children and adults with ADHD includes the use of **CNS stimulants**. These agents work best when used with behavioral therapy. Dosing starts low and is increased until optimal improvement in symptoms is seen without side effects. Immediate-release products are usually tried first. The first dose is often given before school (for children); if a second dose is needed, it will usually be given after school. (See Table 8.8 for more specific dosing information.) If longer effects may be needed, extended-release products may be used. Transdermal patches are applied in the morning, worn for nine hours, and then removed.

Methylphenidate (Concerta, Daytrana, Metadate, Metadate ER, Methylin, Ritalin, Ritalin-SR), a Schedule II agent, is commonly used to treat ADHD. Methylphenidate improves concentration for many patients by increasing levels of neurotransmitters in the brain. It should be used as an adjunct to psychosocial measures. Like amphetamine, it has a paradoxical calming effect in hyperactive children. CBC with differential (number of types of cells) and platelet counts should be monitored during long-term therapy. To help prevent the development of tolerance, the patient can skip methylphenidate doses, especially during times of low stress, such as during weekends and vacations. When the patient resumes medication, he or she may be able to decrease the necessary dosage. Caffeine may decrease this drug's efficacy, so the patient should avoid coffee, tea, and colas. The patient should get plenty of rest. This drug does have abuse potential.

Concerta is dosed once per day, which allows it to be given only in the morning. The outer layer of Concerta dissolves to release part of the dose immediately. The rest of the tablet is an osmotic-release oral delivery system (OROS) tablet (described in Chapter 7 in connection with paliperidone), which releases the drug slowly through pores in the tablet, leaving a ghost tablet that passes through the stool. Daytrana is the patch form of methylphenidate. It is worn for nine hours and then removed.

Caution should be used with administration of the patch, as the drug is contained in the adhesive.

Dexmethylphenidate (Focalin) consists of the dextrorotatory isomer of methylphenidate. An **isomer** is one of two (or more) compounds that contain the same number and type of atoms but have different molecular structures. Many biologically active substances have isomers whose molecules are mirror images of each other, like a pair of gloves. Such isomers are often distinguished by the terms *dextrorotatory* (right) and *levorotatory* (left). Methylphenidate is such a compound, with D (dextrorotatory) and L (levorotatory) isomers. Dexmethylphenidate contains only the more active dextrorotatory isomer of methylphenidate. Because dexmethylphenidate only contains one isomer, it is expected to have fewer side effects than methylphenidate. Like methylphenidate, it is a Schedule II drug.

Dextroamphetamine-amphetamine (Adderall), a Schedule II agent, is an alternative to other stimulants. Its effects can last about six hours, long enough to get some children through the school day. The primary side effect is depression as the drug wears off.

Lisdexamfetamine (Vyvanse) is dextroamphetamine chemically bonded to the amino acid lysine. Enzymes in the GI tract cleave the lysine, leaving dextroamphetamine, an active drug. The attachment to lysine is intended to reduce the abuse potential of the drug, which is a problem with dextroamphetamine. Once the lysine is cleaved, the dextroamphetamine is absorbed rapidly, so this drug is still a Schedule II substance. A medication guide must be distributed with this drug.

Contraindications All stimulant drugs that are mentioned in this chapter for the treatment of ADHD are contraindicated with or within 14 days of the use of MAOIs. Amphetamine salts, dextroamphetamine, and methylphenidate are contraindicated in patients with cardiovascular disease, high blood pressure, hyperthyroidism, glaucoma,

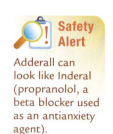

Safety Alert

Adderall can look like Inderal (propranolol, a beta blocker used as an antianxiety agent).

TABLE 8.8   Most Commonly Used Agents for Attention-Deficit Disorders

Generic (Brand)	Pronunciation	Dosage Form	Dispensing Status	Controlled-Substance Schedule
Stimulants				
dexmethylphenidate (Focalin, Focalin XR)	dex-meth-il-FEN-i-date	Capsule, tablet	Rx	C-II
dextroamphetamine-amphetamine (Adderall, Adderall XR)	dex-troe-am-FET-a-meen am-FET-a-meen	Capsule, tablet	Rx	C-II
lisdexamfetamine (Vyvanse)	liss-dex-am-FET-a-meen	Capsule	Rx	C-II
methylphenidate (Concerta, Daytrana, Methylin, Quillivant XR, Ritalin, Ritalin LA, Ritalin-SR)	meth-il-FEN-i-date	Capsule, oral solution, oral suspension, tablet, trans-dermal patch	Rx	C-II
Nonstimulants				
atomoxetine (Strattera)	at-oh-MOX-e-teen	Capsule	Rx	

Note: All of these drugs require a medication guide.

and agitated states, and in patients with a history of drug abuse. Contraindications to dexmethylphenidate include high levels of anxiety, tension, and agitation; glaucoma; and motor tics or a diagnosis of Tourette's syndrome.

Cautions and Considerations The CNS stimulants for ADHD have black box warnings for the potential drug dependence. Dextroamphetamine-amphetamine also carries a boxed warning for associated cardiovascular events. Rare but serious (even fatal) cardiac abnormalities have occurred with the use of all CNS stimulants. All CNS stimulants are controlled substances (Schedule II) and have abuse and addiction potential. Therefore, no refills are allowed, and only a limited supply can be dispensed at each pickup.

Drug Interactions These drugs may enhance the desired effects of analgesics. Stimulants may decrease the desired effects of sedatives. Antipsychotic agents may decrease the desired effects of stimulants. Atomoxetine and MAOIs may increase the hypertensive effects of stimulants.

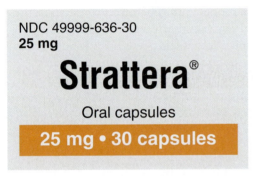

NDC 49999-636-30
25 mg

Strattera®

Oral capsules

25 mg • 30 capsules

Atomoxetine (Strattera) is a drug for ADHD.

Nonstimulant Drugs

Nonstimulant drugs are also used to treat ADHD. **Atomoxetine (Strattera)** may be a good choice for a patient who also has substance abuse problems because it does not have the potential for abuse and, therefore, is not a controlled substance. Other nonstimulant agents, including antidepressants such as bupropion, desipramine, nortriptyline, and venlafaxine, may also be used (see Chapter 7). Clonidine and guanfacine are used when a patient has tics or insomnia as part of ADHD.

Atomoxetine is a nonstimulant medication that selectively inhibits reuptake of norepinephrine, which controls impulsivity and activity. It is the only nonstimulant indicated for the treatment of ADHD in patients six years and older. Atomoxetine has been shown to be as effective as psychostimulants and therefore can be a reasonable alternative with a lower risk for abuse. It is not a controlled substance, so prescriptions can be refilled and called in as a verbal order. Atomoxetine should be used as a first-line agent. Like other drugs for attention-deficit disorders, atomoxetine can cause weight loss and slow growth. Common side effects are nausea, heartburn, fatigue, and decreased appetite.

Contraindications Atomoxetine should be avoided in patients with narrow-angle glaucoma, pheochromocytoma, and heart disorders.

Cautions and Considerations Atomoxetine can cause severe liver injury; therefore, laboratory tests should be conducted and results monitored for patients taking this medication. Patients with preexisting liver problems should avoid atomoxetine, if possible. Finally, atomoxetine has been associated with increased suicidal thoughts and, therefore, has a black box warning regarding this possible event. Children and adolescents who are prescribed atomoxetine should be monitored closely. Patients with depression may not be good candidates for this drug therapy.

Drug Interactions Atomoxetine may prolong the QT interval or enhance the effects of other medications used for this purpose.

Complementary and Alternative Therapies

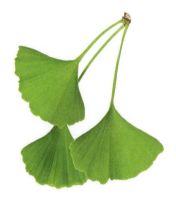

Ginkgo biloba may be used to improve memory.

Yoga, an ancient practice, is used to help patients cope with the effects of many CNS disorders including epilepsy and ADHD. It is generally considered safe for most individuals. Of note, certain yoga breathing techniques should be avoided in patients with lung or heart disease.

Certain complementary and alternative therapies are used in patients with PD. One, **5-hydroxytryptophan**, is the chemical precursor to serotonin and improves motor symptoms in patients with PD. It should be used with caution in patients using antidepressants or other medications for PD. Music therapy may improve motor symptoms, speech, and bradykinesia.

Ginkgo biloba may slightly benefit patients with early Alzheimer's disease, but serious side effects (e.g., bleeding, seizures, and coma) have occurred with its use. Results of studies are inconclusive and do not necessarily show dramatic improvement in memory or thinking. The benefits of taking ginkgo biloba to prevent Alzheimer's disease are questionable, although many patients take it for this purpose. If patients choose to take ginkgo biloba, they should clearly and fully understand the risks and benefits. Typical doses are 120 to 720 mg ginkgo extract, and commercially available products vary in their content. Ginkgo biloba has antiplatelet effects that affect bleeding. Patients taking warfarin or aspirin for coagulation effects should not use ginkgo biloba without medical supervision. This supplement also interacts with several other prescription medications, particularly anticonvulsants. Therefore, patients who take other prescription medications should discuss taking ginkgo biloba with their prescribers and pharmacists before doing so.

CHAPTER SUMMARY

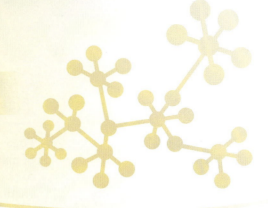

Seizure Disorders

- Epilepsy is a common neurologic disorder defined as paroxysmal seizures. It involves disturbances of neuronal electrical activity that interfere with normal brain function.

- Two major classifications of seizures are generalized and partial.

- The objective of antiepileptic drug therapy is to eliminate seizures without compromising the patient's quality of life because of adverse effects.

- Different seizure types require different drugs.

- All anticonvulsants have very narrow dose/therapeutic ranges. A slight dosage change can result in loss of seizure control or an increase in toxicity; therefore, prescribers often specify the brand-name drug.

- Black box warnings are serious warnings about a drug that are highlighted in a box in the FDA-approved product information.

Parkinson's Disease

- For normal movements to be performed, the two primary neurotransmitters—dopamine (an inhibitor) and acetylcholine (a stimulator)—must be in balance. In PD, these transmitters are not in balance.

- Dopamine will not cross the blood-brain barrier.

- Levodopa-carbidopa is probably the drug that is most often prescribed to treat PD.

- Bromocriptine (Parlodel) is used to treat PD.

- Selegiline (Eldepryl) is an MAOI used to treat PD.

Other Central Nervous System Disorders

- Acetylcholinesterase inhibitors can produce clinical improvement in certain types of myasthenia gravis.

- Interferons are one class of drugs used to treat MS.

- Glatiramer acetate (Copaxone), a drug used to treat MS, must be kept refrigerated but never frozen.

- Alzheimer's disease is a progressive form of dementia.

- Data from clinical trials indicate that memantine (Namenda) slows the progression of Alzheimer's disease.

- Methylphenidate (Concerta, Daytrana, Metadate, Metadate ER, Methylin, Ritalin, Ritalin-SR) is a CNS stimulant and Schedule II controlled substance used primarily for attention-deficit disorders. Improved dosage forms allow the drug to be taken only in the morning, and one form is administered through a patch, improving patient adherence.

- Atomoxetine (Strattera) is the only nonstimulant medication indicated for the treatment of ADHD in patients six years and older.

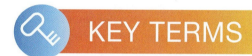 KEY TERMS

absence seizure a type of generalized seizure characterized by a sudden, momentary break in consciousness; formerly called a *petit mal seizure*

Alzheimer's disease a degenerative disorder of the brain that leads to progressive dementia and changes in personality and behavior

amyotrophic lateral sclerosis (ALS) a degenerative disease of the motor nerves; also called *Lou Gehrig's disease*

anticonvulsant a drug used to control seizures

atonic seizure a type of generalized seizure characterized by sudden loss of both muscle tone and consciousness

attention-deficit/hyperactivity disorder (ADHD) a disorder that manifests itself in difficulty in focusing or concentration, overactivity, and difficulty in impulse control

basal nuclei symmetric, subcortical masses of gray matter embedded in the lower portions of the cerebral hemisphere; part of the extrapyramidal system; also called *basal ganglia*

CNS stimulants a common therapy for children and adults diagnosed with ADHD

complex partial seizure a type of seizure in which the patient experiences impaired consciousness, often with confusion, a blank stare, and postseizure amnesia

convulsion involuntary contraction or series of contractions of the voluntary muscles

diplopia the perception of two images of a single object

dysarthria imperfect articulation of speech

dyskinesia impairment of the power of voluntary movement

dysphagia difficulty in swallowing

enzyme biological molecule that catalyzes chemical reactions in the body

epilepsy a neurologic disorder involving sudden and recurring seizures

fibromyalgia a condition characterized by long-term pain throughout the entire body

generalized seizure a seizure that involves both hemispheres of the brain simultaneously and has no local origin; can be a tonic-clonic (grand mal), absence (petit mal), myoclonic, or atonic seizure

grand mal seizure see tonic-clonic seizure

Huntington's disease a neurodegenerative disorder characterized by brief, repetitive, involuntary movements; also known as *Huntington's chorea*

interferon a substance that exerts virus-nonspecific but host-specific antiviral activity by inducing genes coding for antiviral proteins that inhibit the synthesis of viral RNA

isomer one of two or more compounds that contain the same number and type of atoms but have different molecular structures

Lou Gehrig's disease see amyotrophic lateral sclerosis (ALS)

motor end plate the neuromuscular junction, where the nervous system and muscular system meet to produce or stop movement

multiple sclerosis (MS) an autoimmune disease in which the myelin sheaths around nerves degenerate

muscle fasciculation a small, local, involuntary muscular contraction visible under the skin

myasthenia gravis an autoimmune disorder of the neuromuscular junction in which the ACh receptors are destroyed at the motor end plate, preventing muscles from responding to nerve signals to move them

myoclonic seizure a type of generalized seizure characterized by sudden muscle contractions with no loss of consciousness

on-off phenomenon a wide fluctuation between abnormally increased and abnormally diminished motor function, present in many patients with Parkinson's disease after about five years of levodopa therapy

Parkinson's disease (PD) a neurologic disorder characterized by akinesia, resting tremors, and muscular rigidity

paroxysmal something sudden and recurring

partial seizure an abnormal electrical discharge centered in a specific area of the brain; usually caused by trauma

petit mal seizure see absence seizure

phlebitis inflammation of a vein

ptosis paralytic drooping of the upper eyelid

restless leg syndrome (RLS) an overpowering sensation causing the urge to move the legs, especially while at rest

seizures spasms from an overfiring of the neurons of the brain and nervous system; result in a change in behavior of which the patient is not aware

simple partial seizure a type of seizure in which the patient does not lose consciousness and may have some muscular activity manifested as twitching, and sensory hallucinations

sodium channel blockers drugs that make neurons less likely to fire by blocking the flow of positively charged sodium ions

status epilepticus a serious disorder involving tonic-clonic convulsions that last at least 30 minutes

substantia nigra a layer of gray substance separating parts of the brain

tonic-clonic seizure a type of generalized seizure characterized by body rigidity followed by muscle jerks; formerly called a *grand mal seizure*

DRUG LIST

Anticonvulsants

carbamazepine (Epitol, Tegretol)
ethosuximide (Zarontin)
felbamate (Felbatol)
fosphenytoin (Cerebyx)
gabapentin (Horizant, Neurontin)
lacosamide (Vimpat)
lamotrigine (Lamictal)
levetiracetam (Keppra)
oxcarbazepine (Trileptal)
phenobarbital (Luminal)
phenytoin (Dilantin)
pregabalin (Lyrica)
primidone (Mysoline)
tiagabine (Gabitril)
topiramate (Topamax)
valproic acid (Depakene, Depakote)
vigabatrin (Sabril)
zonisamide (Zonegran)

Antiparkinsonian Agents

amantadine (Symmetrel)
apomorphine
benztropine (Cogentin)
bromocriptine (Parlodel)
catechol-O-methyltransferase (COMT)
entacapone (Comtan)
levodopa-carbidopa (Sinemet)
levodopa-carbidopa-entacapone (Stalveo)
pramipexole (Mirapex)
rasagiline (Azilect)
ropinirole (Requip)
selegiline (Eldepryl, Zelapar)
tolcapone (Tasmar)
trihexyphenidyl (Trihexy)

Myasthenia Gravis

azathioprine (Imuran)
cyclophosphamide (Cytoxan)
pyridostigmine (Mestinon)

Amyotrophic Lateral Sclerosis (ALS), Multiple Sclerosis (MS), and Huntington's Disease

dimethyl fumarate (Tecfidera)
fingolimod (Gilenya)
glatiramer acetate (Copaxone)
interferon beta-1a (Avonex, Rebif)
interferon beta-1b (Betaseron, Extavia)
mitoxantrone (Novantrone)
natalizumab (Tysabri)
riluzole (Rilutek)
teriflunomide (Aubagio)
tetrabenazine (Xenazine)

Alzheimer's Disease

donepezil (Aricept)
galantamine (Razadyne)
ginkgo biloba
interferon beta-1a (Avonex, Rebif)
interferon beta-1b (Betaseron, Extavia)
memantine (Namenda)
rivastigmine (Exelon)

Attention-Deficit/Hyperactivity Disorder (ADHD)

atomoxetine (Strattera)
dexmethylphenidate (Focalin)
dextroamphetamine-amphetamine (Adderall)
lisdexamfetamine (Vyvanse)
methylphenidate (Concerta, Daytrana, Metadate, Metadate ER, Methylin, Ritalin, Ritalin-SR)

Restless Leg Syndrome (RLS) and Fibromyalgia

gabapentin (Horizant, Neurontin)
pramipexole (Mirapex)
ropinirole (Requip)

Black Box Warnings

atomoxetine (Strattera)
azathioprine (Imuran)
carbamazepine (Epitol, Tegretol)
dextroamphetamine-amphetamine (Adderall)
fosphenytoin (Cerebyx)
lamotrigine (Lamictal)
lisdexamfetamine (Vyvanse)
methylphenidate (Concerta, Daytrana, Metadate, Methylin, Ritalin)
mitoxantrone (Novantrone)
tetrabenazine (Xenazine)
tolcapone (Tasmar)
valproic acid (Depakene, Depakote)

Medication Guides

dextroamphetamine-amphetamine (Adderall)
divalproex (Depakote)
ethosuximide (Zarontin)
gabapentin (Horizant, Neurontin)
interferon beta-1a (Avonex, Rebif)
interferon beta-1b (Betaseron, Extavia)
lamotrigine (Lamictal)
levetiracetam (Keppra)
lisdexamfetamine (Vyvanse)
methylphenidate (Concerta, Daytrana, Metadate, Methylin, Ritalin)
mitoxantrone (Novantrone)
oxcarbazepine (Trileptal)
phenytoin (Dilantin)
pregabalin (Lyrica)
primidone (Mysoline)
topiramate (Topamax)
valproic acid (Depakene, Depakote)
zonisamide (Zonegran)

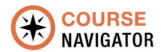

COURSE NAVIGATOR

Access interactive chapter review exercises, practice activities, flash cards, and study games.

9

Respiratory Drugs

Learning Objectives

1 Differentiate between the main pulmonary diseases.

2 Describe the pathophysiology and treatment of asthma.

3 Discuss the pathophysiology and treatment of chronic obstructive pulmonary disease.

4 Summarize the reemergence of tuberculosis and its associated treatments.

5 Describe the mechanism of action and uses of antitussives, expectorants, decongestants, and antihistamines.

6 Paraphrase why some drugs are prescribed for their side effects.

7 Outline smoking cessation plans and supportive therapy.

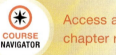 Access additional chapter resources.

The respiratory diseases covered in this chapter include asthma, chronic obstructive pulmonary disease (COPD), and other related disorders. COPD encompasses two major diseases: emphysema and chronic bronchitis. COPD is irreversible, whereas asthma is reversible. Other related obstructive diseases include pneumonia, cystic fibrosis, respiratory distress syndrome, tuberculosis, and histoplasmosis. In addition, the lungs are frequently attacked by less severe upper respiratory tract infections, including the common cold. Allergies are also discussed in this chapter because many of the drugs used to treat respiratory diseases are often used to treat allergies. It is important to remember that asthma and allergies are quite different. Smoking, which is closely linked to many respiratory diseases, is also included in this chapter. Several innovative drugs are available to help smokers quit.

Asthma

Asthma is an inflammatory disorder of the airways and causes coughing, wheezing, breathlessness, and chest tightness. It occurs in intermittent attacks that involve a reversible airway obstruction, and it is precipitated by specific triggering events that vary in severity from patient to patient.

FIGURE 9.1
Upper and Lower Respiratory Tracts

The upper respiratory tract includes structures such as the nasal cavity, pharynx, larynx, and trachea. The lower respiratory tract includes the lungs, bronchi, and bronchioles.

FIGURE 9.2
Exchange of Oxygen and Carbon Dioxide

Oxygen picked up in the lungs is carried by red blood cells to all the cells of the body, while carbon dioxide is returned to the lungs to be expelled during exhalation.

Figure 9.1 shows the upper and lower respiratory tracts (or airways), through which gases pass in the respiratory system. Oxygen flows through and across membrane surfaces, where it is exchanged with carbon dioxide, as shown in Figure 9.2. In asthma, as a result of the obstructed airways, less oxygen is available to exchange with carbon dioxide, or the surface area available for gas exchange is decreased. Bronchioles constrict, mucus production increases, and lung tissue swells (see Figure 9.3), making normal breathing difficult.

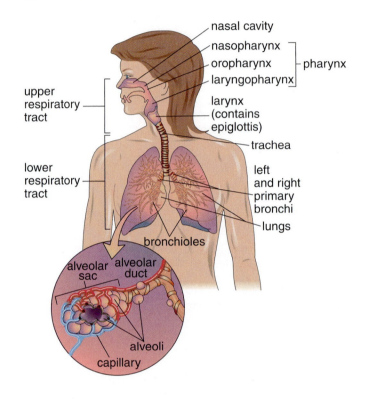

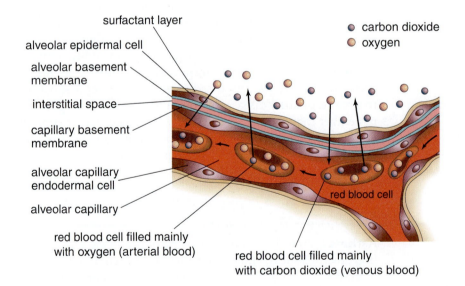

Asthma has the following characteristics: reversible small airway obstruction, progressive airway inflammation, and increased airway responsiveness to a variety of endogenous and exogenous stimuli. These characteristics translate into recurrent episodes of **wheezing** (a whistling respiratory sound), **dyspnea** (labored or difficult breathing), and cough that have both **acute** (short, severe course) and **chronic** (persisting for a long time) manifestations in most patients.

Asthma differs from normal pulmonary defense mechanisms in its severity of **bronchospasm** (spasmodic contraction of the smooth muscles of the bronchioles, or small airways), apparent failure of normal dilator muscle systems, excessive production of mucus that plugs airways, and the presence of sometimes severe long-term inflammatory reactions that may lead to patchy shedding of the linings of small airways.

Asthmatic Response

Asthma is episodic, meaning that times of poor airflow and difficulty with breathing alternate with times of normal function. Acute difficulty with breathing, known as an **asthma attack**, is characterized by hyperreactivity of the airways and bronchospasm, usually in response to allergens or irritants. Common triggers include smoke, dust, exercise, pet dander, cold weather, gastroesophageal reflux disease (GERD), and colds or flu. Other potential triggers include medications, anxiety, laughing, and certain foods.

Immediately after exposure to a trigger, mast cells in the lung tissue release histamine and other chemical mediators that cause bronchoconstriction and increased mucus production. Edema may also result. See Figure 9.3 for an illustration of this process.

Over time, continued release of histamine, bradykinin, prostaglandins, and leukotrienes causes tissues to inflame and airways to constrict and can result in permanent lung tissue damage. Fortunately, in many cases, breathing symptoms and airway constriction can be controlled with proper treatment. Without treatment, lung function can steadily decline.

FIGURE 9.3
Asthmatic Lung

During an asthma attack, the lung "overreacts" to produce excess mucus and swelling. The combination of excess mucus and bronchoconstriction decreases airflow.

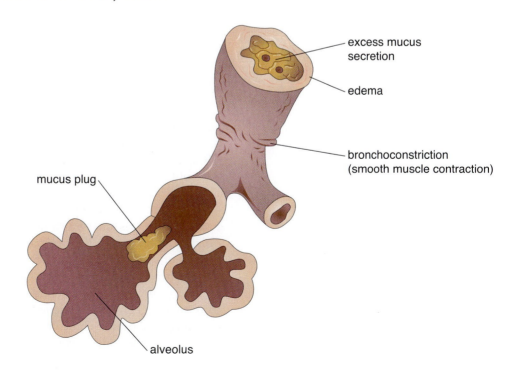

excess mucus secretion

edema

bronchoconstriction (smooth muscle contraction)

mucus plug

alveolus

The most useful means of assessing the severity of asthma is with an instrument known as a **peak flow meter**, which measures **peak expiratory flow rate (PEFR)**. Patients forcefully blow into the peak flow meter, and PEFR is recorded in liters per minute. A measurement below 50% of a patient's personal best PEFR indicates a medical alert; immediate treatment with a bronchodilator and anti-inflammatory agent is needed, and the patient's healthcare provider should be notified.

Asthma Management

Asthma is categorized into levels of severity (intermittent, mild, moderate, and severe) based on how patients' symptoms affect their ability to sleep at night, continue normal daily activities, and breathe freely. Objective **pulmonary function tests** can be done to assess asthma severity. In addition, if a patient is waking up at night more than twice a month because of asthma symptoms or is using relief medication such as an inhaler more than twice a week, asthma is considered "not controlled." Patients should understand that if their asthma is not controlled, they should seek medical treatment and be sure to adhere to prescribed medication schedules. Drug therapy for asthma includes long-term treatment to prevent exacerbations as well as rescue therapies to help once asthma attack symptoms have begun. Many patients need more than simple rescue therapies. Long-term, steady treatment can improve overall lung function, reduce exacerbations, and decrease the need for short-term relief therapies.

As part of good asthma care, the asthmatic patient must learn to manage the disease and its complications and to limit the amount of exposure to irritants that will cause airway inflammation. The patient needs to learn what can trigger asthma attacks and how to control those trigger factors. For example, the patient with asthma should avoid contact with smoke as much as possible because smoke is detrimental to patients with asthma. Also, because many people with asthma are allergic to dust mites, patients should follow simple dust mite control steps, including washing sheets and mattress pads at least once a week in hot (130°F or hotter) water. Asthma patients should also obtain a yearly flu vaccination.

Symptoms alone are not always the best measure of respiratory status. For this reason, patients must learn to use a peak flow meter to measure PEFR. The peak flow meter should be used twice a day and the results recorded in a diary as an aid to better management. Often, simply adjusting asthma medications on the basis of the peak flow meter readings helps manage asthma effectively.

Patients with asthma and their caregivers should be aware of the signs and symptoms of **status asthmaticus**, which is a potentially life-threatening condition. An episode of status asthmaticus begins like any other asthma attack, but, unlike an ordinary attack, it does not respond to normal management. The patient suffering from such an episode experiences increasing difficulty in breathing and exhibits blue lips and nail beds. The patient may lose consciousness. Status asthmaticus

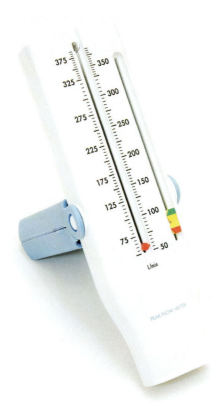

A peak flow meter is a valuable tool for patients to use to measure PEFR and manage symptoms of asthma.

clearly constitutes a medical emergency, and the patient should receive prompt attention. This event may require a visit to the emergency room.

Asthma Drug Therapy

Drug therapy is the mainstay of asthma management. The disease begins with intermittent attacks and may progress from mild to severe, persistent symptoms. Drug therapy depends on the severity of disease.

Drug therapy for asthma has two components: quick-relief medications and long-term persistent medications. **Quick-relief medications** are used intermittently and provide rapid relief, as needed, when asthma symptoms present or when an asthma attack occurs. **Long-term persistent medications** are used regularly to prevent asthma symptoms or attacks. Pharmacy technicians can help patients treat and prevent asthma attacks by promoting correct use of quick-relief medications and adherence to long-term persistent medications.

Asthma management is generally a stepwise process. An important method of administering asthma medications is by a **metered-dose inhaler (MDI)**—sometimes called a "puffer"—that contains medication and compressed gas. The MDI delivers a specific amount of medication with each actuation. The delivery mechanism suspends the medication in particles or droplets that are fine enough to penetrate to the deepest parts of the patient's lungs.

The prescriber usually orders an MDI to be used with a **spacer**. A spacer is recommended to decrease the amount of spray deposited on the back of the throat and swallowed. The spacer chamber holds the drug mist until the patient is ready to breathe. It also allows the patient to breathe the mist in at a slower, more effective rate, which, in turn, provides much better penetration of the drug into the lungs. Side effects are reduced because the drug is delivered to the lower portions of the lungs and fewer particles are left in the mouth and throat to be absorbed. A spacer is extremely useful for children and older adults who may have a hard time coordinating an inhaler. Strong evidence supports the use of spacers.

Historically, the propellant of MDIs has been chlorofluorocarbons (CFCs). Unfortunately, CFCs migrate into the atmosphere, undergo various chemical reactions, and are depleting and destroying the earth's protective ozone layer. CFCs were banned in the late 1980s. In 2008, the US Food and Drug Administration (FDA) required all MDIs to convert to hydrofluoroalkane (HFA) as the propellant; these MDIs are known as *HFA inhalers*. Studies have shown that HFA propellants produce a finer mist that has better pulmonary deposition of particles and does not produce serum or tissue accumulation when given at 12-hour intervals.

MDIs need to be primed (the inhaler should be shaken for five seconds before releasing a spray) before the the first use of the device or if the device is dropped or not used for several weeks. MDIs should also be shaken well before each use.

Most patients with asthma have prescriptions for MDIs. Although it may seem easy, the use of an MDI can be difficult and requires the proper technique to administer the medication effectively. The following describes how to use an MDI with a spacer:

1. Inspect the MDI and prime the inhaler, if necessary.
2. Shake the MDI well.
3. Attach the MDI to the spacer.
4. Breathe out completely.

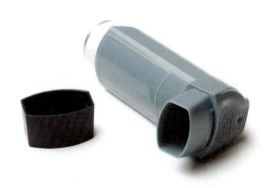

An MDI sprays a controlled amount of drug through the opening when the canister is actuated.

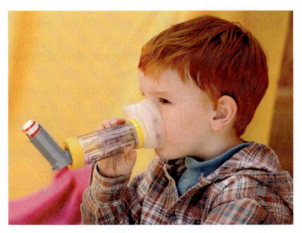

If a spacer is added to an MDI, the medication is more likely to penetrate deeper into the lung tissue than if the MDI is used alone. Spacers come with masks (often used by children, as pictured) and without masks.

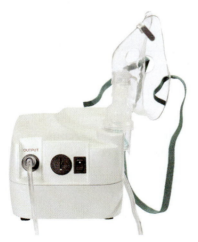

A nebulizer is a common method of administering asthma medication. It is especially effective for children.

5. Put the mouthpiece of the spacer in your mouth and close your lips around the mouthpiece to form a tight seal.

6. Press down on the canister of the MDI.

7. Take a slow, deep breath and breathe in as much air as you comfortably can.

8. Remove the mouthpiece from your mouth and hold your breath for 10 seconds or as long as comfortably possible.

9. If another puff of the inhaler is needed, wait one minute (except during asthma exacerbations) and repeat. During an asthma exacerbation, you may repeat steps immediately.

10. Rinse the plastic portion of the inhaler and the spacer once a week, and allow the devices to air-dry.

If another type of inhaler has been prescribed, the patient should wait five minutes before using it. Patients should always clean the mouthpiece after each use and rinse the mouth if a corticosteroid is used.

The primary difference between an HFA inhaler and a dry-powder inhaler (DPI) is in its actuation. A patient using an HFA inhaler should breathe in *slowly*, whereas a patient using a DPI should breathe in *quickly*. DPIs do not use gas propellants. Many manufacturers are incorporating asthma drugs into dry-powder devices.

Because of the complicated series of steps required to use HFAs and DPIs, they are not recommended for very young children. Asthma medication can be administered to children with a **nebulizer**, a device in which a stream of air flows past a liquid and creates a fine mist, which the patient inhales while breathing normally through a mouthpiece or mask. The drug thus is more likely to be deposited farther into the lungs. This delivery system is quite effective. If not properly cleaned and cared for, however, a home nebulizer can be a source of bronchitis and infections. Therefore, nebulizers should be cleaned regularly.

Short-Acting Beta Agonists

Also known as "rescue medicines," **short-acting beta agonists (SABAs)** are **bronchodilators** (agents that relax smooth-muscle cells of the bronchioles). SABAs work by stimulating beta-2 receptors in the lungs and by producing smooth muscle

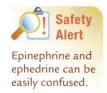

relaxation in the bronchioles. As a result, airway diameter increases, improving the movement of gases into and out of the lungs. Although oral dosage forms are available, most patients use SABAs by inhaling them into the lungs. Because their effects last for only a few hours, these agents may need to be used multiple times a day. Of the available dosage forms, the handheld MDI and nebulizer solution are the most frequently prescribed (see Table 9.1).

The pharmacy technician should be alert to the potential for patient overdependence on short-acting beta agonists. If the patient is using more than one canister per month, the pharmacy technician should alert the pharmacist who, in turn, should notify the prescriber. Such overdependence is generally a sign that the patient's asthma is not being adequately controled and that the prescriber needs to consider alternative treatment regimens.

Albuterol

Albuterol (ProAir, Proventil, Ventolin, VoSpire ER) is a bronchodilator used in the event of airway obstruction, such as asthma or COPD. It relaxes bronchial smooth muscle by acting on pulmonary beta-2 receptors with little effect on heart rate. Albuterol is administered by inhalation or orally for relief of bronchospasms. The duration of inhaled albuterol is typically three to six hours. Side effects include tremors and nervousness.

Contraindications Albuterol does not have contraindications.

Cautions and Considerations Pediatric patients using albuterol MDIs should use spacers if they are under five years of age. For patients younger than four years of age, using a face mask with a spacer may be the best way to deliver the drug.

Drug Interactions SABAs interact with beta blockers, which are frequently used by people with heart disease. Beta blockers inhibit the effect of these beta-agonist drugs. SABAs and beta blockers should not be used together; if they must be, prescribers should carefully adjust the doses.

TABLE 9.1 Most Commonly Used Agents for Asthma

Generic (Brand)	Pronunciation	Dosage Form	Common Dosage	Dispensing Status
albuterol* (ProAir, Proventil, Ventolin, VoSpire ER)	al-BYOO-ter-awl	Aerosol (MDI), nebulizer solution, syrup, tablet	Inhalation: 2.5 mg 3–4 times a day via nebulizer MDI: 1–2 puffs 3–4 times a day PO: 2–4 mg 3–4 times a day	Rx
levalbuterol (Xopenex)	lee-val-BYOO-ter-awl	Aerosol (MDI), nebulizer solution	Inhalation: 0.63–1.25 mg 3 times a day via nebulizer MDI: 2 puffs every 4–6 hr	Rx
metaproterenol* (Alupent)	met-a-proe-TER-e-nawl	Syrup, tablet	PO: 10–20 mg 3–4 times a day	Rx

* These products are produced several dosage forms, such as inhalants, liquids (for use in nebulizers), syrups, and injections. Pharmacists and pharmacy technicians should always carefully read the prescription and select the correct dosage form.

Levalbuterol

Levalbuterol (Xopenex) is similar to albuterol. Albuterol contains two chemical forms of albuterol. Levalbuterol only contains the form of albuterol that is thought to induce bronchodilation. Side effects are similar to albuterol.

Contraindications Levalbuterol is contraindicated in patients with a hypersensitivity to albuterol.

Cautions and Considerations Hypersensitivity reactions have been reported with levalbuterol use.

Drug Interactions SABAs interact with beta blockers, which are frequently used by people with heart disease. Beta blockers inhibit the effect of these beta-agonist drugs. Short-acting beta agonists and beta blockers should not be used together; if they must be, prescribers must carefully adjust the doses.

Metaproterenol

Metaproterenol (Alupent) is a bronchodilator for airway obstruction. It has a rapid onset of action (within minutes), a peak effect (in approximately one hour), and a prolonged effect (approximately four hours). Metaproterenol acts primarily on beta-2 receptors, with little or no effect on heart rate.

Contraindications Metaproterenol does not have contraindications.

Cautions and Considerations Some formulations of metaproterenol contain benzyl alcohol. Benzyl alcohol is associated with toxicities in neonates.

Drug Interactions SABAs interact with beta blockers, which are frequently used by people with heart disease. Beta blockers inhibit the effect of these beta-agonist drugs. Short-acting beta agonists and beta blockers should not be used together; if they must be, prescribers must carefully adjust the doses.

Corticosteroids

Corticosteroids resemble certain chemicals naturally produced by the adrenal gland. Corticosteroids inhibit inflammatory cells by stimulating adenylate cyclase. They act as anti-inflammatory agents to suppress the immune response. Inhaled corticosteroids may be successful when other drugs are not.

The primary side effects of these drugs, if inhaled, are oral candidiasis (a fungal infection), irritation and burning of the nasal mucosa, hoarseness, and dry mouth. This irritation can sometimes lead to episodes of coughing. To reduce the likelihood of these effects, the patient should always be advised to rinse the mouth thoroughly with water after using a corticosteroid inhaler. Improper technique when using an MDI can result in inadequate response, but this problem can be prevented with proper instruction. More information on inhaled corticosteroids can be found in Table 9.2.

If oral corticosteroids are taken for a long period in a dosage exceeding 10 mg of prednisone a day, they can cause growth of facial hair in female patients, breast development in male patients, "buffalo hump," "moon face," edema, weight gain, and easy bruising. A short-term course of high-dose corticosteroids will not cause these side effects.

Another concern is that corticosteroids may stunt a child's growth. Evidence indicates, however, that inhaled steroids do not affect long-term growth in children. Initially, growth may slow down by a half inch in the first year, but children eventually

TABLE 9.2 Common Inhaled Corticosteroids

Generic (Brand)	Pronunciation	Dosage Form	Common Dosage	Dispensing Status
beclomethasone (QVAR, Vanceril)	bek-loe-METH-a-sone	Aerosol (MDI)	40–160 mcg twice a day	Rx
budesonide* (Pulmicort, Rhinocort)	byoo-DES-oh-nide	Powder for inhalation, suspension for inhalation	200–800 mcg twice a day	Rx
flunisolide (Aerospan)	floo-NIS-oh-lide	Aerosol (MDI)	160–320 mcg twice a day	Rx
fluticasone* (Flonase, Flovent)	floo-TIK-a-sone	Aerosol (MDI), powder for inhalation	88–440 mcg twice a day	Rx
mometasone (Asmanex, Asmanex HFA)	moe-MET-a-sone	Aerosol (MDI), powder for inhalation	110–440 mcg 1–2 times a day	Rx
Combinations				
budesonide-formoterol (Symbicort)	byoo-DES-oh-nide for-MOE-ter-awl	Aerosol (MDI)	160/9–320/9 mg twice a day	Rx
fluticasone-salmeterol (Advair Diskus, Advair HFA)	floo-TIK-a-sone sal-ME-te-role	Aerosol (MDI), powder for inhalation	Advair Diskus: 100 mcg/50 mcg to 500 mcg/50 mcg twice a day Advair HFA: 45 mcg/21 mcg–230 mcg/21 mcg, two inhalations, twice a day	Rx

* These products are produced in several dosage forms, such as inhalants, liquids (for use in nebulizers), syrups, and injections. Pharmacists and pharmacy technicians should always carefully read the prescription and select the correct dosage form.

reach normal adult height. The benefits of controlling asthma may outweigh the risks of achieving normal growth and development.

Patients should always use the lowest effective dose of a corticosteroid. A beta agonist should be added to inhaled corticosteroids if needed to decrease the steroid dose necessary for control. The beta agonist helps open the airway, thus allowing more of the inhaled steroid to reach its site of action in the lungs.

Beclomethasone

Beclomethasone (QVAR) is a commonly used inhaled corticosteroid. Patients should rinse their mouth after using beclomethasone, as they should with any steroid inhaler.

Contraindications Inhaled corticosteroids are contraindicated during acute asthma attacks.

Cautions and Considerations Beclomethasone is delivered with an MDI and should not be confused with DPIs.

Drug Interactions Beclomethasone interacts with immunosuppressants, efalizumab, natalizumab, and tacrolimus.

Budesonide

Budesonide (Pulmicort Flexhaler, Pulmicort Respules) is a corticosteroid with unique administration techniques. Pulmicort Flexhaler uses a dry-powder, propellant-free inhalant that is breath activated. As a result, it may be easier to use. Moreover, the Flexhaler needs to be primed only prior to the initial use rather than before each dose, as is necessary with other corticosteroid inhalers. As with other drugs in this class, patients should be instructed to rinse the mouth after each dose. Inadequate response to budesonide is often the result of improper inhalation technique. Pulmicort is associated with a lower frequency of coughing episodes than other inhaled corticosteroids. Pulmicort Respules was the first formulation of budesonide for use in home nebulizers. This formulation has made it possible to treat children as young as 12 months with budesonide.

Contraindications These inhalers are contraindicated during acute asthma attacks.

Cautions and Considerations DPIs should not be shaken prior to use. Patients should carefully follow instructions for puncturing the powder packet or capsule and then placing the device in the mouth before forceful inhalation.

Drug Interactions Budesonide is a cytochrome P-450 3A4 (CYP 3A4) substrate, and metabolism decreases with concomitant administration with CYP 3A4 inhibitors, such as ketoconazole, itraconazole, and ritonavir. Budesonide doses must be decreased when patients are using one of these drugs.

Fluticasone

Fluticasone (Flovent) is the same drug found in the nasal spray Flonase and is available as a topical product. For respiratory disorders, fluticasone is available as an aerosol for inhalation (MDI) and as a DPI. It may be used once or twice daily, depending on the product, and may take up to two weeks to reach maximum benefit.

Contraindications Inhaled corticosteroids are contraindicated during acute asthma attacks. Fluticasone powder for inhalation contains lactose and should not be used in those patients with a hypersensitivity to milk proteins or lactose. That same patient population should also avoid the combined product, fluticasone-salmeterol.

Cautions and Considerations MDIs should be shaken before each use. DPIs should not be shaken prior to use. Patients should carefully follow instructions for puncturing the powder packet or capsule and then placing the device in the mouth before forceful inhalation.

Drug Interactions Fluticasone is a CYP 3A4 substrate, and metabolism decreases with concomitant administration with CYP 3A4 inhibitors, such as ketoconazole, itraconazole, and ritonavir. Fluticasone doses must be decreased when patients are using one of these drugs.

Mometasone

Mometasone (Asmanex) is a dry powder for inhalation. It should be dosed once daily in the evening or twice daily. The dispenser is called a Twisthaler, and it has a dose counter. When the dose counter gets to 00 or the package has been opened for 45 days, the patient should throw the dispenser away. Pharmacy technicians should write the date opened on the dispenser and make sure the patient knows when to dispose of the drug. Mometasone can be used for prophylactic therapy, but maximum benefit may take two weeks or longer. Headache is the major side effect. Mometasone has high potency and little systemic bioavailability.

Contraindications Inhaled corticosteroids are contraindicated during acute asthma attacks.

Mometasone powder for inhalation contains lactose and should not be used in those patients with a hypersensitivity to milk proteins or lactose.

Cautions and Considerations DPIs should not be shaken prior to use. Patients should carefully follow instructions for puncturing the powder packet or capsule and then placing the device in the mouth before forceful inhalation.

Drug Interactions Mometasone is a CYP 3A4 substrate, and metabolism decreases with concomitant administration with CYP 3A4 inhibitors, such as ketoconazole, itraconazole, and ritonavir. Mometasone doses must be decreased when patients are using one of these drugs.

Other inhaled steroids include **triamcinolone (Azmacort)**, **ciclesonide (Alvesco)**, and **flunisolide (AeroBid)**. Oral steroids include prednisone (Deltasone), hydrocortisone (Solu-Cortef), methylprednisolone (Medrol Dosepak, Solu-Medrol), dexamethasone (Decadron), and prednisolone (Orapred, Pediapred).

Leukotriene Inhibitors

Used for long-term control of moderate to severe asthma, **leukotriene inhibitors** (see Table 9.3) are often prescribed when short-acting beta agonists and inhaled corticosteroids are not adequately controlling breathing symptoms. Leukotrienes increase accumulation of mucus and fluid in the spaces between cells; they also increase vascular permeability, permitting substances to pass through the blood vessels. A leukotriene inhibitor blocks either the synthesis of, or the body's inflammatory responses to, the leukotrienes. Blocking leukotriene receptors also blocks tissue inflammatory responses.

Montelukast

Montelukast (Singulair) is a leukotriene receptor antagonist. This drug is indicated for the prophylaxis and chronic treatment of asthma. Montelukast has been shown to reduce the incidence of daytime asthma and nocturnal awakenings due to asthma attacks. It can also decrease the need for beta-adrenergic agonists. Unlike the other leukotriene inhibitors, which can be prescribed only for adults or older children, montelukast has been approved for use in children over the age of 12 months. Montelukast also has the benefit of a once-daily dosage, as opposed to the other leukotriene inhibitors, which must be dosed two to four times per day. A headache is the most common side effect associated with the use of montelukast. This drug is also approved to treat seasonal allergic rhinitis (inflammation of the nasal membrane). Asthma and allergic rhinitis are treated with the same dose.

Contraindications Montelukast does not have contraindications.

Cautions and Considerations Leukotriene inhibitors are not to be used for reversal of bronchospasm in acute asthma attacks. Leukotriene inhibitors have been associated with liver problems, eosinophilia, vasculitis, and behavioral changes (such as unusual dreams, agitation, anxiety, and hallucinations).

Drug Interactions Gemfibrozil may increase serum concentrations of montelukast. Loxapine's adverse effects may be potentiated by montelukast.

TABLE 9.3 Common Leukotriene Inhibitors

Generic (Brand)	Pronunciation	Dosage Form	Common Dosage	Dispensing Status
montelukast (Singulair)	mon-te-LOO-kast	Chewable tablet, granules, tablet	4–10 mg once a day (4 mg pediatric dose)	Rx
zafirlukast (Accolate)	za-FEER-loo-kast	Tablet	10–20 mg twice a day (10 mg pediatric dose)	Rx
zileuton (Zyflo)	zye-LOO-ton	Tablet	600–1,200 mg twice a day	Rx

Zafirlukast

Zafirlukast (Accolate), like montelukast, antagonizes leukotriene receptors, thus reducing edema, mucus, and vascular permeability. It is intended for prophylaxis and long-term treatment in patients five years of age or older. Side effects are headache, rhinitis, and cough.

Contraindications Zafirlukast is contraindicated in patients with liver impairment, and patients using it will need periodic liver tests.

Cautions and Considerations Leukotriene inhibitors are not to be used for reversal of bronchospasm in acute asthma attacks. Leukotriene inhibitors have been associated with liver problems, eosinophilia, vasculitis, and behavioral changes (such as unusual dreams, agitation, anxiety, and hallucinations).

Drug Interactions Loxapine's adverse effects may be potentiated by zafirlukast.

Zileuton

Zileuton (Zyflo) is a leukotriene inhibitor that reduces the production of leukotrienes rather than blocking leukotriene receptors. It is approved only for patients 12 years of age or older.

Contraindications Zileuton is contraindicated in patients with liver impairment, and patients using the drug will need periodic liver tests.

Cautions and Considerations Leukotriene inhibitors are not to be used for reversal of bronchospasm in acute asthma attacks. Leukotriene inhibitors have been associated with liver problems, eosinophilia, vasculitis, and behavioral changes (such as unusual dreams, agitation, anxiety, and hallucinations).

Drug Interactions Zileuton may enhance the toxic effects of loxapine.
    Serum concentrations of pimozide, theophylline, and tizanadine may be increased by zileuton use.

Mast Cell Stabilizer

A **mast cell stabilizer** may be used for mild persistent or more severe asthma. A mast cell stabilizer protects mast cell membranes against rupture caused by antigenic substances. As a result, less histamine, leukotrienes, and prostaglandins are released in airway tissue. More information can be found in Table 9.4.

Cromolyn Sodium

Cromolyn sodium works topically in the airways. It is a prophylactic drug with no benefit for acute reactions. Cromolyn sodium stabilizes mast cell membranes and directly inhibits other inflammatory cells. The airways must be open before administration, so a bronchodilator is often given first. This drug can be effective, but patient adherence can be problematic. Cromolyn sodium is dosed four times a day, and most patients have difficulty fitting the four doses into their daily routine. Moreover, cromolyn sodium has an unpleasant taste after inhalation, and side effects include hoarseness, dry mouth, and stuffy nose. The drug has many dosage forms, so care must be taken to select the correct one.

Contraindications Acute asthma attack is a contraindication to the use of cromolyn sodium.

Cautions and Considerations Use cromolyn sodium with caution in patients with kidney or liver dysfunction.

Drug Interactions There are no known drug interactions.

Monoclonal Antibody

A **monoclonal antibody** is an antibody produced in a laboratory from an isolated specific lymphocyte that produces a pure antibody against a known specific antigen.

Omalizumab

Omalizumab (Xolair) is a monoclonal antibody for the treatment of asthma that is not controlled with the use of inhaled steroids. It is used for adults and children older than 12 years. It is not to be used for an acute event, as in status asthmaticus or asthma exacerbations. Omalizumab blocks the immunoglobulin IgE, which is a major cause of allergic asthma. This drug should be reserved for cases that have proven difficult to treat with other medications. It is administered subcutaneously.

Contraindications Omalizumab does not have contraindications.

Cautions and Considerations Omalizumab has a black box warning for hypersensitivity and anaphylactic reactions. These reactions can be immediate or delayed.

Drug Interactions Omalizumab may increase the toxicities of belimumab and loxapine.

Xanthine Derivative

A **xanthine derivative** is structurally similar to caffeine and causes relaxation of airway smooth muscle. This leads to airway dilation and better air movement. See Table 9.4 for additional information.

Theophylline

Theophylline (Elixophyllin, Theo-24, Theochron) is a phosphodiesterase inhibitor that reverses early bronchospasm associated with antigens or irritants. Theophylline improves the contractility of the fatigued diaphragm. It can be used as a bronchodilator in reversible airway obstruction due to asthma, chronic bronchitis, or emphysema. Blood levels should be maintained at 5 to 20 mcg/mL. Theophylline has many interactions, however, and blood levels can become elevated quickly. Consequently, it is

TABLE 9.4 Other Asthma Therapies

Generic (Brand)	Pronunciation	Dosage Form	Common Dosage	Dispensing Status
Mast Cell Stabilizer				
cromolyn sodium*	KROE-moe-lin SOE-dee-um	Nebulizer solution	20 mg 3–4 times a day	Rx
Monoclonal Antibody				
omalizumab (Xolair)	oh-mah-lye-ZOO-mab	Solution for subcutaneous injection	150–300 mg every 4 weeks	Rx
Xanthine Derivative				
theophylline (Elixophyllin, Theo-24, Theochron, Theolair)	thee-OFF-i-lin	Capsule, elixir, oral solution, solution for injection, tablet	Varies based on patient specific factors and therapeutic drug levels	Rx

* These products are produced in several dosage forms, such as inhalants, liquids (for use in nebulizers), syrups, and injections. Pharmacists and pharmacy technicians should always carefully read the prescription and select the correct dosage form.

used only for lung disease unresponsive to other drugs. Theophylline should be taken one hour before or two hours after a meal. Theophylline can also be used for neonatal (the first four weeks after birth) apnea and bradycardia.

Contraindications The premixed injection formulation may contain corn-derived dextrose, and its use is contraindicated in patients with allergies to corn-related products.

Cautions and Considerations Theophylline toxicity is a concern with use. Drug levels should be monitored in all patients using theophylline.

Drug Interactions Drug interactions with theophylline are numerous. Drugs that may interact with theophylline include adenosine; adrenaline-like drugs (e.g., ephedrine, phenylephrine, pseudoephedrine); allopurinol; antiarrhythmic drugs (e.g., mexiletine, propafenone); antiseizure drugs (e.g., carbamazepine, phenobarbital, phenytoin); benzodiazepines (e.g., diazepam, flurazepam); beta blockers (e.g., propranolol); cimetidine; digoxin; disulfiram; fluvoxamine; interferons; isoproterenol; oral contraceptives; pentoxifylline; rifampin; riociguat; St. John's wort; sulfinpyrazone; tacrine; thiabendazole; ticlopidine; verapamil; and zileuton.

Chronic Obstructive Pulmonary Disease

Chronic obstructive pulmonary disease (COPD) refers to a group of chronic lung diseases that impede airflow and cause breathing difficulty. COPD is a long-term, progressive condition in which airflow is limited by an abnormal inflammatory response. COPD is irreversible, which means lung function does not significantly improve with administration of bronchodilators. COPD progressively worsens, even with treatment.

On the positive side, COPD is largely preventable. Although some patients are genetically predisposed to developing COPD, most patients with COPD have a history of smoking or exposure to pollution or occupational hazards. Repeated respiratory infections can also contribute to this condition. COPD has several subtypes, including emphysema and chronic bronchitis.

Emphysema

Emphysema is characterized by destruction of the tiny alveoli, or air sacs, of the lungs (shown in Figure 9.1). As a result, air accumulates in tissues and organs. Typically, air spaces distal to (farther away from) the terminal bronchioles are enlarged. Inflammation destroys these air sacs, which then lose their ability to expand and contract as well as to pass oxygen into the blood and remove carbon dioxide (see Figure 9.4). In the early stages, shortness of breath occurs only after heavy exercise. As the disease progresses, walking even a short distance can make the patient gasp for air. Patients with emphysema have **tachypnea** (very rapid respiration), which gives them a flushed appearance. Major risk factors are cigarette smoking (which destroys the walls of the lungs), occupational exposure, air pollution, and genetic factors.

Bronchitis

Bronchitis is a condition in which the lining of the bronchial airways becomes inflamed, which obstructs airflow during expiration (see Figure 9.4). This disease is characterized by a cough that produces sputum (phlegm) that may be purulent (containing pus), green, or blood streaked. *Acute bronchitis* is caused by an infection, usually viral; it runs a brief course and is usually terminated by the body's immune responses, often with the aid of antibiotics to prevent or treat secondary bacterial infections. The infection that caused the acute bronchitis generally does not return. *Chronic bronchitis* is a serious disease, defined as excessive production of tracheobronchial mucus sufficient to cause cough with expectoration of at least 30 mL of sputum per 24 hours, for 3 months of the year and for more than 2 consecutive years. Patients usually are overweight, have a barrel chest, and tend to retain carbon dioxide. Most individuals have a morning cough resulting from irritation to the lungs.

FIGURE 9.4
Chronic Bronchitis and Emphysema

Chronic bronchitis and emphysema are the two main types of COPD.

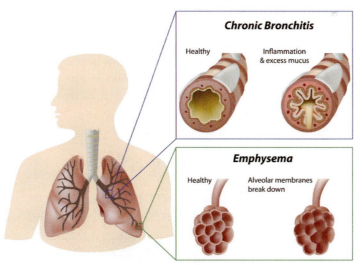

Chronic Obstructive Pulmonary Disease (COPD)

Several factors can contribute to the development of chronic bronchitis. The most prominent factors include cigarette smoke; exposure to occupational dusts, fumes, and environmental pollution; and bacterial infection. Studies of lungs from smoking and nonsmoking subjects clearly demonstrate that those individuals who smoke cigarettes have more bronchial inflammation and substantially increased numbers of alveolar macrophages.

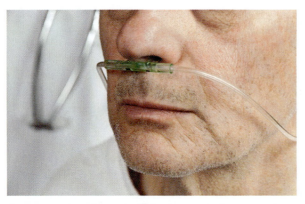

Oxygen can be a key part of the treatment for any patient who has COPD.

Drug Treatments for COPD

To understand the treatment for emphysema and chronic bronchitis, you must also understand the lungs' natural defense system. When this system is functioning properly, the host defenses of the respiratory tract provide good protection against pathogen invasion, and they remove potentially infectious agents from the lungs. The lungs are normally sterile below the first branch, and when organisms breach this region, infection and inflammation are initiated.

The lung's defenses include a number of different types of cells:

- The ciliary carpet consists of minute hairlike processes, called *cilia*, that move rhythmically to propel fluid or mucus. Any inhaled particles that have become trapped in the fluid are pushed over the inner surface of the airway, then upward and out.
- Goblet cells secrete mucus.
- Clara cells, unciliated cells at the branching of the alveolar ducts into the bronchioles, secrete enzymes that break down airborne toxins.
- Epithelial cells produce a protein-rich exudate in the small bronchi and bronchioles.
- Type I pneumocytes in the alveolar membranes act as the phagocytes of the lung. They clear waste and organisms from the lung.
- Type II pneumocytes synthesize and secrete surfactant.

Figure 9.5 demonstrates the locations of various cells in the alveolus and its blood supply.

Emphysema and chronic bronchitis sometimes occur together, and their pharmacologic treatment is similar. The pharmacologic management of emphysema and bronchitis is still largely empirical, with beta agonists, anticholinergics, corticosteroids, and methylxanthines forming the foundation of therapy. Oxygen administration and physical therapy play an important role in treating both lung diseases. In both

FIGURE 9.5
Cellular Makeup of an Alveolus and Capillary Supply

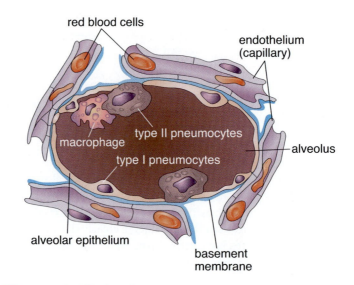

red blood cells

endothelium (capillary)

type II pneumocytes

macrophage

type I pneumocytes

alveolus

alveolar epithelium

basement membrane

emphysema and chronic bronchitis, antibiotic therapy is sometimes needed if signs and symptoms of infection are present. Expectorants (discussed in greater detail later in the chapter) are sometimes used to stimulate respiratory secretions and counter dryness, which stimulates irritation and coughing. Drinking large amounts of water helps to break up mucus and enables the patient to cough up secretions; water is the expectorant of choice. Patients with COPD should always be encouraged to get influenza and pneumococcal vaccinations annually because this disease state predisposes them to flu and pneumonia.

Anticholinergics

Used as a first-line treatment for bronchoconstriction related to COPD, **anticholinergic agents** (see Table 9.5) work by inhibiting acetylcholine, a neurotransmitter that stimulates smooth muscle in the lungs to constrict. Anticholinergics are used when long-term bronchodilation is needed. The purpose of these agents is to prevent frequent COPD exacerbations, not to treat acute breathing problems after they begin. These agents improve the quality of life for patients with COPD and can reduce the need for hospitalization.

Side effects of anticholinergics include headache, flushed skin, blurred vision, tachycardia, and palpitations.

Ipratropium

Ipratropium (Atrovent) blocks the action of acetylcholine in bronchial smooth muscle, causing bronchodilation. It is derived from atropine and is used for prevention, not for acute management. Ipratropium is a short-acting agent and is not absorbed into general circulation when inhaled, so it usually does not cause arrhythmias. It is FDA approved for the treatment of COPD; however, it is sometimes used for emergency treatment of acute asthma exacerbations in combination with other drugs.

Contraindications Ipratropium is contraindicated in patients with a hypersensitivity to atropine.

Put Down Roots

It can be difficult to remember which medication is an anticholinergic and which medication is a long-acting beta agonist. The anticholinergic agents that target the respiratory system end in –ium. The long-acting beta agonists that are used for respiratory disorders end in –erol.

Cautions and Considerations Ipratropium is not indicated for the initial treatment of acute episodes of bronchospasm where rescue therapy is required for a rapid response.

Drug Interactions Ipratropium should not be used with other anticholinergic products. The potential of orally administered potassium chloride to cause ulcers is increased with concurrent use.

Aclidinium

Aclidinium (Tudorza Pressair) is indicated for long-term maintenance treatment of bronchospasm associated with COPD. It is available as a DPI with a dose counter. Unlike some other DPIs, aclidinium does not involve loading capsules into an inhaler.

Contraindications Aclidinium does not have any contraindications.

Cautions and Considerations Aclidinium is not for the initial treatment of acute episodes of bronchospasm. The DPI contains lactose and should not be used by patients with severe milk protein allergy.

TABLE 9.5 Commonly Used Anticholinergic Drugs

Generic (Brand)	Pronunciation	Dosage Form	Common Dosage	Dispensing Status
aclidinium (Tudorza Pressair)	a-kli-DIN-ee-um	Powder for inhalation	400 mcg twice a day	Rx
ipratropium (Atrovent)	i-pra-TROE-pee-um	Aerosol (MDI), nebulizer solution	MDI: 2 puffs 4 times a day Nebulizer: 500 mcg 3–4 times a day	Rx
ipratropium-albuterol (DuoNeb, Respimat)	i-pra-TROE-pee-um al-BYOO-ter-awl	Nebulizer solution, oral inhalation solution	Nebulizer: 3 mL treatment 4 times a day Oral inhalation solution: 1 inhalation 4 times a day	Rx
tiotropium (Spiriva HandiHaler)	tye-oh-TROE-pee-um	Powder for inhalation	Inhale contents of 1 capsule a day	Rx
tiotropium (Spiriva)	tye-oh-TROE-pee-um	Oral inhalation solution	2 puffs once daily	Rx
umeclidinium (Incruse Ellipta)	ue-MEK-li-DIN-ee-um	Powder for inhalation	1 inhalation once a day	Rx
umeclidinium-vilanterol (Anoro Ellipta)	ue-MEK-li-DIN-ee-um vye-LAN-ter-ol	Powder for inhalation	1 inhalation once a day	Rx

Drug Interactions Aclidinium should not be used with other anticholinergic drugs. The potential of orally administered potassium chloride to cause ulcers is increased with concurrent use.

Umeclidinium

Umeclidinium (Incruse Ellipta) is the newest member of the long-acting anticholinergic COPD treatments. It is available alone (Incruse Ellipta) or combined with the long-acting beta agonist vilanterol as Anoro Ellipta. Both products are indicated for maintenance treatment of airflow obstruction in patients who have COPD.

Contraindications Umeclidinium is contraindicated in patients with a hypersensitivity to milk proteins.

Cautions and Considerations Umeclidinium should not be used for acute episodes of COPD. It should not be started in patients with significantly worsening COPD. Umeclidinium may worsen symptoms in patients with glaucoma and benign prostatic hyperplasia.

Drug Interactions Anticholinergic agents may enhance the anticholinergic effects of umeclidinium. The adverse effects of glucagon may be enhanced with umeclidinium use. The ulcer-causing effects of oral potassium chloride may be enhanced with the use of anticholinergic agents such as umeclidinium.

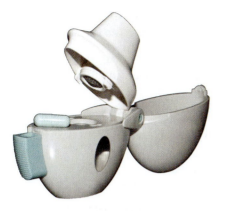

Tiotropium comes in both a powder for inhalation and an MDI. The powder for inhalation requires the use of an inhaler. The capsules containing the powdered medication are punctured, and the powder is placed in the inhaler. Warn patients that tiotropium capsules are not to be swallowed.

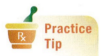

Practice Tip

Tiotropium is dispensed as a capsule for INHALATION that is administered using a DPI. Patients can find this confusing and have been reported to erroneously swallow the capsules. Swallowing the capsules will not have the intended therapeutic effect.

Tiotropium

Tiotropium (Spiriva) is a long-acting anticholinergic and is dosed only once daily, although it works for approximately 36 hours. It is indicated only for long-term maintenance therapy for bronchospasms associated with emphysema and chronic bronchitis. Dry mouth is a common side effect. Tiotropium is provided by the manufacturer in two forms. One is a capsule for inhalation (Spiriva HandiHaler). In this form, one capsule should be placed in the HandiHaler and the button pressed to disperse the powder into the inhaler. After the inhaler is used, the empty capsule should be disposed of in a proper container. The dry powder should not be touched. This drug is sensitive to moisture and heat, and the capsule should not be exposed before the patient is ready to use it. Therefore, the patient needs to know that the package should be peeled back only to the STOP mark. The second form of tiotropium is an MDI (Spiriva Respimat).

Contraindications Tiotropium should not be used by patients who have lactose sensitivity.

Cautions and Considerations Tiotropium capsules are used only with an inhaler device; they should not be swallowed. Patients should take care to follow instructions for puncturing the capsule and inhaling the powder using the inhaler device.

Drug Interactions Tiotropium should not be used with other anticholinergic drugs. The potential of orally administered potassium chloride to cause ulcers is increased with concurrent use.

Long-Acting Beta Agonists

Used for both COPD and asthma, **long-acting beta agonists (LABAs)** work in a way that is similar to the action of short-acting beta agonists (discussed earlier in this chapter); they simply do not have to be administered as frequently. Used more frequently for COPD, the long-acting agents can also be used for severe asthma, where short-acting bronchodilator therapy is needed multiple times a day on a regular basis. For a list of common long-acting beta agonists, see Table 9.6.

Common side effects for LABAs include dizziness, heartburn, nausea, and tremors. LABAs can cause cardiac effects including increased blood pressure and tachycardia. Patients with high blood pressure or heart problems should discuss the side effects of these beta agonists with their physicians before using them.

Arformoterol

Arformoterol (Brovana) is a LABA indicated for long-term COPD therapy. Structurally, it is similar to formoterol; it is the active isomer of formoterol. Arformoterol only comes in a nebulizer solution.

Contraindications Arformoterol is contraindicated in patients with a hypersensitivity to formoterol.

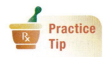

Practice Tip

Arformoterol nebulizer solution comes in 2 mL unit-dose containers. Be mindful of this packaging when figuring days of use for insurance billing purposes. Most nebulizer solutions are manufactured in 3 mL packets; however, arformoterol is dispensed in a 2 mL packet.

LABAs should not be used as monotherapy for patients with asthma. Patients with asthma should always take an inhaled corticosteroid, such as fluticasone, concurrently with the LABA.

Cautions and Considerations LABAs carry a black box warning for an increased risk of asthma-related deaths.

Patients should not take LABAs with beta blockers.

Drug Interactions Patients should not take arformoterol with other LABAs because there is an increased risk of toxicities.

Formoterol

Formoterol (Foradil) is a long-acting bronchodilator approved for the long-term maintenance of asthma and COPD, for preventing bronchospasms, and for the prevention of exercise-induced asthma. It is a selective beta-2 agonist, which means that it acts locally in the lungs to relax smooth muscle and inhibit the release of mast cells. It has a faster onset than salmeterol, working within minutes. Formoterol is supplied in a capsule that is to be loaded into a DPI, not taken orally. Formoterol must be refrigerated until dispensed, but it does not need to be refrigerated after dispensing, at which time it is good for four months. The pharmacy technician must mark on the box the date after which the drug should not be used. This date is either the expiration date or four months after the drug was dispensed, whichever comes first.

Proper administration of formoterol is important. A capsule is placed in the chamber of the inhaler, and the mouthpiece is closed. The capsule is pierced by pressing and releasing the buttons on the side. The patient should then inhale quickly and deeply, which causes the capsule to spin, dispensing the drug. The patient should then hold his or her breath as long as possible. The capsule should be checked to ensure that all of the powder was released; if it was not, then it should be inhaled again. The most common side effects are tremors. Even though this drug has a quick onset, it should not be used to treat acute asthma. If it is being used to prevent exercise-induced asthma, it should be used 15 minutes before exercise. No more than one capsule should be used in 12 hours.

TABLE 9.6 Common Long-Acting Beta Agonists

Generic (Brand)	Pronunciation	Dosage Form	Common Dosage	Dispensing Status
arformoterol (Brovana)	ar-for-MOE-ter-awl	Nebulizer solution	15 mcg twice a day	Rx
formoterol* (Foradil Aerolizer, Perforomist)	for-MOE-ter-awl	Nebulizer solution, powder capsule for inhalation	Foradil Aerolizer: 12 mcg every 12 hr; Perforomist: 20 mcg twice a day	Rx
indacaterol (Arcapta Neohaler)	in-da-KAT-e-role	Powder capsule for inhalation	75–300 mcg a day	Rx
olodaterol (Striverdi Respimat)	oh-loh-DAT-er-ole	Solution for inhalation	2 inhalations a day	Rx
salmeterol* (Serevent Diskus)	sal-ME-te-role	Powder for inhalation	1 inhalation twice a day	Rx

*This drug has an FDA indication for COPD and asthma.

Contraindications The Foradil brand of formoterol should not be used in acute episodes of asthma or exacerbations of COPD.

LABAs should not be used as monotherapy for patients with asthma. Patients with asthma should always take an inhaled corticosteroid, such as fluticasone, concurrently with the LABA.

Cautions and Considerations LABAs carry a black box warning for an increased risk of asthma-related deaths. Foradil Aerolizer carries an additional boxed warning for the risk of asthma-related hospitalization in pediatric and adolescent patients.

Formoterol powder for inhalation contains lactose. Patients with lactose allergies should avoid this formulation.

Patients should not take LABAs with beta blockers.

Drug Interactions Patients should not take formoterol with other LABAs because there is an increased risk of toxicities.

Indacaterol

Indacaterol (Arcapta Neohaler) is a once-daily maintenance drug that has been approved by the FDA for treatment of COPD. It is a hard gelatin capsule containing a powder that should be inhaled, and, because it is a LABA, it is to be used daily and not for rescue therapy. The once-daily dosing is an advantage of this drug.

Contraindications LABAs should not be used as monotherapy for patients with asthma. Patients with asthma should always take an inhaled corticosteroid, such as fluticasone, concurrently with the LABA.

Cautions and Considerations LABAs carry a black box warning for an increased risk of asthma-related deaths.

Patients should not take LABAs with beta blockers.

Drug Interactions Patients should not take indacaterol with other LABAs because it increases the risk of toxicities.

Olodaterol

Olodaterol (Striverdi Respimat) is another LABA indicated for COPD. It is formulated as a soft-mist inhaler that is used once daily. Olodaterol may be a convenient choice for COPD patients because it is dosed once a day, and unlike indacaterol, it does not require a separate device for delivery.

Contraindications LABAs should not be used as monotherapy for patients with asthma. Patients with asthma should always take an inhaled corticosteroid, such as fluticasone, concurrently with the LABA.

Cautions and Considerations LABAs carry a black box warning for an increased risk of asthma-related deaths.

Patients should not take LABAs with beta blockers.

Drug Interactions Patients should not take olodaterol with other LABAs because it increases the risk of toxicities.

Salmeterol

Salmeterol (Serevent Diskus) is indicated for maintenance therapy of asthma and COPD. It has a long duration of action, and its onset of action is 30 to 60 minutes.

Salmeterol is taken twice a day. When used for asthma, it should be reserved for patients with more serious cases and for those individuals who are already receiving anti-inflammatory therapy. Its long duration of action makes it particularly useful for nocturnal symptoms of asthma. Salmeterol is available as a DPI.

Contraindications LABAs should not be used as monotherapy for patients with asthma. Patients with asthma should always take an inhaled corticosteroid, such as fluticasone, concurrently with the LABA.

Cautions and Considerations LABAs carry a black box warning for an increased risk of asthma-related deaths. Salmeterol carries an additional boxed warning for the risk of asthma-related hospitalization in pediatric and adolescent patients.

Patients should not take LABAs with beta blockers.

Salmeterol should not be used to treat rescue situations. Improper use of this drug has been implicated in deaths.

Drug Interactions Patients should not take salmeterol with other LABAs because it increases the risk of toxicities.

Drugs that should not be used with salmeterol include darunavir, fosamprenavir, indinavir, lopinavir, nelfinavir, and ritonavir.

Other COPD Therapies

Some COPD therapies are less commonly used. These therapies include **phosphodiesterase-4 inhibitors** and mucolytics as discussed below.

Phosphodiesterase-4 Inhibitors

Alpha-1 proteinase inhibitor (Aralast NP, Glassia, Prolastin-C, Zemaira), also known as alpha-1 antitrypsin, is indicated for the treatment of emphysema in patients with alpha-1 antitrypsin deficiency. It is an intravenous (IV) drug that works by inhibiting phosphodiesterase-4 (antitrypsin), thereby preventing leukocytes and neutrophils from infiltrating the lungs. Pharmacy technicians should be mindful of infusion rates. Aralast NP and Glassia should be infused at a rate of ≤ 0.2 mL/kg/minute. Prolastin-C and Zemaira should be infused at approximately 0.08 mL/kg/minute.

Contraindications This drug should be used only in patients who have emphysema due to a congenital deficiency of alpha-1 proteinase inhibitor. It is administered once weekly.

Cautions and Considerations Alpha-1 proteinase inhibitor is made from human plasma and therefore carries the risk of transmitting infectious agents. It cannot be mixed with other agents or diluting solutions. Alpha-1 proteinase inhibitor can be infused at home. The most common side effects are headache and dizziness.

Drug Interactions There are no known significant interactions.

Roflumilast

Roflumilast (Daliresp), which is made in tablet form, is used to treat severe COPD. It reduces lung inflammation. It should only be used to treat severe COPD, because in less serious cases, the side effects may not outweigh the benefit of the drug. It is an add-on therapy to decrease exacerbations. It also has several interactions with other medications and serious side effects, including mental health problems such as suicidal thoughts.

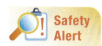
Mucolytics

Another treatment for chronic bronchitis is the use of a **mucolytic** (an agent that destroys or dissolves mucus), such as **acetylcysteine (Acetadote, Mucomyst)**, which breaks apart glycoproteins, thereby reducing viscosity and promoting easier movement and removal of secretions. Another mucolytic, **dornase alfa (Pulmozyme)**, is discussed in the section concerning cystic fibrosis.

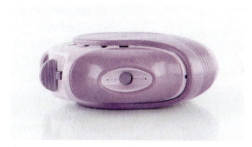

Some DPIs look like a discus and are actuated by breathing in deeply at the opening.

Combination Products for Asthma and/or COPD

To improve patient adherence and ease of administration, several LABAs are available as **combination products** (see Table 9.7). Pharmacy technicians should keep in mind that combination products have the side effects, contraindications, cautions, and drug interactions of both drugs that comprise them.

   Budesonide-formoterol (Symbicort) is indicated for maintenance therapy for asthma and COPD. The drug is approved for acute symptoms in Canada, but not in the United States. The budesonide-formoterol inhaler must be primed, and patients are directed to take two puffs twice daily, with mouth rinsing afterward. The combination may work better than either drug alone.

TABLE 9.7   Commonly Used Combination Products for Asthma and/or COPD

Generic (Brand)	Pronunciation	Dosage Form	Common Dosage	FDA Indication	Dispensing Status
budesonide-formoterol (Symbicort)	byoo-DES-oh-nide for-MOE-ter-awl	Aerosol (MDI)	2 inhalations twice a day	Asthma	Rx
fluticasone-salmeterol (Advair Diskus, Advair HFA)	floo-TIK-a-sone sal-MEte-rawl	Aerosol (MDI), powder for inhalation	MDI 100 mcg/50–500 mcg/50 mcg twice a day HFA: 2 inhalations twice a day	Asthma, COPD	Rx
ipratropium-albuterol (Combivent Respimat, DuoNeb)	i-pra-TROE-pee-um al-BYOO-ter-awl	Nebulizer solution, oral inhalation solution	Nebulizer: 3 mL treatment 4 times a day Oral inhalation: 1 inhalation 4 times a day	COPD	Rx
mometasone-formoterol (Dulera)	moe-MET-a-sone for-MOE-ter-ol	Aerosol (MDI)	2 inhalations twice a day	Asthma	Rx

Fluticasone-salmeterol (Advair Diskus, Advair HFA) is an anti-inflammatory and beta-2 adrenergic agonist used for maintenance treatment of asthma and COPD for patients older than 12 years. It is available in two forms: a dry powder for oral inhalation and an aerosol (MDI). Fluticasone, a corticosteroid, is a potent vasoconstrictor and anti-inflammatory. Salmeterol is a LABA and relaxes bronchial smooth muscle with little effect on heart rate. Together, the two drugs act synergistically to improve pulmonary function.

Ipratropium-albuterol (Combivent Respimat, DuoNeb) is a combination inhaler that should be used for COPD patients who require a second inhaler. The pharmacy technician should determine whether the patient has a peanut allergy if this drug is prescribed because the propellant is based on soy lecithin, which can trigger a cross-reaction in patients who have a peanut allergy. The drug combination is also available as DuoNeb, a solution for nebulizer use.

Mometasone-formoterol (Dulera) is a combination LABA for maintenance treatment of asthma. Mometasone is the same corticosteroid used in asthma treatment and for seasonal allergies, which will be discussed later in the chapter. Prior to the first use, a mometasone-formoterol inhaler must be primed by actuating four sprays. If it has been more than five days since the last use, the inhaler must be primed again. This product contains a dose counter. Do not remove the drug canister from the actuator because it may cause inhaler malfunction.

Other Lung Diseases

In addition to the diseases previously discussed in this chapter, there are many other lung disorders. Several measures can be taken to prevent and control lung disease and infection. Not smoking is one way to prevent lung disease. Avoiding secondhand smoke and air pollution is also important. Influenza and pneumococcal pneumonia can be prevented with vaccination. Most infections occur when people are exposed to fluids or droplets produced by sneezing or coughing that contain bacteria, viruses, or fungi. It has long been thought that respiratory infections are transmitted through inhalation, but recent studies have shown that hand contact is the most frequent culprit. Thus, frequent handwashing and avoiding close contact with infected hosts are the best defense.

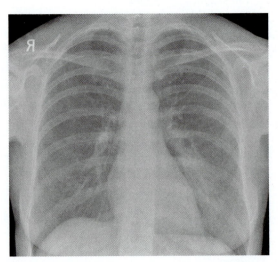

This image is an example of an X-ray of a patient with pneumonia.

Pneumonia

Pneumonia is a common lung infection that affects individuals of all ages. The microorganisms that cause pneumonia gain access to the lower respiratory tract by the following three routes:

- inhalation of aerosolized particles
- entry through the bloodstream
- aspiration of oropharyngeal contents

Aspiration, which involves inhalation of fluids from the mouth and throat, is a common occurrence in both healthy and ill individuals during sleep. It is the major mechanism by which pulmonary pathogens gain access to the normally sterile lower airways and alveoli.

Pneumonia is treated with antibiotics, depending on the causative organism. Patients who get pneumonia from exposure outside of an inpatient facility have **community-acquired pneumonia (CAP)**. Pneumonia that is acquired while an individual is hospitalized or living in a long-term care facility is called **nosocomial pneumonia**. Nosocomial pneumonia is severe and difficult to treat because it is usually caused by pathogens that are more virulent than those that cause CAP. Patients in the hospital setting encounter such pathogens because they are near other sick patients who have these infections.

Cystic Fibrosis

Cystic fibrosis (CF) is a hereditary disease that involves the gastrointestinal (GI) and respiratory systems. CF can be a fatal disease, with some patients dying in early adulthood. Many health consequences associated with CF are a result of pulmonary manifestations of the disease. The GI involvement is due to increased viscosity of secreted mucus, which blocks the bile ducts, and a relative deficiency of pancreatic digestive enzymes.

Patients with CF experience hypoxia (lack of adequate oxygen), resulting in cyanosis, and, in some cases, digital clubbing (enlarged fingertips with loss of normal angle at the nail bed). A patient's respiratory status follows a cyclic pattern, from a state of relative well-being to one of acute pulmonary deterioration. Management of the pulmonary aspect of this disease requires two approaches: respiratory therapy and antibiotic therapy.

A critical part of respiratory therapy is **percussion**, a tapping movement to induce cough and expectoration of sputum from the lungs. Percussion is often used with nebulizer therapy, during which bronchodilators, hypertonic saline, acetylcysteine, and other specialized medications are inhaled to liquefy pulmonary secretions.

Bronchodilators, such as beta-2 agonists and anticholinergics, may be used to improve airflow obstruction in CF. Other agents may be used to help clear airway secretions such as inhaled dornase alfa (Pulmozyme), hypertonic saline, and N-acetylcysteine (Mucomyst). Oral Mucomyst has an unpleasant taste and odor and some patients prefer not to use it. Theophylline may be of benefit; however, theophylline clearance in patients who have CF may differ from that of patients with asthma. Consequently, clearance and dosage should be carefully monitored.

TABLE 9.8 Commonly Used Drugs for Cystic Fibrosis

Generic (Brand)	Pronunciation	Dosage Form	Common Dosage	Dispensing Status
aztreonam (Cayston)	AZ-tree-oh-nam	Inhalation solution	75 mg 3 times a day	Rx
dornase alfa (Pulmozyme)	DOOR-nase AL-fa	Inhalation solution	2.5 mg daily	Rx
tobramycin (Bethkis, Kitabis Pak, Tobi, Tobi Podhaler)	toe-bra-MYE-sin	Capsule for inhalation, inhalation solution	Capsule for inhalation: 112 mg twice a day	Rx
			Inhalation solution: 300 mg twice a day	

Antibiotics for Cystic Fibrosis

Several **antibiotics** are used to combat the pathogens that take root in the respiratory mucous secretions. The infectious organism(s) must be identified so that the appropriate antibiotic can be prescribed. Possible systemic antibiotics given intravenously include amikacin, aztreonam, cefazolin, cefepime, ceftazidime, ciprofloxacin, colistin, imipenem-cilastin, linezolid, meropenem, nafcillin, piperacillin-tazobactam, tobramycin, and vancomycin.

Regular treatment with nebulized antibiotics directed against *Pseudomonas aeruginosa* appears to improve lung function and is recommended for many patients who have CF. Inhaled antibiotics commonly used in the treatment of CF include aztreonam (Cayston) and tobramycin (Bethkis, Kitabis Pak, Tobi, Tobi Podhaler).

Aztreonam (Cayston) is an inhaled antibiotic used to improve respiratory symptoms in patients who have CF. It is for adults and children seven years and older who have certain bacteria in their lungs. It may be used only with an Altera nebulizer. Like other antibiotics, even if symptoms improve, it must be used for the full length of the prescription. Aztreonam is a powder that must be mixed with a provided diluent prior to nebulization. The reconstituted solution must be used immediately after it is mixed. Doses must be spaced at least four hours apart. A patient may need to use a bronchodilator preceding the inhalation treatment of this drug. It must be stored in the refrigerator in the pharmacy.

Tobramycin (Bethkis, Kitabis Pak, Tobi, Tobi Podhaler) is an aminoglycoside antibiotic that is available in multiple dosage forms. The capsule for inhalation and nebulization solution are indicated for the management of patients who have CF and have been infected with *P. aeruginosa*. The Bethkis, Kitabis Pak, and Tobi products should be inhaled over 15 minutes using a particular handheld reusable nebulizer (PARI LC PLUS) with a PARI Vios air compressor (Bethkis) or a DeVilbiss Pulmo-Aide air compressor (Kitabis Pak, Tobi). If multiple different nebulizer treatments are required, the bronchodilator should be administered first, followed by chest physiotherapy, any other nebulized medications, and then tobramycin last. The tobramycin should not be mixed with other nebulizer medications. The Tobi Podhaler is a DPI with capsules that should be administered by oral inhalation via the Podhaler device, following manufacturer recommendations for use and handling. Capsules should be removed from the blister packaging immediately prior to use and should not be swallowed.

Mucolytics for Cystic Fibrosis

Dornase alfa (Pulmozyme) selectively breaks down deoxyribonucleic acid (DNA) that is released by degenerating leukocytes. The leukocytes collect in response to infection. By destroying DNA in the mucus, dornase alfa helps reduce secretion viscosity (resistance to flow, thickness).

Pancreatic Enzymes for Cystic Fibrosis

Because the GI system and pancreas are also affected, providers often prescribe special vitamins and **pancreatic enzyme supplements** for patients with CF. These supplements help prevent ductal obstructions and **steatorrhea** (fatty, foul-smelling diarrhea that occurs when dietary fat is not absorbed). They improve growth and life expectancy for children with CF. The number of pancreatic enzyme supplements is large and is beyond the scope of this text. However, they all contain varying amounts of **lipase**, **protease**, and **amylase**. Pancreatic dysfunction also contributes to **malabsorption**, especially of fat-soluble vitamins. Therefore, many patients with CF take supplements containing vitamins A, D, E, and K.

Respiratory Distress Syndrome

Respiratory distress syndrome (RDS) occurs in neonates during the first few hours of life. It is characterized by inadequate production of pulmonary **surfactant**—a fluid that, like a soap bubble, lowers the surface tension between the air and alveolar surfaces. Lack of surfactant leads to collapse of the alveoli along with acute asphyxia with hypoxia and acidosis. Prematurity and maternal diabetes are two known causative factors of RDS. If RDS occurs, a replacement surfactant is administered. Table 9.9 lists the most commonly used agents to treat RDS.

Beractant (Survanta) is a natural bovine lung extract and is supplied as a suspension for intratracheal administration. Beractant replaces deficient or ineffective endogenous lung surfactant in neonates. It prevents the alveoli from collapsing during expiration by lowering the surface tension between the air and alveolar surfaces. Beractant is used for prophylactic therapy in high-risk infants and for rescue therapy within eight hours of birth.

Calfactant (Infasurf) replaces deficient endogenous lung surfactant and is indicated for neonates who are less than 72 hours of age. When taking this drug, infants may require less oxygen than with other RDS drugs. The drug should be stored in the refrigerator. The suspension settles and should be swirled gently but not shaken to redisperse the medication. It is not necessary to warm calfactant before administration. Vials that have been stored unopened at room temperature for less than 24 hours may be safely returned to the refrigerator.

Lucinactant (Surfaxin) was FDA approved as the first synthetic surfactant for neonates with RDS. Like the other surfactants, lucinactant is for intratracheal administration. Prior to administration, the suspension needs to be properly warmed, shaken vigorously, and visually inspected (to ensure the suspension is uniform, free-flowing, and opaque white to off-white). Vials are for single use only; discard any unused portion. If not used immediately after warming, the suspension may be stored for up to two hours at room temperature in an area protected from light. Warmed vials should not be returned to the refrigerator and should be discarded if not used within two hours.

Poractant alfa (Curosurf) may be preferred for very tiny babies because it requires much less fluid than the other RDS drugs and can be administered in one dose. With some of the other drugs, a partial dose must be administered, and then another partial dose is given two to three hours later.

TABLE 9.9 Most Commonly Used Surfactants for Respiratory Distress Syndrome

Generic (Brand)	Pronunciation	Dosage Form	Common Dosage	Dispensing Status
beractant (Survanta)	ber-AKT-ant	Intratracheal suspension	4 mL/kg	Rx
calfactant (Infasurf)	kal-FAK-tant	Intratracheal suspension	3 mL/kg	Rx
lucinactant (Surfaxin)	loo-sin-ACT-ant	Intratracheal suspension	5.8 mL/kg	Rx
poractant alfa (Curosurf)	por-AKT-ant AL-fa	Intratracheal suspension	2.5 mL/kg	Rx

Tuberculosis

Tuberculosis (TB) is caused by the bacterium *Mycobacterium tuberculosis*. The disease most commonly affects the lungs, but it may also infect other body tissues and organs. TB is transmitted by respiratory droplets inhaled into the lungs of individuals at risk. Respiratory droplets are produced when infected persons with active TB cough, sneeze, speak, kiss, or spit. Suspended in the air, these droplets descend under the influence of gravity at the relatively slow rate of one to two inches (2.5–5 cm) per hour. Once inhaled, *M. tuberculosis* may spread throughout the body in the bloodstream and in lymphatic fluids. A follicle forms and is surrounded by epithelial cells. The mass may spread or liquefy, forming a cavity filled with fluid and teeming with organisms. The fluid may move in the direction of least resistance, spreading organisms and disease within the organ, and thereby destroying more tissue (called fibrosis). *M. tuberculosis* thrives in areas of high oxygen, so resulting lesions concentrate primarily in the lung. However, lesions may also occur in bone and kidney tissue.

Tuberculosis is seen primarily in alcoholics, prison populations, immunocompromised individuals, and older adults. It should be included in the differential diagnosis of patients with fever of unknown origin, subacute meningitis, or chronic infection at any site.

Two groups of tuberculosis patients are distinguished by their disease symptoms and antibody production:

- Exposed but showing no disease: If time has elapsed since exposure, these patients produce TB antibodies and may have a positive tuberlin skin test (TST). This test result does not mean they have active disease.

- Exposed and having active organisms: These patients may or may not produce antibodies, depending on the competence of their immune systems. Significant signs and symptoms of active disease include weight loss, blood in the sputum, night sweats and night fever, chest pain, and malaise.

The agent used for TST is **purified protein derivative (PPD)** from killed bacteria. This product is injected intradermally. Individuals who have been exposed to or have the disease show a circular area of hardened tissue (**induration**) at the injection site within 48 to 72 hours. A false-negative reaction may occur in individuals recently exposed and in older adults who have delayed-type hypersensitivity. If the reading is positive, the patient should have a chest X-ray taken to check for a lung shadow, which may indicate active disease.

Tuberculosis generally develops slowly and may take as long as 20 years to develop from the time of exposure. The highest incidence of infection occurs one to two years after exposure. Even if the disease is arrested early (4 to 10 weeks after exposure), a patient still has a risk of reactivity for the remainder of his or her life. The organism can lie dormant for years, until the immune system is depressed, when it will reemerge as an active infection. The medical history of the patient should be watched for disease symptoms such as weight loss, fever, night sweats, malaise, and loss of appetite.

The goals of TB therapy are to initiate treatment promptly, convert the sputum culture from positive to negative, achieve cure without relapse, and prevent emergence of drug-resistant strains. Table 9.10 describes the most commonly used agents for treating TB. The primary agents used are ethambutol, isoniazid, pyrazinamide, and rifampin or rifapentine.

TABLE 9.10 Commonly Used Agents for Tuberculosis

Generic (Brand)	Pronunciation	Dosage Form	Dispensing Status
ethambutol (Myambutol)	e-THAM-byoo-tawl	Tablet	Rx
isoniazid (Rifamate, IsonaRif)	eye-soe-NYE-a-zid	Injection, oral liquid, tablet	Rx
isoniazid-pyrazinamide-rifampin (Rifater)	eye-soe-NYE-a-zid peer-a-ZIN-a-mide rif-AM-pin	Tablet	Rx
pyrazinamide	peer-a-ZIN-a-mide	Tablet	Rx
rifampin (Rifadin)	rif-AM-pin	Capsule, injection	Rx
rifapentine (Priftin)	RIF-a-pen-teen	Tablet	Rx

A strain of *M. tuberculosis* that is highly resistant to many currently used drugs, and therefore very difficult to treat, has emerged. Defined as **multidrug-resistant tuberculosis (MDR-TB)**, this strain is a serious health problem. The organisms show resistance to the commonly used therapeutic agents. Risk factors include being exposed to MDR-TB, failing to complete TB therapy, being prescribed inappropriate agents, having immune deficiencies, and having a recurrence of TB. Successful therapy for MDR-TB may require 18 to 24 months of treatment.

Patient adherence is a major problem in treating TB. The severe side effect profile, the length of time required for treatment, and the number of medications required all contribute to nonadherence. Patients being treated for active TB should avoid alcohol.

Ethambutol

Ethambutol (Myambutol) is an antitubercular agent that is administered as a single daily oral dose. It works by impairing synthesis of the mycobacterial cell wall and is usually well tolerated. The major side effect is optic neuritis, which is relatively uncommon with standard dosing.

Isoniazid

Isoniazid (Rifamate, IsonaRif) is a bactericidal agent that works by inhibiting synthesis of the mycobacterium cell wall synthesis. Isoniazid tends to be easily tolerated orally in a single daily dose, and it is inexpensive. Hepatitis is the most serious side effect associated with isoniazid use, and there is a black box warning about this complication. Peripheral neuropathy may also occur. Neuropathy may be minimized with pyridoxine use.

Pyrazinamide

Pyrazinamide is a bactericidal for TB that may be given once daily. The most common side effects are nausea and vomiting. Hepatoxicity is also a concern.

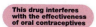

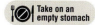

Rifampin

Rifampin (Rifadin) is an antitubercular agent that inhibits bacterial RNA synthesis. Side effects include the discoloration of urine, tears, sweat, and other body fluids, which turn reddish orange. This discoloration can permanently stain soft contact lenses.

Rifampin interferes with oral contraceptives; thus, female patients taking this drug must be advised to seek alternative forms of birth control. Rifampin must be taken on an empty stomach.

Rifapentine

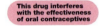

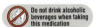

Rifapentine (Priftin) has a longer duration of action than rifampin and, therefore, has the advantage of a less frequent administration schedule, leading to improved patient adherence. However, it can still decrease the effectiveness of oral contraceptives such as rifampin can. Rifapentine is always used as an adjunctive therapy. This drug has the same side effect profile as rifampin, but it must be taken with food.

Patient adherence is a major problem in treating TB. The severe side effect profile, the length of time required for treatment, and the number of medications required all contribute to nonadherence. Patients being treated for active TB should avoid alcohol.

Histoplasmosis

Another pulmonary disease, **histoplasmosis**, is caused by a fungus that most commonly occurs in accumulated droppings from bats and various birds including chickens, pigeons, and starlings. When the fungus-bearing dust is inhaled, spores are transported into the bronchial tubes. The lymph tissue reacts to this invasion and sensitivity develops; as a result, tissue becomes inflamed. This disease is most prevalent in the valleys of the Missouri and Ohio Rivers.

Histoplasmosis is often referred to as the *summer flu* because it produces flulike symptoms. Although the disease mimics tuberculosis, most patients recover on their own without treatment. Histoplasmosis is usually self-limiting and is serious only if there are high levels of fungi. In the disseminated form, however, it can be fatal without treatment. Amphotericin B and itraconazole appear to be the only effective drugs for the more serious disseminated form. Surgery may sometimes be indicated.

Cough, Cold, and Allergy

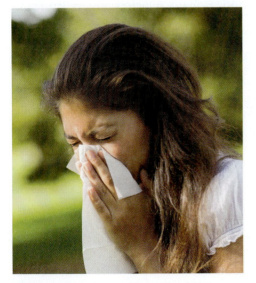

Millions of people are affected by allergies, including hay fever.

The most prevalent form of respiratory tract infection is the **common cold**, which is a mild, self-limited viral infection. Symptoms are readily recognized by the patient and include mild malaise, rhinorrhea (runny nose), sneezing, scratchy throat, and fever. Bacterial sinusitis and otitis media are frequent complications necessitating antimicrobial therapy. Antibiotics and sometimes antivirals are used in treating these problems. However, many different viruses are often the most common cause of infections in the respiratory system.

Symptoms of some allergies are the same as those of colds—runny nose and itchy eyes—so these allergies can be misidentified as a cold. In contrast to the viral cause of the common cold, an allergy results from a state of hypersensitivity induced by exposure to a particular antigen. Both colds and many allergies are treated with the same medications.

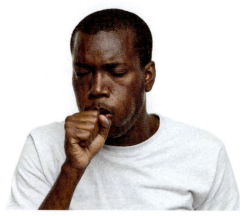

Stimulating receptors in the airways and lungs produces a cough.

The vast majority of colds are self-limiting, but people seek self-treatment to relieve the symptoms and often to prevent complications. Ordinarily, the common cough and cold are treated with four groups of drugs, either alone or in combination: antitussives, expectorants, decongestants, and antihistamines. Many of these drugs are available as over-the-counter (OTC) products. Knowledge of OTC products is an area in which pharmacy technicians can assist individuals who are looking for symptom relief. Technicians can teach patients how to read OTC product labels to find the product that will address their needs. Although recommendations should not be made, the technician can certainly make the patient aware of the proper uses and side effects of these drugs.

For the most part, colds can be successfully prevented if a few simple precautions are taken. Colds can be directly transmitted from an infected person to other people when an infected person sneezes or coughs, or they may be passed along indirectly by contact with surfaces such as telephones, doorknobs, or toys. A sneeze or cough should be covered by turning the head and coughing into the elbow, *not the hand*. Many people contract a cold by rubbing their eyes or nose after touching contaminated surfaces or people with colds. Using a telephone right after an infected person has used it is often how a cold is transmitted. In the pharmacy, it is very important to regularly wipe the phones with disinfectant. However, frequent hand washing is the best preventative measure against the common cold—this cannot be stressed enough.

Antitussives

Coughing is a mechanism for clearing the airways of excess secretions and foreign materials, but intense, frequent coughing with lack of sputum production can be annoying to the patient. In these instances, an **antitussive** can be therapeutic. An antitussive is an agent that suppresses coughing and is indicated when cough frequency needs to be reduced, especially when the cough is dry and nonproductive. The mechanism by which the narcotic and nonnarcotic antitussive agents affect the intensity and frequency of a cough depends on the principal site of action: (1) central nervous system (CNS) depression of the cough center in the medulla (cough reflex), or (2) suppression of the nerve receptors within the respiratory tract.

The **cough reflex** involves two types of receptors found in the lungs and airways. These receptors, when stimulated, can initiate the events leading to a cough:

- A **stretch receptor** responds to elongation of muscle.
- An **irritant receptor** responds to coarse particles and chemicals.

Theoretically, the cough reflex can be stopped at several points. The antitussive products are formulated to act on one or more of the events in the following series:

- correcting or blocking the irritation of receptors
- blocking transmission to the brain
- increasing the cough center threshold
- blocking the action of the expiratory muscles

Table 9.11 lists the most commonly used antitussive medications.

TABLE 9.11 Most Commonly Used Antitussive Medications

Generic (Brand)	Pronunciation	Dosage Form	Common Dosage	Dispensing Status	Controlled-Substance Schedule
benzonatate (Tessalon Perles, Zonatuss)	ben-ZOE-na-tate	Capsule	100–200 mg 3 times a day as needed; not to exceed 600 mg a day	Rx	
codeine (various combinations)	KOE-deen	Oral liquid	15–30 mg every 6–8 hrs as needed; not to exceed 120 mg a day	OTC	C-II, C-III, or C-V
dextromethorphan (Delsym, various brands)	dex-troe-meth-OR-fan	Capsule, gel, lozenge, oral liquid, oral strip	Regular release: 10–20 mg every 4 hrs or 30 mg every 6–8 hrs Extended release: 60 mg 2 times a day Not to exceed 120 mg a day	OTC	
hydrocodone-chlorpheniramine (TussiCaps, Tussionex Pennkinetic, Vituz)	hye-droe-KOE-done klor-fen-EER-a-meen	Capsule, oral solution, oral suspension	Varies based on dosage form	Rx	C-II
promethazine-codeine (Phenergan with codeine)	proe-METH-a-zeen KOE-deen	Oral liquid	Promethazine 6.25 mg/codeine 10 mg every 4–6 hrs	Rx	C-V
Dextromethorphan Combinations					
dextromethorphan-pseudoephedrine-brompheniramine (Bromfed DM)	dex-troe-meth-OR-fan soo-doe-e-FED-rin brom-fen-EER-a-meen	Oral liquid	Varies based on dosage form	Rx	
guaifenesin-dextromethorphan (Mucinex DM)	gwye-FEN-e-sin dex-troe-meth-OR-fan	Capsule, oral liquid, tablet	Varies based on dosage form	OTC	
promethazine-dextromethorphan	proe-METH-a-zeen dex-troe-meth-OR-fan	Oral liquid	Varies based on dosage form	Rx*	

* Dispensing status per federal law. Individual states may have different dispensing statuses.

Codeine

Codeine is the traditional agent used to treat a cough. Codeine is a controlled substance, and its schedule depends on its concentration, strength, and the other medications used in its combination product. Codeine may be a Schedule-II, Schedule-III, or Schedule-V drug. Codeine-derivative cough suppressants may be available over the counter but are restricted. Many states limit the quantities of these drugs that can be purchased at one time. The most common side effects are nausea, drowsiness, light-headedness, and constipation, especially if the recommended dose is exceeded. Codeine should be taken with food to decrease stomach upset.

Contraindications Contraindications to codeine include respiratory depression, acute or severe asthma, presence of or suspicion of paralytic ileus, and postoperative pain management in children who have undergone tonsillectomy.

Cautions and Considerations Codeine has a black box warning for respiratory depression and death in children who received codeine after a tonsillectomy or adenoidectomy.

Codeine is also thought to have a drying effect on the respiratory mucosa; this effect would be detrimental to patients with asthma or emphysema.

Drug Interactions Codeine is a CNS depressant, and this effect is additive if taken with other CNS depressants, such as alcohol. Codeine may enhance the constipating effect of eluxadoline.

When used at the recommended dosage, codeine has a low potential for dependency. However, codeine products are frequently misused, so now there are more stringent controls regarding their dispensing. They may be purchased without a prescription in some states, but the purchaser must sign for them, be an adult according to state law, and show identification. The products may be dispensed only by the pharmacist because the pharmacist is required to place his or her initial by the patient's signature.

Hydrocodone-Chlorpheniramine

Hydrocodone-chlorpheniramine (TussiCaps, Tussionex Pennkinetic, Vituz) is a popular medication. Hydrocodone is a derivative of codeine with many of the same qualities and side effects. It is prescribed for cough and upper respiratory symptoms of allergies and colds. This drug has abuse potential and is a Schedule-II substance. It has a high potential for psychological and physical dependence. A prescription for this drug should be checked carefully to make sure it is legal. Side effects include blurred vision, drowsiness, constipation, and mood changes.

Contraindications The extended-release (ER) capsule and suspension should not be used in children younger than six years of age because of the increased risk of fatal respiratory depression.

The oral solution should not be used with or within 14 days of monoamine oxidase inhibitor (MAOI) therapy or in patients who also have narrow-angle glaucoma, urinary retention, severe hypertension, or severe coronary artery disease.

Cautions and Considerations Hydrocodone-chlorpheniramine may cause CNS and respiratory depression. It should be used with caution in older adults. Some formulations contain polysorbate 80 and propylene glycol.

Drug Interactions Hydrocodone-chlorpheniramine interacts with the following drugs: aclidinium, azelastine, conivaptan, eluxadoline, glucagon, MAOIs, paraldehyde, potassium chloride, thalidomide, tiotropium, and umeclidinium. Consequently, concurrent use should be avoided.

Benzonatate

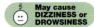

Benzonatate (Tessalon, Zonatuss) is a prescription drug used to treat a nonproductive cough. It locally anesthetizes the stretch receptors in the airways, lungs, and pleura (membrane that lines the thoracic cavity), but it does not affect the respiratory center. Benzonatate should carry a warning label telling the patient not to chew the capsule because chewing the drug would cause a very unpleasant effect with pronounced salivation. Fluid intake is especially encouraged to help liquefy sputum. The main side effects are sedation, headache, and dizziness.

Contraindications This drug is contraindicated in patients who are known to be hypersensitive to benzonatate or related compounds (such as tetracaine).

Cautions and Considerations There are reports of abnormal behavior (mental confusion and hallucinations) with benzonatate use.

Drug Interactions Benzonatate has no known drug interactions.

Dextromethorphan

Dextromethorphan (Delsym) has similar efficacy to codeine; however, it does not have its analgesic properties and does not depress respiration. Furthermore, dextromethorphan acts on the same receptors as codeine, which is why it is a good cough suppressant. Dextromethorphan is a nonopioid derivative of morphine and acts on the cough center to suppress the cough reflex. Dextromethorphan may be the most common nonopioid agent used for cough. If a patient is allergic to morphine, the pharmacy database on the technician's computer will flag the patient as also being allergic to dextromethorphan. If large quantities of dextromethorphan are consumed, it can produce hallucinations; this is known as "robo-tripping," which is popular with teenagers. For this reason, dextromethorphan has become a recreational drug. Because of the potential for misuse, anyone purchasing dextromethorphan must be able to prove that he or she is older than 18 years.

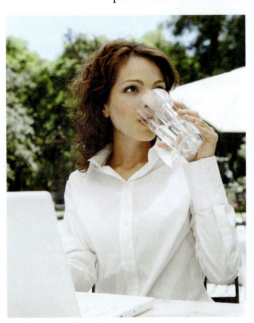

Sometimes maintaining good fluid intake is all that is needed to allow the respiratory tract to clear itself through coughing.

Contraindications Dextromethorphan should not be used with an MAOI or within two weeks of discontinuing an MAOI.

Cautions and Considerations Some forms of liquid dextromethorphan contain benzyl alcohol, which can result in neonatal toxicity.

Drug Interactions Dextromethorphan, which is commonly combined with other drugs, interacts with MAOIs. It also interacts with other drugs that affect serotonin levels (such as selective serotonin reuptake inhibitors).

Expectorants

The purpose of an **expectorant** is to enable the patient to rid the lungs and airway of mucus when coughing. Expectorants decrease the thickness and viscosity (stickiness) of mucus, so that a cough will eject mucus and other fluids from the bronchi. Such a cough is called a *productive cough*. Expectorants are used for both dry, unproductive coughs and productive coughs.

TABLE 9.12 Most Commonly Used Expectorants

Generic (Brand)	Pronunciation	Dosage Form	Common Dosage	Dispensing Status	Controlled-Substance Schedule
guaifenesin (Mucinex, various brands)	gwye-FEN-e-sin	Caplet, granules, oral liquid, syrup, tablet	Regular release: 200-400 mg every 4 hrs, not to exceed 2.4 g a day Extended release: 600-1,200 mg every 12 hrs, not to exceed 2.4 g a day	OTC	
Guaifenesin Combinations					
guaifenesin-codeine (Robitussin A-C)	gwye-FEN-e-sin KOE-deen	Oral liquid	Varies based on dosage form	OTC, Rx	C-V
guaifenesin-pseudoephedrine (Mucinex D)	gwye-FEN-e-sin soo-doe-e-FED-rin	Tablet	Varies based on dosage form	Behind the counter	

If a patient is well hydrated, coughing up mucus is not a problem. Hydration can be accomplished by drinking six to eight glasses of water a day, which by itself can be as effective as an expectorant. Fluid intake and adequate humidity in the inspired air are important to liquefy mucus in the respiratory tract and, therefore, are essential in cold therapy. Table 9.12 lists commonly used expectorants.

Guaifenesin

The most commonly used OTC expectorant is **guaifenesin (Mucinex)**, which can be taken in caplet, capsule, granules, liquid, syrup, tablet, or sustained-release form. This drug is also frequently combined with other drugs. It is derived from tree bark extract and is a common component of many cough and cold remedies. It loosens phlegm (mucus) and thins bronchial secretions to make coughs more productive and rid the respiratory tract of mucus. Guaifenesin is especially indicated in patients with a persistent or chronic cough (from smoking, asthma, or emphysema) with excessive secretions. The side effects include vomiting, nausea, GI upset, and drowsiness.

Contraindications There are no contraindications associated with guaifenesin use.

Cautions and Considerations Some guaifenesin products contain benzyl alcohol (which is implicated in neonatal toxicities) and phenylalanine.

Drug Interactions Guaifenesin has no known significant interactions.

Decongestants

Vasodilation of blood vessels in the nasal mucosa allows fluids to leak into these tissues, resulting in swelling and stuffiness. A **decongestant** stimulates the alpha-adrenergic receptors of the vascular smooth muscle, constricting the dilated arteriolar network within the nasal mucosa. This constriction shrinks the engorged mucous membranes, which promotes drainage, improves nasal ventilation, and relieves the feeling of stuffiness. Shrinking the mucous membranes not only makes breathing easier but also permits the sinus cavities to drain. Topical agents are more immediately effective but of shorter duration than systemic agents. Decongestants should not be given to patients who cannot tolerate sympathetic nervous system stimulation. Sympathetic nervous system stimulation increases heart rate and blood pressure and heightens CNS stimulation. Decongestants are often combined with antihistamines in an effort to offset the antihistamine side effect of drowsiness. Most decongestants are OTC drugs.

Following the label directions regarding the frequency and duration of use is very important when using decongestants. Topical nasal application of these drugs over prolonged periods is often followed by a phenomenon called **rhinitis medicamentosa** more commonly known as *rebound congestion*. It is thought to be caused by severe nasal edema and reduced receptor sensitivity. Patients with this condition use more spray more often, but it is less effective. Patients should be counseled on the use of topical decongestants to prevent rhinitis medicamentosa. Duration of therapy of a nasal decongestant should be limited to three to five days.

These drugs should be used with caution in older adults and in patients with hypertension, diabetes, or cardiovascular disease. They can be dangerous if overdosed. They directly stimulate the alpha-adrenergic receptors of respiratory mucosa, causing vasoconstriction to relieve congestion. Their mechanism of action also affects blood pressure and the heart.

TABLE 9.13   Most Commonly Used Decongestants

Generic (Brand)	Pronunciation	Dosage Form	Dispensing Status
pseudoephedrine (Sudafed)	soo-doe-e-FED-rin	Oral liquid, tablet	Behind the counter
phenylephrine (Neo-Synephrine, Sudafed PE, various brands)	fen-il-EFF-rin	Oral liquid, suppository, tablet	OTC
Pseudoephedrine Combinations			
cetirizine-pseudoephedrine (Zyrtec-D)	se-TEER-a-zeen soo-doe-e-FED-rin	Tablet	Behind the counter
fexofenadine-pseudoephedrine (Allegra-D)	fex-o-FEN-a-deen soo-doe-e-FED-rin	Tablet	Rx
guaifenesin-pseudoephedrine (Mucinex D)	gwye-FEN-e-sin soo-doe-e-FED-rin	Tablet	Behind the counter
ibuprofen-pseudoephedrine (Advil Cold and Sinus, Sine-aid IB)	eye-byoo-PROE-fen soo-doe-e-FED-rin	Liquid-filled capsule, tablet	Behind the counter
ibuprofen-pseudoephedrine-chlorpheniramine (Advil Allergy Sinus)	eye-byoo-PROE-fen soo-doe-e-FED-rin klor-fen-EER-a-meen	Tablet	Behind the counter
loratadine-pseudoephedrine (Claritin D)	lor-AT-a-deen soo-doe-e-FED-rin	Tablet	Behind the counter
naproxen-pseudoephedrine (Aleve Cold and Sinus)	na-PROX-en soo-doe-e-FED-rin	Tablet	Behind the counter
triprolidine-pseudoephedrine (Actifed Cold and Allergy)	trye-PROE-li-deen soo-doe-e-FED-rin	Oral solution, tablet	Behind the counter

Table 9.13 describes the most commonly used decongestants. Decongestants can be administered topically or orally. Topical administration takes the form of drops, sprays, and vapors that are applied nasally. Oral administration takes the form of capsules, syrups, and tablets. Administering a decongestant orally distributes the drug through the systemic circulation to the vascular bed of the nasal mucosa.

Therapeutic Uses of Decongestants

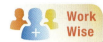

Work Wise

Spend some time in the cough and cold aisle of a pharmacy near you. Familiarize yourself with the active ingredients of products available for purchase.

Decongestants are used for temporary symptomatic relief of nasal congestion due to the common cold, upper respiratory allergies, and sinusitis. Decongestants should *not* be taken if the patient is using other sympathomimetic drugs. They should also be avoided if the patient has any of the following conditions:

- diabetes
- heart disease
- uncontrolled hypertension
- hyperthyroidism
- benign prostatic hypertrophy
- Tourette's syndrome

Both oral and topical agents have side effects, which are listed in Table 9.14. Some of these are unpleasant but relatively minor, whereas others can be serious. Side effects differ for oral agents and topical agents.

Pseudoephedrine

Pseudoephedrine (Sudafed) is a commonly used and effective decongestant. It may be combined with many other drugs. In the past, patients with hypertension were advised to avoid this drug. Current evidence shows that if the hypertension is controlled, by whatever means, then pseudoephedrine is not contraindicated for short-term use. The results of clinical trials cited in the scientific literature indicate that pseudoephedrine works best when combined with an antihistamine.

Pseudoephedrine has strong abuse potential because it is a derivative of ephedrine, which is a controlled substance in some states. In addition, it can be made into methamphetamine. Because of illegal methamphetamine production, the amount

TABLE 9.14 Side Effects of Decongestants

Oral Agents	Topical Agents
Anxiety	Burning sensation
CNS stimulation (can be used to prevent sleep)	Contact dermatitis
Dizziness	Dry mouth
Hallucinations	Rhinitis medicamentosa
Headache	Sneezing
Increased blood pressure	Stinging sensation
Increased heart rate	
Insomnia	
Tremors	

of pseudoephedrine a consumer may purchase at one time is limited. Products containing pseudoephedrine are kept behind the counter, and the consumer must specifically ask for them and present identification.

Contraindications Pseudoephedrine should not be used with or within 14 days of MAOI therapy.

Cautions and Considerations As discussed previously, chronic use may lead to rebound congestion.

Some formulations contain sodium and should be used with caution in patients following a diet with sodium restrictions. Other formulations contain benzyl alcohol, which is associated with neonatal toxicities.

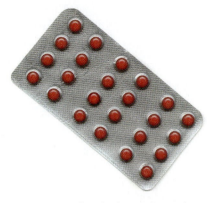

Because pseudoephedrine (pictured above) is a key ingredient in manufacturing methamphetamines, laws have been passed to restrict access to this medication.

Drug Interactions Pseudoephedrine should not be used with ergot alkaloids or MAOIs.

Phenylephrine

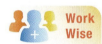

Work Wise

Combinations of ingredients in OTC preparations change frequently without notice to consumers or healthcare professionals. When purchasing any OTC medications, it is important to read the labels.

Phenylephrine (Neo-Synephrine, Sudafed PE) is used over-the-counter, primarily to treat symptoms of colds and allergies and itchy, watery eyes. It has replaced pseudoephedrine in many decongestant combinations because it cannot be made into methamphetamine and, therefore, does not require special security measures. Phenylephrine is, however, less effective than pseudoephedrine as a decongestant. Both drugs seem to work better in combination with an antihistamine. Phenylephrine is often administered intravenously to treat hypotension because of the vasoconstriction it causes. It is also used in eyedrops and nasal sprays. To prevent rebound congestion, the sprays should not be used more than three days in a row. The eyedrops are also used extensively in the treatment of allergies.

Contraindications Phenylephrine contraindications include high blood pressure and ventricular tachycardia.

Cautions and Considerations IV phenylephrine has a black box warning that indicates it should only be used by experienced and adequately trained providers. Phenylephrine should be diluted prior to administration and is known as a vesicant. Some phenylephrine products contain sulfites and can, therefore, cause reactions in allergic individuals.

Drug Interactions Phenylephrine should not be used with ergot alkaloids, hyaluronidase, and MAOIs.

Antihistamines

Histamine is found in all body tissue. It induces capillary dilation and increases capillary permeability, both of which help to decrease blood pressure. It contracts most smooth muscle, increases gastric acid secretion, increases heart rate, and mediates hypersensitivity. Basically, two types of drugs block the histamine receptors. The drugs commonly referred to as **antihistamines** block the H_1 receptors in the upper respiratory system.

TABLE 9.15 Commonly Used Antihistamines

Generic (Brand)	Pronunciation	Dosage Form	Dispensing Status	Controlled-Substance Schedule
First Generation				
chlorpheniramine (Chlor-Trimeton)	klor-fen-EER-a-meen	Oral liquid, oral suspension, tablet	OTC	
chlorpheniramine-hydrocodone (Tussionex Pennkinetic, Vituz)	klor-fen-EER-a-meen hye-droe-KOE-doan	Oral liquid	Rx	C-II
chlorpheniramine-hydrocodone-pseudoephedrine (Zutripro)	klor-fen-EER-a-meen hye-droe-KOE-doan soo-doe-e-FED-rin	Capsule, oral solution, oral suspension	Rx	C-II
clemastine (Tavist)	KLEM-as-teen	Oral liquid, tablet	OTC	
diphenhydramine (Benadryl)	dye-fen-HYE-dra-meen	Injection	Rx	
		Capsule, tablet	OTC	
Second Generation				
azelastine (Astelin, Astepro, Optivar)	a-ZEL-a-steen	Nasal spray, ophthalmic	Rx	
cetirizine (Zyrtec)	se-TEER-a-zeen	Oral liquid, tablet	OTC	
desloratadine (Clarinex)	des-lor-AT-a-deen	Oral liquid, tablet	Rx	
fexofenadine (Allegra)	fex-o-FEN-a-deen	Oral liquid, tablet	OTC	
loratadine (Claritin)	lor-AT-a-deen	Capsule, oral liquid, tablet	OTC	
olopatadine (Pataday, Patanase, Patanol, Pazeo)	o-lo-PAT-a-deen	Nasal solution, ophthalmic solution	Rx	

The other type of antihistamines are referred to as H_2 blockers, and they affect the cells in the GI tract. This chapter discusses the H_1 blockers.

Antihistamines are well absorbed in tissues and widely distributed across the blood-brain barrier and placenta. Sedation occurs when they penetrate the blood-brain barrier. Pregnant mothers are warned not to take antihistamines because these products can cross the placenta and may adversely affect the fetus. Table 9.15 lists the most commonly used antihistamines.

Therapeutic Uses of Antihistamines

The drugs typically thought of as antihistamines (H_1 blockers) provide symptomatic relief by acting on the H_1 receptors to prevent histamine binding. Among the many uses of antihistamines are the following:

- treatment of allergies and rashes
- treatment of insomnia
- symptomatic relief of urticarial lesions (rash), edema, and hay fever
- control of cough
- alleviation of vertigo
- alleviation of nausea and vomiting
- relief of serum sickness (hypersensitivity reaction that may occur several days to two to three weeks after receiving antisera or following drug therapy)
- control of venom reactions (venom contains histamine and other substances causing histamine release)
- mitigation of the extrapyramidal side effects of antipsychotic medication
- prophylaxis for certain drug reactions
- prophylaxis for certain drug allergies

Antihistamines can also be used in the treatment of hypersensitivity reactions. **Hypersensitivity** is a state of altered reactivity in which the body reacts with an exaggerated immune response to a foreign agent. This response can range from quite serious, as in serum sickness, to a slight rash or low-grade fever. **Promethazine (Phenergan)** and **meclizine (Antivert)** are the antihistamines used most frequently for nausea and motion sickness. (In low doses, promethazine is an antihistamine, even though it is a derivative of phenothiazine. In high doses, promethazine can function as an antipsychotic; however, it is rarely used this way.) Some antihistamines are promoted for specific indications, even though the therapeutic uses of these drugs overlap considerably. The side effect profile is also the same even though there may be varying degrees for each drug. Antihistamines are more effective at preventing some allergic reactions from occurring than in reversing these actions once they have taken place.

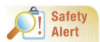

Safety Alert

Zantac (gastric acid reducer) and Zyrtec (antihistamine) could easily be misread, one for the other.

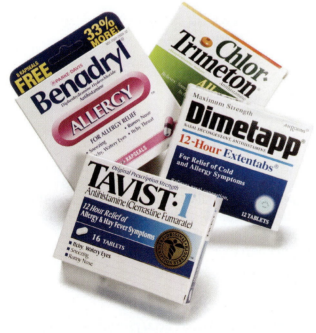

Many antihistamines, such as the ones pictured, are available as OTC products.

First-Generation Antihistamines

First-generation antihistamines for cold and allergy were developed before second-generation varieties. They include chlorpheniramine (used for upper respiratory symptoms), clemastine (used for the common cold and allergies), and diphenhydramine (for allergic reactions and sleep promotion). These drugs, unless combined with a controlled substance, are available OTC and are similar in efficacy.

The most common side effects of the currently available antihistamines include anticholinergic responses, hyperactivity (in children), and sedation. The anticholinergic responses include dry mouth, drying of the mucosa of the upper respiratory tract, blurred vision, constipation, and urinary retention. Sedation is the most common side effect of antihistamines. Some antihistamines are actually prescribed to induce sleep. In fact, many

OTC sleep aids contain the antihistamine diphenhydramine. This effect is synergistic with alcohol use. Dizziness is also a common side effect. The newer drugs on the market have fewer side effects.

Chlorpheniramine and Products Containing Chlorpheniramine

Chlorpheniramine (Chlor-Trimeton) is a first-generation antihistamine that is available by itself and in combination with other drugs.

Chlorpheniramine-hydrocodone (Tussionex Pennkinetic, Vituz) is a popular drug and an effective treatment for cough. However, it is a drug with a high potential for abuse.

Chlorpheniramine-hydrocodone-pseudoephedrine (Zutripro) also has become a very popular drug. However, it may impair thinking and slow reaction time. Alcohol increases these side effects. It works well for treating coughs, but it is a drug that must be used cautiously because of the potential for abuse.

Contraindications Contraindications to chlorpheniramine include narrow-angle glaucoma, bladder-neck obstruction, prostate enlargement, acute asthma attacks, stenosing peptic ulcer, and pyloroduodenal obstruction.

Cautions and Considerations Chlorpheniramine may cause CNS depression. It should be used with caution in older adults because of the increased risk of confusion, dry mouth, and constipation. Because of these side effects, this drug is on the Beers Criteria of potentially inappropriate drugs for older adults.

Drug Interactions Chlorpheniramine may potentiate the effects of CNS depressants (such as alcohol and opioids) and anticholinergics.

Clemastine

Clemastine (Tavist) is a first-generation antihistamine used for colds and allergies. Of the first-generation antihistamines, it is the least likely to cause sedation.

Contraindications Clemastine is contraindicated in narrow-angle glaucoma.

Cautions and Considerations Clemastine may cause CNS depression. Older adults may have increased confusion, dry mouth, and constipation. Because of these side effects, clemastine is on the Beers Criteria of potentially inappropriate drugs for older adults.

Drug Interactions Clemastine may potentiate the effects of CNS depressants (such as alcohol and opioids) and anticholinergics.

Diphenhydramine

Diphenhydramine (Benadryl) is an antihistamine that also has antitussive properties. The usual adult dose is 25 mg every four hours. The main side effect is drowsiness, which is additive if the drug is taken with other CNS depressants.

Contraindications Diphenhydramine should not be used in patients with acute asthma, neonates or premature infants, or breast-feeding mothers.

Cautions and Considerations CNS depression may occur with diphenhydramine use. Older adults may have increased confusion, dry mouth, and constipation. Because of these side effects, diphenhydramine is on the Beers Criteria of potentially inappropriate drugs for older adults.

Some formulations may contain alcohol, benzyl alcohol, phenylalanine, polysorbate 80, propylene glycol, and soy protein. Soy protein products should not be used in patients with soy or peanut allergies.

Drug Interactions Diphenhydramine may potentiate the effects of CNS depressants (such as alcohol and opioids) and anticholinergics.

Second-Generation Antihistamines

This drug class includes azelastine, cetirizine, desloratadine, fexofenadine, loratadine, and olopatadine. These agents were developed to provide antihistamine therapy without the unwanted side effects of the first-generation drugs. In general, second-generation antihistamines have fewer CNS side effects and cause less sedation. For that reason, second-generation antihistamines are popular options for patients compared with their first-generation counterparts. Second-generation antihistamines, however, may cause dry eyes.

Azelastine

Azelastine (Astelin, Astepro, Optivar) was the first antihistamine nasal spray. It is indicated in seasonal allergic rhinitis and seems to work as well as the oral antihistamines for itchy, runny nose and sneezing. It has a bitter taste to many patients. Even though the drug has a low incidence of sedative side effects, the bottle should carry an auxiliary label warning patients of potential drowsiness with the use of this drug. Azelastine is stable for three months after the bottle is opened.

Contraindications There are no contraindications for the use of azelastine.

Cautions and Considerations Azelastine may cause CNS depression.

Drug Interactions Azelastine may potentiate the effects of CNS depressants (such as alcohol and opioids) and anticholinergics.

Cetirizine

Cetirizine may be confused with sertraline (an antidepressant) or stavudine (an antiviral). The brand name Zyrtec may be confused with Zantac (used to treat gastroesophageal reflux disease).

Cetirizine (Zyrtec), while effective, is the second-generation antihistamine with the highest potential for drowsiness. It is administered once daily and is available as an OTC product.

Contraindications Cetirizine does not have contraindications.

Cautions and Considerations Use with caution in patients with renal or hepatic dysfunction. Dose reduction may be required. Use with caution in older adults, as they may be more sensitive to adverse reactions.

Drug Interactions Cetirizine may increase side effects associated with anticholinergic agents and CNS depressants.

Fexofenadine

Fexofenadine (Allegra) is a second-generation antihistamine and is generally not as sedating as many of the other antihistamines. Studies have not reported any arrhythmias or other serious reactions in patients who use this drug.

Contraindications Fexofenadine does not have contraindications.

Cautions and Considerations This drug should be used with caution in patients with kidney impairment. Dose adjustments may be needed.

The oral disintegrating tablet formula contains phenylalanine.

Drug Interactions Fexofenadine may increase the side effects associated with anticholinergic agents and CNS depressants.

Loratadine and Desloratadine

Loratadine (Claritin) has been an OTC drug since 2002, but **desloratadine (Clarinex)** does require a prescription. Desloratadine is a long-acting metabolite of loratadine. It has additional anti-inflammatory properties and should not be given with erythromycin or ketoconazole.

Contraindications Neither loratadine nor desloratadine have contraindications.

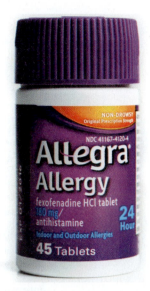

Fexofenadine is sold under the brand name, Allegra, and is now available as an OTC drug.

Cautions and Considerations Both drugs should be used with caution in patients with liver or kidney disease. Pharmacy technicians should be aware that some formulations contain benzyl alcohol or phenylalanine.

Drug Interactions Loratadine and desloratadine may increase the side effects associated with anticholinergic agents and CNS depressants.

Olopatadine

Olopatadine (Pataday, Patanase, Patanol, Pazeo) is a second-generation antihistamine for allergic rhinitis in patients six years and older. This drug is available in nasal and ophthalmic forms, and nasal form can leave a bitter taste in the mouth. It should be used as rescue therapy for symptoms of allergies. Because it is an antihistamine, it can also cause sleepiness.

Contraindications There are no contraindications for the use of olopatadine.

Cautions and Considerations The ophthalmic product should not be used to treat lens-related irritation. If the patient wears contact lenses, he or she should remove the lenses prior to administration and wait at least 10 minutes before reinserting them.

Drug Interactions Olopatadine has no known drug interactions.

Nasal Corticosteroids

A new group of drugs has emerged to treat allergies: **nasal corticosteroids**. These medications must be used daily for maximum benefit. Administration (spray) should be directed away from the septum to prevent nasal irritation and bleeding. Other side effects of nasal allergy products include cough, sore throat, headache, and runny nose. Typically, these effects are mild and tolerable. Local infections of *Candida albicans* may occur in the nose of patients using nasal steroids on a long-term basis. Nasal steroids are now the most effective monotherapy for allergic rhinitis. These drugs have also shown some value in the treatment of otitis media (earaches) in children. The most commonly prescribed nasal corticosteroids are listed in Table 9.16.

TABLE 9.16   Most Commonly Used Nasal Corticosteroids

Generic (Brand)	Pronunciation	Dosage Form	Common Dosage	Dispensing Status
beclomethasone (Beconase AQ)	be-kloe-METH-a-sone	Nasal spray	1–2 sprays in each nostril twice a day	Rx
budesonide (Rhinocort Aqua)	byoo-DES-oh-nide	Nasal spray	1–4 sprays in each nostril once a day	Rx
ciclesonide (Omnaris, Zetonna)	sye-KLES-oh-nide	Nasal spray	1–2 sprays in each nostril once a day	Rx
flunisolide (Nasarel)	floo-NISS-oh-lide	Nasal spray	1–2 sprays in each nostril 2–3 times a day	Rx
fluticasone furoate (Veramyst)	floo-TIK-a-sone fur-oh-ate	Nasal spray	2 sprays in each nostril once a day	Rx
fluticasone propionate (Flonase)	floo-TIK-a-sone PRO-pee-oh-nate	Nasal spray	2 sprays in each nostril once a day	OTC, Rx
mometasone (Nasonex)	moe-MET-ah-sone	Nasal spray	1–2 sprays in each nostril once a day	Rx
triamcinolone (Nasacort AQ)	trye-am-SIN-oh-lone	Nasal spray	1–2 sprays in each nostril once a day	OTC, Rx

Ciclesonide (Alvesco, Omnaris, Zetonna) is a prodrug that is converted to the active form (desisobutyryl ciclesonide) by an enzyme in the nasal mucosa. This process is known as *target activation*. Theoretically, target activation should reduce side effects; however, systemic exposure is negligible after nasal inhalation. Alvesco appears to cause less hoarseness and oral thrush than other nasal steroids because it is dispersed in very small particles.

Fluticasone is used in two different forms. The furoate formulation **(Veramyst)** is dispensed via a device that may be easier for patients use. The propionate formulation **(Flonase)** is available as an OTC product.

Mometasone (Nasonex) depresses the release of endogenous chemical mediators of inflammation (histamine, kinin, and prostaglandins). It reverses the dilation and permeability of vessels in the area and decreases access of cells to the site of injury. It may be used in children who are over 12 years of age to prevent symptoms of allergic rhinitis. Nasal corticosteroids are administered intranasally. Patients should use the following instructions to instill these medications:

1. Shake product well before use.

2. Clear nasal passages by either blowing the nose or using a saline irrigation system.

3. Sit in an upright position with the head tilted slightly forward.

4. Close one nostril by pressing it with a finger, and insert the sprayer tip into the other nostril, with the tip pointing away from the nasal septum. Breathe in and depress the applicator to deliver a metered dose.

5. Breathe out from the mouth.

6. Repeat the procedure for the other nostril.

It is not necessary for patients to breathe in quickly or forcefully or to hold their breath. The site of action is in the nose, not deep in the sinuses or lungs. Patients should be aware that postnasal drip may occur and that they may taste the nasally administered medication. Patients should avoid sneezing or blowing their nose just after using the spray.

Contraindications Flunisolide is contraindicated in infections of the nasal mucosa, such as bacterial or viral infections. The other nasal corticosteroids listed in Table 9.16 do not have contraindications.

Cautions and Considerations To ensure proper dosing, patients should shake these products well before administration. The pharmacy technician should affix an auxiliary warning label to the drug container to remind patients to shake the container prior to using the medication.

The spray application bottle should be primed when new and whenever it has not been used for a while. **Priming** a nasal spray means that the patient should pump the sprayer a few times away from the nose until an even amount of spray exits the applicator.

Drug Interactions Systemic corticosteroids may enhance the hyperglycemic potential of nasal corticosteroids.

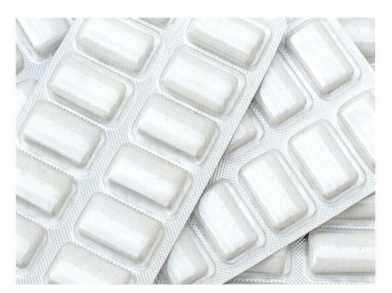

Nicotine replacement therapy is available in multiple forms, including chewing gum.

Smoking Cessation

According to the Centers for Disease Control and Prevention, smoking causes nearly a half million deaths each year in the United States and increases the risk of death from all causes. Its impact on the respiratory system is especially destructive, resulting in damaged airways and alveoli. In fact, cigarette smoking causes the most cases of lung cancer in the United States and is responsible for nearly 80% of all deaths from COPD. Asthma can also be caused or exacerbated by smoking or by exposure to cigarette smoke. In addition, smoking harms other organs in the body, increasing the risk for heart disease and stroke, cancer, Type 2 diabetes mellitus, rheumatoid arthritis, reproductive difficulties, and decreased bone health. On average, cigarette smokers live approximately 15 years less than non-smokers. Cigarette smoke contains more than 4,000 identified chemical compounds, including at least 43 carcinogens. Lung cancer, leukemia, and cancers of the mouth, pharynx, larynx, esophagus, pancreas, cervix, kidney, and bladder are associated with smoking. Evidence also links smoking with other cancers, such as ovarian, uterine, and prostate. Tobacco is the single largest cause of preventable death.

Environmental (secondhand) tobacco smoke also poses a substantial health threat because it contains all the carcinogens and toxins present in inhaled cigarette smoke. Children living in a household with smokers have a higher risk of respiratory infection, asthma, and middle-ear infection than those who live with nonsmokers. Birth defects may be related to the mother's smoking during pregnancy.

The physical benefits of smoking cessation include a longer life and better health (i.e., decreased risk of lung, laryngeal, esophageal, oral, pancreatic, bladder, and cervical cancers; coronary heart disease; and other diseases aggravated by smoking). A few personal benefits from smoking cessation are listed in Table 9.17.

TABLE 9.17 Personal Benefits from Smoking Cessation

Improved performance in athletic endeavors

Improved sexual function

Better-smelling home, car, clothing, and breath

Economic savings

Freedom from addiction

Healthier babies

Improved health

Improved self-esteem

Improved sense of taste and smell

Lack of guilt about exposing others to smoke

Opportunity to set a good example for children and young adults

Nicotine, the addictive component of tobacco, is readily absorbed in the lungs from inhaled smoke. Nicotine from smokeless tobacco products, such as chewing tobacco and snuff, is absorbed across the oral or nasal mucosa, respectively. In the body, nicotine is extensively metabolized in the liver and, to a lesser extent, in the kidneys and lungs. One major urinary metabolite, **cotinine**, has a longer half-life (15 to 20 hours) and a tenfold higher concentration than nicotine. Presence of this metabolite indicates that a person is a smoker.

Nicotine and polycyclic aromatic hydrocarbons in cigarette smoke induce the production of hepatic (liver) enzymes responsible for metabolizing caffeine, theophylline, imipramine, and other drugs. Smoking increases plasma cortisol (a major natural glutocorticoid) and catecholamine (sympathomimetic amines, including dopamine, epinephrine, and norepinephrine) concentrations, which affect treatment with adrenergic agonists and adrenergic-blocking agents.

Nicotine is an agonist of ganglionic cholinergic receptors with dose-related, pharmacologic effects. These effects include CNS and peripheral nervous system stimulation and depression, respiratory stimulation, skeletal muscle relaxation, catecholamine release by the adrenal medulla, peripheral vasoconstriction, and increases in blood pressure, heart rate, cardiac output, and oxygen consumption. Chronic nicotine ingestion leads to physical and psychological dependence. Consequently, smoking cessation results in withdrawal symptoms, usually within 24 hours. These symptoms are listed in Table 9.18.

TABLE 9.18 Symptoms of Nicotine Withdrawal

Anxiety	Gastrointestinal disturbances
Craving for tobacco	Headache
Decreased blood pressure and heart rate	Hostility
Depression	Increased appetite and weight gain
Difficulty in concentrating	Increased skin temperature
Drowsiness	Insomnia
Frustration, irritability, impatience, restlessness	

Planning to Stop Smoking

One of the reasons it is so difficult to stop smoking is that nicotine has many properties that reinforce various behaviors. These properties include relaxation, increased alertness, decreased fatigue, improved cognitive performance, and a "reward" effect (pleasure or euphoria). Increased alertness and improved cognitive performance result from stimulation of the cerebral cortex, which can occur at low doses. The "reward" effect, mediated by the limbic system, occurs at high doses.

To combat these properties, smoking cessation treatment involves three main elements: behavior modification, social support from the clinician, and nicotine replacement therapy. Nicotine replacement therapy is recommended as first-line pharmacotherapy for smokers without contraindications to therapy (myocardial infarction in the previous four weeks, serious arrhythmias, severe or worsening angina pectoris). Patients must understand, however, that nicotine replacement therapy is not a substitute for behavior modification and that success is greatest when both are used concomitantly. Individual or group counseling is highly recommended.

The steps in establishing a plan for quitting are as follows:

1. Set a date.
2. Inform family, friends, and coworkers of the decision and request understanding and support.
3. Remove cigarettes from the environment and avoid spending a lot of time in places where smoking is prevalent.
4. Review previous attempts to quit, if applicable, and analyze the factors that caused relapse.
5. Anticipate challenges, particularly during the critical first few weeks.

The key to smoking cessation is total abstinence. Patients should reward themselves for abstaining and avoid situations that serve as smoking triggers. Because drinking alcohol is strongly associated with relapse to tobacco use, smokers should reduce their alcohol consumption or abstain from drinking altogether during the quitting process.

One major reason smokers are reluctant to quit is fear of weight gain. Although weight gain does occur, most smokers gain less than 10 pounds. The weight gain is caused by both increased caloric intake and metabolic adjustments; it can occur even if caloric intake remains constant or is restricted.

Smoking Cessation Drug Therapy

The most commonly used agents for smoking cessation are listed in Table 9.19. Patients must be strongly advised to stop smoking when initiating nicotine replacement therapy. Those individuals who continue to smoke may show signs of nicotine excess. The symptoms of nicotine excess are listed in Table 9.20; note that they often overlap with withdrawal symptoms. Dizziness and perspiration are more often associated with excessive nicotine levels; anxiety, depression, and irritability are common symptoms of nicotine withdrawal.

All of the listed drugs except the nicotine nasal spray and inhalant (**Nicotrol**), **varenicline (Chantix)**, and the antidepressant **bupropion (Wellbutrin SR, Zyban)** have been approved for OTC drug use. More information on bupropion can be found in Chapter 7.

TABLE 9.19 Commonly Used Agents for Smoking Cessation

Generic (Brand)	Pronunciation	Dosage Form	Common Dosage	Dispensing Status
bupropion (Wellbutrin SR, Zyban)	byoo-PROE-pee-on	Tablet	150 mg twice a day	Rx
nicotine (Commit, Nicoderm CQ, Nicorette, Nicotrol)	NIK-oh-teen	Gum, inhaler, lozenge, nasal solution, transdermal patch	Varies based on product and patient	OTC
varenicline (Chantix)	var-EN-i-kleen	Tablet	1 mg twice a day	Rx

Nicotine Supplements

Nicotine supplements are used to reduce absorbed nicotine slowly over time, thereby reducing many withdrawal symptoms. They are available in several OTC dosage forms, including gum, inhaler, lozenge, and patch.

Nicotine gum works best for users of smokeless tobacco products. These forms are chewed briefly and then "parked" in the cheek until the craving for nicotine returns. Inhaled forms mimic the use and effects of smoking while eliminating the harmful toxins from inhaling smoke. In the patch form, nicotine is absorbed transdermally and provides the most continuous nicotine delivery. However, this form does not allow the smoker to adjust nicotine exposure throughout the day. Nicotine nasal spray is administered intranasally and results in more rapid absorption compared to oral dosage forms. Its use is limited because of its side effects, such as rhinitis, sneezing, tearing, and nose and throat irritation.

The dose of nicotine supplements usually depends on the number of cigarettes smoked daily. Doses should be tapered gradually as nicotine withdrawal symptoms subside.

Contraindications Nicotine supplements are contraindicated in patients who smoke after a recent heart attack and in patients who have life-threatening arrhythmias or worsening chest pain. These supplements should be avoided by pregnant patients as well. Nicotine gum should not be used by patients with active temporomandibular joint disease.

TABLE 9.20 Symptoms of Nicotine Excess

Abdominal pain	Hypersalivation
Confusion	Nausea
Diarrhea	Perspiration
Dizziness	Visual disturbances
Headache	Vomiting
Hearing loss	Weakness

Cautions and Considerations Nicotine can increase heart rate and blood pressure. Risk-benefit analysis should be performed for patients who require nicotine replacement and who have concurrent heart disease, hypertension, or arrhythmias. Dental problems may worsen with the gum form of nicotine. Airway irritation may result from the inhaled form of nicotine, and caution must be used in patients with airway disease. Nicotine patches should be used cautiously in patients who are allergic to adhesive tape or in those individuals who have skin problems. Nicotine nasal spray is not recommended for patients with chronic nasal disorders, such as allergy, rhinitis, nasal polyps, and sinusitis.

Drug Interactions Nicotine may enhance cardiac effects related to adenosine use. Cimetidine and varenicline may enhance adverse effects of nicotine.

Bupropion

Bupropion (Wellbutrin SR, Zyban) is an antidepressant used to combat the mood changes and emotional instability associated with smoking cessation. It can also reduce cravings for nicotine. Bupropion is available only by prescription. Side effects of bupropion include drowsiness, dizziness, blurred vision, and insomnia. To reduce these effects, patients should avoid drinking alcohol while taking this medication and take the medication in the morning.

Contraindications Contraindications to bupropion include seizure disorder, history of anorexia or bulimia, abrupt discontinuation of ethanol or sedatives, use of MAOIs, and use of linezolid or IV methylene blue.

Cautions and Considerations When discontinuing bupropion therapy, doses must be tapered to avoid a rebound of depressive symptoms. Patients should not stop taking bupropion abruptly.

As with starting any antidepressant therapy, patients using bupropion should talk with their healthcare prescribers if they notice symptoms of depression or suicidal ideation. The FDA-approved labeling for bupropion includes a black box warning that alerts users of serious mental health events. Patients should be observed for signs of agitation, hostility, depression, and behavioral changes.

Drug Interactions Bupropion should not be used with MAOIs.

Varenicline

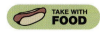

Varenicline (Chantix) blocks nicotine binding to pleasure receptors and reduces the severity of craving and withdrawal symptoms. Smoking while taking Chantix does not provide the same sense of satisfaction. Foods also do not provide as much satisfaction while a patient is taking varenicline, so weight gain is usually not a problem while using this drug for smoking cessation. This advantage is important because weight gain is a common side effect of smoking cessation that causes many patients to resume smoking. Varenicline needs to be started a week before the quit date. It should be taken with food and a full glass of water to help prevent or decrease nausea, which is one of the primary side effects. Varenicline should be taken for 24 weeks, and the patient should attend a smoking-cessation program. The most prominent side effect is unusual dreams.

Contraindications Varenicline does not have any contraindications.

Cautions and Considerations The FDA-approved labeling for varenicline includes a black box warning that alerts users to serious neuropsychiatric events. Patients should be observed for agitation, hostility, depression, and changes in behavior. Patients with suicidal ideation should stop taking varenicline immediately and talk with their healthcare prescribers.

Drug Interactions Individuals taking varenicline with ethanol, famotidine, inhaled nicotine, intranasal nicotine, nizatidine, ranitidine, tobramycin, or vandetanib should be monitored.

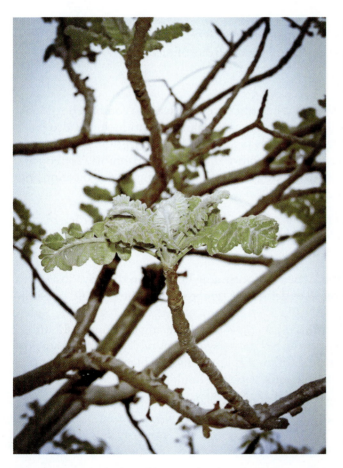

Boswellia serrata is the branching tree that has anti-inflammatory properties.

Complementary and Alternative Therapies

Boswellia serrata (or Indian frankincense) is a branching tree that is native to India, Northern Africa, and the Middle East. It possesses anti-inflammatory properties and has been used for centuries to treat chronic inflammatory diseases, such as asthma. Of note, *Boswellia serrata* is for chronic treatment and should be avoided in acute asthma exacerbations. It is usually consumed as the powdered form of the plant resin. In this form, *Boswellia serrata* is usually taken as 300 mg three times daily. The most common GI side effects are diarrhea, stomach pain, and acid reflux. It should be avoided in patients with acid reflux and liver dysfunction.

Choline is a nutrient related to B vitamins. It is naturally consumed through diet (in sources such as egg yolk, liver, peanuts, fish, soybeans, cabbage, and cauliflower) and can be synthesized by the body. Choline may be effective when used orally for chronic management of asthma. Typical choline doses range from 500–1,000 mg three times daily. Side effects include decreased blood pressure, nausea, dizziness, and headache.

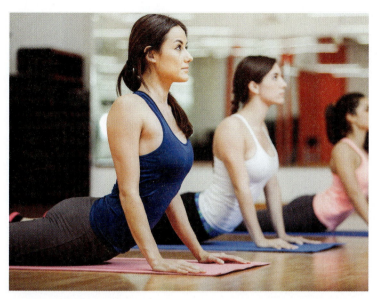

Yoga can benefit patients who have mild-to-moderate asthma or COPD.

Yoga may be used to improve symptoms of mild-to-moderate asthma and COPD. It is generally considered safe in healthy individuals. Patients with intervertebral disk and back ailments, high or low blood pressure, glaucoma, or severe osteoporosis should avoid inverted poses. Certain breathing techniques should be avoided in patients with asthma and COPD.

Nasal irrigation may effectively relieve allergies and sinusitis. It is generally well tolerated. However, it is important to use clean irrigation dispensers and to use water that is sterile or has been boiled. Patients can purchase kits that include water dispensers and powders for dilution.

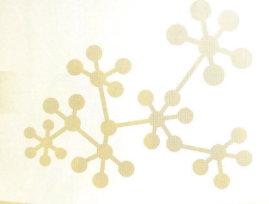

CHAPTER SUMMARY

Asthma

- Asthma is a disease in which inflammation causes the airways to tighten; asthma is a reversible condition in that it can improve or be controlled with the use of appropriate medications.

- Asthma is a pulmonary condition with the following characteristics: reversible small airway obstruction, progressive airway inflammation, and increased airway responsiveness to stimuli.

- Drug therapy is the mainstay of asthma management.

- A rescue course of corticosteroids may be needed at any time.

- Individuals who have asthma should not use antihistamines in acute attacks and should avoid beta blockers. Other drugs to be avoided include aspirin, NSAIDs, penicillins, cephalosporins, and sulfa drugs.

- With an MDI, the patient inhales slowly, whereas with a DPI, the patient breathes in quickly to activate the inhaler.

- Nebulizers are effective delivery systems for children too young to use inhalers.

- Home nebulizers can easily become contaminated if not cleaned properly.

- A spacer is recommended for use with an MDI to decrease the amount of spray that is deposited on the back of the throat and then swallowed. It increases drug penetration into the lungs.

- Short-acting inhaled bronchodilators are albuterol, levalbuterol, and metaproterenol.

- Levalbuterol, one of two isomers of albuterol, may be more effective than the other isomer and has fewer side effects.

- Inhaled corticosteroids are often used for asthma treatment. They should not be used for the treatment of acute attacks.

- Inhaled corticosteroids include beclomethasone, budesonide, flunisolide, fluticasone, and mometasone. Combination products that include inhaled corticosteroids include budesonide-formoterol and fluticasone-salmeterol.

- Zafirlukast (Accolate) is a leukotriene receptor antagonist that has been shown to be effective for asthma in adults and children.

- Zileuton (Zyflo) is a leukotriene inhibitor that carries strong warnings about liver toxicity and can increase theophylline levels.

- Montelukast (Singulair) is indicated for prophylaxis and chronic treatment of asthma. It is approved for use in adults and children 12 months and older.

- Cromolyn sodium is a mast cell stabilizer used to treat asthma.

- Omalizumab is a monoclonal antibody that can be used to treat asthma that is not controlled with an inhaled corticosteroid.

- Theophylline interacts with many drugs, so it should be used only when a patient's lung disease is unresponsive to other drugs.

Chronic Obstructive Pulmonary Disease

- COPD encompasses emphysema and chronic bronchitis. COPD is irreversible.

- Emphysema is characterized by destruction of the tiny alveoli, or air sacs, of the lungs.

- Chronic bronchitis can be caused by cigarette smoke; exposure to occupational dusts, fumes, and environmental pollution; and bacterial infection.

- Pharmacologic management of bronchitis and emphysema is still largely empirical, and anticholinergics and LABAs are used most frequently.

- Anticholinergics include aclidinium, ipratropium, tiotropium, and umeclidinium.

- Anticholinergic side effects include dry mouth, nervousness, dizziness, headache, cough, and bitter taste.

- LABAs include arformoterol, formoterol, indacaterol, olodaterol, and salmeterol. These agents are more frequently used for COPD, but may also be used for asthma.

Other Lung Diseases

- Pneumonia is a common lung infection that affects individuals of all ages, and is treated with antibiotics.

- Cystic fibrosis (CF) is a hereditary disease that involves the gastrointestinal (GI) and respiratory systems. CF can be a fatal disease, with some patients dying in early adulthood.

- RDS occurs in neonates and is treated with surfactants.

- The treatment regimen for TB varies depending on the patient's symptoms.

- Histoplasmosis is often referred to as the *summer flu*. It is usually benign, but some rare cases can be life-threatening. The only drug that is effective in the treatment of histoplasmosis is amphotericin B.

Cough, Cold, and Allergy

- Antitussives, expectorants, decongestants, and antihistamines each have a different mechanism of action and purpose. Most are OTC products.

Antitussives

- Antitussives are indicated to reduce the frequency of a cough, especially when it is dry and nonproductive.
- The cough reflex can be stopped at several points in the reflex pathway.
- Dextromethorphan is the most commonly used OTC antitussive.
- Dextromethorphan may only be sold to individuals who show proof that they are least 18 years old.

Expectorants

- Expectorants decrease the thickness and stickiness of mucus by decreasing its viscosity.
- Guaifenesin is the most commonly used expectorant, but drinking several glasses of water may work as well.

Decongestants

- Decongestants stimulate the alpha-adrenergic receptors of the vascular smooth muscle, constricting the dilated arteriolar network and shrinking the engorged mucous membranes. This mechanism of action promotes drainage of the sinus cavities and makes breathing easier. Stimulation of the sympathetic nervous system also increases heart rate and blood pressure and heightens CNS stimulation. Patients sometimes take decongestants to overcome drowsiness; these drugs should not be taken by those individuals who cannot tolerate sympathetic stimulation.
- Topical application of decongestants (nasal sprays and drops) can cause a phenomenon called rhinitis medicamentosa or rebound congestion.
- Pseudoephedrine is the most effective decongestant, but it may be purchased only in limited quantities. The consumer must show proof that he or she is at least 18 years old.

Antihistamines

- Antihistamines are used primarily to combat allergic reactions, nausea, vertigo, and insomnia. They prevent binding of histamine to the receptor sites.
- The most common side effects of antihistamines are sedation and anticholinergic responses (dry mouth, constipation, urinary retention).
- Many antihistamines are sold over the counter.

- Diphenhydramine is the major ingredient in OTC sleep medications.
- Second-generation antihistamines may cause fewer side effects.

Nasal Corticosteroids

- The most effective treatment for allergic rhinitis is application of nasal steroids.

Smoking Cessation

- Benefits of smoking cessation include a longer life and better health. The key to smoking cessation is total abstinence.
- Most nicotine cessation drugs are over the counter.
- Chantix is a prescription drug that has been successful in helping patients quit smoking.

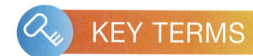

KEY TERMS

acute short, severe course

amylase an enzyme that catalyzes the hydrolysis of starch into sugars

antibiotics chemical substances with the ability to kill or inhibit the growth of bacteria by interfering with bacteria life processes

anticholinergic agents that inhibit acetylcholine, a neurotransmitter that stimulates smooth muscle in the lungs to constrict

antihistamines drugs that block the H_1 receptors

antitussives drugs that block or suppress the act of coughing

aspiration inhalation of fluids from the mouth and throat

asthma a reversible lung disease with intermittent attacks in which inhalation is obstructed; provoked by airborne allergens

asthma attack an acute difficulty with breathing

beta agonists agents that relax smooth-muscle cells of the bronchioles

bronchitis a condition in which the inner lining of the bronchial airways becomes inflamed, which obstructs exhalation

bronchodilator an agent that relaxes smooth muscle cells of the bronchioles, thereby increasing airway diameter and improving the movement of gases into and out of the lungs

bronchospasm spasmodic contraction of the smooth muscles of the bronchiole

chronic persisting for a long time

chronic obstructive pulmonary disease (COPD) a lung disease, often attributed to smoking, that narrows the airways and leads to shortness of breath and lack of oxygen; two types are chronic bronchitis or emphysema

codeine the traditional agent used to manage heavy coughs

combinations drugs used for similar effects that get a greater effect when used together

common cold a mild, self-limited viral infection

community-acquired pneumonia (CAP) pneumonia infection that results from exposure outside of an inpatient facility

corticosteroid steroid hormone produced by the adrenal cortex; often used to reduce inflammation and pain

cotinine a major metabolite of nicotine

cough reflex a coordinated series of events, initiated by stimulation of receptors in the lungs and airways, that results in a cough

cystic fibrosis (CF) a hereditary disorder of infants, children, and young adults that involves widespread dysfunction of the gastrointestinal and pulmonary systems

decongestant an agent that causes the mucous membranes to shrink, thereby allowing the sinus cavities to drain

dyspnea labored or difficult breathing

emphysema an irreversible lung disease characterized by destruction of the alveoli in the lungs, which allows air to accumulate in tissues and organs

expectorant an agent that decreases the thickness and stickiness of mucus, enabling the patient to rid the lungs and airway of mucus by coughing

histoplasmosis a respiratory tract infection caused by a fungus, most often found in accumulated droppings from birds and bats; often called the *summer flu*

induration a circular area of hardened tissue that indicates a positive reaction to a skin test in people who have been exposed to or have the disease that the test is for (e.g., tuberculosis)

irritant receptor a nerve cell in the lungs and airways that responds to coarse particles and chemicals to trigger a cough

leukotriene inhibitor an agent that blocks the body's inflammatory responses to leukotrienes or blocks their synthesis

lipase an enzyme that catalyzes the hydrolysis of fats (lipids)

long-acting beta agonists (LABAs) drugs that are similar to short-acting beta agonists but do not have to be administered as frequently

long-term persistent medications drugs used regularly to prevent asthma symptoms or attacks

malabsorption imperfect absorption of food material by the small intestine

mast cell stabilizer an agent that stabilizes mast cell membranes against rupture caused by antigenic substances and thereby reduces the amount of histamine and other inflammatory substances released in airway tissues

metered-dose inhaler (MDI) a device that delivers a specific amount of medication (as for asthma) in a fine spray in order to reach the innermost parts of the lungs

monoclonal antibody an antibody produced in a laboratory from an isolated specific lymphocyte that produces a pure antibody against a known, specific antigen

mucolytic an agent that destroys or dissolves mucus

multidrug-resistant tuberculosis (MDR-TB) strains of tuberculosis that are highly resistant to many currently used drugs

nasal corticosteroids drugs that are taken daily to treat allergies

nasal irrigation a flushing of the nasal cavity to remove excess mucus and debris from the nose and sinuses

nebulizer a device that creates a mist from air flowing over a liquid and is used in the administration of inhaled medications

nicotine the addictive component of tobacco

nicotine supplements agents that are used to reduce absorbed nicotine slowly over time

nosocomial pneumonia pneumonia acquired while a patient is hospitalized

pancreatic enzyme supplements pancreatic enzymes given to patients with cystic fibrosis; they help prevent ductal obstructions

peak expiratory flow rate (PEFR) the maximum flow rate generated during a forced expiration, measured in liters per minute

peak flow meter a device used to measure the PEFR as an indication of respiratory status; usually used twice a day by patients who have asthma

percussion a therapy used for patients who have cystic fibrosis that involves a tapping movement to induce cough and expectoration of sputum from the lungs; usually preceded by nebulizer therapy during which nebulized sterile water or normal saline is inhaled to liquefy pulmonary secretions

phosphodiesterase-4 inhibitors drugs that prevent leukocytes and neutrophils from infiltrating the lungs

pneumonia a common lung infection caused by microorganisms that gain access to the lower respiratory tract

priming the act of pumping a nasal sprayer a few times, away from the nose, until the correct amount of spray is dispensed by the applicator

protease an enzyme that begins protein catabolism by hydrolysis of the peptide bonds that link amino acids together

pulmonary function test a test done to assess asthma severity

purified protein derivative (PPD) an agent used in a tuberculosis test

quick-relief medications drugs used intermittently to provide rapid relief as needed

respiratory distress syndrome (RDS) a syndrome occurring in neonates that is characterized by acute asphyxia with hypoxia and acidosis

rhinitis medicamentosa a condition of decreased response that results when nasal decongestants are used over prolonged periods; also known as *rebound congestion*

short-acting beta agonists (SABAs) bronchodilators that relieve acute asthma symptoms

spacer a device used with a metered-dose inhaler (MDI) to decrease the amount of spray deposited on the back of the throat and swallowed

status asthmaticus a medical emergency that begins as an asthma attack but does not respond to normal management; can result in loss of consciousness and death

steatorrhea fatty, foul-smelling diarrhea that occurs when fatty foods are not properly absorbed in the gastrointestinal tract

stretch receptor a nerve cell in the lungs and airways that responds to elongation of muscle to trigger a cough

surfactant a fluid that reduces surface tension between the air in the alveoli and the inner surfaces of the alveoli, allowing gas to be exchanged between the lung and the air

tachypnea very rapid respiration causing a flushed appearance; a characteristic of emphysema

tuberculosis (TB) a disease of the lungs and other body tissues and organs caused by *Mycobacterium tuberculosis*

wheezing a whistling respiratory sound

xanthine derivative a drug that causes relaxation of airway smooth muscle, thus causing airway dilation and better air movement

yoga an ascetic discipline in which breath control, simple meditation, and the adoption of bodily postures is practiced for health and relaxation

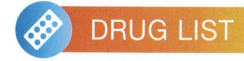 DRUG LIST

Antiasthma Agents

Bronchodilators

albuterol (ProAir, Proventil, Ventolin, VoSpire ER)
levalbuterol (Xopenex)
metaproterenol (Alupent)

Inhaled Corticosteroids

beclomethasone (QVAR, Vanceril)
budesonide (Pulmicort Respules, Pulmicort Turbuhaler, Rhinocort)
budesonide-formoterol (Symbicort)

flunisolide (Aerospan)
fluticasone (Flonase, Flovent)
fluticasone-salmeterol (Advair Diskus, Advair HFA)
mometasone (Asmanex, Asmanex HFA)
triamcinolone (Azmacort)

Xanthine Derivative

theophylline (Elixophyllin, Theo-24, Theochron, Theolair)

Leukotriene Inhibitors

montelukast (Singulair)
zafirlukast (Accolate)
zileuton (Zyflo)

Monoclonal Antibody

omalizumab (Xolair)

Mast Cell Stabilizer

cromolyn sodium

Combinations

budesonide-formoterol (Symbicort)
fluticasone-salmeterol (Advair Diskus, Advair HFA)
ipratropium-albuterol (Combivent Respimat, DuoNeb)
mometasone-formoterol (Dulera)

COPD Agents

Long-Acting Beta Agonists

arformoterol (Brovana)
formoterol (Foradil Aerolizer, Perforomist)
indacaterol (Arcapta Neohaler)
olodaterol (Striverdi Respimat)
salmeterol (Serevent Diskus)

Mucolytics

acetylcysteine (Acetadote, Mucomyst)
dornase alfa (Pulmozyme)

Antibiotics

aztreonam (Cayston)
tobramycin (Bethkis, Kitabis Pak, Tobi, Tobi Podhaler)

Anticholinergic

aclidinium (Tudorza Pressair)
ipratropium (Atrovent)
ipratropium-albuterol (Combivent Respimat, DuoNeb)
olodaterol (Striverdi Respimat)
salmeterol (Serevent Diskus)
tiotropium (Spiriva, Spiriva Handihaler)
umeclidinium (Incruse Ellipta)
umeclidinium-vilanterol (Anoro Ellipta)

Phosphodiesterase-4 Inhibitors

alpha-1 proteinase inhibitor (Aralast NP, Glassia, Prolastin-C, Zemaira)
roflumilast (Daliresp)

Cystic Fibrosis Drugs

aztreonam (Cayston)
dornase alfa (Pulmozyme)
tobramycin (Bethkis, Kitabis Pak, Tobi, Tobi Podhaler)

Surfactants

beractant (Survanta)
calfactant (Infasurf)
lucinactant (Surfaxin)
poractant alfa (Curosurf)

Tuberculosis Agents

ethambutol (Myambutol)
isoniazid
isoniazid-pyrazinamide-rifampin (Rifater)
pyrazinamide
rifampin (Rifadin)
rifapentine (Priftin)

Antitussives

benzonatate (Tessalon Perles, Zonatuss)
codeine (various combinations)
dextromethorphan (Delsym, various brands)
hydrocodone-chlorpheniramine (TussiCaps, Tussionex Pennkinetic, Vituz)
promethazine-codeine (Phenergan AC)

Dextromethorphan Combinations

dextromethorphan-pseudoephedrine-brompheniramine (Bromfed DM)
guaifenesin-dextromethorphan (Mucinex DM)
promethazine-dextromethorphan

Expectorants

guaifenesin (Mucinex, various brands)

Guaifenesin Combinations

guaifenesin-codeine (Robitussin A-C)
guaifenesin-pseudoephedrine (Mucinex D)

Decongestants

cetirizine-pseudoephedrine (Zyrtec-D)
fexofenadine-pseudoephedrine (Allegra-D)
guaifenesin-pseudoephedrine (Mucinex D)
ibuprofen-pseudoephedrine (Advil Cold and Sinus, Sine-Aid IB)
ibuprofen-pseudoephedrine-chlorpheniramine (Advil Allergy Sinus)
loratadine-pseudoephedrine (Claritin D)
naproxen-pseudoephedrine (Aleve Cold and Sinus)
phenylephrine (Neo-Synephrine, Sudafed PE)
pseudoephedrine (Sudafed)
triprolidine-pseudoephedrine (Actifed Cold and Allergy)

Antihistamines

azelastine (Astelin, Astepro, Optivar)
cetirizine (Zyrtec)
clemastine (Tavist)
chlorpheniramine (Chlor-Trimeton)
chlorpheniramine-hydrocodone (Tussicaps, Tussionex, Vituz)
chlorpheniramine-hydrocodone-pseudoephedrine (Zutripro)
desloratadine (Clarinex)
diphenhydramine (Benadryl)
fexofenadine (Allegra)

loratadine (Claritin)
meclizine (Antivert)
olopatadine (Pataday, Patanase, Patanol, Pazeo)
promethazine (Phenergan)

Nasal Corticosteroids

beclomethasone (Beconase AQ)
budesonide (Rhinecort Aqua)
ciclesonide (Omnaris, Zetonna)
flunisolide (Nasarel)
fluticasone furoate (Veramyst)
fluticasone propionate (Flonase)
mometasone (Nasonex)
triamcinolone (Nasacort AQ)

Smoking Cessation Agents

bupropion (Wellbutrin SR, Zyban)
nicotine (Commit, Nicoderm CQ, Nicorette, Nicotrol)
varenicline (Chantix)

Black Box Warnings

acetylcysteine (Acetadote, Mucomyst)
budesonide (Rhinocort)
bupropion (Wellbutrin SR, Zyban)
fluticasone-salmeterol (Advair Diskus, Advair HFA)
isoniazid (Rifamate, IsonaRif)
isoniazid-pyrazinamide (Rifampin)
promethazine (Phenergan)
promethazine-codeine (Phenergan AC)
promethazine-dextromethorphan
varenicline (Chantix)

Medication Guides

budesonide-formoterol (Symbicort)
bupropion (Wellbutrin SR, Zyban)
fluticasone-salmeterol (Advair Diskus, Advair HFA)
mometasone-formoterol (Dulera)
omalizumab (Xolair)
varenicline (Chantix)

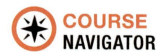

COURSE NAVIGATOR

Access interactive chapter review exercises, practice activities, flash cards, and study games.

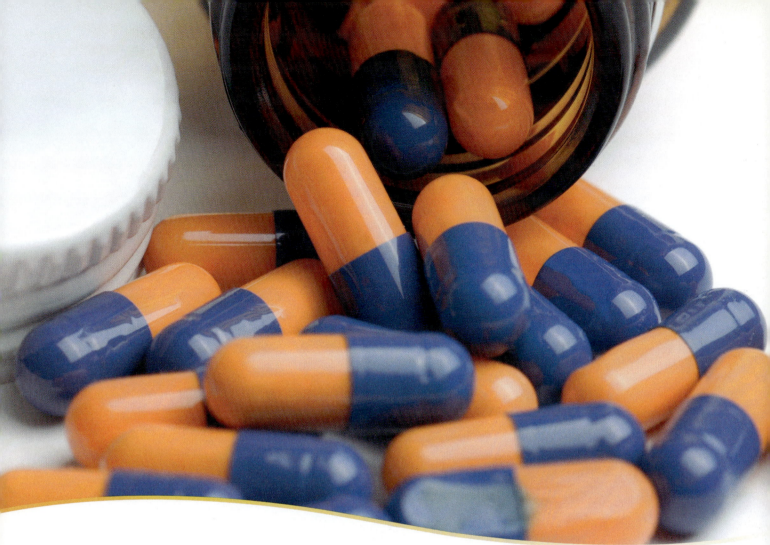

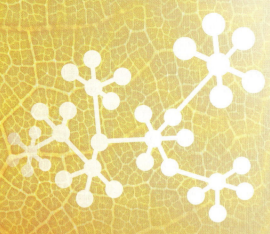

10

Drugs for Gastrointestinal and Related Diseases

Learning Objectives

1 Describe gastrointestinal (GI) physiology.

2 Describe drug treatments for GI diseases.

3 Describe gastroesophageal reflux disease and its ramifications.

4 Discuss antidiarrheal agents, and explain their mechanisms of action.

5 Describe the role of fiber in the digestive process.

6 Discuss laxatives and their mechanisms of action.

7 Identify the chemoreceptor trigger zone (CTZ), and discuss its role in nausea.

8 State the antiemetics that act on the CTZ and their mechanisms of action.

9 Describe the measures to prevent and treat hepatitis.

COURSE NAVIGATOR

Access additional chapter resources.

This chapter will discuss the diseases and disorders of the gastrointestinal (GI) system. Disorders examined range from gastroesophageal reflux disease (GERD) to hepatitis. Among the GI disorders discussed are ulcers and their causes; peptic disease, ulcerative colitis, and Crohn's disease; GERD and the lifestyle factors that may contribute to it; gallstones and their dissolution; diarrhea, including traveler's diarrhea; and constipation and its association with a low-fiber diet. Next, the chapter examines vomiting and explains how the chemoreceptor trigger zone in the brain can initiate it. The chapter concludes with an examination of the drugs used to treat hepatitis.

The Gastrointestinal System

The **gastrointestinal (GI) system** is the group of organs that process food and liquids. These actions include **digestion** (breakdown of large food molecules to smaller ones) and **absorption** (uptake of essential nutrients into the bloodstream). The GI system is composed of the **GI tract** (also known as the **alimentary tract**) and a number of supportive organs. Specifically, the GI tract includes the

mouth, **esophagus**, **stomach**, **small intestine**, **colon**, and **rectum** (see Figure 10.1). The GI tract is a continuous tube that begins in the mouth, extends through the pharynx, esophagus, stomach, small intestine, and large intestine, and ends at the anus. The GI tract varies considerably in diameter. The major function of the GI tract is to convert complex food substances into simple compounds that can be absorbed into the bloodstream and used by the cells of the body. It also excretes solid waste from the body.

GI transit time also known as *bowel transit time* is the time it takes for material to pass from the mouth to the anus. This time frame is subdivided into gastric emptying time and small intestine and colon transit time. Reducing transit time by speeding the movement of material through the intestines decreases the absorption of nutrients and water. Slowing intestinal transit time increases absorption because nutrients and water spend more time at the absorptive surfaces.

FIGURE 10.1 The Gastrointestinal System

The mouth, esophagus, and stomach are part of the upper GI system, and the intestines, colon, and rectum are part of the lower GI system.

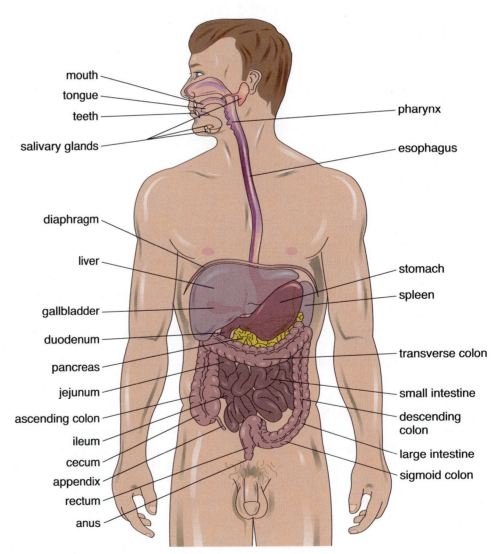

The stomach is composed of layers of smooth muscle lined with glands that secrete gastric juice. Gastric juice contains enzymes and hydrochloric acid that help break down food and mucus. Most absorption takes place in the small intestine. In the large intestine, the material that has not been absorbed is exposed to bacteria, which continue some limited digestion. Mucous membranes protect the entire GI system against abrasion and strong digestive enzymes.

Other Organs of the GI System

Other components of the GI system include the salivary glands, gallbladder, pancreas, and liver (see Figures 10.1 and 10.2). These organs release secretions that help the body digest food and absorb nutrients. **Saliva** provides lubrication for food, making swallowing easier, and contains enzymes that begin the process of digesting sugars. The gallbladder is a holding area where bile is stored. **Bile**, an alkaline fluid, is produced by the liver and aids digestion and absorption of fat and cholesterol from the small intestine. The pancreas produces many enzymes that help digest carbohydrates, fats, and proteins. The pancreas is also important because it releases secretions that neutralize the acid from the stomach.

FIGURE 10.2
Auxiliary Organs of the GI System

Without neutralization by pancreatic secretions, acid from the stomach would damage the small intestine.

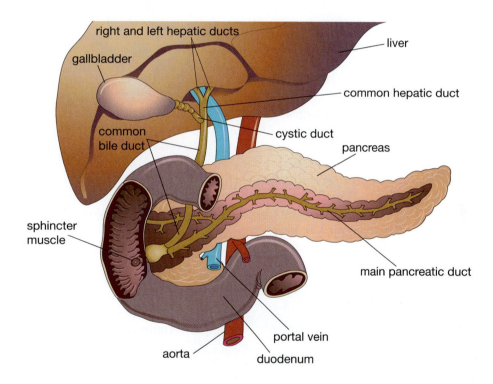

After being absorbed from the small intestine, molecules travel in the blood via the portal vein directly to the liver. The liver produces bile and removes harmful substances before they reach the general circulation. Before orally administered drugs enter the circulation, they must pass through the liver. The liver metabolizes drugs before they reach their target in the body; this is called the **first-pass effect** (see Figure 10.3).

FIGURE 10.3
Liver Function and First-Pass Effect

Alternatives to oral administration are necessary for drugs that will lose their efficacy if they undergo the first-pass effect.

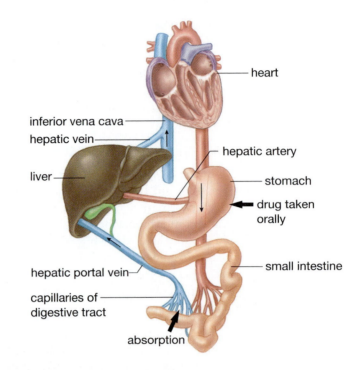

- heart
- inferior vena cava
- hepatic vein
- hepatic artery
- liver
- stomach
- drug taken orally
- small intestine
- hepatic portal vein
- capillaries of digestive tract
- absorption

Gastroesophageal Reflux Disease

Gastroesophageal reflux disease (GERD), also called *heartburn*, is a common problem. Symptoms include radiating burning or pain in the upper abdomen and chest and an acid taste. GERD patients also have recurrent abdominal pain, which may move about in the epigastric area. They may have nonspecific epigastric discomfort (gnawing or burning) that is worse before meals and may awaken them from sleep.

The primary mechanism responsible for meal-related symptoms of esophagitis (irritation of the esophagus) is the **reflux** (backflow) of acidic stomach contents through an incompetent lower esophageal sphincter. In its normal state, the sphincter is contracted. During swallowing, it relaxes enough to allow the forward passage of food and drink into the stomach; then it contracts again, preventing the reflux of the stomach contents. Heartburn occurs when the sphincter becomes incompetent (unable to keep itself sufficiently contracted). Figure 10.4 shows a normal sphincter retaining the stomach contents and an incompetent sphincter allowing reflux of the stomach contents up into the esophagus. Even with a competent sphincter, the likelihood of reflux increases during pregnancy as the uterus exerts upward pressure on abdominal organs. When this pressure occurs, the gastric contents are pushed toward the lower esophageal sphincter and up into the esophagus. GERD may also result from physical conditions such as a hiatal hernia.

GERD not only produces bothersome symptoms for patients, but also, over time, causes

Millions of Americans suffer from various types of GI ailments, including GERD.

FIGURE 10.4
Function of the Esophageal Sphincter

(a) The normal esophageal sphincter closes between swallowings. (b) The incompetent esophageal sphincter does not close completely, allowing the gastric contents (both food and stomach acids) to be ejected upward into the esophagus.

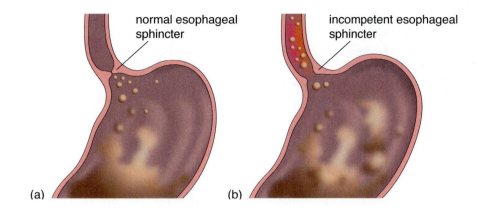

normal esophageal sphincter

incompetent esophageal sphincter

(a)   (b)

permanent changes in the tissue lining of the esophagus. These changes have been linked to narrowing of the esophagus (esophageal stricture) and esophageal cancers, so repeated bouts of GERD indicate a condition the patient should not ignore. Long-term treatment involves reducing the acidity of the stomach contents to limit damage to the esophagus.

Factors that may contribute to the malfunctioning of the lower esophageal sphincter include overeating, eating on the run, eating late at night, drinking alcohol, smoking tobacco, using nicotine, and consuming certain foods (see Table 10.1). Foods known to trigger reflux symptoms include those with a high fat content and those containing caffeine (in particular, chocolate, coffee, tea, and colas), citric and other acids, and certain spices. Gas-producing foods may also contribute to heartburn. Alcohol, caffeine, and smoking are complicating and precipitating factors in GERD. Alcohol is the most common cause of **gastritis** (irritation and erosion of stomach lining), mucosal irritation, and esophageal varices (swollen veins). Caffeine stimulates acid secretion. Smoking reduces the production of acid-neutralizing bicarbonate in the pancreatic juices. Nicotine can decrease sphincter pressure, resulting in reflux.

Symptomatic relief of mild-to-moderate GERD can be obtained by using a combination of lifestyle modifications and medications. The main premise underlying treatment is that many patients have a lifelong problem. Ideally, persons prone to reflux will adopt preventive behavior, but adherence is difficult to achieve. Patient education remains the cornerstone of therapy. Medications that promote reflux (e.g., theophylline and nifedipine) should be avoided. Patients should be advised to stop smoking. To reduce discomfort, patients should be advised not to lie down for at least three hours after a meal and, if necessary, to sleep with their head propped up.

Although the underlying problems of GERD and GI ulcers relate to damage in the GI tract from stomach acid, most treatments for these conditions do not directly

TABLE 10.1   Foods and Medications That May Worsen GERD

Foods		Medications	
• Alcohol	• Garlic	• Alendronate	• Iron
• Caffeine	• Onions	• Anticholinergics	• Nicotine (from smoking)
• Chocolate	• Orange juice	• Aspirin	• Nitrates
• Coffee or soft drinks	• Peppermint and spearmint	• Barbiturates	• Nonsteroidal anti-inflammatory drugs (NSAIDs)
• Fatty foods	• Spicy foods	• Dopamine	• Tetracycline

fix this problem. Antacids, proton pump inhibitors (PPIs), and histamine H_2 receptor blockers relieve symptoms of GERD by decreasing acid production in the stomach. However, stomach contents may still be regurgitated into the esophagus or come into contact with an ulcer in the stomach or intestines, but less damage will occur because the gastric juices are less acidic.

Antacids

Name Exchange

OTC antacids are commonly used products. Technicians may find it helpful to learn the generic and brand names of antacids, as patients often refer to these products by their brand names. Calcium carbonate is commonly known by the brand names Tums or Maalox; calcium carbonate-magnesium hydroxide is sold under the brand names Mylanta Supreme and Rolaids.

Mild-to-moderate GERD can be treated with antacids. **Antacids** contain special ions that react with hydrogen ions in the stomach and neutralize acid. They are effective for only a few hours, so it may be necessary to take these medications after every meal. Antacids are available over the counter (OTC). See Table 10.2 for information on antacids.

Antacid therapy has several shortcomings, including the need for frequent dosing and low patient adherence. For patients with active GI bleeding, antacids must be given every hour between meals for six to eight weeks. If there is no active bleeding, these medications must be dosed one hour before meals and at bedtime. Patient adherence is a major problem. Common side effects of antacids include constipation, diarrhea, stomach pain, nausea, and vomiting. These effects are generally mild. Calcium- and aluminum-containing antacids tend to cause constipation, whereas magnesium-containing antacids tend to cause diarrhea.

Contraindications There are no contraindications to the use of antacids.

Cautions and Considerations Antacids provide short-term relief for patients with heartburn. Patients requiring repeated or constant use of antacids should see their prescribers and discuss other treatment options. Continuous use of calcium-containing antacids can cause acid hypersecretion, particularly when the medication is discontinued, so long-term use of calcium products should be discouraged.

Antacids must be used with caution in patients with renal failure because aluminum and magnesium can accumulate in the blood. Patients should let their pharmacists or physicians know if they have kidney failure.

Antacid suspensions need to be shaken well before use to ensure adequate mixing of contents and proper dosing.

Drug Interactions Antacids bind to several other orally administered drugs, decreasing their absorption. For this reason, antibiotics such as isoniazid, quinolones, and tetracyclines should not be taken with antacids. Other interacting medications include iron supplements containing ferrous sulfate, and the sulfonylureas (treatment for diabetes). Antacids should be taken more than two hours before or after the other medication.

Histamine H_2 Receptor Antagonists

Gastric acid secretion and pepsin (a digestive enzyme) secretion occur in response to histamine, gastrin, foods, stomach distension, caffeine, or cholinergic stimulation. When these processes are due to excess histamine release, they can be blocked by a **histamine H_2 receptor antagonists**. These medications work by competitively binding H_2 receptors on the stomach's gastric acid secreting cells. All of these antagonists are available in OTC strengths, but some doses are by prescription only. The bedtime dose is the most important dose for H_2 receptor antagonists.

TABLE 10.2 Commonly Used Agents for GERD

Generic Name	Pronunciation	Dosage Form	Brand Name	Dispensing Status
Antacids				
aluminum hydroxide	a-LOO-mi-num hye-DROX-ide	Oral liquid	AlternaGel	OTC
aluminum hydroxide-magnesium carbonate	a-LOO-mi-num hye-DROX-ide mag-NEE-zhum KAR-bon-ate	Oral liquid, tablet	Gaviscon Extra Strength	OTC
aluminum hydroxide-magnesium hydroxide-simethicone	a-LOO-mi-num hye-DROX-ide mag-NEE-zhum hye-DROX-ide si-METH-i-kone	Oral liquid, tablet	Mylanta	OTC
calcium carbonate	KAL-see-um KAR-bo-nate	Capsule, chewable tablet, oral liquid, powder	Maalox, Tums	OTC
calcium carbonate-famotidine-magnesium hydroxide	KAL-see-um KAR-bon-ate fa-MOE-ti-deen mag-NEE-zhum hye-DROX-ide	Tablet	Pepcid Complete	OTC
calcium carbonate-magnesium hydroxide	KAL-see-um KAR-bo-nate mag-NEE-zhum hye-DROX-ide	Liquid, tablet	Mylanta, Rolaids	OTC
magnesium hydroxide	mag-NEE-zhum hye-DROX-ide	Oral liquid, tablet	Phillips Milk of Magnesia	OTC
Histamine H$_2$ Receptor Antagonists				
cimetidine	sye-MET-i-deen	Tablet	Tagamet	Rx
			Tagamet HB	OTC
famotidine	fa-MOE-ti-deen	Injection, oral liquid, tablet	Pepcid	Rx
			Pepcid AC	OTC
nizatidine	ni-ZAT-i-deen	Capsule, oral liquid, tablet	Axid	Rx
			Axid AR	OTC
ranitidine	ra-NIT-i-deen	Capsule, injection, oral liquid, tablet	Zantac	Rx
			Zantac 75	OTC
Proton Pump Inhibitors				
dexlansoprazole	deks-lan-SOE-pra-zole	Capsule	Dexilant	Rx
esomeprazole	es-oh-MEP-ra-zole	Capsule, granules, powder for reconstitution	Nexium	OTC, Rx
lansoprazole	lan-SOE-pra-zole	Capsule, oral suspension, oral disintegrating tablet	Prevacid	OTC, Rx
omeprazole	oh-MEP-ra-zole	Capsule, oral liquid, oral packet, tablet	Prilosec	Rx
			Prilosec OTC	OTC
omeprazole-sodium bicarbonate	oh-MEP-ra-zole soe-dee-um by-KAR-bo-nate	Capsule, powder for reconstitution	Zegerid	OTC
pantoprazole	pan-TOE-pra-zole	Injection, oral packet, tablet	Protonix	Rx
rabeprazole	ra-BEP-ra-zole	Oral sprinkle capsule, tablet	Aciphex	Rx
Coating Agent				
sucralfate	soo-KRAL-fate	Oral liquid, tablet	Carafate	Rx
Prostaglandin E Analog				
misoprostol	mye-soe-PROS-tawl	Tablet	Cytotec	Rx

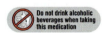

Cimetidine

Cimetidine (Tagamet, Tagamet HB) is indicated for treating ulcers, gastric hypersecretory states, GERD, postoperative ulcers, and upper GI bleeds, and for preventing stress ulcers. It reduces hydrogen ion concentration in gastric secretions by 70%. Four to six weeks of therapy are required for ulcers to heal. Reduced doses are necessary in patients with renal disease. Use may be limited by the quantity of drug interactions. Side effects include headache, dizziness, drowsiness, diarrhea, agitation, and gynecomastia.

Contraindications A hypersensitivity to other H_2 receptor antagonists contraindicates the use of cimetidine.

Cautions and Considerations Prolonged treatment (at least two years) may lead to malabsorption of dietary vitamin B_{12} and its subsequent deficiency.

H_2 blockers decrease the absorption of drugs that require an acidic environment to dissolve. Ketoconazole (an antifungal) is an acid-soluble drug that may not be effective if used with H_2 blockers. For that reason, an alternative should be sought for patients taking ketoconazole.

Drug Interactions Because it can inhibit the cytochrome P-450 system, cimetidine has many drug interactions. Avoid concurrent use with dasatinib, delavirdine, dofetilide, epirubicin, pazopanib, pimozide, risedronate, or thioridazine.

Nizatidine

Nizatidine (Axid, Axid AR) is used for treating duodenal ulcers and GERD. It may take several days before the medication provides the patient with relief from symptoms. If an antacid is added to the regimen, the doses of the two agents should be taken at least 30 minutes apart. A 100 mg dose of nizatidine is approximately equivalent to 300 mg of cimetidine. Patients should avoid aspirin, alcohol, caffeine, cough and cold preparations, and black pepper and other spices while taking this drug. Drowsiness is a side effect.

Contraindications A hypersensitivity to other H_2 receptor antagonists contraindicates the use of nizatidine.

Cautions and Considerations Prolonged treatment (at least two years) may lead to malabsorption of dietary vitamin B_{12} and its subsequent deficiency.

H_2 blockers decrease the absorption of drugs that require an acidic environment to dissolve. Ketoconazole (an antifungal) is an acid-soluble drug that may not be effective if used with H_2 blockers. For that reason, an alternative should be sought for patients taking ketoconazole.

Drug Interactions Avoid concurrent use with dasatinib, delavirdine, pazopanib, or risedronate.

Ranitidine

Ranitidine (Zantac, Zantac 75) is used for treating active duodenal ulcers and benign gastric ulcers, long-term prophylaxis of duodenal ulcers, gastric hypersecretory states, GERD, postoperative ulcers, and upper GI bleeding and for preventing stress ulcers. It has fewer interactions than some of the other H_2 blockers. Antacids should be administered 30 to 60 minutes before or after the administration of ranitidine. Constipation is the primary side effect.

Contraindications Patients with hepatitis should not take ranitidine. Although rare, reports of liver failure and death have occurred in patients with hepatitis who are taking ranitidine. A hypersensitivity to other H$_2$ receptor antagonists contraindicates the use of ranitidine.

Cautions and Considerations Prolonged treatment (at least two years) may lead to malabsorption of dietary vitamin B$_{12}$ and its subsequent deficiency.

H$_2$ blockers decrease the absorption of drugs that require an acidic environment to dissolve. Ketoconazole (an antifungal) is an acid-soluble drug that may not be effective if used with H$_2$ blockers. For that reason, an alternative should be sought for patients taking ketoconazole.

Drug Interactions Ranitidine tends to have fewer drug interactions than the other drugs in this class. However, it should still not be prescribed for patients taking dasatinib, delavirdine, pazopanib, or risedronate.

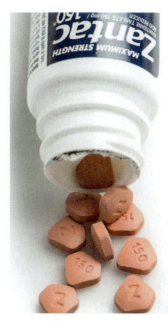

Ranitidine is sold over-the-counter in a generic form and brand (Zantac).

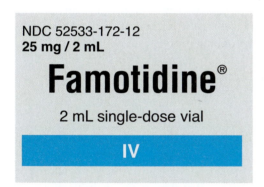

The H$_2$ blocker famotidine is available in oral dosage forms and intravenously (as pictured).

Famotidine

Famotidine (Pepcid, Pepcid AC) is used for treating duodenal ulcers, gastric ulcers, stress ulcers, GERD, and hypersecretory conditions. It relieves heartburn, acid indigestion, and sour stomach. The dose should be modified if the patient's kidney function is impaired, and it should be used cautiously in patients taking a calcium channel blocker. **Calcium carbonate-famotidine-magnesium hydroxide (Pepcid Complete)** is indicated for heartburn due to acid indigestion.

Contraindications A hypersensitivity to other H$_2$ receptor antagonists contraindicates the use of famotidine.

Cautions and Considerations Prolonged treatment (at least two years) may lead to malabsorption of dietary vitamin B$_{12}$ and its subsequent deficiency.

Drug Interactions Avoid concurrent use with dasatinib, delavirdine, pazopanib, or risedronate.

Proton Pump Inhibitors

Acidity in gastric secretions is maintained by an enzyme known as the *parietal cell H⁺, K⁺-ATPase pump (hydrogen ion–potassium ion pump)*. The term indicates that this enzyme pumps acidic hydrogen ions (H⁺), or protons, into the stomach; pumps nonacidic potassium (K⁺) ions out; and uses energy (ATP) to do so. A **proton pump inhibitor (PPI)**, a drug that blocks this enzyme, reduces stomach acidity. PPIs must be taken daily, not as needed, in order for them to work properly.

Dexlansoprazole

Dexlansoprazole (Dexilant) is the R-isomer of lansoprazole. It is indicated for the treatment of GERD for eight weeks and for the treatment of erosive esophagitis for up to six months. The drug has two releases of medicine in one pill. The first is within an hour of taking the drug, and the second 4-5 hours later. It must be taken daily rather than as needed. It should be taken first thing in the morning before breakfast. To reduce side effects and interactions, dexlansoprazole should be taken with a full glass of water. Side effects include headache, nausea, vomiting, and diarrhea.

Contraindications A hypersensitivity to one PPI contraindicates the use of all PPIs.

Cautions and Considerations Dexlansoprazole should be used with caution in patients who have liver dysfunction.

Drug Interactions PPIs may decrease the absorption of drugs that need an acidic environment to dissolve. Ketoconazole (an antifungal drug) is an acid-soluble drug that may not work if used simultaneously with PPIs. For that reason, alternatives to PPIs should be sought for patients taking ketoconazole.

Esomeprazole

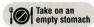

Esomeprazole (Nexium) is the S-isomer of omeprazole, and is thus very similar to it. Esomeprazole is metabolized more slowly, which leads to higher and more prolonged drug concentrations and longer acid suppression. It relieves heartburn faster than omeprazole and is slightly more effective for healing erosive esophagitis. Esomeprazole is used to treat GERD and in combination with amoxicillin and clarithromycin to treat *Helicobacter pylori (H. pylori)*. It should be taken on an empty stomach. The capsules can be opened and mixed with a small amount of applesauce if patients have difficulty swallowing pills. Side effects include headache, nausea, vomiting, and diarrhea.

Contraindications A hypersensitivity to one PPI contraindicates the use of all PPIs.

Cautions and Considerations Esomeprazole should be used cautiously in pediatric patients. The esomeprazole strontium product may be incorporated into bone.

Drug Interactions PPIs may decrease the absorption of drugs that need an acidic environment to dissolve. Ketoconazole (an antifungal drug) is an acid-soluble drug that may not work if used simultaneously with PPIs. For that reason, alternatives to PPIs should be sought for patients taking ketoconazole.

Lansoprazole

Lansoprazole (Prevacid) has the same mechanism of action and indications as omeprazole (see next section). It is used for short-term treatment of ulcers (four weeks) and esophagitis (eight weeks). It is also used in long-term treatment of hypersecretory conditions and Zollinger-Ellison syndrome (hypersecretion from a tumor). H_2 blockers and other PPIs can also be used to treat this syndrome. Side effects include headache, nausea, vomiting, and diarrhea.

Contraindications A hypersensitivity to one PPI contraindicates the use of all PPIs.

Cautions and Considerations Lansoprazole is available as tablets that are placed on the tongue and allowed to dissolve (oral disintegrating tablets). The dissolved particles must be swallowed without chewing.

Drug Interactions Lansoprazole may decrease serum concentrations of clopidogrel. PPIs may decrease the absorption of drugs that need an acidic environment to dissolve. Ketoconazole (an antifungal drug) is an acid-soluble drug that may not work if used simultaneously with PPIs. For that reason, alternatives to PPIs should be sought for patients taking ketoconazole.

Omeprazole

Omeprazole (Prilosec, Prilosec OTC) is indicated for the short-term treatment of severe erosive esophagitis, GERD, and hypersecretory conditions. It should be taken before meals. It is also indicated for peptic disease caused by the bacterium *H. pylori*, in which case it is used in combination with other drugs such as tetracycline, clarithromycin, and an H_2 receptor antagonist. Side effects include headache, nausea, vomiting, and diarrhea. **Omeprazole-sodium bicarbonate (Zegerid)** is an OTC medication for the short-term treatment of ulcer and GERD.

Contraindications A hypersensitivity to one PPI contraindicates the use of all PPIs.

Cautions and Considerations OTC omeprazole should be used for only 14 days. If symptoms have not resolved after two weeks, patients should consult their healthcare practitioners.

Drug Interactions Omeprazole may diminish the antiplatelet effect of clopidogrel. PPIs may decrease the absorption of drugs that need an acidic environment to dissolve. Ketoconazole (an antifungal drug) is an acid-soluble drug that may not work if used simultaneously with PPIs. For that reason, alternatives to PPIs should be sought for patients taking ketoconazole.

Pantoprazole

Pantoprazole (Protonix) is a prescription-only PPI. Many hospitals have pantoprazole on formulary because it has an intravenous (IV) form, which facilitates switching a patient from an IV to an oral dosage form. Side effects include headache, nausea, vomiting, and diarrhea.

Contraindications A hypersensitivity to one PPI contraindicates the use of all PPIs.

Cautions and Considerations Some pantoprazole formulations contain polysorbate 80, which can cause hypersensitivity reactions. Safety of pantoprazole in children younger than five years has not been established.

Drug Interactions Pantoprazole may decrease concentrations of clopidogrel. PPIs may decrease the absorption of drugs that need an acidic environment to dissolve. Ketoconazole (an antifungal drug) is an acid-soluble drug that may not work if used simultaneously with PPIs. For that reason, alternatives to PPIs should be sought for patients taking ketoconazole.

Rabeprazole

Rabeprazole (Aciphex) is a PPI supplied as a delayed-release tablet. It works best if taken in the morning before breakfast. Side effects include headache, nausea, vomiting, and diarrhea.

Contraindications A hypersensitivity to one PPI contraindicates the use of all PPIs.

Cautions and Considerations Use with caution in patients with severe liver dysfunction.

Drug Interactions PPIs may decrease the absorption of drugs that need an acidic environment to dissolve. Ketoconazole (an antifungal drug) is an acid-soluble drug that may not work if used simultaneously with PPIs. For that reason, alternatives to PPIs should be sought for patients taking ketoconazole.

Coating Agents

Coating agents adhere to proteins at the ulcer site, forming a protective coat or shield over the ulcer that resists degradation by gastric acid, pepsin, and bile salts. It also inhibits pepsin, exhibits a cytoprotective effect (protecting cells from noxious chemicals), and forms a viscous, adhesive barrier on the surface of the intact intestinal mucosa and stomach.

Sucralfate

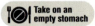

Sucralfate (Carafate) is a complex of aluminum hydroxide and sulfated sucrose with an affinity for proteins. It is used to treat duodenal ulcers. Sucralfate is dosed every six hours (the duration of the coating action's effectiveness). Patients are often awakened from sleep by the ulcer, so around-the-clock dosing is recommended for the first few days. Once the symptoms of the ulcer are relieved, dosing can be reduced to twice daily for better patient adherence. Sucralfate should be taken on an empty stomach and should not be taken within two hours of other medications.

Contraindications Sucralfate does not have contraindications.

Cautions and Considerations Use with caution in patients with renal dysfunction.

Drug Interactions Simultaneous sucralfate administration may decrease the absorption of cimetidine, digoxin, fluoroquinolone antibiotics, ketoconazole, l-thyroxine, phenytoin, quinidine, ranitidine, tetracycline, and theophylline.

Prostaglandin E$_1$ Analog

As described in more detail in Chapter 13, nonsteroidal anti-inflammatory drugs (NSAIDs) inhibit the production of prostaglandins. This prostaglandin inhibition may lead to gastric ulcers. **Prostaglandin E$_1$ analogs** replace the protective prostaglandins inhibited by NSAIDs.

Misoprostol

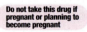

Misoprostol (Cytotec) is a synthetic prostaglandin E$_1$ analog for NSAID-induced gastric ulcers. The primary side effects of this drug are diarrhea and abdominal pain. In other countries, misoprostol is used for ulcers other than those caused by NSAIDs.

Contraindications Pregnant women should not use or handle misoprostol. Misoprostol is also used to induce labor. Patients with prostaglandin allergy are contraindicated from using misoprostol.

Cautions and Considerations Misoprostol is a hazardous agent and should be handled and disposed of appropriately. This drug should not be given to women of childbearing age unless they can comply with effective contraception. Misoprostol may cause abortion, birth defects, or premature birth. Patients should not share their medication with others.

Drug Interactions Antacids may enhance the toxicities of misoprostol. Misoprostol may enhance the therapeutic effects of carbetocin. Misoprostol may enhance the effects of oxytocin.

Peptic Disease

The term **peptic disease** is used to refer to a broad spectrum of disorders of the upper GI tract caused by the action of acid and pepsin. An **ulcer** is a local lesion or lesion of the surface of an organ or tissue. A **peptic ulcer** is an ulcer formed along any part of the GI tract exposed to acid and the enzyme pepsin (see Figure 10.5). There are three common types of peptic ulcers: gastric, duodenal, and stress ulcers. Many factors, including bacterial infection and severe physiologic stress, can contribute to the development of ulcers. Certain medications can also cause ulcers.

A **gastric ulcer** is a local excavation in the gastric mucosa. These lesions have malignant potential, occur more often in men than women, and become more frequent with aging. They are prevalent in smokers and in certain populations in the Western Hemisphere. Gastric ulcers do not necessarily occur in individuals who are high acid secretors. A family history of gastric ulcers represents a risk factor. As discussed later, a contributing factor for many patients is the presence of the bacterium *H. pylori*.

A **duodenal ulcer** is a peptic lesion situated in the duodenum. Duodenal ulcers occur more frequently in hypersecretors and are more difficult to treat than gastric ulcers because medications are usually absorbed in the stomach before they reach the duodenum.

A **stress ulcer** is a peptic ulcer, usually gastric, that occurs in the clinical setting in patients who are under severe physiologic stress from serious illness, such as sepsis, burns, major surgery, chronic disease, or chronic infection. Usually, the patient is in

FIGURE 10.5
Peptic Ulcers

Peptic ulcers are erosions of the mucosal lining of the GI tract. PPIs are commonly used to treat these ulcers.

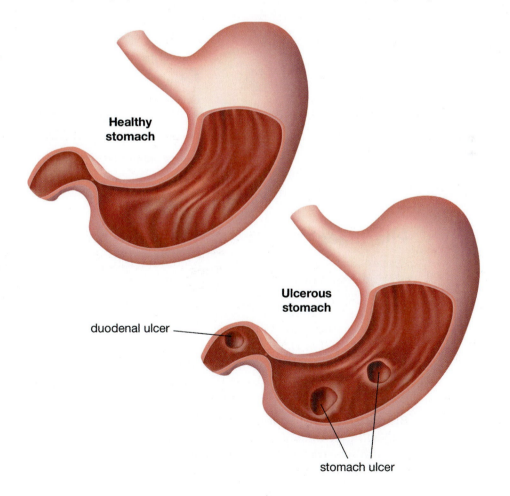

Healthy stomach

Ulcerous stomach

duodenal ulcer

stomach ulcer

the intensive care unit (ICU). Stress ulcers are caused by the breakdown of natural mucosal resistance. The patient usually has no clinical symptoms but can experience acute hemorrhage. Inserting a nasogastric tube yields blood in the aspirate of the stomach contents. Perforations of the stomach wall occur in 8%–18% of patients, with severe pain radiating toward the back. Therapy includes antacids, histamine H$_2$ receptor antagonists, or blockers. Alternatively, PPIs may be administered through an IV or a feeding tube. The potential for developing stress ulcers is why many patients in the ICU receive drugs typically used for treating GERD.

NSAIDs such as **ibuprofen** and **aspirin** can cause ulcers (see Table 10.3). These drugs can irritate and erode GI tissue. More importantly, they inhibit production of prostaglandins. Prostaglandins produce inflammation and pain throughout most of the body, but in the stomach, they protect the lining from acid secretion. Prolonged use of NSAIDs removes the protective effects of prostaglandins in the stomach and can result in GI ulceration. When ulceration erodes into a blood vessel, a **GI bleed** can occur. GI bleeds may be asymptomatic for many patients and are particularly dangerous for older adults or those patients who are critically ill. Patients taking long-term NSAIDs, aspirin, and anticoagulation therapy are at high risk for developing ulcers and life-threatening bleeding.

TABLE 10.3 Drugs That May Cause Ulcers

Drug	Adverse Effect
Alcohol	Irritates the GI tract
Aspirin	Irritates the GI tract
Corticosteroids	Reduce the mucosal barrier
Iron	Causes esophageal ulceration (must be taken with food, milk, or copious amounts of water)
Methotrexate	Irritates the GI tract, causes ulceration or hemorrhage
NSAIDs (such as ibuprofen, ketorolac, naproxen)	Reduce production of prostaglandins
Potassium chloride (KCl)	Irritates the GI tract

Pharmacologic Treatment of *Helicobacter pylori*

Research has shown that *H. pylori*, a bacterium, is responsible for the majority of peptic ulcers. It may also play a role in chronic active gastritis and gastric cancer. If a patient with peptic ulcer disease has a positive (+) test result for *H. pylori*, a multidrug regimen is prescribed (see Table 10.4). These drug combinations treat the ulcer, reduce symptoms, and kill *H. pylori* in the GI tract at the same time. All regimens consist of a PPI or H$_2$ receptor blocker to heal the ulcer and antibiotics to destroy the bacteria. Combination products are also available.

Bismuth Subcitrate Potassium-Metronidazole-Tetracycline

Bismuth subcitrate potassium-metronidazole-tetracycline (Pylera), combined with a PPI, an antibiotic, and an antacid, is approved to treat *H. pylori*. An advantage of bismuth subcitrate is that it is not a salt of salicylic acid and therefore can be used in people who have an aspirin allergy.

TABLE 10.4 Commonly Used *Helicobacter Pylori* Regimens

PPI	Plus Antibiotic	Plus Antacid	Brand Names of Combination Products
Esomeprazole (Nexium) Lansoprazole (Prevacid) Omeprazole (Prilosec) Pantoprazole (Protonix) Rabeprazole (AcipHex)	Clarithromycin* 500 mg twice a day Amoxicillin* 1 g twice a day or Metronidazole* 500 mg twice a day		Prevpac (lansoprazole-amoxicillin-clarithromycin)
PPI listed above	Metronidazole* 250–500 mg 4 times a day	Bismuth subsalicylate (Pepto-Bismol) 525 mg 4 times a day	Pylera (bismuth subcitrate potassium-metronidazole-tetracycline)

*Antibiotics discussed in detail in Chapter 4

Safety Alert

Metronidazole and macrodantin (nitrofurantoin, prescribed for urinary tract infections) can be confused with one and the other.

Contraindications A hypersensitivity to bismuth, metronidazole, tetracycline, or any component of the formulation contraindicates the use of this combination product. Patients with severe renal impairment should not use Pylera. Concomitant use with disulfiram or within the previous two weeks, and use with methoxyflurane, alcohol, or products containing propylene glycol are contraindications.

Cautions and Considerations This product contains a tetracycline and should not be used in pediatric patients. Pylera may cause QT-interval prolongation. Bismuth may be neurotoxic. Patients should be monitored for neurotoxicity.

Drug Interactions Pylera may enhance adverse cardiac effects of other QT-prolonging medications.

Lansoprazole-Amoxicillin-Clarithromycin

Lansoprazole-amoxicillin-clarithromycin (Prevpac) is a combination product containing a PPI and two antibiotics for the treatment of *H. pylori*. It is taken for 7 to 14 days. Headache, diarrhea, and taste perversion are side effects.

Contraindications Contraindications include severe hypersensitivity to lansoprazole, PPIs, any penicillin or cephalosporin, macrolide antibiotics, or any component of the formulation. Concurrent use with pimozide, cisapride, ergotamine, dihydroergotamine, astemizole, terfenadine, colchicine, lovastatin, or simvastatin contraindicates use. Patients with a history of cholestatic jaundice or hepatic dysfunction with prior clarithromycin use or those individuals with a history of QT-interval prolongation or ventricular arrhythmia should not use Prevpac.

Cautions and Considerations Use with caution in older adults due to an increased risk of cardiac side effects and in patients with renal dysfunction.

Drug Interactions Prevpac may decrease concentrations of clopidogrel. Citalopram, fluticasone-salmeterol, sildenafil, simvastatin, and tamsulosin should not be used concurrently with Prevpac.

Ulcerative Colitis and Crohn's Disease

Ulcerative colitis and Crohn's disease are two conditions that cause chronic diarrhea.

Ulcerative colitis involves excessive inflammation of the GI tract, causing ulcers. This damage causes abdominal pain and weight loss as well as diarrhea. The damage tends to be limited to specific portions of the colon or large intestine, and some patients can be cured surgically by removing the affected portion. Months can go by without symptoms. This is known as remission. When symptoms return, this is known as a flare. This disease can be eliminated through a surgical resection, in which physicians remove the diseased part of the colon.

Crohn's disease is similar to ulcerative colitis in that it involves inflammation of the GI tract and causes chronic diarrhea. It also manifests outside the GI tract. However, it is different in that it is an autoimmune disease in which the immune system malfunctions and attacks the tissue lining of the entire GI tract. Although surgery is sometimes performed, it cannot cure Crohn's disease. Despite these differences, ulcerative colitis and Crohn's disease share similar symptoms and many of the same treatments. Symptoms flare up unexpectedly, can be mild to severe, and vary widely from person to person. Common symptoms are diarrhea, vomiting, bloating, fatigue, and abdominal pain.

Table 10.5 lists the agents commonly used to treat these GI diseases. In some cases, disease-modifying antirheumatic drugs (DMARDs) may be used for ulcerative colitis and Crohn's disease. More information on DMARDs can be found in Chapter 13. Specific treatments will be discussed in greater detail in the following sections.

Corticosteroids

Corticosteroids are used for their anti-inflammatory and **immunosuppressive** properties. Patients with ulcerative colitis and Crohn's disease typically use corticosteroids orally or intravenously. (Refer to Chapter 14 for additional information concerning corticosteroids.)

Common side effects of corticosteroids include headache, dizziness, insomnia, and hunger. Taking oral corticosteroids first thing in the morning will lessen the effects of insomnia. Long-term use can affect metabolism in the body and cause facial swelling (typically referred to as "moon facies" or "moon face"), significant weight gain, fluid retention, and fat redistribution to the back and shoulders ("buffalo hump").

Other side effects include high blood pressure, loss of bone mass, electrolyte imbalance, cataracts and glaucoma, and insulin resistance (diabetes). Patients taking corticosteroids for an extended period will need to work with their healthcare practitioners to monitor these effects. If possible, therapy with corticosteroids should be used on a short-term basis and only when needed.

Contraindications Prednisone and methylprednisolone are contraindicated in patients who have systemic fungal infections. Live or live-attenuated vaccines should not be administered when immunosuppressive doses of prednisone are used. Hydrocortisone use is contraindicated in patients with systemic fungal infection, serious infections, and tubercular skin lesions. Contraindications to budesonide include primary treatment of status asthmaticus, acute episodes of asthma, and acute bronchospasm.

TABLE 10.5　Commonly Used Agents for Ulcerative Colitis and Crohn's Disease

Generic (Brand)	Pronunciation	Dosage Form	Common Dosage	Dispensing Status
Aminosalicylates				
mesalamine (Apriso, Asacol, Canasa, Delzicol, Lialda, Pentasa)	me-SAL-a-meen	Capsule, enema, suppository, tablet	PO: dose varies Rectal: administered once a day	Rx
sulfasalazine (Azulfidine, Sulfazine)	sul-fa-SAL-a-zeen	Tablet	2–4 g a day, divided	Rx
Corticosteroids				
budesonide (Entocort EC)	byoo-DES-oh-nide	Capsule, tablet	2 mg twice a day	Rx
hydrocortisone (A-Hydrocort, Cortef, Solu-Cortef)	hye-droe-KOR-ti-sone	Cream, enema, foam, suppository, tablet	PO: 100–500 mg a day Rectal: apply/instill twice a day	Rx
methylprednisolone (A-MethaPred, Depo-Medrol, Medrol, Solu-Medrol)	meth-ill-pred-NISS-oh-lone	Tablet	4–48 mg a day	Rx
prednisone (Sterapred)	PRED-ni-sone	Oral solution, tablet	5–60 mg a day	Rx
Immunosuppressant				
azathioprine (Imuran)	ay-za-THYE-oh-preen	Tablet	2–3 mg/kg a day	Rx

Cautions and Considerations Because corticosteroids suppress the immune system, patients taking them are at an increased risk of infection. With prolonged use, corticosteroids have been found to stunt growth in children. Patients who are taking budesonide should be instructed to swallow the capsule whole rather than crush or chew it.

Drug Interactions Corticosteroids may render anticoagulants less effective. Diabetes medications may be less effective when patients are using corticosteroids. Risk of infections with live vaccines increases with concurrent corticosteroid use.

Aminosalicylates

Aminosalicylates are used for both induction and maintenance of remission in patients with Crohn's disease and ulcerative colitis. Although their exact mechanism is unknown, it is thought that aminosalicylates modulate chemical mediators of the inflammatory response. Aminosalicylates can be administered orally or rectally, depending on the product. Common side effects of aminosalicylates include upset stomach, headache, arthralgia, and pharyngitis. Ulcerative colitis may worsen in patients, particularly children, using aminosalicylates.

Mesalamine

Mesalamine (Apriso, Asacol, Canasa, Delzicol, Lialda, Pentasa) is an aminosalicylate that is available in multiple dosage forms. It can be administered orally or rectally. Rectal administration is by enema or suppository. The enema product should be maintained for eight hours or as long as practical; the suppository should be retained for one to three hours.

Contraindications A hypersensitivity to one aminosalicylate contraindicates the use of all others.

Cautions and Considerations Intolerance or worsening of ulcerative colitis may occur with use. Patients should be monitored for this response. There are reports of hypersensitivity in patients using aminosalicylates. In some cases, this reaction can be rash and in others, organ involvement occurs (liver, kidney, and heart). Hepatic failure has been reported. Patients with hepatic or renal impairment should be monitored closely when using aminosalicylates. There are reports of myocarditis associated with the use of mesalamine as well.

The enema formulation of mesalamine may contain sulfites. Patients with a sulfite allergy should not use this formulation of mesalamine.

Drug Interactions Mesalamine has no documented drug interactions.

Sulfasalazine

Sulfasalazine (Azulfidine, Sulfazine) is a commonly used aminosalicylate. It is available as an oral product only. Sulfasalazine should be administered in evenly divided doses, preferably after meals. The delayed-release tablets should be swallowed whole, not crushed or chewed.

Contraindications A hypersensitivity to one aminosalicylate contraindicates the use of all others. Sulfasalazine should be avoided in patients with a sulfa hypersensitivity.

Cautions and Considerations Sulfasalazine may cause a discoloration of urine, perspiration, tears, and semen (orange-yellow).

There are reports of hypersensitivity in patients using aminosalicylates. In some cases, this reaction can be rash and, in others, organ involvement occurs (liver, kidney, and heart). These medications should be used cautiously in patients predisposed to heart conditions. Hepatic failure has been reported. Patients with hepatic or renal impairment should be monitored closely when using aminosalicylates. There are reports of myocarditis associated with the use of sulfasalazine. Use with caution in patients with severe asthma.

Drug Interactions Sulfasalazine may decrease the concentration of cardiac glycosides. The adverse effects of heparin, low-molecular-weight heparin, methotrexate, nitric oxide, and prilocaine may be enhanced by sulfasalazine use.

Immunosuppressants

Medications that suppress the immune system are called **immunosuppressants**. These medications may induce response and remission in patients with Crohn's disease or ulcerative colitis. Common side effects of immunosuppressants include sore throat, cough, dizziness, nausea, muscle aches, fever, chills, itching, and headache. These effects are usually mild to moderate. Taking acetaminophen can alleviate some of these effects if they are bothersome.

Azathioprine

Azathioprine (Imuran) is an **immunosuppressive agent** that interferes with nucleic acid synthesis in both normal and precancerous cells. The overall action is suppression of the immune system. This drug is approved to treat severe arthritis and to prevent the rejection of transplanted organs. It is also used as an **anti-inflammatory agent** in Crohn's disease, ulcerative colitis, and chronic active hepatitis. It can cause serious but reversible forms of bone marrow depression. Side effects include chills, fever, arthralgias, rash, alopecia (hair loss), hepatotoxicity, and increased risk of infection.

Contraindications Azathioprine is contraindicated during pregnancy and in patients with rheumatoid arthritis and a history of treatment with alkylating agents.

Cautions and Considerations Azathioprine has a black box warning for increased risk of malignancy (such as lymphoma). Patients should be warned of this risk prior to starting therapy.

Because immunosuppressants suppress the immune system, patients taking them are at an increased risk of infection. Patients are often instructed to take special precautions to minimize exposure to infection. They may be directed to wear face masks and stay out of crowded public areas. Of course, frequent hand washing to prevent disease is recommended.

Drug Interactions Febuxostat may increase concentrations of azathioprine. The side effects of mercaptopurine, natalizumab, and tofacitinib may be enhanced by azathioprine. Toxic effects of azathioprine may be enhanced by pimecrolimus and tacrolimus.

Gallstones

Gallstones are pebble-like structures that obstruct the **cystic duct** (see Figure 10.6). The cystic duct connects the gallbladder to the common hepatic duct. It then joins the common bile duct. Classic symptoms of gallstones include intense and dull abdominal discomfort. Sweating, nausea, and vomiting are other signs.

Gallstone Dissolution Agent

Gallstones may be recurrent and are most commonly treated with **cholescystectomy** (surgical removal of the gallbladder). However, there are pharmacologic options. Gallstones can be dissolved with **gallstone dissolution agents**.

Ursodiol

Ursodiol (Actigall) is a naturally occurring bile acid that is administered orally to dissolve cholesterol gallstones in the gallbladder or common bile duct (see Figure 10.6). It decreases the cholesterol content of bile and bile stones by reducing the secretion of cholesterol from the liver and the fractional reabsorption of cholesterol by the intestines. Frequent blood tests are necessary to monitor the drug's effects. Persistent nausea, vomiting, and abdominal pain should be reported. Gallstone dissolution can take several months; for some patients, however, gallstones never dissolve. Even in cases of successful dissolution, recurrence of stones within five years has been observed in 50% of patients.

FIGURE 10.6

The Gallbladder and Bile Duct

The gallbladder is connected to the common hepatic duct, and the common bile duct via the cystic duct.

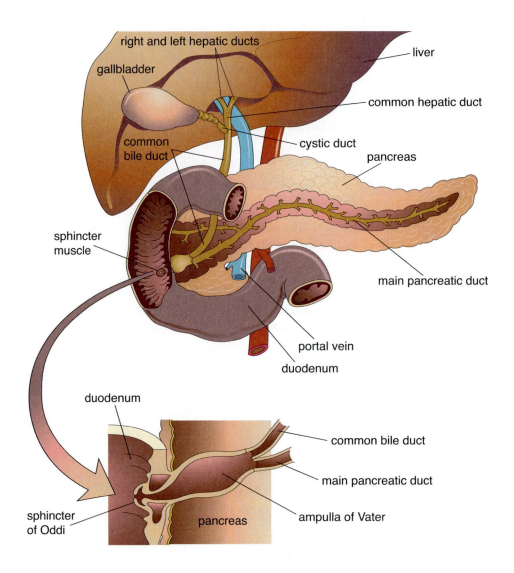

right and left hepatic ducts

liver

gallbladder

common hepatic duct

common bile duct

cystic duct

pancreas

sphincter muscle

main pancreatic duct

portal vein

duodenum

duodenum

common bile duct

main pancreatic duct

sphincter of Oddi

pancreas

ampulla of Vater

Contraindications Ursodiol is contraindicated in patients with complete biliary obstruction. It should not be used in patients with calcified bile stones, as it is ineffective in these cases. Patients who have compelling reasons for cholecystectomy should not receive ursodiol. An allergy to bile acids contraindicates the use of ursodiol.

Cautions and Considerations Gallstone dissolution can take months, and patients should expect a longer period of therapy. Use with caution in patients with liver dysfunction.

Drug Interactions Antacids and bile acid may decrease concentrations of ursodiol. Clofibrate and estrogens may encourage the formation of gallstones and may counteract the benefits of ursodiol.

Diarrhea

Diarrhea is defined as excessive, soft, or watery stools. Excessive stool can mean large stool volume or larger number of bowel movements than normal. In diarrhea, increased GI motility leads to frequent bowel movements.

Acute diarrhea is a common condition that can be caused by infections such as **traveler's diarrhea** and **food poisoning**, as well as certain drugs (see Table 10.6). Infectious causes of diarrhea include bacterial infections such as **salmonella** and *Escherichia coli (E. coli)*, protozoal infections such as giardiasis, or viral infections such as **Norwalk virus** and **rotavirus**. Drugs used to treat infections are discussed in Chapter 4. Chronic diarrhea is less common and can be caused by irritable bowel syndrome, ulcerative colitis, or Crohn's disease.

Diarrhea can be dangerous because it can quickly lead to dehydration. It decreases GI transit time and will impair absorption of drugs, vitamins, nutrients, and toxins. The most commonly used antidiarrheal agents are listed in Table 10.7. Specifically, the antimotility drugs should be used in managing chronic disease states, such as inflammatory bowel disease, postvagotomy diarrhea, and ileostomy. They should not be used to manage short-term, self-limiting diarrhea. These agents can also be hazardous in infectious diarrhea by prolonging fever and delaying clearance of organisms.

Adsorbents

Adsorbents are a class of **antidiarrheals**. They are thought to work by binding to (and therefore neutralizing) diarrhea-causing toxins. This mechanism of action prevents the adherence of infectious pathogens to the walls of the GI tract.

Bismuth Subsalicylate

Bismuth subsalicylate (Kaopectate, Pepto-Bismol) is generally safe to use as an antidiarrheal. This OTC product acts as an adsorbent, instead of reducing GI motility. Bismuth subsalicylate has both antibacterial and antisecretory actions. In addition, it has anti-inflammatory effects, making it beneficial in treating *H. pylori* infection and traveler's diarrhea.

Bismuth subsalicylate may cause constipation, nausea, vomiting, and darkening of the tongue and/or stools. Taking bismuth subsalicylate with food and plenty of water may relieve nausea symptoms. Although rare, neurotoxic symptoms such as tinnitus (ringing in the ears), confusion, and generalized weakness are also potential side effects. To prevent these more serious side effects, patients should not take excessive doses of bismuth subsalicylate. Bismuth subsalicylate is available OTC as a chewable tablet and an oral suspension.

TABLE 10.6   Drugs That Can Cause Diarrhea

• Alcohol	• H$_2$ receptor antagonists
• Angiotensin-converting enzyme (ACE) inhibitors	• Magnesium-containing laxatives or antacids
• Antibiotics	• Nonsteroidal anti-inflammatory drugs
• Certain chemotherapy agents (fluoropyrimidines, irinotecan)	(NSAIDs)
• Digoxin	• Proton pump inhibitors (PPIs)

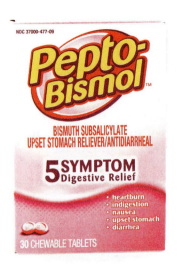

The OTC adsorbent bismuth subsalicylate is sold under the brand name Pepto-Bismol.

Contraindications Bismuth subsalicylate should not be used in patients with a history of severe GI bleeding or coagulation problems. In addition, patients with aspirin hypersensitivity should avoid products containing bismuth subsalicylate because such products may trigger an allergic type of reaction.

Cautions and Considerations Patients should be warned that their tongue and stools might darken while taking this medication. These changes are harmless and temporary. Patients should also be told to stop taking bismuth subsalicylate if they experience confusion, dizziness, or vision changes and to report these problems to their healthcare practitioners.

Bismuth subsalicylate may decrease the effectiveness of tetracycline antibiotics, so patients should not take the two medications concurrently. In addition, bismuth subsalicylate products may enhance the anticoagulant effects of warfarin, thereby increasing a patient's risk of bleeding. To prevent or limit these potential drug interactions, patients should tell their physicians and pharmacists about all prescription and nonprescription products they are taking. Patients with renal failure or gout should consult their healthcare practitioners before using bismuth subsalicylate.

Parents should consult their pharmacists or physicians before giving this product to children. Children and adolescents are at risk of a condition known as Reye's syndrome, a potentially life-threatening disorder caused by salicylate use for viral infections.

Oral suspensions must be shaken well before ingestion to ensure adequate mixing and proper dosing.

Drug Interactions Anticoagulants may increase the risk of bleeding when used with bismuth subsalicylate. Methotrexate concentrations may be increased by bismuth subsalicylate use. Tetracycline levels may decrease with bismuth subsalicylate administration.

TABLE 10.7 Most Commonly Used Antidiarrheal Agents

Generic (Brand)	Pronunciation	Dosage Form	Dispensing Status	Control Schedule
Adsorbent				
bismuth subsalicylate (Kaopectate, Pepto-Bismol)	BIS-muth sub-sa-LISS-i-late	Oral liquid, tablet	OTC	
Antimotility Drugs				
difenoxin-atropine (Motofen)	dye-fen-OX-in AT-roe-peen	Tablet	Rx	C-IV
diphenoxylate-atropine (Lomotil)	dye-fen-OX-i-late AT-roe-peen	Oral liquid, tablet	Rx	C-V
loperamide (Imodium, Imodium A-D)	loe-PAIR-a-mide	Capsule, oral solution, tablet	OTC	
Drugs for Infectious Diarrhea				
nitazoxanide (Alinia)	nye-tah-ZOX-ah-nide	Oral liquid, tablet	Rx	
rifaximin (Xifaxan)	rye-FAX-i-min	Tablet	Rx	

Antimotility Drugs

Antimotility drugs for diarrhea work by slowing **peristalsis**, the smooth muscle contractions that propel fecal matter along the colon. Water absorption from the feces is increased as the colon contents spend more time in GI transit. Most of these drugs contain opiates and, therefore, are controlled substances. Recall that long-term use of narcotics for pain leads to constipation; the use of narcotics to control diarrhea is an example of using a drug for its side effects to treat another condition.

Diphenoxylate-Atropine

Diphenoxylate-atropine (Lomotil) is a combination of 2.5 mg of diphenoxylate and 0.025 mg of atropine. Diphenoxylate is derived from the narcotic meperidine, which is why the medication is a Schedule V controlled substance. Atropine is added to discourage abuse; it also reduces peristalsis, but in excessive doses it produces anticholinergic side effects (dry mouth, blurred vision, flushing, and urinary retention). Additional side effects include constipation, paralytic ileus, respiratory depression, and sedation. Care should be taken in patients who have infectious diarrhea with fever; acute diarrhea; toxic megacolon, which can result in perforation; and advanced liver disease. Both of these drugs slow peristaltic action, which produces bulking of fecal matter.

Contraindications Diphenoxylate-atropine is contraindicated in children younger than two years. This drug is also contraindicated in patients with obstructive jaundice and diarrhea associated with pseudomembranous enterocolitis or enterotoxin-producing bacteria.

Cautions and Considerations Diphenoxylate can cross the blood-brain barrier and cause euphoria, which increases its potential for abuse. Atropine is added to diphenoxylate to discourage misuse because it has undesirable side effects, including blurred vision, urinary retention, and dry mouth. Still, pharmacies must follow state laws regarding controlled substance dispensing. In some states, special restrictions apply to the purchase of these products, and all sales are documented in a logbook.

Opiate derivatives are not appropriate for treating all types of diarrhea. If fever or bloody stool is present, the patient should consult a physician. In addition, if diarrhea continues for 48 hours after use of an opiate derivative, the patient needs further evaluation by a medical professional.

Because opiate derivatives may cause dizziness and drowsiness, patients should be reminded that activities such as driving might not be safe while taking these medications. Caution patients to take careful note of the effects of these drugs before attempting such activities.

Drug Interactions Diphenoxylate-atropine may enhance the adverse effects of anticholinergic agents, glucagon, thalidomide, and zolpidem. Central nervous system (CNS) depressant side effects may be increased with concurrent diphenoxylate-atropine use. Diphenoxylate-atropine may enhance the ulcer-causing effects of potassium chloride.

Difenoxin-Atropine

Difenoxin-atropine (Motofen) contains a metabolite of diphenoxylate and is classified as a Schedule IV controlled substance. The side effect profile and usage are the same as for **diphenoxylate-atropine (Lomotil)**.

Contraindications A hypersensitivity to difenoxin, atropine, or any component of the formulation contraindicates use. Patients with severe liver disease, jaundice, dehydration, or angle-closure glaucoma should not use difenoxin-atropine. This medication is not for use in children younger than two years, patients with diarrhea associated with organisms that penetrate the intestinal mucosa, and patients with pseudomembranous colitis associated with broad-spectrum antibiotics.

Cautions and Considerations Difenoxin-atropine may cause CNS depression. Use with caution in patients with liver or hepatic disease.

Drug Interactions Difenoxin-atropine may enhance the adverse effects of CNS depressants and anticholinergics.

Loperamide

Loperamide (Imodium, Imodium A-D) is a synthetic opioid similar to diphenoxylate. It acts on the intestinal nerves and reduces peristaltic activity, but it does not act on the CNS. Loperamide has been used for prolonged periods (18 months or longer) without loss of efficacy or signs of toxicity. Side effects are drowsiness, constipation, and dry mouth. Being an OTC product is an advantage of loperamide as well as its lack of addictive side effects.

Contraindications Loperamide should be avoided in children younger than two years and in patients who have abdominal pain without diarrhea.

Cautions and Considerations If diarrhea lasts longer than two days, symptoms worsen, or abdominal swelling or bulging develops, patients should discontinue use and consult a healthcare practitioner.

Drug Interactions Loperamide does not have any major drug interactions.

Drugs for Infectious Diarrhea

Food- and water-borne illnesses can cause significant morbidity, and even death. These illnesses result from the ingestion of food or water contaminated with infectious pathogens. Some cases occur domestically, whereas others occur with travel.

Giardia lamblia is a **protozoan** (single-celled animal) that can cause infection (called giardiasis). It is a microscopic parasite that is found worldwide in water. Streams, lakes, wells, and swimming pools can all contain *G. lamblia*. It can also be transmitted through food and person-to-person contact. Symptoms of *G. lamblia* infection include abdominal cramps, bloating, nausea, and bouts of watery diarrhea.

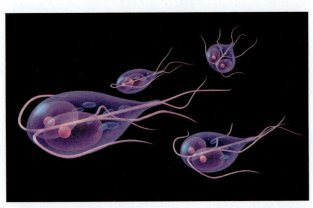

G. *lamblia* is a protozoan that can cause intestinal infection.

Traveler's diarrhea (TD) is a condition that poses a significant risk to US citizens who travel to some foreign countries; it is acquired through ingestion of food or water contaminated with the fecal bacterium *E. coli*. TD may affect 30%–70% of travelers after arrival at their destination. To prevent contamination, travelers should limit their consumption to well-cooked foods, peeled fruits and vegetables, and bottled water. Previously, systemic antibiotics were commonly prescribed, but because of increased antibiotic resistance, this practice is no longer recommended. Prophylactic antibiotics may be used for travelers who are high-risk (such as those who are immunosuppressed) or who are taking critical trips. If prophylaxis is warranted, some physicians recommend taking a quinolone antibiotic (see Chapter 4) and loperamide after the first loose stool.

Nitazoxanide

Nitazoxanide (Alinia) is indicated for the treatment of infectious diarrhea caused by the water-borne parasites *G. lamblia* and *Cryptosporidium parvum*. It may be used in patients age one year or older. Nitazoxanide interferes with an enzyme-dependent electron transfer that is essential for anaerobic energy metabolism. Nitazoxanide available as a tablet and as a powder that is to be mixed with water. Both the powder and oral suspension should be refrigerated. The reconstituted suspension should be discarded after seven days. Other drugs used against GI parasites are described in a later section of this chapter.

Contraindications There are no manufacturer-reported contraindications to the use of nitazoxanide.

Cautions and Considerations Patients with renal or hepatic dysfunction should use nitazoxanide with caution. The safety of this medication has not been established in patients who have human immunodeficiency virus (HIV). Patients who have diabetes should be informed that this drug contains 1.48 g of sucrose per 5 mL.

Drug Interactions There are no known significant interactions associated with nitazoxanide use.

Rifaximin

Rifaximin (Xifaxan) is indicated for the treatment of TD. Rifaximin works by inhibiting bacterial ribonucleic acid (RNA) synthesis. The significant advantage of this drug is that it is not absorbed into the body, so there is little risk of developing long-term resistance. It is indicated for patients 12 years and older. It should not be used in diarrhea complicated by fever or blood in stool.

Contraindications Hypersensitivity to rifamycin antibiotics contraindicates use.

Cautions and Considerations Hypersensitivity reactions have occurred with use. Prolonged use may result in bacterial superinfection. Rifaximin should not be used for systemic infections, as it is not efficacious.

Drug Interactions Cyclosporine may increase the concentrations of rifaximin. Rifaximin may diminish the therapeutic effects of sodium picosulfate.

Constipation and Flatulence

Constipation is the opposite of diarrhea. It is characterized by infrequent bowel movements, small stool size, hard stools, or the feeling of incomplete bowel evacuation. Most people pass at least three stools a week, so fewer stools could constitute constipation. However, diagnosis depends on the individual patient. Many episodes of constipation are related to a diet low in fiber or fluid intake. Constipation can also be caused by certain foods or drugs (see Table 10.8). Although many drugs have the potential to cause diarrhea or constipation, the ones most associated with constipation include antacids and pain medications such as opiates. Stress may also exacerbate constipation, whereas light exercise promotes GI motility.

TABLE 10.8 Drugs That May Cause Constipation

- Antiemetics
- Antihistamines
- Calcium- and aluminum-containing laxatives or antacids
- Calcium channel blockers
- Diuretics
- Iron
- Nonsteroidal anti-inflammatory drugs (NSAIDs)
- Opiates (morphine, hydrocodone, oxycodone, etc.)
- Tricyclic antidepressants (TCAs)

Dietary modification and lifestyle changes should accompany pharmacologic treatment of constipation. Adequate dietary intake of fiber (including fruits, vegetables, and cereals) and regular exercise (even light walking) regulate GI motility. Patients with repeat bouts of constipation should drink plenty of fluids, eat adequate fiber, and exercise regularly.

Drugs that relieve constipation are known as **laxatives**. Typically, laxatives are used only as needed on a short-term basis. Electrolyte abnormalities may occur if laxatives are used too frequently. If patients are regularly using laxatives, they should consult their physicians for a full evaluation.

In addition to oral dosage forms, many laxatives are available as suppositories or enemas. These dosage forms are used for rapid treatment of moderate-to-severe constipation. Rectal suppositories take 15 to 60 minutes to work. They are useful for hospitalized patients who are unable to swallow oral laxatives. Before inserting a rectal **suppository**, the patient can squat or lie on his or her side with one leg straight and the other bent. The patient should remove the foil wrapping from the suppository and insert the pointed end first into the rectum (see Figure 10.7). It needs to be inserted far enough into the rectum so that it does not slip out. Afterward, the patient should wash his or her hands.

An enema is a liquid solution that is delivered directly into the rectum. Enemas are used to rapidly empty the bowels prior to surgery or diagnostic procedures, such as a colonoscopy or barium enema. They also can remove excessive fecal matter that is blocking the GI tract. To use an enema, the patient should lie down. The enema tip is inserted into the rectum, and the liquid is allowed to drain into the rectum via gravity or by squeezing the bottle. The patient should hold the enema liquid in the rectum for a specific period (2 to 60 minutes, depending on the product) and then defecate normally.

FIGURE 10.7
Suppository Insertion

A suppository must be inserted past the rectal sphincter so that it does not slip out.

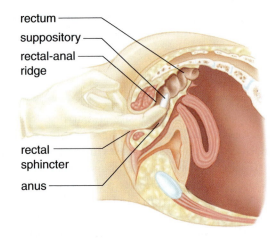

rectum
suppository
rectal-anal ridge
rectal sphincter
anus

Fiber

Fiber is defined as the undigested residue of fruits, vegetables, and other foods of plant origin after digestion by the human GI enzymes. The most important classification of fiber is by water solubility. Fruits, vegetables, and grains contain both soluble and insoluble fibers. Total fiber is the sum of soluble and insoluble fiber. Dietary fiber consists of relatively large carbohydrate molecules. The term "fiber" is a bit misleading, as many of these molecules are not actually *fibrous*. Figure 10.8 illustrates the colon, or large intestine, an organ that depends on dietary fiber to function normally.

In addition to solubility, fiber is characterized by fermentability (ability to be converted into other compounds by bacteria in the colon), water-holding capacity, and stool-bulking capacity. The bacteria in the colon are able to ferment some types of fiber. Soluble fibers are fermented to a greater extent than insoluble ones. The end products of fermentation are short-chain fatty acids, gases, water, and energy. The water-holding and stool-bulking capacities of fiber are related in that absorbing and holding water is how fiber increases the bulk (volume) of fecal material. Insoluble fibers hold less water than soluble ones. Bacterial growth in the colon provides additional bulking. Most dietary fiber reaches the colon unaltered; it increases colon content, reduces colon pressure, and increases propulsive motility (forward motion). These effects account for fiber's role in preventing or relieving constipation. Chronic constipation has often been associated with low-fiber diets. It is a common problem among older adults in the United States and other Western countries, but it does not appear to be a problem in less-developed countries.

Extended transit time in the colon permits more water to be absorbed from the GI tract into the body, thus producing smaller, harder stools. Shortening the transit time produces looser, more watery stools because less water is absorbed.

Insoluble fibers reduce GI transit time. Some soluble fibers, such as psyllium (the common name of a group of plants whose seeds yield fiber), regulate the speed at which waste moves through the colon. Soluble fibers form gels when mixed with water. In the GI tract, they act more like solids than like liquids and thus delay emptying. This action explains why psyllium can be used as an antidiarrheal as well as a laxative. Inactivity or confinement to bed can actually cause constipation when combined with soluble fibers.

Dietary fiber offers benefits aside from those associated with constipation. Soluble fibers exert metabolic effects that can lower the risk of diabetes and coronary artery disease. In addition to delaying emptying, natural soluble fibers slow the absorption of glucose from the small intestine. Fiber may also increase tissue sensitivity to insulin by increasing the number of insulin receptors on target cells. For these reasons, high-fiber diets or fiber supplements can have a positive effect on diabetes.

In addition, psyllium, fruit and vegetable fiber, and other soluble fibers bind to bile acids in the small intestine. The liver makes bile acids from cholesterol and other circulating lipids and stores the acids in the gallbladder. From that site, the acids are released into the duodenum, where they help to break masses of dietary fats into small droplets that can be absorbed. Most of the bile acids are reabsorbed in the ileum (the lowest section of the small

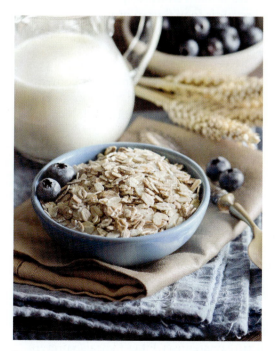

Foods that contain large amounts of fiber include oats and fruit (pictured), as well as beans, vegetables, and flaxseed.

FIGURE 10.8
Large
Intestine

The large intestine, also known as the colon, is an organ that depends on dietary fiber for its normal function.

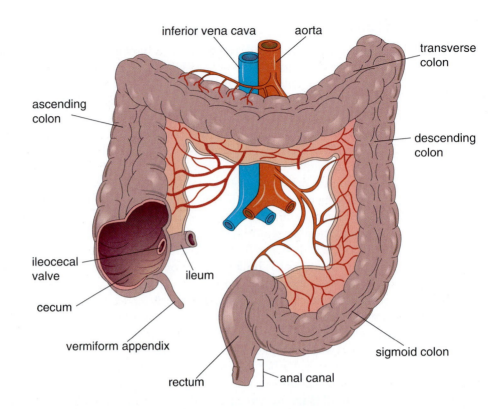

intestine) and recycled in a process known as *enterohepatic circulation*. By binding bile acids and transporting them onward into the stool, fiber interrupts the enterohepatic circulation. The removed bile acids must be replaced to ensure that fat continues to be metabolized. Making more bile acids removes cholesterol from the pool of lipoproteins circulating in the bloodstream. The end result is to maintain or increase blood levels of high-density lipoproteins and to reduce blood levels of low-density lipoproteins—an effect that lowers the risk of coronary artery disease.

Fiber also plays a role in lowering the risk of colorectal cancer. Colon cancer is more likely to develop when the diet has a high fat content and a low fiber content (the latter raises the risk even more). As dietary fiber increases, risk of colon cancer is reduced. Average-risk patients age 50 and older should be screened for colorectal cancer.

Fiber Supplementation

The most widely accepted therapeutic use of high-fiber foods is in managing constipation, but fiber supplementation is also widely used to suppress appetite and achieve weight loss. Fiber helps to produce feelings of satiety (fullness). The most effective diets are low-calorie, high-residue (high-fiber) ones. The beneficial fiber intake threshold is approximately 40 g/day. Most Americans consume only 15 to 20 g/day. Doubling the daily fiber intake could yield significant health benefits.

The adverse effects of fiber are distension, and flatulence, but these symptoms usually subside after the first few weeks of increased fiber consumption. These symptoms may also be associated with esophageal, gastric, or small-bowel or rectal obstruction, especially in patients with intestinal stricture or stenosis. Fiber may also prevent absorption of some drugs and nutrients.

Bulk-Forming Laxatives

Mild constipation can be treated with bulk-forming laxatives. As with dietary fiber, **bulk-forming agents** are poorly absorbed and remain in the GI tract, drawing water and other electrolytes into the GI system. Increased volume in the GI tract triggers peristalsis and facilitates bowel movements. In general, these agents take between one and three days to work. Bulk-forming laxatives work best for preventing constipation rather than as acute treatment. Patients with repeated problems with constipation may consider daily use of a bulk-forming laxative to remain regular. These laxatives may also have beneficial effects in patients who have diabetes or high cholesterol because they absorb fat and reduce glucose. Bulk-forming laxatives are available over the counter. Table 10.9 contains information on commonly used laxatives.

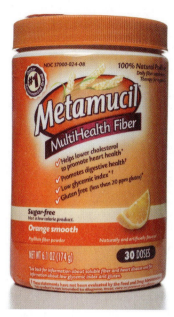

Metamucil is a brand-name product for psyllium.

Although rare, obstruction of the esophagus or bowels is possible with bulk-forming laxatives. To avoid obstruction, patients should take bulk-forming laxatives with a full glass of liquid (at least eight ounces).

Contraindications Bulk-forming laxatives are contraindicated in patients with impaired intestinal motility and in patients with intestinal stenosis.

Cautions and Considerations Bulk-forming laxatives should be used with caution in patients with esophageal strictures, ulcers, and intestinal adhesions, or who have difficulty swallowing. Products should be taken with at least eight ounces of water to prevent choking or obstruction.

Drug Interactions Because they increase GI motility, bulk-forming laxatives can affect drug absorption. Patients should separate doses of these laxatives from other medications by at least two hours to ensure that other drugs are absorbed properly.

Methylcellulose

Methylcellulose (Citrucel, Maltsupex, Unifiber) is a bulk-forming laxative. It works by increasing the amount of water in the stool. It can be taken as a powder for solution or as a tablet. Methylcellulose needs to be taken with adequate water (eight ounces per dose). The powder for oral solution should be mixed with a cold, noncarbonated beverage.

Polycarbophil

Polycarbophil (Equalactin, FiberCon, Fiber-Lax, Konsyl Fiber) is a laxative that is available in tablet form. Polycarbophil tablets should be taken with plenty of water (eight ounces). Without drinking enough water, polycarbophil may swell and block the esophagus and result in choking. Patients who have difficulty swallowing should not use polycarbophil.

TABLE 10.9 Most Commonly Used Agents to Treat Constipation

Generic (Brand)	Pronunciation	Dosage Form	Common Dosage	Dispensing Status
Bulk-Forming Laxatives				
methylcellulose (Citrucel, Maltsupex, Unifiber)	meth-il-SELL-yoo-los	Powder for solution, tablet	See individual product; taken 3–4 times a day	OTC
polycarbophil (Equalactin, FiberCon, Fiber-Lax, Konsyl Fiber)	pol-i-KAR-boe-fil	Chewable tablet, tablet	2 tablets 1–4 times a day	OTC
psyllium (Fiberall, Metamucil, Perdiem Fiber Therapy)	SIL-ee-um	Capsule, oral packet, oral powder for solution	Varies based on formulation	OTC
wheat dextrin (Benefiber)	weat DEX-trin	Chewable tablet, powder for solution	3 g up to 3 times a day	OTC
Surfactants Laxatives				
docusate (Colace, Ex-Lax Stool Softener, Surfak)	DOK-yoo-sate	Capsule, enema, oral liquid, syrup, tablet	Varies based on formulation	OTC
docusate-senna (Senokot-S)	DOK-yoo-sate SEN-na	Tablet	2 tablets once daily	OTC
Osmotic Laxatives				
glycerin (Fleet Glycerin Suppositories)	GLIS-er-in	Suppository	1 suppository (2–3 g) for 15 mins once a day	OTC
lactulose (Enulose)	LAK-tu-los	Oral liquid	10–20 g (15–30 mL) every other day. May increase up to 2 times a day	Rx
magnesium hydroxide (Phillips Milk of Magnesia)	mag-NEE-zhum hye-DROX-ide	Oral liquid, tablet	Tablet: 8 tablets once a day Liquid: 2,400–4,800 mg once per day	OTC
magnesium sulfate (Epsom salts)	mag-NEE-zhum SUL-fate	Granules	5–10 g dissolved in 240 mL of water once a day	OTC
polyethylene glycol 3350 (MiraLax)	pol-ee-ETH-il-een GLYE-kawl 3350	Powder for oral solution	8.5–34 g in 240 mL of (8 oz) liquid	OTC
Stimulant Laxatives				
bisacodyl (Dulcolax)	bis-a-KOE-dil	Suppository, tablet	PO: 10–30 mg once a day Rectal: 10 mg suppository once a day	OTC

senna (ExLax, Fletcher's Castoria, various brands)	SEN-na	Chewable tablet, oral solution, syrup, tablet	2–4 tablets (8.6 mg per tablet) or 1–2 tablets (15 mg per tablet) as a single daily dose or divided twice daily	OTC
Antiflatulents				
aluminum hydroxide–magnesium hydroxide–simethicone (Mylanta, Mylanta Maximum Strength)	a-LOO-mi-num hye-DROX-ide mag-NEE-zhum hye-DROX-ide si-METH-i-kone	Oral liquid, tablet	Tablet: 1–4 tablets up to 4 times daily Liquid: 10–20 mL between meals and at bedtime	OTC
calcium carbonate–simethicone (Maalox)	kal-SEE-um KAR-bun-ate si-METH-i-kone	Tablet	40–125 mg, 4 times daily	OTC
simethicone (Gas Aid, Mylicon Drops)	si-METH-i-kone	Oral liquid, tablet	40–360 mg 4 times daily	OTC
Bowel Evacuants				
polyethylene glycol 3350 with electrolytes (Colyte, GaviLyte-C, GaviLyte-G, GaviLyte-N, GoLYTELY, MoviPrep, NuLYTELY, TriLyte)	pol-ee-ETH-il-een GLYE-kawl 3350 and ee-LEK-tro-lytes	Powder	Varies based on formulation	Rx
sodium phosphate (Fleet Phospho-Soda, Visicol)	SOE-dee-um FOS-fate	Enema, oral liquid, tablet	Varies based on formulation	Rx
Miscellaneous Agents				
lubiprostone (Amitiza)	loo-bi-PROS-tone	Capsule	24 mcg twice daily	Rx
methylnaltrexone (Relistor)	meth-il-nal-TREKS-own	Injection	12 mcg once daily	Rx

Psyllium

Psyllium (Fiberall, Metamucil, Perdiem Fiber Therapy) increases nonabsorbable bulk to promote soft stools and easy defecation in patients who should avoid straining (e.g., postoperative, postmyocardial infarction, older adults, and pregnant patients). Patients should drink six to eight glasses of water a day. Psyllium is classified as an antidiarrheal as well as a laxative. It absorbs water in the intestine, producing a viscous liquid that promotes peristalsis and reduces transit time. Patients must be active for it to work; as mentioned earlier, psyllium can cause constipation in a bedridden patient. It is also an effective cholesterol-lowering agent.

Wheat Dextrin

Wheat dextrin (Benefiber) is a clear fiber supplement. It can be added to beverages or soft foods prior to administration. However, adding it to carbonated beverages is not recommended. Additional fluid intake is encouraged with use.

Surfactant Laxatives

A **surfactant laxative** is a substance that acts as a detergent, helping fatty and watery components of the intestinal contents to mix, thus making the stool soft and mushy. These laxatives are not as effective for treatment of acute constipation as they are for helping reduce or prevent constipation when it is likely to occur. Surfactant laxatives are typically taken daily.

Docusate

Docusate (Colace, Ex-Lax Stool Softener, Surfak) is a surfactant laxative. Docusate is commonly used and is available over the counter. It can be taken as a capsule, enema, oral liquid, or tablet. Docusate may cause throat irritation (oral formulations), abdominal pain, diarrhea, and intestinal obstruction. Drinking plenty of fluids each day can reduce these effects. Docusate is also available as a combination product, **docusate-senna (Senokot-S)**.

Contraindications Docusate is contraindicated for patients with intestinal obstruction, acute abdominal pain, nausea, or vomiting. This drug should not be used concomitantly with mineral oil.

Cautions and Considerations The oral liquid dosage form has a bitter taste. Taking these products with eight ounces of milk or juice can mask the bad taste. Drinking plenty of fluids while taking surfactants enhances their effects. As with many laxatives, excessive or long-term use may lead to electrolyte imbalance.

Drug Interactions There are no known drug interactions associated with docusate.

Osmotic Laxatives

Osmotic laxatives (for example, **glycerin [Fleet Glycerin Suppositories]**) are organic substances that draw water into the colon and thereby stimulate evacuation of the lower bowel. This mechanism of action allows the retention of nutrients. Glycerin suppositories are a fairly quick, effective method to relieve constipation.

Lactulose

Lactulose (Enulose) is metabolized by bacteria in the colon; this metabolic process reduces fecal pH, reduces absorption of ammonia and toxic nitrogenous substances, and has a cathartic effect (empties the bowel). Lactulose delivers osmotically active molecules to the colon. It is used to prevent and treat hepatic-induced encephalopathy. Normally, the liver removes nitrogen waste by-products that the blood has picked up from the intestines. When the liver is not functioning properly, as in alcoholism, these nitrogen by-products build up in the blood, destroying brain cells, which results in encephalopathy. Lactulose is thought to offset this process by reducing ammonia production and increasing absorption from the GI tract. The side effects include nausea and vomiting, cramps, diarrhea, and anorexia.

Contraindications Lactulose is not for use in patients requiring a low-galactose diet.

Cautions and Considerations Electrolyte abnormalities can occur with lactulose use. Patients with diabetes should use lactulose with caution, as the product contains lactose and galactose.

Drug Interactions There are no known drug interactions associated with the use of lactulose.

Polyethylene Glycol 3350

Polyethylene glycol 3350 (MiraLax) is an OTC stool softener. This product contains the same active ingredient as GoLYTELY, discussed later in the section on bowel evacuants, but in a much smaller quantity (17 g). It is taken daily to maintain soft stools and to prevent constipation. MiraLax is frequently used in children.

Contraindications There are no contraindications to polyethylene glycol 3350.

Cautions and Considerations Avoid use in patients with bowel obstruction. Use with caution in patients with kidney dysfunction.

Drug Interactions Propylene glycol 3350 may decrease digoxin levels.

Saline Laxatives

A **saline laxative** is an inorganic salt that, like an osmotic laxative, draws water into the intestinal lumen (the hollow portion of the bowel through which fecal material passes) and increases intraluminal pressure.

    Magnesium hydroxide (Phillips Milk of Magnesia) is a laxative as well as an antacid. Magnesium is supplied as citrate, hydroxide, and sulfate (**Epsom salts**) forms. It promotes evacuation of the bowel by causing osmotic retention of fluid, which distends the colon and increases peristaltic activity. It also reacts with hydrochloric acid in the stomach, producing the antacid effects. Caution should be used in patients with renal disorders.

Stimulant Laxatives

Acute constipation can be treated with **stimulant laxatives**. These medications work by stimulating parasympathetic neurons that control bowel muscles, thereby enhancing peristalsis and GI motility. To prevent electrolyte imbalances, stimulant laxatives are taken only when needed on a short-term basis. These drugs are commonly used to treat opiate-induced constipation. Common side effects of stimulant laxatives include mild abdominal pain, nausea, vomiting, and rectal burning. Patients should take these agents at bedtime to prevent these side effects. Serious electrolyte abnormalities are very rare but can occur with chronic use. For this reason, long-term use is not recommended.

Bisacodyl

Bisacodyl (Dulcolax) and **senna (ExLax, Fletcher's Castoria)** are stimulant laxatives. These products are commonly prescribed concurrently for patients who have been taking long-term narcotic pain medications, which can cause constipation. Pharmacy technicians should question any orders for long-term narcotic pain medications that are not accompanied by orders for stimulant laxatives, and bring these observations to the attention of a pharmacist.

Contraindications Bisacodyl is contraindicated in patients with abdominal pain or obstruction, nausea, or vomiting. Senna should not be taken by patients with intestinal obstruction, acute intestinal inflammation, colitis, ulcerative colitis, appendicitis, and abdominal pain of unknown origin.

Cautions and Considerations Patients should take bisacodyl with a full glass of water on an empty stomach to achieve the best effect. Dairy products and antacids can decrease the effects of bisacodyl, so patients should not ingest these substances simultaneously.

Drug Interactions Antacids may diminish the therapeutic effect of delayed-release bisacodyl tablets by causing the tablets to release the drug before it reaches the large intestine. Gastric irritation and/or cramps may occur.

Miscellaneous Constipation Agents

The agents used for constipation thus far in the chapter are fiber and laxatives. There are, however, other mechanisms of action to treat constipation. One such mechanism involves chloride channels in the gastrointestinal system.

Lubiprostone

Lubiprostone (Amitiza) is a drug approved for the treatment of chronic idiopathic constipation. It is a prostaglandin derivative that activates chloride channels locally in the small intestine, which increases intestinal fluid secretion. Nausea is the primary side effect. Patients may want to take this drug with food to minimize this side effect.

Contraindications Known or suspected bowel obstruction contraindicates use.

Cautions and Considerations **Dyspnea** (shortness of breath), and chest tightness, has occurred with lubiprostone use. Patients with moderate-to-severe liver dysfunction should use it with caution.

Drug Interactions Methadone may decrease the therapeutic effect of lubiprostone.

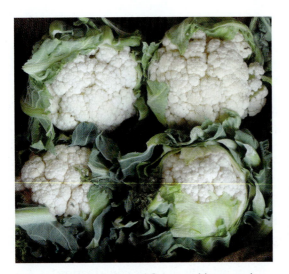

Brassica plants include cauliflower, cabbage, and broccoli, all foods that can cause flatulence.

Antiflatulent Agents

Flatulence (stomach or intestinal gas) is a condition that affects many patients. Complaints of excess gas often represent a hyperawareness of or sensitivity to gas.

Intestinal gas is typically caused by the fermentation of undigested food in the colon. Gas can also form when food isn't completely broken down. Other causes of gas include intestinal bacteria changes when taking antibiotics or other medications, poor carbohydrate absorption, swallowed air, and constipation. Food sources of intestinal gas include beans, legumes, cabbage, onions, broccoli, cauliflower, beer, and carbonated drinks.

Simethicone

Simethicone (Gas Aid, Mylicon Drops) is an inert silicone polymer for gastric defoaming. By reducing surface tension, the drug causes gas bubbles to break or to coalesce into a foam that can be eliminated more easily by belching or passing flatus. Simethicone relieves flatulence, functional gastric bloating, and postoperative gas pains. Dosage recommendations should not be exceeded, especially in children.

Contraindications Simethicone does not have contraindications.

Cautions and Considerations Some dosage forms contain benzyl alcohol. These dosage forms should not be used by pediatric patients.

Drug Interactions Simethicone has no known drug interactions.

Bowel Evacuants

In contrast to laxatives, which are used to restore normal bowel function, a **bowel evacuant** is used to cleanse the bowel prior to GI examination (colonoscopy or X-ray with barium enema), or, in rare cases, following ingestion of toxic substances.

Polyethylene Glycol 3350 with Electrolytes

Polyethylene glycol 3350 with electrolytes (Colyte, GaviLyte-C, GaviLyte-G, GaviLyte-N, GoLYTELY, HalfLYTELY, MoviPrep, NuLYTELY, TriLyte) increases the osmolarity of bowel contents, thus drawing large amounts of water into the lumen to flush out the bowel contents. The recommended dose is dissolved in 4 L of fluid. The patient should fast three to four hours prior to administration and for two hours following administration; 240 mL (8 oz) should be consumed every 10 minutes until the solution is gone. The physician or manufacturer usually supplies a printed informational sheet for the patient with explicit instructions. HalfLYTELY is sometimes used instead of GoLYTELY. It consists of 2 L (half the amount of GoLYTELY) of solution that is to be combined with bisacodyl (a stimulant laxative) delayed-release tablets.

Contraindications Ileus, GI obstruction, gastric retention, bowel perforation, toxic colitis, and toxic megacolon all contraindicate the use of polyethylene glycol 3350 with electrolytes.

Cautions and Considerations Serious cardiac arrhythmias have occurred in patients using polyethylene glycol 3350 with electrolytes. Use with caution in patients with renal dysfunction.

Drug Interactions Polyethylene glycol 3350 with electrolytes has no known significant drug interactions.

Sodium Phosphate

Sodium phosphate (Fleet Phospho-Soda, Visicol) is indicated for evacuation of the colon and for treating and preventing hypophosphatemia. Like saline laxatives, sodium phosphate draws water into the colon. Visicol is a sodium phosphate tablet indicated for bowel preparation prior to colonoscopy. The tablets are tasteless and can be taken with any clear liquid such as water, lemonade, or ginger ale. This drug has been proven to cause significantly less nausea, vomiting, and bloating than other bowel preparation products. It may be much better tolerated by patients than other bowel evacuants.

Contraindications The enema product is contraindicated in patients with kidney impairment, ascites, heart failure, known or suspected GI obstruction, or megacolon. Sodium phosphate tablets should not be used in patients with phosphate nephropathy, bowel obstruction or perforation, gastric bypass surgery, toxic colitis, or megacolon.

Cautions and Considerations Sodium phosphate has a black box warning for the development of acute phosphate nephropathy.

Drug Interactions Drugs with kidney toxicity (such as angiotensin-converting enzyme [ACE] inhibitors or NSAIDs) increase the nephrotoxic effects of sodium phosphate.

Other Gastrointestinal Diseases That May Accompany Constipation

Low amounts of fiber in the diet not only produce a state of constipation; they can also increase the likelihood that a patient will encounter a number of other GI diseases. Several of these diseases are discussed here.

Diverticular Disease

Diverticular disease occurs when an outpocketing (diverticulum) from the bowel wall forms (diverticulosis) and/or becomes inflamed (diverticulitis; see Figure 10.9). It is believed to result from a deficiency of fiber over time. Vegetarians, whose average daily intake of fiber (40 g) is about twice that of nonvegetarians, have approximately one-third the incidence of diverticular disease. Diverticular disease seems to be related to the predominance of more highly refined carbohydrates and other processed foods in the modern diet. **Colonic segmentation** (in which the colon acts as if it is divided into small parts that move independently of each other rather than contributing to an integrated overall motion) is accompanied by an increase in pressure inside the colon, prolonged GI transit time, and low fecal weight. All of these factors contribute to **herniation** (protrusion through a weakened muscular wall) of the colon lining, with accompanying inflammation and pain. Fiber may reduce the pressure generated in the colon.

Hiatal Hernia

Hiatal hernia is related to chronic constipation. Straining to pass small, firm stools can significantly raise intra-abdominal pressures. Over a period of several years, daily straining to pass stools can force the gastroesophageal junction upward into the thoracic cavity through the **esophageal hiatus** (the opening in the diaphragm through which normally only the esophagus passes).

FIGURE 10.9
Portion of the Colon with Diverticula

In diverticular disease, herniations form along the mucous membranes, and the muscular layers of the colon wall may become inflamed, causing pain.

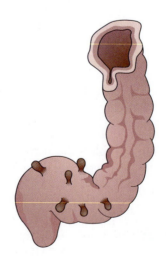

Irritable Bowel Syndrome

Irritable bowel syndrome (IBS) is the most common of the GI disorders. Many patients with GI complaints are diagnosed with IBS. IBS is a functional disorder in which the lower GI tract does not have the appropriate tone or spasticity to regulate bowel activity. Some evidence also suggests that patients with presenting symptoms of IBS have an abnormal sensitivity to a neurotransmitter within the GI tract. This disorder affects twice as many women as men. Patients with IBS have an increased rate of hospital stays, abdominal surgery, and absenteeism from work. Criteria for diagnosis include the following:

- abdominal distension
- gas
- increased colonic mucus
- irregular bowel habits (diarrhea or constipation more than 25% of the time)
- pain

Hemorrhoids

Hemorrhoids result from pressure exerted on anal veins while straining to pass a stool, which causes engorgement of the vascular cushions within the sphincter muscles. Passing a small, hard stool through the anal canal can abrade the overlying mucosa, causing hemorrhoidal bleeding. Prolapse (displacement) of the vascular cushions may occur from rupture of their attachments to the surrounding sphincter.

Hydrocortisone

Hemorrhoids are treated with suppositories, ointments, and, sometimes, surgery. Most medications for hemorrhoids include **hydrocortisone (Anusol HC, Cortifoam)**, a synthetic preparation used to treat inflammation (see Table 10.10). Modifying the diet by increasing fiber can help prevent hemorrhoids.

Contraindications The rectal enema formulation of hydrocortisone is contraindicated in patients with systemic fungal infections and ileocolostomy during the immediate or early postoperative period. Cortifoam is also contraindicated in patients with obstruction, abscess, perforation, peritonitis, fresh intestinal anastomoses, and extensive fistulas and sinus tracts.

TABLE 10.10 Most Commonly Used Hemorrhoidal Agents

Generic (Brand)	Pronunciation	Dosage Form	Dispensing Status
hydrocortisone (Anusol HC, Cortifoam)	hye-droe-KOR-ti-sone	Enema, foam, rectal cream, suppository	Rx
nitroglycerin (Rectiv)	nye-troe-GLI-ser-in	Rectal ointment	Rx

Cautions and Considerations The rectal enema formulation may damage the rectal wall if the applicator is inserted improperly.

Drug Interactions Although hemorrhoidal agents are inserted through the rectal route (considered a systemic route of administration), these drugs are formulated for local activity. However, some systemic absorption may occur through the mucosal lining of the rectum. Hydrocortisone may diminish the therapeutic effects of aldesleukin.

Nitroglycerin

A tear or fissure in the anal canal can also cause pain and bleeding. **Nitroglycerin (Rectiv)**, a vasodilator that causes smooth muscle relaxation, reduces resting pressure on the anal canal and permits healing. A 2%–4% ointment is inserted into the anal canal with the finger. Before instilling nitroglycerin, the patient should place the tube of medication in a container of warm water to soften the tube's contents and allow for an accurate amount of medication to be dispersed. The patient should also don gloves before instillation and wash the hands after the procedure. The primary side effect is headache, and the patient should make sure to take 12-hour breaks from the drug to minimize this effect.

Contraindications Use of phosphodiesterase-5 (PDE-5) inhibitors (such as sildenafil) are contraindicated, as these drugs have been shown to potentiate the hypotensive effects of nitroglycerin. Other contraindications include severe anemia, increased intracranial pressure, and known hypersensitivity to nitrates or nitrites.

Cautions and Considerations Severe hypotension can result from the use of nitroglycerin rectal ointment. Patients with hypotension or those known to be at risk for it should use with caution.

Drug Interactions Antihypertensives and PDE-5 inhibitors may increase the hypotensive effects of nitroglycerin. Aspirin may increase nitroglycerin levels. Heparin's anticoagulant effect may be decreased by the use of nitroglycerin.

Nausea and Vomiting

The vomiting center in the brain is located in the medulla. It receives input from the **chemoreceptor trigger zone (CTZ)** via the vagus nerve or the tenth cranial nerve. The CTZ, which is located below the floor of the fourth ventricle of the brain, receives its input from the cerebral cortex and hypothalamus and also from blood-borne stimuli (such as bacterial toxins and drugs that have access to the brain via the vascular system). The main neurotransmitters that cause nausea and vomiting are acetylcholine, dopamine, histamine, and serotonin.

Vomiting (also referred to as **emesis**) can be initiated in two ways: by stimulating the CTZ, which in turn stimulates the GI tract via the vomiting center (e.g., narcotics stimulate brain receptors); or by stimulating the vagal receptors in the stomach with no CTZ involvement (see Figure 10.10).

Vomiting can cause dehydration, electrolyte imbalance leading to alkalosis (loss of acid from the body), and possible aspiration pneumonia. It may also cause bradycardia or other arrhythmias resulting from an electrolyte imbalance.

Emesis often results from narcotic intake and is dose related. Morphine and its derivatives stimulate the CTZ. Narcotics also increase the vomiting center's sensitivity to stimuli from the vestibular nuclei of the ear, which is near the vomiting center.

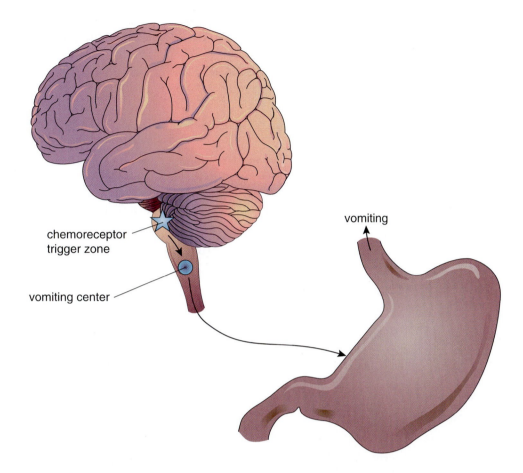

FIGURE 10.10
Chemoreceptor Trigger Zone and Vomiting Center

The vomiting center in the brain receives input from the chemoreceptor trigger zone (CTZ).

chemoreceptor trigger zone

vomiting center

vomiting

Stimulating the labyrinth system of the inner ear produces impulses that are transmitted via cholinergic and adrenergic tracts to the vestibular nuclei. This is the pathway that commonly underlies car sickness. **Vertigo**, the sensation of the room spinning when one gets up or changes positions, is treated with anticholinergic agents.

An **antiemetic** is a drug that works primarily in the vomiting center to inhibit impulses that travel to the stomach, thus preventing vomiting. Table 10.11 presents the most commonly used antiemetics.

Antihistamines and Anticholinergics

Antihistamines and **anticholinergics** are antiemetics that share a similar chemical structure. They are used to treat mild motion sickness. They work by blocking histamine and acetylcholine, two neurotransmitters in the CTZ and vomiting center (see Table 10.11 for more information). Side effects of antihistamine and anticholinergic antiemetics are drowsiness, dry mouth, and urinary retention. Patients who take other medications that also cause drowsiness should be careful because sedation could be excessive. Patients should avoid drinking alcohol and take care when driving until they know how the medication affects them. Patients who have an enlarged prostate should not use anticholinergic antiemetics because they can make urination even more difficult.

In some children, anticholinergic antiemetics have a paradoxical effect, where excitation occurs rather than drowsiness. Parents should be aware of the potential for this side effect.

TABLE 10.11 Most Commonly Used Antiemetic Medications

Generic (Brand)	Pronunciation	Dosage Form	Dispensing Status
Antihistamines and Anticholinergics			
diphenhydramine (Benadryl)	dye-fen-HYE-dra-meen	Capsule, injection, oral liquid, tablet	OTC, Rx
dimenhydrinate (Dramamine)	dye-men-HYE-druh-nate	Chewable, injection, oral liquid, tablet	OTC, Rx
hydroxyzine (Atarax, Vistaril)	hye-DROX-i-zeen	Capsule, injection, oral liquid, tablet	Rx
meclizine (Antivert)	MEK-li-zeen	Tablet	Rx
scopolamine (Scopace, Transderm Scop)	scoe-POL-a-meen	Injection, transdermal patch	Rx
Serotonin Receptor Antagonists			
dolasetron (Anzemet)	dol-AS-e-tron	Injection, tablet	Rx
granisetron (Kytril)	gra-NI-se-tron	Injection, oral solution, tablet, transdermal patch	Rx
ondansetron (Zofran)	on-DAN-se-tron	Injection, oral film, oral solution, tablet	Rx
palonosetron (Aloxi)	pa-lone-O-se-tron	Injection	Rx
Phenothiazines			
prochlorperazine (Compazine)	proe-klor-PAIR-a-zeen	Injection, suppository, tablet	Rx
promethazine (Phenergan)	proe-METH-a-zeen	Oral liquid, suppository, tablet	Rx
Benzamides			
aprepitant, fosaprepitant (Emend)	ap-REP-i-tant	Capsule (aprepitant), injection (fosaprepitant)	Rx
Neurokinin-1 Receeotpr Antagonist			
metoclopramide (Reglan)	met-oh-KLOE-pra-mide	Injection, oral solution, tablet	Rx

NDC 63323-373-02
4 mg / 2 mL (2mg/2 mL)

Ondansetron®

2 mL single-dose vial

IM or IV

There are times when patients experiencing nausea and vomiting are unable to tolerate oral antiemetics. In these cases, intramuscular or IV administration is used. This label shows the injectable form of the 5-HT3 receptor antagonist, ondansetron.

Contraindications Anticholinergic and antihistamine antiemetics should not be given to infants or mothers who are breastfeeding. In addition, patients with glaucoma or those individuals using monoamine oxidase inhibitors (MAOIs) should not take these agents. Hydroxyzine should not be used in early pregnancy, and it should not be injected via subcutaneous, intra-arterial, or IV routes. Contraindications to scopolamine include a hypersensitivity to belladonna alkaloids and narrow-angle glaucoma. The injectable form of scopolamine should not be used repeatedly in patients with chronic lung disease. Meclizine does not have contraindications.

Cautions and Considerations Patients who have high blood pressure or heart problems should talk with their prescribers before taking anticholinergic or antihistamine antiemetics.

Drug Interactions Drugs with anticholinergic properties will intensify the anticholinergic properties of these drugs.

Serotonin Receptor Antagonists

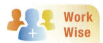

Work Wise

A few of the 5-HT3 receptor antagonist medications are expensive. For a patient's insurance plan to cover these drugs, the prescriber may need to complete a prior authorization request. As a pharmacy technician, you may be asked to prepare the documentation needed for such a request.

Serotonin (5-HT) receptor antagonists are potent antiemetics used to prevent and treat severe nausea and vomiting associated with chemotherapeutic medications, radiation treatment, or anesthesia. 5-HT receptor antagonists work by blocking serotonin type 3 (5-HT3) receptors in the brain and GI tract. Blocking these receptors stops nausea signals traveling from the brain to the stomach. These powerful antiemetics are prescription-only products (see Table 10.11) that pharmacy technicians in the inpatient and oncology specialty clinics will encounter.

Dolasetron

Dolasetron (Anzemet) was designed to be used for the prevention of chemotherapy-induced nausea. 5-HT is released from the GI cells, which stimulates those receptors that cause vomiting when chemotherapy is administered. Dolasetron is also used for the prevention of surgery-related nausea. The IV form can be given IV push over 30 seconds or diluted in 50 mL of compatible fluid and infused over 15 minutes. Dolasetron can also be diluted in apple or apple-grape juice and taken orally. If given for the prevention of chemotherapy-induced nausea, it should be administered one hour before administration of the chemotherapy agent; if given for postsurgery nausea, it should be given 15 minutes before stopping anesthesia. Dolasetron can also be given to treat postsurgery nausea on an as-needed basis.

Contraindications Dolasetron is contraindicated via the IV route when used for the prevention of chemotherapy-associated nausea and vomiting.

Cautions and Considerations Because 5-HT3 receptor antagonists may cause dizziness and drowsiness, patients should be reminded that activities such as driving may not be safe while taking these medications.

Drug Interactions 5-HT receptor antagonists may enhance the hypotensive effects of apomorphine. 5-HT receptor antagonists may also enhance the QT-prolonging effects of other QT-prolonging agents.

Granisetron

Granisetron (Kytril) binds to 5-HT receptors with little or no affinity for dopamine D_2, benzodiazepine, or opiate receptors. It blocks the 5-HT receptors both peripherally on vagal nerve terminals and centrally in the CTZ. Side effects of granisetron include headache, asthenia (weakness), drowsiness, and diarrhea. It is usually given by the IV route. Granisetron must be protected from light.

Contraindications Granisetron does not have contraindications.

Cautions and Considerations Because 5-HT receptor antagonists may cause dizziness and drowsiness, patients should be reminded that activities such as driving may not be safe while taking these medications.

Drug Interactions 5-HT receptor antagonists may enhance the hypotensive effects of apomorphine. 5-HT receptor antagonists may enhance the QT-prolonging effects of other QT-prolonging agents.

Ondansetron

Ondansetron (Zofran) blocks 5-HT receptors in either the CTZ or vagal nerve terminals in the small bowel. It is used for chemotherapy-induced emesis. Headache is a major side effect. Ondansetron can also cause either constipation or diarrhea.

Contraindications Ondansetron does not have contraindications.

Cautions and Considerations Because 5-HT receptor antagonists may cause dizziness and drowsiness, patients should be reminded that activities such as driving may not be safe while taking these medications.

Drug Interactions 5-HT receptor antagonists may enhance the hypotensive effects of apomorphine. 5-HT receptor antagonists may enhance the QT-prolonging effects of other QT-prolonging agents.

Palonosetron

Palonosetron (Aloxi) is an injectable 5-HT receptor antagonist that is indicated for chemotherapy-related and postoperative nausea and vomiting. It is injected prior to chemotherapy or surgical procedures.

Contraindications Palonosetron does not have contraindications.

Cautions and Considerations Because 5-HT receptor antagonists may cause dizziness and drowsiness, patients should be reminded that activities such as driving may not be safe while taking these medications.

Drug Interactions 5-HT receptor antagonists may enhance the hypotensive effects of apomorphine. 5-HT receptor antagonists may enhance the QT-prolonging effects of other QT-prolonging agents.

Dopamine Receptor Antagonists

Dopamine receptor antagonists include phenothiazines and benzamides. Phenothiazine compounds, related to the typical antipsychotics described in Chapter 7, inhibit the CTZ. **Phenothiazines** are potent antiemetic drugs that work by blocking dopamine. They are first-generation antipsychotics when used in higher doses. Pharmacy technicians working in an inpatient setting will likely dispense phenothiazines daily because they are frequently ordered in that setting. **Benzamides** cause dopamine antagonism and, at higher doses, 5-HT3 antagonism.

These medications are available in many different dosage forms (see Table 10.11), an important feature because patients with nausea and vomiting may not be able to swallow a pill or oral solution. Patients can receive an intramuscular (IM) or IV injection, or a rectal suppository to relieve symptoms.

They act as a sedative, antiemetic, and anticholinergic (causing dry mouth, blurred vision, and urinary retention). Movement disorders such as tardive dyskinesia and dystonia (called extrapyramidal side effects or EPS effects) are possible with dopamine receptor antagonists, particularly at high doses. EPS effects include uncontrollable movements of the eyes, face, and limbs that may become permanent. Patients, especially older adults, have to be closely monitored for the appearance of EPS effects. If EPS effects appear, patients should stop taking the antiemetic. To prevent hypotension, these drugs should not be given by an IV push.

Prochlorperazine

Prochlorperazine (Compazine) is a phenothiazine that can be administered by oral, rectal, IM, or IV routes. It must be used with caution in children and is easily overdosed, precipitating seizures.

Contraindications Prochlorperazine should not be used in patients with severe CNS depression or coma. In addition, prochlorperazine is contraindicated in pediatric surgery and in children younger than two years or weighing less than 9 kg.

Cautions and Considerations Patients with liver problems cannot eliminate these agents from the bloodstream properly, increasing the risk for EPS effects. Patients should inform their prescribers if they have liver problems so that this risk can be assessed and other therapy chosen if necessary.

Drug Interactions Prochlorperazine can cause QT-interval prolongation and can enhance the effects of other QT-interval prolonging agents.

Promethazine

Promethazine (Phenergan), a phenothiazine, is probably the most widely used anti-emetic. It is usually given as an IV push, but if the dose is greater than 100 mg, it should be diluted *in the pharmacy* to a maximum concentration of 25 mg/mL and infused over 15 to 30 minutes. Side effects are much more unpleasant than the 5-HT receptor antagonists. Suppositories are stored in the refrigerator.

Contraindications Promethazine is contraindicated for patients who are in a coma or experiencing lower respiratory tract symptoms. Promethazine is also contraindicated in children younger than two years, and for intra-arterial or subcutaneous administration.

Cautions and Considerations Promethazine has a black box warning regarding the use of the drug in children younger than two years.

Drug Interactions CNS depressants may enhance the CNS side effects of promethazine. Anticholinergic agents may enhance the anticholinergic side effects of promethazine. Promethazine may enhance the toxic effects of glucagon. The ulcerogenic effects of potassium chloride may be enhanced by promethazine.

Metoclopramide

Metoclopramide (Reglan), a benzamide, is used in **gastric stasis** (lack of stomach motility), GI reflux, and chemotherapy-induced emesis. It inhibits or reduces nausea and vomiting by blocking dopamine receptors in the CTZ. Metoclopramide relieves esophageal reflux by improving the tone of the lower esophageal sphincter and reduces gastric stasis by stimulating motility of the upper GI tract, thus reducing gastric emptying time.

The side effects are drowsiness, depression, and EPS effects (which are parkinsonian, especially in children). Diphenhydramine is used to reduce the EPS effects. Metoclopramide should not be used longer than 12 weeks.

Contraindications Metoclopramide is contraindicated in patients with GI obstruction, perforation, or hemorrhage; pheochromocytoma; and a history of seizures. It should not be used with other agents that are likely to increase EPS effects.

Cautions and Considerations Metoclopramide has a black box warning for causing tardive dyskinesia. Metoclopramide should be discontinued in patients with any signs or symptoms of dyskinesia.

Drug Interactions Metoclopramide may increase the adverse effects of antipsychotics, droperidol, and tetrabenazine.

Neurokinin-1 Receptor Antagonists

As the name suggests, neurokinin-1 (NK-1) receptor antagonists work on the NK-1 receptor. The NK-1 receptor is the preferred receptor for substance P, a neuropeptide involved in the induction of nausea and vomiting. The NK-1 receptor antagonists prevent both acute and delayed vomiting.

Aprepitant

Aprepitant (Emend) is an oral medication used to treat postoperative and chemotherapy-related nausea. The injectable form of Emend is **fosaprepitant**, which has the same indication. Aprepitant should be administered within three hours prior to surgery or chemotherapy. Fosaprepitant is usually given 30 minutes prior to surgery or chemotherapy. Common side effects of aprepitant and fosaprepitant include fatigue, muscle weakness, and constipation. Hypotension, slow heart rate, diarrhea, GI pain, kidney and liver dysfunction, and blood abnormalities are rare but significant side effects. If a patient experiences severe side effects while taking aprepitant, he or she should call for medical help immediately.

Contraindications Aprepitant is contraindicated in patients using cisapride or pimozide.

Cautions and Considerations Use with caution in patients with renal impairment.

Drug Interactions Aprepitant may increase the concentration of bosutinib, ibrutinib, ivabradine, lomitapide, naloxegol, olaparib, pimozide, simeprevir, tolvaptan, trabectedin, and ulipristal. Conivaptan, fusidic acid, and idelalisib may increase the serum concentration of aprepitant.

Hepatitis

Hepatitis is a liver disease that has several forms, distinguished by the letters A through G. The three most common (A, B, and C) will be discussed. Each can damage liver cells and cause the liver to become swollen and tender. Some can cause permanent damage. Hepatitis has many causes. Some forms are viral, but others are caused by medications, long-term alcohol use, or exposure to certain industrial chemicals.

Types of Hepatitis

Hepatitis A is a viral infection that can be spread from one person to another. It is present worldwide and can be transmitted through blood and body fluids. Incidence has decreased dramatically in the United States since vaccination was targeted in high-risk populations, children in states with high incidence, and infants. Hepatitis A often produces epidemics due to its feces-to-mouth route of transmission. The highest rates occur in children. Treatment is supportive (no drugs, just food and rest).

Hepatitis A can be prevented by the hepatitis A vaccine, also known as HAV. If individuals know they have been exposed, they should be protected with immune globulin (IG) within two weeks of exposure. IG can be given by either an IM or IV injection. If it is ordered as an IV injection, it will be written **IVIG**. IG provides passive immunity by increasing the antibody titer and antigen-antibody reaction potential.

Hepatitis B is a virus transmitted parenterally, through bodily fluids, from sexual contact, and perinatally. There are two types of hepatitis B: acute and chronic. *Acute hepatitis B* usually clears up on its own without treatment. The patient develops antibodies that provide lifelong protection. *Chronic hepatitis B*, which is the most dangerous form of hepatitis, continues to be present for six months or more. It can be the cause of serious liver disease, such as cirrhosis or liver cancer. The patient may require a liver transplant. Chronic hepatitis B is treated with antiviral medications, depending on antigens in the blood. The vaccines for hepatitis B, **Energix-B** and **Recombivax HB** are given in a three-dose series over six months. Most healthcare workers, including pharmacy technicians, should receive these vaccines. These vaccines are stored in the refrigerator.

Hepatitis C is an infection that cannot be spread from one person to another by casual contact. It is most commonly transmitted through blood transfusions or illicit drug use. The acute form should be treated to prevent the disease from becoming chronic. It can progress to liver fibrosis and end-stage liver disease. The virus genotype is determined in patients who have hepatitis C. There are several genotypes, with Type 1 being the most common. Treatments for Type 1 are included in the following sections.

Pharmacologic Treatment and Prevention of Hepatitis

Prevention of hepatitis is achieved through vaccination. Anyone who works in a hospital must be vaccinated against hepatitis B. The Centers for Disease Control and Prevention now recommends that travelers who are going to endemic areas or who are otherwise high-risk patients should be vaccinated against hepatitis B in two to three doses over the six months prior to travel. They should also receive hepatitis A vaccine two to four weeks before travel. It is sometimes recommended that babies and schoolchildren have the hepatitis B vaccine with their other immunizations. Anyone who is immunocompromised should also be vaccinated against hepatitis. Table 10.12 lists the drugs used to treat hepatitis B.

Entecavir

Entecavir (Baraclude) is indicated for the treatment of chronic hepatitis B. It blocks an enzyme responsible for replication of the virus in the body. The major advantage of entecavir is that it can be used in HIV-positive patients. It is taken once a day on an empty stomach; that is, two hours before or after eating.

Contraindications There are no contraindications for the use of entecavir.

Cautions and Considerations There are three black box warnings associated with entecavir. The first is for lactic acidosis, severe liver enlargement, and fatty liver. Use entecavir with caution in patients with risk factors for liver disease. The second black box warning is for severe exacerbation of hepatitis B upon drug discontinuation. Patients should be monitored for several months after stopping treatment. The third boxed warning is for HIV resistance to some antiretrovirals in patients using entecavir with unrecognized or untreated HIV.

Drug Interactions Entecavir's adverse effects may be enhanced by ganciclovir, ribavirin, and valganciclovir.

TABLE 10.12 Most Commonly Used Drugs to Treat Hepatitis B

Generic (Brand)	Pronunciation	Dosage Form	Dispensing Status
entecavir (Baraclude)	en-TEK-a-vir	Oral liquid, tablet	Rx
lamivudine (Epivir, Epivir-HBV)	la-MIV-yoo-deen	Oral liquid, tablet	Rx
ledipasvir-sofosbuvir (Harvoni)	le-DIP-as-vir soe-FOSS-bue-vir	Tablet	Rx
ombitasvir-paritaprevir-ritonavir-dasabuvir (Viekira Pak)	om-BIT-as-vir par-i-TA-pre-vir rit-OH-na-vir da-SA-bue-vir	Tablet	Rx
peginterferon alfa-2a (Pegasys)	peg-in-ter-FEER-on AL-fa 2A	Injection	Rx
ribavirin (Copegus, Moderiba, Rebetol, Ribasphere, Ribasphere RibaPak, Virazole)	rye-ba-VYE-rin	Capsule, oral liquid, tablet	Rx
simeprevir (Olysio)	sim-E-pre-vir	Capsule	Rx
sofosbuvir (Sovaldi)	soe-FOS-bue-vir	Tablet	Rx
tenofovir (Viread)	te-NOE-fo-veer	Oral powder, tablet	Rx

Lamivudine

Lamivudine (Epivir, Epivir-HBV) is a nucleoside reverse transcriptase inhibitor (NRTI) that is used for the treatment of hepatitis B. Lamivudine is also used to treat HIV (see Chapter 5). Lamivudine tends to be less expensive than other hepatitis B treatments. However, because there are more potent viral suppressors (such as entecavir and telbivudine), the use of lamivudine is decreasing. Lamivudine must be taken exactly as prescribed. It has the fewest side effects of any of the NRTIs.

Contraindications There are no manufacturer-reported contraindications to the use of lamivudine.

Cautions and Considerations Lamivudine is indicated to treat HIV and chronic hepatitis B. When used for the treatment of hepatitis B, lamivudine has several black box warnings. The first warning is about product selection. The hepatitis B product should not be used to treat HIV. The second warning is about medication discontinuation. After therapy stops, patients should be monitored closely for hepatitis exacerbations. The third boxed warning addresses HIV resistance. Healthcare practitioners need to be aware that HIV resistance may emerge when patients who have hepatitis B and an undiagnosed HIV infection use lamivudine. Lamivudine may precipitate pancreatitis.

Drug Interactions Emtricitabine and lamivudine should not be used together. Ganciclovir, ribavarin, and valganciclovir may enhance the toxic effects of lamivudine.

Pegylated Interferon

Pegylated Interferon is a class of drugs that includes Pegylated interferon-alpha-2a, Pegylated interferon-alpha-2b, and Pegylated interferon-beta-1a. **Peginterferon alfa-2a (Pegasys)** is interferon linked to a high-molecular-weight branched polyethylene glycol (PEG) molecule. This linkage increases the half-life, allowing once-weekly dosing. It is indicated for patients who have hepatitis C and chronic hepatitis B. Peginterferon alfa-2a requires a medication guide when dispensed from an outpatient pharmacy. The advantage of peginterferon alfa-2a over regular interferon is its long half-life. The most serious adverse events associated with this drug include neuropsychiatric disorders (suicidal ideation).

The prefilled syringes should be stored in the refrigerator. They can safely be left out for 24 hours, but no longer. The drug should be injected subcutaneously into the abdomen or thigh, using a different site each time to prevent tissue damage or irritation.

Contraindications Contraindications to the use of peginterferon alfa-2a include a hypersensitivity to other interferons, autoimmune hepatitis, and decompensated cirrhosis. It should not be used in neonates and infants because the formulation includes benzyl alcohol. When combined with ribavirin, peginterferon alfa-2a is contraindicated in pregnant women and men whose female partners are pregnant.

Cautions and Considerations Peginterferon alfa-2a has a black box warning for causing or aggravating fatal or life-threatening neuropsychiatric, autoimmune, ischemic, and infectious disorders. Therapy should be discontinued immediately in patients with signs or symptoms of these disorders.

Drug Interactions Peginterferon alfa-2a may enhance the adverse effects of clozapine, telbivudine, and zidovudine.

Tenofovir

Tenofovir (Viread) is a nucleotide reverse transcriptase inhibitor (NtRTI) that is used to treat hepatitis B and HIV (see Chapter 5). Tenofovir can be dosed once daily without regard to food. Tenofovir's limiting toxicity is renal dysfunction. Other side effects include dizziness, depression, skin rash, and dyslipidemia.

Contraindications Tenofovir does not have contraindications.

Cautions and Considerations Tenofovir carries two black box warnings. One is for the risk of lactic acidosis and severe hepatomegaly. The other is for the risk of severe and acute exacerbation of hepatitis B upon discontinuation. Kidney toxicity is a concern with tenofovir use. Patients should not take other drugs that could also damage the kidneys while using tenofovir. Use should be discontinued in patients who experience subsequent decline in renal function.

Drug Interactions Adefovir may decrease the effectiveness of tenofovir. Tenofovir may increase levels of adefovir. Concomitant use is not recommended.

Ledipasvir-Sofosbuvir

Ledipasvir, a nonstructural protein 5A (NS5A) inhibitor, is available as a combination product with sofosbuvir **(Harvoni)**. **Sofosbuvir (Sovaldi)**, a nonstructural protein 5A (NS5B) inhibitor, is also available by itself. The sofosbuvir-only product needs to be taken in combination with other drugs. Common adverse reactions to both drugs are fatigue and headache.

Contraindications There are no contraindications to either drug or the combination product.

Cautions and Considerations Significant drug interactions may exist, and screening should occur prior to starting either drug. These drugs should be prescribed by an experienced healthcare practitioner. The ledipasvir-sofosbuvir combination product may contain lactose. Use with caution in patients with lactose intolerance.

Drug Interactions Sofosbuvir blood levels can be decreased by carbamazepine, oxcarbazepine, phenobarbital, phenytoin, and St. John's wort.

Ombitasvir-Paritaprevir-Ritonavir-Dasabuvir

Ombitasvir-paritaprevir-ritonavir-dasabuvir (Viekira Pak) is a combination product used for the treatment of chronic hepatitis C infection. Each fixed-dose tablet contains ombitasvir 12.5 mg, paritaprevir 75 mg, and ritonavir 50 mg; these are co-packaged with dasabuvir 250 mg tablets. Viekira Pak should be administered with a meal. Adverse reactions include headache, fatigue, and nausea.

Contraindications Contraindications include hypersensitivity to any component of the combination product and severe hepatic impairment. Other contraindications are related to drug interactions. Concurrent use of drugs that are highly dependent on cytochrome P-450 3A4 for clearance, concurrent use of strong inducers of cytochrome P-450 3A4 and 2C8, or strong inhibitors of 2C8 are contraindicated. Alfuzosin, carbamazepine, ergot derivatives (dihydroergotamine, ergonovine, ergotamine, and methylergonovine), efavirenz, ethinyl estradiol-containing products, gemfibrozil, lovastatin, midazolam (oral), phenobarbital, phenytoin, pimozide, rifampin, sildenafil (when used for the treatment of pulmonary arterial hypertension), simvastatin, St. John's wort, and triazolam are specific drug contraindications.

Cautions and Considerations Elevation of hepatic enzymes has occurred with use. Women using ethinyl estradiol products (often oral contraceptives) are at an increased risk. Ritonavir, a component of the product, is also used to treat HIV. HIV resistance to ritonavir may occur in patients using Viekira Pak with undiagnosed or untreated HIV. Use with caution in patients with moderate liver impairment.

Drug Interactions There are many drug interactions with this combination product. See the Contraindications section for specific drugs that should never be used with Viekira Pak.

Ribavirin

Ribavirin (Copegus, Moderiba, Rebetol, Ribasphere, Ribasphere RibaPak, Virazole) can be used for the treatment of respiratory syncytial virus (RSV) infections as well as hepatitis C. It is administered by inhalation for RSV, and orally for hepatitis C. For hepatitis C, it should always be taken concurrently with interferon therapy. Ribavirin inhibits the replication of RNA and DNA in the virus. It is known to cause bothersome side effects, including anxiety, emotional lability, irritability, fatigue, fever, headache, injection-site inflammation/reaction, myalgia, nausea, and rigor.

Contraindications Ribavirin is contraindicated in patients who have hemoglobinopathies (such as sickle-cell anemia), women who are or who may become pregnant, men whose female partners are pregnant, patients using didanosine, and patients who have renal impairment.

Cautions and Considerations Ribavirin has several black box warnings. The first warning states that ribavirin monotherapy is not effective for the treatment of chronic hepatitis C. It should be used in combination with other therapies. Another warning is for the risk of hemolytic anemia, which may result in worsening cardiac disease. A third boxed warning focuses on the severe teratogenic and embryocidal effects associated with the use of ribavarin. Ribavirin should not be used in women who are pregnant or in men whose female partners are pregnant. Extreme measures to prevent pregnancy should be taken during therapy (by the patient or male partners of patients) and for six months after therapy.

Drug Interactions Ribavirin may enhance the adverse effects of didanosine. Ribavirin may decrease the effect of live vaccines.

Simeprevir

Simeprevir (Olysio) is a protease inhibitor for the treatment of chronic hepatitis C. It is not meant to be used as monotherapy; simeprevir should be used in combination with other agents. Simeprevir should be taken with food. Common adverse effects include rash and photosensitivity.

Contraindications No contraindications have been reported by the manufacturer.

Cautions and Considerations Simeprevir doses should not be missed. Skipped doses may lead to viral resistance. Simeprevir should not be used in patients with moderate-to-severe hepatic dysfunction.

Drug Interactions Simeprevir may increase concentrations of bosutinib, cisapride, pazopanib, protease inhibitors, topotecan, and vincristine. Conivaptan, cyclosporine, erythromycin, fusidic acid, idelalisib, ledipasvir, and milk thistle may increase the concentrations of simeprevir. St. John's wort may decrease the serum concentrations of simeprevir.

Complementary and Alternative Therapies

Shiatsu acupressure or massage has been used to treat nausea. Shiatsu acupressure involves finger pressure at certain points along body.

Ginger *(Zingiber officinale)* can be used to reduce nausea associated with surgery, vertigo, and motion sickness. It also has demonstrated benefits in pregnant women with morning sickness, but it has not undergone rigorous safety testing in this patient population. The mechanism of action of ginger is still poorly defined, but it may exert its effects by blocking 5-HT in the same way that other antiemetics do. The standard dose for preventing nausea and vomiting is 500 to 1,000 mg. Ginger may cause heartburn, gas, bloating, mouth and throat irritation, and diarrhea. Because ginger has antiplatelet effects, its use should be avoided in patients taking aspirin, warfarin, or other anticoagulants.

Probiotics are products that contain live cultures of yeast or bacteria. They are not herbal products or dietary supplements. Probiotics are used as nonpharmacologic adjunctive treatment for diarrhea, constipation, *H. pylori* infection, and antibiotic-induced diarrhea. They may even be used to treat diarrhea associated with rotavirus, Crohn's disease, ulcerative colitis, and IBS. Probiotic organisms are not pathogenic and are commonly available in capsules, powders, beverages, and yogurts, some of which need to be refrigerated to keep the microorganisms alive. These products are used to colonize the GI tract with beneficial organisms for digestion and regular GI motility. These bacteria compete with harmful bacteria, hopefully replacing or displacing them. They may enhance the immune response to pathogenic organisms and break down toxins. Patients with poor immune system function should not use probiotic products. Doses vary based on the product and indication.

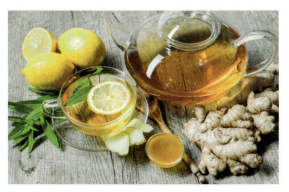

Ginger may be used for nausea.

Lactobacilli are Gram-positive bacteria that are normal flora of the human GI tract. Common lactobacilli products contain *Lactobacillus acidophilus*, *Lactobacillus helveticus*, *Lactobacillus bulgaricus*, and *Lactobacillus rhamnosus*. Lactobacilli products are taken each day, divided into three or four doses. They are usually well tolerated with few side effects, the most common of which are gas and bloating.

Saccharomyces boulardii (S. boulardii) is a yeast organism that lives in the human GI tract. Florastor is the brand name of a product that is used to prevent antibiotic-associated diarrhea. Typically, 250–500 mg of Florastor is taken two to four times a day. *S. boulardii* can cause gas, bloating, and constipation.

Bifidobacteria agents are not as well studied as lactobacilli and *S. boulardii* products. However, they might be effective for diarrhea associated with a variety of causes. Doses vary with products and indications. As with other probiotics, bifidobacteria are well tolerated in general but have the potential to cause gas and bloating.

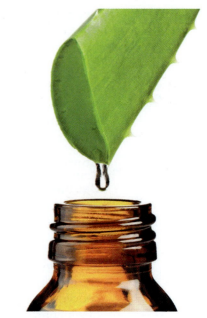

Aloe ingested orally is used to treat constipation.

Aloe ingested orally may be used to treat patients with constipation. It appears to work as a stimulant laxative. Dosing may range from 40–170 mg of dried juice. Caution is advised when taking aloe supplements, as adverse effects including diarrhea and drug interactions are possible. Aloe supplements should not be used by pregnant or breastfeeding women, unless directed by a healthcare practitioner.

CHAPTER SUMMARY

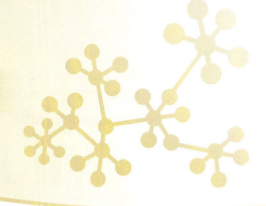

Gastrointestinal System

- The GI tract is a tube that begins in the mouth; extends through the pharynx, esophagus, stomach, small intestine, and large intestine; and ends at the anus.

- The digestive and absorptive processes take place in the GI tract.

- Mucous membranes protect the entire digestive system against abrasion and strong digestive chemicals.

Gastrointestinal Diseases

- GERD is commonly known as *heartburn*. Alcohol, nicotine, and caffeine exacerbate GERD.

- Antacids can be used to treat GERD; they neutralize the acidic stomach contents so that, if reflux does occur, the contents will be less irritating to the esophageal lining.

- H_2 blockers can be used to treat GERD. The bedtime dose of the H_2 blockers is the most important one. PPIs may also be used for GERD.

- The three types of ulcers are *gastric ulcer*, *duodenal ulcer*, and *stress ulcer*.

- There are drug regimens for the treatment of the bacterium *H. pylori*, which contributes to the development of ulcers.

- Gastritis is an irritation and superficial erosion of the stomach lining. Ulcerative colitis is an inflammation of the large bowel.

- Azathioprine (Imuran) is used to treat GI diseases as well as other autoimmune diseases.

- Mesalamine (Apriso, Asacol, Canasa, Delzicol, Lialda, Pentasa) and sulfasalazine (Azulfidine, Sulfazine) are used to treat ulcerative colitis.

- Sulfasalazine (Azulfidine, Sulfazine) decreases inflammatory response in the colon. It can change the color of urine and stain soft contact lenses.
- Ursodiol (Actigall) is used to dissolve gallstones, but it can take several months.

Diarrhea

- Diphenoxylate-atropine (Lomotil) is a combination drug and a controlled substance used to treat diarrhea.
- Loperamide (Imodium) may be as effective as diphenoxylate-atropine and is available over the counter.

Constipation and Flatulence

- Dietary fiber increases colon content and propulsive motility.
- Chronic constipation is often associated with low-fiber diets.
- Aluminum hydroxide-magnesium hydroxide-simethicone is a gastric defoaming antiflatulent agent. It reduces surface tension, causing bubbles to be broken or to coalesce into a foam that can be eliminated more easily by belching or passing flatus.
- Constipation can be relieved with bulk-forming laxatives, surfactant laxatives, osmotic laxatives, and stimulant laxatives.
- Patients taking opioids should take a stimulant laxative.
- Constipation and lack of dietary fiber increase the likelihood of other diseases, including diverticular disease, hiatal hernia, and hemorrhoids.

Nausea and Vomiting

- The CTZ, when stimulated, may trigger vomiting.
- Some antiemetics bind to serotonin (5-HT) receptors to prevent nausea.

Hepatitis

- Hepatitis A, hepatitis B, and hepatitis C are the most common hepatitis viruses.
- Hepatitis C can be transmitted only through blood and body fluids.
- Vaccines have been developed to prevent infection by hepatitis A and hepatitis B, but not hepatitis C.

absorption the uptake of essential nutrients and drugs into the bloodstream

adsorbents a class of antidiarrheals

alimentary tract the GI tract, made up of the mouth, esophagus, stomach, small intestine, colon, and rectum

aloe plant that, when ingested orally, may be used to relieve constipation

aminosalicylates drugs used for both induction and maintenance of remission in patients with Crohn's disease and ulcerative colitis

antacids medications preventing or correcting acidity, especially in the stomach

anticholinergic antiemetics drugs used as antiemetics for mild motion sickness

antidiarrheals drugs that prevent or alleviate diarrhea symptoms

antiemetic a drug that prevents or controls nausea and vomiting

antiflatulents drugs that prevent or alleviate excessive intestinal gas

antihistamines drugs used to relieve the symptoms of allergies

anti-inflammatory agent a drug that reduces inflammation in the body, such as swelling, tenderness, fever, and pain

benzamides drugs that cause dopamine antagonism and, at higher doses, 5-HT3 antagonism

bifidobacteria not yet thoroughly studied agents that may be effective for diarrhea management

bile an alkaline fluid produced by the liver; assists in the digestion and absorption of fat and cholesterol

bowel evacuant an agent used to empty the colon prior to GI examination or after ingestion of toxic substances

bulk-forming agent medication used to treat constipation; a type of laxative

chemoreceptor trigger zone (CTZ) an area below the floor of the fourth ventricle of the brain that can trigger nausea and vomiting when certain signals are received

cholescystectomy surgical removal of the gallbladder

coating agent an agent used to treat duodenal ulcers

colon part of the lower GI system

colonic segmentation when the colon acts as if it is divided into small parts that move independently of each other rather than contributing to an integrated overall motion

constipation a condition in which an individual has difficulty emptying their bowels

corticosteroids drugs used for their anti-inflammatory and immunosuppressive properties

Crohn's disease an inflammatory bowel disease affecting the entire GI tract from mouth to anus

cystic duct connection between the gallbladder and the common bile duct

diarrhea excessive, soft, or watery stool

digestion breakdown of large food molecules to smaller ones

diverticular disease formation and inflammation of an outpocketing from the colon wall

duodenal ulcer a peptic lesion situated in the duodenum

dyspnea shortness of breath

emesis vomiting

enema procedure in which liquid or gas is introduced into the rectum

Escherichia coli (E. coli) a bacterial cause of diarrhea

esophageal hiatus the opening in the diaphragm through which normally only the esophagus passes

esophagus part of the upper GI system

fiber the undigested residue of fruits, vegetables, and other foods of plant origin that remains after digestion by the human GI enzymes; characterized by fermentability and may be either water soluble or insoluble

first-pass effect process where the liver metabolizes drugs before they reach their target sites in the body

flatulence gas from the GI system

food poisoning an infectious cause for acute diarrhea

gallstone dissolution agent drug that assists in removing gallstones from the GI and urinary tracts

gastric stasis lack of stomach motility

gastric ulcer a local excavation in the gastric mucosa

gastritis irritation and superficial erosion of the stomach lining

gastroesophageal reflux disease (GERD) a GI disease characterized by radiating burning or pain in the chest and an acid taste; caused by backflow of acidic stomach contents through an incompetent lower esophageal sphincter; also referred to as *heartburn*

gastrointestinal (GI) system the system of organs that processes foods and liquids

gastrointestinal (GI) tract a continuous tube that begins in the mouth and extends through the pharynx, esophagus, stomach, small intestine, and large intestine to end at the anus

GI bleed condition where ulceration erodes into a blood vessel

GI transit time the time it takes for material to pass from the mouth to the anus; the slower the GI transit time, the greater the amounts of nutrients and water absorbed

herniation a protrusion through a weakened muscular wall

Helicobacter pylori (H. pylori) a bacterium that contributes to the development of many gastric ulcers

hemorrhoids a condition marked by engorgement of the vascular cushions situated within the anal sphincter muscles; result from pressure exerted on anal veins while straining to pass a stool

hepatitis a disease of the liver that causes inflammation, can be acute or chronic, and has several forms, A through G

hepatitis A a viral form of hepatitis that is usually mild and transient and can be spread from one person to another

hepatitis B a viral form of hepatitis that can be acute or chronic; transmitted parenterally, through body fluids, from sexual contact, and perinatally

hepatitis C an infection of the liver that cannot be spread from one person to another by contact; most commonly transmitted by blood transfusions or illicit drug use

hiatal hernia a protrusion through the esophageal hiatus of the diaphragm

histamine H$_2$ receptor antagonist an agent that blocks acid and pepsin secretion in response to histamine, gastrin, foods, abdominal distension, caffeine, or cholinergic stimulation; used to treat GERD and *H. pylori*

immunosuppressive reducing the ability of the immune system to function

immunosuppressive agent drug that interferes with nucleic acid synthesis in both normal and precancerous cells; the overall action is suppression of the immune system

irritable bowel syndrome (IBS) a functional disorder in which the lower GI tract does not have appropriate tone or spasticity to regulate bowel activity

IVIG the notation for immune globulin that is given intravenously

lactobacilli Gram-positive bacteria that are normally found in the GI tract

laxatives drugs that relieve constipation

mouth part of the upper GI system where food enters the system

Norwalk virus viral infection that causes diarrhea

osmotic laxative an organic substance that draws water into the colon and thereby stimulates evacuation

peptic disease disorder of the upper GI tract caused by the action of acid and pepsin; includes mucosal injury, erythema, erosions, and frank ulceration

peptic ulcer an ulcer formed at any part of the GI tract exposed to acid and pepsin

peristalsis muscle contractions that propel fecal matter along the colon

phenothiazine a drug that controls vomiting by inhibiting the CTZ

probiotics live bacteria and yeasts that are good for a healthy GI system

prostaglandin E analog drug used in the treatment of ulcers

proton pump inhibitor (PPI) a class of drugs that works to stop stomach acid; blocks acid secretion by inhibiting the enzyme that pumps hydrogen ions into the stomach

protozoan a single-celled organism that inhabits water and soil

rectum part of the lower GI system

reflux backflow; specifically in GERD, the backflow of acidic stomach contents through an incompetent lower esophageal sphincter

rotavirus a viral infection that causes diarrhea

Saccharomyces boulardii (S. boulardii) yeast organism that lives in the human GI tract

saline laxative an inorganic salt that attracts water into the hollow portion (lumen) of the colon, increasing intraluminal pressure to cause evacuation

saliva lubrication for food

salmonella infectious cause of diarrhea

serotonin (5-HT) receptor antagonist antiemetic used to prevent and treat severe nausea and vomiting associated with chemotherapeutic medications

shiatsu acupressure the application of pressure to the discrete points on the body in order to provide therapeutic effects

small intestine part of the lower GI system; the site where most digestion and nutrient absorption occur

stimulant laxative a laxative that increases gut activity by irritating the mucosa

stomach part of the upper GI system

stress ulcer a peptic ulcer, usually gastric, that occurs in a clinical setting; caused by a breakdown of natural mucosal resistance

suppository medication inserted into the rectum, vagina, or urethra where it dissolves or melts and is absorbed into the bloodstream

surfactant laxative a stool softener that has a detergent activity that facilitates mixing of fat and water, making the stool soft and mushy

traveler's diarrhea diarrhea caused by ingesting contaminated food or water; so called because it is often contracted by travelers in countries where the water supply is contaminated

ulcer a local defect or excavation of the surface of an organ or tissue

ulcerative colitis irritation and inflammation of the large bowel, causing it to look scraped; characterized by bloody mucus leading to watery diarrhea containing blood, mucus, and pus

vertigo the sensation of the room spinning when one gets up or changes positions; can be treated with anticholinergic agents

DRUG LIST

GERD

Antacids

aluminum hydroxide (AlternaGel)
aluminum hydroxide-magnesium carbonate (Gaviscon Extra Strength)
aluminum hydroxide-magnesium hydroxide-simethicone (Mylanta)
calcium carbonate (Maalox, Tums)
calcium carbonate-famotidine-magnesium hydroxide (Pepcid Complete)
magnesium hydroxide (Phillips Milk of Magnesia)

Histamine H₂ Receptor Antagonists

cimetidine (Tagamet, Tagamet HB)
famotidine (Pepcid, Pepcid AC)
nizatidine (Axid, Axid AR)
ranitidine (Zantac, Zantac 75)

Proton Pump Inhibitors

dexlansoprazole (Dexilant)
esomeprazole (Nexium)
lansoprazole (Prevacid)
omeprazole (Prilosec, Prilosec OTC)
omeprazole-sodium bicarbonate (Zegerid)
pantoprazole (Protonix)
rabeprazole (Aciphex)

Coating Agent

sucralfate (Carafate)

Prostaglandin E Analog

misoprostol (Cytotec)

H. pylori

Antibiotics

amoxicillin (Amoxil, Trimox)
clarithromycin (Biaxin)
metronidazole (Flagyl, Flagyl IV)

Combinations

bismuth subcitrate-metronidazole-tetracycline (Pylera)
lansoprazole-amoxicillin-clarithromycin (Prevpac)

Gastrointestinal Diseases

Aminosalicylates

mesalamine (Apriso, Asacol, Canasa, Delzicol, Lialda, Pentasa)
sulfasalazine (Azulfidine, Sulfazine)

Corticosteroids

budesonide (Entocort EC)
hydrocortisone (A-Hydrocort, Cortef, Solu-Cortef)
methylprednisolone (A-MethaPred, Depo-Medrol, Medrol, Solu-Medrol)
prednisone (Sterapred)

Immunosuppressant

azathioprine (Imuran)

Gallstone Dissolution Agent

ursodiol (Actigall)

Antidiarrheals

Adsorbent

bismuth subsalicylate (Kaopectate, Pepto-Bismol)

Antimotility Drugs

difenoxin-atropine (Motofen)
diphenoxylate-atropine (Lomotil)
loperamide (Imodium, Imodium A-D)

Drugs for Infectious Diarrhea

nitazoxanide (Alinia)
rifaximin (Xifaxan)

Antiflatulent Agents

aluminum hydroxide-magnesium hydroxide-simethicone (Mylanta, Mylanta Maximum Strength)
calcium carbonate-simethicone (Maalox)
simethicone (Gas Aid, Mylicon Drops)

Bowel Evacuants

polyethylene glycol 3350 with electrolytes (Colyte, GaviLyte-C, GaviLyte-G, GaviLyte-N, GoLYTELY, HalfLYTELY, MoviPrep, NuLYTELY, TriLyte)
sodium phosphate (Fleet Phospho-Soda, Visicol)

Bulk-Forming Laxatives

methylcellulose (Citrucel, Maltsupex, Unifiber)
polycarbophil (Equalactin, FiberCon, Fiber-Lax, Konsyl Fiber)
psyllium (Fiberall, Metamucil, Perdiem Fiber Therapy)
wheat dextrin (Benefiber)

Osmotic Laxatives

glycerin (Fleet Glycerin Suppositories)
lactulose (Enulose)
magnesium hydroxide (Phillips Milk of Magnesia)
magnesium sulfate (Epsom Salts)
polyethylene glycol 3350 (MiraLax)

Stimulant Laxatives

bisacodyl (Dulcolax)
senna (ExLax, Fletcher's Castoria, various brands)

Surfactant Laxatives

docusate (Colace, Ex-Lax Stool Softener, Surfak)
docusate-senna (Senokot-S)

Miscellaneous

lubiprostone (Amitiza)
methylnaltrexone (Relistor)

Hemorrhoidal Agent

hydrocortisone (Anusol HC, Cortifoam)
nitroglycerin (Rectiv)

Antiemetic Medications

Antihistamines and Anticholinergics

diphenhydramine (Benadryl)
hydroxyzine (Atarax, Vistaril)
meclizine (Antivert, Dramamine)
scopolamine (Scopace, Transderm Scop)

Serotonin Receptor Antagonists

dolasetron (Anzemet)
granisetron (Kytril)
ondansetron (Zofran)
palonosetron (Aloxi)

Phenothiazines

prochlorperazine (Compazine)
promethazine (Phenergan)

Other Antiemetic Medications

aprepitant, fosaprepitant (Emend)
metoclopramide (Reglan)

Hepatitis Drugs

entecavir (Baraclude)
hepatitis B vaccine (Energix B, Recombivax HB)
immune globulin (Gamunex)
lamivudine (Epivir, Epivir-HBV)
ledipasvir-sofosbuvir (Harvoni)
ombitasvir-paritaprevir-ritonavir-dasabuvir (Viekira Pak)
peginterferon alfa-2a (Pegasys)
ribavirin (Copegus, Moderiba, Rebetol, Ribasphere, Ribasphere RibaPak, Virazole)
simeprevir (Olysio)
sofosbuvir (Sovaldi)
tenofovir (Viread)

Black Box Warnings

bismuth subcitrate-metronidazole-tetracycline (Pylera)

entecavir (Baraclude)
immune globulin (Gamunex)
lamivudine (Epivir, Epivir-HBV)
peginterferon alfa-2a (Pegasys)
metoclopromide (Reglan)
metronidazole (Flagyl)
misoprostol (Cytotec)
promethazine (Phenergan)
ribavirin (Copegus)
sodium phosphate (Fleet Phospho-Soda,
   Visicol)
tenofovir (Viread)

Medication Guides

metoclopramide (Reglan)
peginterferon alfa-2a (Pegasys)
ribavirin (Copegus, Moderiba, Rebetol,
   Ribasphere, Ribasphere RibaPak,
   Virazole)

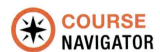

COURSE NAVIGATOR

Access interactive chapter review exercises, practice activities, flash cards, and study games.

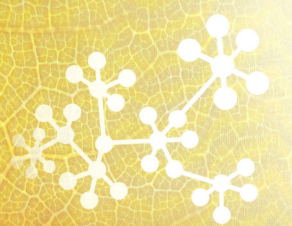

11

Renal System Drugs

Learning Objectives

1 Explain the renal system, its importance, and how it works.

2 Differentiate the parts of the renal system.

3 Describe the drugs used to treat renal disease.

4 State the causes and treatment of urinary tract infections.

5 Explain the classes of diuretics and how they work.

COURSE NAVIGATOR

Access additional chapter resources.

The kidneys, ureters, bladder, and urethra are all part of the renal system, also known as the urinary system. Disorders of the renal system can upset the delicate balance of the body and result in many serious health problems. When the kidneys are not functioning properly waste products and fluid can build up in the body, leading to swelling, vomiting, weakness, and eventually could lead to kidney failure or death. Although the kidneys are most often thought of as excretory organs, most of their metabolic work is directed toward the reclamation of filtered solutes. In addition, the kidneys play an important role in the metabolism of various peptide hormones and are active biosynthetically in the production of renin, ammonia, erythropoietin, and 1-alpha, 25-dihydroxyvitamin D_3.

Function and Anatomy of the Renal System

The primary function of the kidneys is to maintain the balance of water, electrolytes, and acids and bases in the extracellular fluid (plasma and tissue fluid) of the body. They accomplish this function through the formation of urine, which is a modified filtrate of plasma. Urine formation is essential for normal body function because it enables the blood to reabsorb necessary nutrients, water, and electrolytes. Large molecules, such as plasma proteins, cannot cross the glomerular membranes to be filtered from the blood, whereas small molecules, such as water, ions, and glucose, do pass through the membranes, later to be reabsorbed into the blood. Figure 11.1 illustrates the urinary system and renal anatomy. In the process of urine formation, the kidneys regulate (1) the volume of blood plasma (thus contributing significantly to the regulation of blood pressure); (2) the concentration of waste products in the blood; (3) the concentration of electrolytes—sodium (Na^+), potassium (K^+), bicarbonate (HCO_3^-), calcium (Ca^{2+}), and phosphate (PO_4^{3-})—in the plasma; and (4) the pH, or acid-base balance, of plasma.

FIGURE 11.1
Renal System

The urinary system includes the kidneys, important organs that maintain the balance of water, electrolytes, and acids and bases in the extracellular fluid.

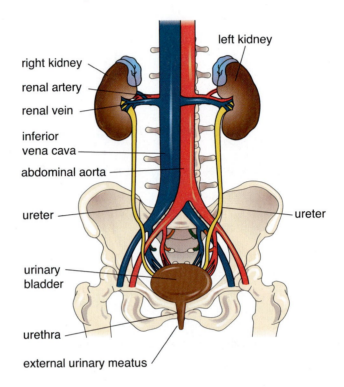

Kidneys

The **kidneys** are bean-shaped organs located in the rear upper torso, just inferior to the ribs. Although they are in the abdominal region, they are not inside the peritoneal cavity, where the stomach, pancreas, and intestines are located. The adrenal glands are on top of the kidneys, almost like two little caps, and they produce hormones. The **renal artery** branches off the abdominal aorta and brings blood into the kidneys. Blood that has been filtered in the kidneys returns to the bloodstream via the **renal vein** (see Figure 11.2).

The **renal cortex** is the outer layer of the kidneys and is responsible for filtration. The renal medulla, in the body of each kidney, also performs filtration. The renal cortex and **renal medulla** are made up of thousands of microscopic **nephrons**, the functional filtering units of the kidney. Urine formation, a multistep process including glomerular filtration, tubular reabsorption, and tubular secretion, begins in the nephron.

The normal human kidney contains two million microscopic nephrons (see Figure 11.3). The nephrons work in a highly consistent manner to produce urine and thereby maintain constancy in the body's internal environment. The renal tubules of the nephrons produce urine through three processes: filtration, reabsorption, and secretion.

FIGURE 11.2

FIGURE 11.2
Anatomy of the Kidney

The kidney contains two million microscopic nephrons that produce urine and maintain constancy in the body's internal environment.

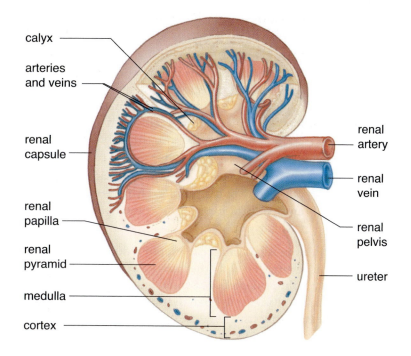

FIGURE 11.3
Anatomy of the Nephron

Each part of the microscopic-sized nephron performs specific functions: filtration, reabsorption, and secretion of select electrolytes, fluids, and other substances.

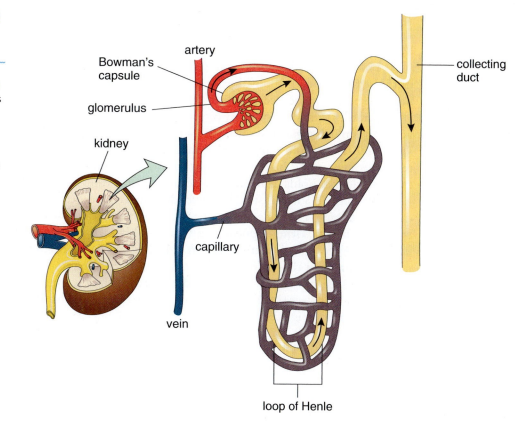

- **Filtration**, or the removal of substances from the blood, takes place in the glomeruli.

- During **reabsorption**, filtered substances are selectively pulled back into the blood. Sodium is the principal (99%) cation (positively charged ion) of extra-cellular fluid transported (exchanged for hydrogen and potassium ions), and chloride is the principal anion (negatively charged ion) transported. In the loop of Henle, sodium is absorbed along with chloride. In the distal tubule, potassium is secreted into the urine in exchange for sodium. This exchange is promoted by aldosterone.

- **Secretion** of hydrogen ions, potassium ions, weak acids, and weak bases also takes place in the tubules. Hydrogen ion secretion regulates acid-base balance and acidification of urine (blood pH is normally between 7.32 and 7.42, which is slightly basic).

Acute renal failure is a rapid reduction in kidney function, resulting in accumulation of nitrogen and other waste. It may be caused by renal ischemia, trauma, pregnancy, volume depletion, hemorrhage, surgery, or shock. **Uremia** is the clinical syndrome resulting from renal dysfunction. In this syndrome, excessive products of protein metabolism (e.g., urea) are retained in the blood, and the toxic condition produced is marked by nausea, vomiting, vertigo, convulsions, and coma.

Ureters and Urinary Bladder

The **ureters** are paired muscular ducts that extend from the renal pelvis to the bladder. The main function of the ureters is to move urine from the kidney to the bladder. Movement is facilitated by smooth muscle contraction in the ureter wall.

The **urinary bladder** is located in the pelvic region. It collects and holds urine until the fluid exits the body during urination. The bladder is made of stretchy epithelial and smooth muscle cells, which allow it to expand and hold up to 1 L of fluid. However, the functional capacity of the bladder (the volume held before voluntary voiding) is much smaller—around 300–400 mL in adults. The **internal urinary sphincter** is an involuntary muscle that keeps urine from flowing back into the ureters once it enters the bladder. In contrast, the **external urinary sphincter** is a voluntary muscle that holds urine in the bladder before it exits the body.

When the bladder is full and distended, stretch receptors sense the pressure and cause the **detrusor muscles** in the bladder to contract and the external urinary sphincter to relax. Urine is pushed out, and the bladder empties (see Figure 11.4). This urination process is called **micturition**. **Urinary retention** occurs when the kidneys produce urine, but the micturition process does not function properly, and consequently, urine accumulates in the bladder. This problem is a malfunction of the bladder. The inability to control the external urinary sphincter, thus allowing urine to leak out of the bladder, is called **incontinence**.

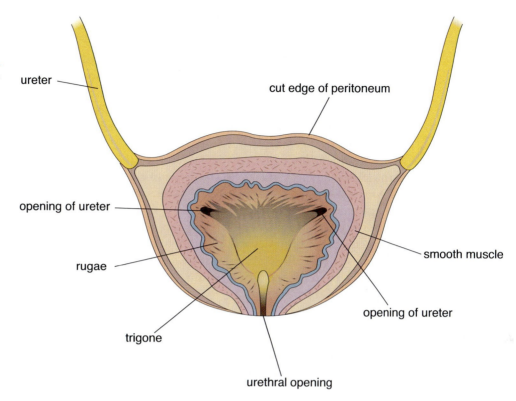

ureter

cut edge of peritoneum

opening of ureter

smooth muscle

rugae

opening of ureter

trigone

urethral opening

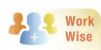
Work Wise

Learning healthcare jargon is an important communication skill. Abbreviations used to describe kidney function are pronounced in different ways. For example, the abbreviations *BUN* and *GFR* are generally pronounced by saying the letters individually. The abbreviation *CrCl* is generally spoken by saying "creatinine clearance."

Assessing Kidney Function

Laboratory blood tests are used to diagnose and monitor kidney function. The most common tests are **blood urea nitrogen (BUN)** and **serum creatinine (SCr)**. When kidney function is impaired, the elimination of urea, nitrogen, and creatinine (a byproduct of muscle metabolism) is also impaired, and the concentrations of these substances increase in the blood. Although results of these tests vary according to age, weight, and gender, as well as other factors such as exercise, these tests are good markers for kidney function.

Typically, the normal range for SCr is 0.5–1.5 mg/dL. SCr can be used to calculate **creatinine clearance (CrCl)**, which estimates **glomerular filtration rate (GFR)**. A low CrCl (<60 mL/min) is a sign of impaired kidney function. CrCl and GFR estimate the level of kidney function while taking into account such factors as age, ideal body weight, and gender. A common formula used to calculate CrCl is the **Cockcroft and Gault equation**:

$$\text{Men: CrCl in mL/min} = \frac{(140 - \text{age}) \times \text{weight in kilograms (kg)}}{\text{SCr in mg/dL} \times 72}$$

$$\text{Women: CrCl in mL/min} = \frac{(140 - \text{age}) \times \text{weight in kilograms (kg)} \times 0.85}{\text{SCr in mg/dL} \times 72}$$

Although other formulas for estimating kidney function exist, the Cockcroft and Gault equation is used most often when adjusting drug dosing for impaired renal function. For instance, the dose is decreased or the interval between doses is increased for many drugs when CrCl drops below 30 mL/min or 60 mL/min.

Acute Kidney Injury and Chronic Kidney Disease

Kidney disease or **renal disease** can be acute or chronic. **Acute kidney injury** is a decrease in kidney function or GFR that occurs over hours, days, or even weeks. If supportive care is provided and the cause of failure resolved, kidney function may return to normal. If the insult is sufficiently severe, acute kidney injury can be life-threatening and might result in some level of permanent damage. Table 11.1 presents commonly used agents in renal disease.

Chronic kidney disease (CKD), on the other hand, involves progressive damage to the kidney tissue, resulting in the death of this tissue over time. Common causes of CKD include diabetes and untreated hypertension. CKD is more common than acute kidney injury and cannot be reversed. As it worsens, it can be categorized into stages that guide the approach and degree of urgency for treatment (see Table 11.2). Drug therapies, such as diuretics and other renal protective medications, can help slow the progression of the disease in early stages, but in later stages, these agents are of no use. Eventually, in end-stage kidney failure, dialysis and kidney transplantation are the only means of treatment.

TABLE 11.1 Most Commonly Used Agents in Renal Disease

Generic (Brand)	Pronunciation	Dosage Form	Dispensing Status
Anemia Therapies			
darbepoetin alfa (Aranesp)	dar-be-POE-e-tin AL-fa	Injection	Rx
epoetin alfa, erythropoietin (Epogen, Procrit)	eh-POE-e-tin AL-fa ah-rith-RO-poy-tin	Injection	Rx
Dialysis Therapies			
cinacalcet (Sensipar)	sin-a-KAL-set	Tablet	Rx
sevelamer (Renagel, Renvela)	se-VEL-a-mer	Tablet	Rx
Supplemental Therapies			
ergocalciferol, vitamin D (Deltalin, Drisdol)	er-goe-kal-SIF-e-rawl VYE-ta-min D	Capsule, oral liquid, tablet	Rx
ferumoxytol (Feraheme)	fer-u-MOX-ee-tole	Injection	Rx
folic acid, vitamin B_9 (various brands)	FOE-lik AS-id VYE-ta-min B-nine	Injection, tablet	OTC, Rx
iron dextran (INFeD)	EYE-ern DEX-tran	Injection	Rx
iron sucrose (Venofer)	EYE-ern SOO-krose	Injection	Rx
levocarnitine (Carnitor)	lee-voe-KAR-ni-teen	Capsule, injection, oral liquid, tablet	Rx
multiple vitamin complex (various brands)	MUL-ti-ple VYE-ta-min KOM-plex	Injection, oral liquid, tablet	OTC, Rx
pyridoxine, vitamin B_6 (various brands)	peer-i-DOX-een VYE-ta-min B six	Injection, tablet	OTC, Rx
sodium ferric gluconate (Ferrlecit)	SOE-dee-um FERR-ic GLOO-ko-nate	Injection	Rx

TABLE 11.2 Stages of Chronic Kidney Disease

Stage	GFR (mL/min/1.73 m²)	Description
I	≥90	Normal kidney function, but urine findings, structural abnormalities, or a genetic trait point to kidney disease
II	60–89	Mildly reduced kidney function, but urine findings, structural abnormalities, or a genetic trait point to kidney disease
IIIa	45–59	Moderately reduced kidney function
IIIb	30–44	Moderately reduced kidney function
IV	15–29	Severely reduced kidney function
V	<15	End-stage kidney failure (sometimes called *established renal failure*)

Kidney Disease Treatments

Acute kidney injury typically improves or reverses as its cause is resolved. Therefore, drug treatment for acute kidney injury is limited and short-term. CKD is more frequently treated with medication. Therapy is aimed at reestablishing an appropriate intravascular fluid volume and pressure and treating underlying problems. Treatment for advanced stages of CKD often includes dialysis or kidney transplant.

In patients who have CKD, hypertension management is a key to prevent disease progression. In order to decrease hypertension, angiotensin-converting enzyme (ACE) inhibitors and angiotensin receptor blockers (ARBs) are given initially (discussed in Chapter 12), followed by diuretics (discussed later in this chapter).

Anemia is a condition characterized by deficiency in red blood cells (RBCs) or hemoglobin that is common in patients who have CKD. Anemia due to kidney disease is caused by reduction in **erythropoietin**. Erythropoietin is a hormone secreted by the kidneys that stimulates the production of red blood cells. Most patients with kidney disease have erythropoietin deficiency. Treatments for anemia will be discussed in the following section.

Dialysis is an artificial method of filtering blood and correcting the electrolyte imbalances caused by kidney failure. When indicated, dialysis is accomplished by one

FIGURE 11.5
Hemodialysis

In hemodialysis, a patient is connected to a machine in a dialysis center and must remain at the center for several hours.

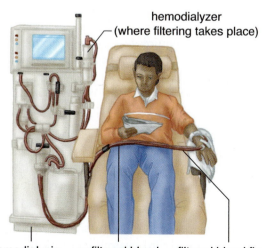

hemodialyzer
(where filtering takes place)

hemodialysis machine   unfiltered blood flows to hemodialyzer   filtered blood flows back to body

of two common methods: hemodialysis or peritoneal dialysis. **Hemodialysis** is accomplished by diverting blood flow through a machine that mechanically filters the blood and returns the blood to the body (see Figure 11.5). **Peritoneal dialysis** is accomplished by putting **dialysate** (a special fluid that draws toxins from the body into itself) into the abdominal cavity and leaving it there for a certain period—typically, a few hours (see Figure 11.6). During this time, toxins and electrolytes diffuse into the dialysate fluid from the many capillaries in the abdominal cavity.

FIGURE 11.6
Peritoneal Dialysis

In peritoneal dialysis, a patient has the freedom to receive treatment at home, at work, or while traveling.

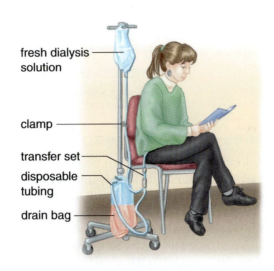

fresh dialysis solution

clamp

transfer set

disposable tubing

drain bag

Kidney transplantation is the treatment of choice for stage V, or *end-stage*, kidney disease. The process involves surgically implanting a kidney from a living or deceased donor into a recipient. Kidney transplantation is one of the most common transplant operations in the United States.

Anemia Therapies

Name Exchange

Procrit is one of the two brand names for epoetin alfa. It is pronounced PRO-krit.

As discussed previously, patients who have kidney disease often are deficient in erythropoietin. Erythropoietin-stimulating agents (ESAs) are used to induce red blood cell production by activating the release of **reticulocytes** (immature red blood cells). The side effects of ESAs include hypertension, seizures, increased risk of blood clots, and allergic reactions.

Darbepoetin alfa (Aranesp) is similar to epoetin alfa but is longer acting, which means it requires less frequent administration. Darbepoetin is administered once a week or every two weeks. Like epoetin alfa, it is approved for treating anemia associated with CKD.

Epoetin alfa (Epogen, Procrit) is an ESA that is used to treat anemia associated with CKD. It is available as an injectable product only. Epoetin alfa needs to be administered three times a week.

Contraindications Both darbepoetin alfa and epoetin alfa are contraindicated in patients with uncontrolled hypertension and pure red cell aplasia. Epoetin multidose vials contain benzyl alcohol, which is contraindicated in neonates and infants, as well as in pregnant and breast-feeding women.

Cautions and Considerations ESAs have black box warnings. One warning is for the risk of serious cardiovascular events, thromboembolic events, stroke, and death when ESAs are prescribed for patients with hemoglobin levels greater than 11 mg/dL. Another boxed warning recommends blood clot prophylaxis in patients using ESAs who are due for surgery. Still another warns of shortened survival and increased risk of tumor progression in patients who have cancer and are taking ESAs. For that reason, this patient population must obtain the drug through a Risk Evaluation and Mitigation Strategies (REMS) program.

Drug Interactions ESAs may stimulate the blood-clotting effects of lenalidromide and thalidomide.

Dialysis Therapy

Dialysis can be a lifesaving intervention. However, it is not without adverse effects. Patients who have CKD and are undergoing dialysis therapy may experience imbalances in electrolytes and hormones. Patients undergoing dialysis will have their electrolytes and hormones monitored, and often use drug therapy to balance levels.

    Cinacalcet (Sensipar) lowers parathyroid hormone, calcium, and phosphate levels and is indicated for the treatment of secondary hyperparathyroidism in adult patients receiving dialysis. It is also indicated for **hypercalcemia**. Cinacalcet can be given alone or in combination with vitamin D. It reduces serum calcium, so calcium levels should be monitored.

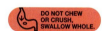

    Sevelamer (Renagel, Renvela) binds phosphate in the intestinal lumen, limiting its absorption. The drug has the ability to decrease serum phosphate concentrations without altering calcium, aluminum, or bicarbonate concentrations. Sevelamer can interfere with the absorption of other drugs. Therefore, patients should take other medications at least one hour before or three hours after the administration of this drug. Serum calcium, bicarbonate, and chloride concentrations should be monitored. Sevelamer is available as a powder and as tablets. Tablets should be taken whole and not crushed or broken.

    Renagel is in the form of a hydrochloride salt. Renvela has the advantage of being a carbonate salt, which serves as a buffer and may be better tolerated.

Contraindications Cinacalcet is contraindicated in patients who have **hypocalcemia** (below normal levels of calcium). Sevelamer is contraindicated in patients who have a bowel obstruction.

Cautions and Considerations Cinacalcet should only be used by CKD patients undergoing dialysis. Cinacalcet decreases calcium levels. Hypocalcemia can be dangerous and life-threatening. For example, lowered calcium levels can increase the likelihood of seizures. Calcium levels should be monitored in patients using cinacalcet. Sevelamer should be used with caution in patients who have gastrointestinal (GI) disorders.

Drug Interactions Cinacalcet interacts with multiple drugs. It may increase the concentrations of aripiprazole, atomoxetine, brexpiprazole, doxorubicin, eliglustat, iloperidone, metoprolol, pimozide, tamoxifen, thioridazine, tricyclic antidepressants (TCAs), and vortioxetine. It may decrease the effects of codeine and tamoxifen. Cinacalcet concentrations may be increased by idelalisib.

    Sevelamer may decrease concentrations of calcitriol, cholic acid, cyclosporine, levothyroxine, mycophenolate, quinolone antibiotics, and tacrolimus.

Supplemental Therapies

CKD and its treatments (such as dialysis) are associated with altered levels of vitamins and minerals. Hence, many patients who have CKD use vitamin and mineral supplements.

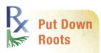

Put Down Roots

The elemental abbreviation for iron is *Fe*. Remembering this abbreviation may help you identify the brand names of parenteral iron: Feraheme, Ferrlecit, INFeD, and Venofer.

Use of **ergocalciferol (Deltalin, Drisdol)**, a vitamin D supplement, is determined by serum calcium concentrations. Ergocalciferol is not routinely given to patients until they begin dialysis.

Folic acid (vitamin B_9) should be administered daily to patients with renal disease, because it is required for forming new erythrocytes. Nephrocaps is a vitamin supplement especially formulated for patients receiving dialysis. It has folic acid, other B vitamins, and vitamin C.

Parenteral iron supplementation is used in patients who have CKD to replenish iron body stores when levels are deficient. Compared with oral iron supplementation, parenteral or intravenous (IV) administration restores iron levels much more rapidly.

There are several forms of iron that are administered parenterally. One form of parenteral iron is **iron dextran (INFeD)**. Iron dextran releases iron from the plasma and eventually replenishes the iron stores in bone marrow, where it is incorporated into hemoglobin. This drug must be used with caution, and a test dose should be given before the full dose is administered.

Ferumoxytol (Feraheme) is a newer, parenterally administered iron formulation. It is compatible with NS.

Iron sucrose (Venofer) is used to replenish iron body stores and is eliminated mainly by urinary excretion. A significant amount of the iron is concentrated in the liver, spleen, and bone marrow. Iron sucrose is administered one to three times a week, either by slow injection or by slow IV infusion. Most IV iron supplements need a test dose, but iron sucrose does not. It appears to be a safer alternative than the other iron supplements, especially for those patients who have had a reaction to iron dextran. Patients still need to be monitored for hypotension, which is the most common side effect.

Sodium ferric gluconate (Ferrlecit) seems to have fewer adverse reactions than iron dextran. Sodium ferric gluconate is compatible with NS, but it should not be mixed with other infusions.

Levocarnitine (Carnitor) is an amino acid derivative involved in metabolism. It is a cofactor needed for the transformation of long-chain fatty acids. A deficiency of levocarnitine leads to fatigue. It is thought that dialysis reduces circulating levels of levocarnitine. The most common GI side effects include nausea, vomiting, cramps, and diarrhea. It is used primarily for deficiency states and hemo-dialysis patients.

Multiple vitamin complexes are necessary because of the imbalance of electrolytes (and other substances) that coincides with renal disease, which depletes vitamin stores. **Pyridoxine**, vitamin B_6, should also be administered daily. It is removed by dialysis and must be replaced.

Kidney Transplant Therapy

Potential kidney transplant recipients undergo an evaluation to determine if they are eligible candidates for the procedure. If so, patients are placed on a **national waiting list**. Waiting list priority depends on key factors such as the type of kidney problem, disease severity, and likelihood of transplant success. Kidney transplant surgery takes approximately three hours. After the procedure, patients can expect to stay in the hospital for several days. Procedure recovery time varies, but the average is six months.

Almost all patients who undergo kidney transplantation will require maintenance immunosuppression with **renal transplant drugs** to help prevent organ rejection (see Table 11.3). Common side effects of immunosuppressants include sore

TABLE 11.3 Most Commonly Used Renal Transplant Drugs

Generic (Brand)	Pronunciation	Dosage Form	Dispensing Status
cyclosporine (Gengraf, Neoral, Sandimmune)	SYE-kloe-spor-een	Capsule, injection, oral liquid	Rx
mycophenolate mofetil (CellCept)	my-koe-FEN-oh-late MOE-fi-til	Capsule, injection, oral liquid, tablet	Rx
mycophenolic acid (Myfortic)	my-koe-fen-AW-lik AS-id	Tablet	Rx
tacrolimus (Astagraf XL, Prograf)	ta-KROE-li-mus	Capsule, injection	Rx

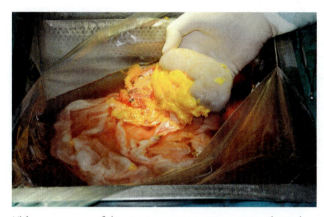

Kidneys are one of the most common organs transplanted.

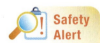

Safety Alert

The oral liquid formulation of cyclosporine should not be consumed out of a plastic or Styrofoam cup. Cyclosporine binds to plastic, and using a plastic container may result in receiving a smaller dose than intended.

throat, cough, dizziness, nausea, muscle aches, fever, chills, itching, and headache. Most of the time, these effects are mild to moderate. Taking acetaminophen can alleviate some of these effects if they are bothersome. Close follow-up care with a healthcare practitioner is necessary for many years after the procedure.

Cyclosporine (Gengraf, Neoral, Sandimmune) is an immunosuppressant that can prevent organ rejection. It can also be used for rheumatoid arthritis (see Chapter 13). Cyclosporine has a small therapeutic window, and blood levels are often monitored. Grapefruit juice may increase cyclosporine levels and should not be consumed concurrently. Cyclosporine is available in modified and unmodified formulations. The two formulations are not bioequivalent and should not be used interchangeably. Cyclosporine has a black box warning that addresses this caution. Cyclosporine also has several other black box warnings. Warnings include an increased risk of hypertension, infections, malignancies such as lymphomas, kidney impairment, and skin cancer. Another warning states that patients taking cyclosporine should be supervised only by experienced healthcare practitioners.

Tacrolimus (Astagraf XL, Prograf) is an immunosuppressant that is used to prevent transplanted organ rejection. Alcohol can increase the rate of release of the extended-release formulation. Orally administered tacrolimus cannot be taken with antacids. Tacrolimus has a black box warning warning for the increased risk of infection, and another warning addresses the possible development of malignancies (such as lymphoma). Extended-release tacrolimus formulations are associated with an increased mortality in female liver transplant recipients, and its use is not recommended after liver transplant. Another warning states that only experienced healthcare practitioners should be supervising patients taking tacrolimus. The Astagraf XL formulation must be dispensed with an FDA medication guide.

Mycophenolate is an immunosuppressant used to prevent the body from rejecting a kidney transplant. It is available in two forms: one is **mycophenolic acid (Myfortic)** and the other is **mycophenolate mofetil (CellCept)**. Mycophenolic acid is available for oral administration; mycophenolate mofetil is available for both oral and IV administration. When preparing mycophenolate mofetil for IV use, make sure to only use D5W for dilution. Mycophenolate has several black box warnings. There is a boxed warning stating that mycophenolic acid and mycophenolate mofetil are not interchangeable.

In terms of pregnancy, there is a warning for the increased risk of congenital malformations and first-trimester pregnancy loss when used by pregnant females. Additional black box warnings address the risk of infections and the risk of malignancies (such as lymphoma and skin cancer). The last warning says that only experienced healthcare practitioners should be supervising patients taking mycophenolate.

Contraindications Cyclosporine is contraindicated in patients with a hypersensitivity to polyoxyethylated castor oil.

Tacrolimus does not have contraindications.

CellCept, a brand name for mycophenolate mofetil, should not be used in patients with a hypersensitivity to polysorbate 80.

Cautions and Considerations Because these agents suppress the immune system, patients taking immunosuppressants are at an increased risk of infection. Patients are often instructed to take special precautions to minimize exposure to infection, such as wearing face masks and avoiding crowded public areas. Frequent handwashing to prevent disease is always recommended.

These drugs are considered hazardous agents, and appropriate handling and disposal precautions should be taken.

Drug Interactions These drugs have many drug interactions. Only drugs that should be avoided with concurrent use will be addressed. Consult a pharmacist or other drug information specialist for specific drug interaction queries.

Cyclosporine may increase the concentration of aliskiren, atorvastatin, bosutinib, cholic acid, dronedarone, lovastatin, pimozide, pitavastatin, silodosin, simeprevir, simvastatin, topotecan, and vincristine. Cyclosporine levels may be increased by conivaptan, crizotinib, idelalisib, and mifepristone. Cyclosporine levels may be decreased by enzalutamide. Eplerenone and potassium-sparing diuretics may enhance the hyperkalemic effect of cyclosporine. Foscarnet and tacrolimus may enhance the nephrotoxic effects of cyclosporine. Cyclosporine may enhance the adverse effects of natalizumab, pimecrolimus, and tofacitinib.

Tacrolimus may increase the levels of bosutinib, pazopanib, silodosin, topotecan, and vincristine. Tacrolimus levels may be increased by conivaptan, crizotinib, grapefruit juice, and idelalisib. Tacrolimus levels may be decreased by enzalutamide. Tacrolimus may enhance the adverse effects of clozapine, cyclosporine, and tofacitinib. The adverse effects of tacrolimus may be enhanced by eplerenone, foscarnet, mifepristone, natalizumab, pimecrolimus, potassium-sparing diuretics, sirolimus, and temsirolimus.

Mycophenolate concentrations may be decreased by bile acid sequestrants, cholestyramine, natalizumab, rifamycin derivatives, and tacrolimus. Pimecrolimus may enhance mycophenolate's adverse reactions.

Immunosuppressants may enhance the adverse effects of live vaccines and should not be used concurrently.

Urinary Tract Disorders

In addition to renal disease, the **urinary tract** can be affected by several other disorders. These disorders include urinary problems such as urinary incontinence caused by spastic bladder and frequent urination, urinary tract infections caused by bacteria, and benign prostatic hyperplasia, an abnormal enlargement of the prostate gland that occurs in men as they age. The symptoms in each case may include bothersome urination, but they are treated with different classes of drugs. Postmenopausal women and elderly men are frequently prone to incontinence (inability to control urination).

Urinary Incontinence

Urinary incontinence is the complaint of involuntary loss of urine. Incontinence affects one-third of adults and one-half of older adults. The primary symptoms are urgency, frequency, and incontinence. Common types of urinary incontinence include *urge* or *overactive bladder* and *overflow incontinence*. The prevalence of urinary incontinence is correlated with age. In addition to involuntary loss of urine, patients may feel pain and the urge to urinate often. Urinary incontinence can limit travel; long trips where bathrooms are not available for several hours can become a serious problem. There are numerous medications available to treat urinary incontinence; behavioral techniques for treating this condition should also be considered. Table 11.4 lists the most commonly used agents for urinary incontinence.

TABLE 11.4   Most Commonly Used Agents for Urinary Incontinence

Generic (Brand)	Pronunciation	Dosage Form	Dispensing Status
darifenacin (Enablex)	dar-i-FEN-a-sin	Tablet	Rx
fesoterodine (Toviaz)	fes-oh-TER-oh-deen	Tablet	Rx
flavoxate (Urispas)	fla-VOX-ate	Tablet	Rx
oxybutynin (Ditropan, Oxytrol)	ox-i-BYOO-ti-nin	Oral liquid, patch, tablet, transdermal gel	Rx
solifenacin (Vesicare)	sol-i-FEN-a-sin	Tablet	Rx
tolterodine (Detrol)	tole-TAIR-oh-deen	Capsule, tablet	Rx
trospium (Sanctura)	TROSE-pee-um	Capsule, tablet	Rx

Darifenacin (Enablex) blocks the cholinergic receptor in the bladder and limits contractions, which reduces the symptoms of urgency and frequency. The drug must be protected from light. As with all other agents in this class, the primary side effect is dry mouth.

Fesoterodine (Toviaz) prevents the bladder muscle from contracting too frequently. In this way, it prevents leaks, strong sudden urges to void, and voiding too often. If the patient cannot completely empty the bladder, he or she should not take Toviaz.

Flavoxate (Urispas) exerts a direct spasmolytic effect on smooth muscle, primarily in the urinary tract. Acting on the detrusor muscle by cholinergic blockage, this agent increases bladder capacity in patients with bladder spasticity. It also has local anesthetic and analgesic effects. It can cause drowsiness, blurred vision, and GI upset.

May Cause **DROWSINESS**

Oxybutynin (Ditropan, Oxytrol) is a urinary antispasmodic agent used to decrease frequent urination. The antispasmodic works to inhibit the action of acetylcholine. It decreases spasms in smooth muscle without affecting skeletal muscles. This drug also increases bladder capacity and decreases urgency and frequency. Dry mouth and drowsiness are common side effects. Oxytrol is a transdermal patch composed of three layers: (1) backing film that protects the middle adhesive/drug layer; (2) the adhesive/drug layer; and (3) the release liner that is pulled off prior to application. The patch is applied twice a week to dry, intact skin on the abdomen, hip, or buttock. The site should be rotated with each application, and a patch should not be reapplied to the same site within seven days. It should be stored away from humidity and moisture at room temperature. The transdermal form minimizes the side effects of dry mouth and constipation, possibly because the transdermal patch is constantly releasing the drug. Thus, first-pass metabolism is prevented. The patch also prevents high peak concentration.

Solifenacin (Vesicare) is an anticholinergic agent used for the treatment of overactive bladder. It is more selective for the muscarinic receptors and should have fewer side effects (including reduced occurrence of dry mouth). The maximum dose should not exceed 5 mg a day.

Tolterodine (Detrol) is a competitive muscarinic receptor antagonist similar to oxybutynin. It differs in its selectivity for urinary bladder receptors over salivary receptors. As a result, dry mouth effects of tolterodine are significantly less than those of oxybutynin. This drug also decreases detrusor muscle pressure.

Trospium (Sanctura) is an antispasmodic agent. It does not cross the blood-brain barrier, so it will not cause drowsiness, which is a common side effect of most of the drugs in this class. It should be taken on an empty stomach. It is dosed twice a day, whereas most of the other agents have once-daily dosing. It relaxes the smooth muscle tissue in the bladder, decreasing bladder contractions.

Contraindications The urinary incontinence agents discussed previously are contraindicated in patients with gastric retention and narrow-angle glaucoma.

Cautions and Considerations Urinary incontinence drugs should be used with caution in older adults. This patient population may be particularly susceptible to adverse effects such as hallucinations, dry mouth, blurred vision, and constipation.

Drug Interactions The urinary incontinence agents have anticholinergic side effects that may potentiate side effects of other drugs with anticholinergic properties.

Urinary Tract Infections

A **urinary tract infection (UTI)** occurs when bacteria, most often *Escherichia coli (E. coli),* enter the opening of the urethra and multiply. The infection usually begins in the lower urinary tract (urethra and bladder) and, if not treated, progresses to the upper urinary tract (ureters and kidneys). Even when the urinary tract is healthy, bacteria may enter. In UTIs, many more organisms than normal are found. The presence of bacteria in the urine with localized symptoms is considered diagnostic of a UTI. Blood may appear in the urine, and urination may be difficult or painful. Fever is common. Community-acquired UTIs account for more than five million physician visits yearly.

The highest incidence of UTIs occurs in sexually active women. Incidence is related to the ability of intestinal bacteria to colonize the vagina, ascend the short urethra, and gain access to the bladder. UTIs become a problem for men older than 50 years because of prostatic obstruction, catheter use, or surgery.

TABLE 11.5 Most Commonly Used Medications to Treat UTIs

Generic (Brand)	Pronunciation	Dosage Form	Dispensing Status
Antibiotics			
amoxicillin (Amoxil)	a-mox-i-SIL-in	Capsule, oral liquid, tablet	Rx
amoxicillin-clavulanate (Augmentin)	a-mox-i-SIL-in klav-yoo-LAN-ate	Oral liquid, tablet	Rx
ampicillin (Principen)	am-pi-SIL-in	Capsule, injection, oral liquid	Rx
ciprofloxacin (Cipro)	sip-roe-FLOX-a-sin	Injection, oral liquid, tablet	Rx
methenamine (Cystex, Hiprex, Urex)	meth-EN-a-meen	Tablet	Rx
nitrofurantoin (Macrobid, Macrodantin)	nye-troe-fyoor-AN-toe-in	Capsule	Rx
sulfamethoxazole-trimethoprim (Bactrim, Bactrim DS, Cotrim, Cotrim DS, Septra, Septra DS, Sulfatrim)	sul-fa-meth-OX-a-zole try-METH-oh-prim	Injection, oral liquid, tablet	Rx
Urinary Analgesic			
phenazopyridine (Azo-Standard, Pyridium, Uristat)	fen-az-oh-PEER-i-deen	Tablet	OTC

UTIs are classified according to their anatomic locations in the urinary tract. The classifications are as follows:

- cystitis (lower urinary tract infection)
- pyelonephritis (upper urinary tract infection)

UTIs are most commonly treated with antibiotics or **urinary analgesics** listed in Table 11.5. Treatment may involve a single dose of medication or a 3- to 14-day regimen, depending on the extent of infection and the treatment agent selected. If several infections occur in sequence, an antibiotic may be prescribed for 6 to 12 months to prevent recurrence. A female patient with recurrent UTIs may be instructed to urinate and take one dose of an antibiotic immediately after sexual intercourse.

Amoxicillin (Amoxil) is taken without regard for food; the primary side effect is skin rash. It is dosed three times a day.

Amoxicillin-clavulanate (Augmentin) should be taken with food to prevent an upset stomach. Diarrhea is the primary side effect.

Ampicillin should be taken on an empty stomach; the primary side effects are diarrhea and skin rash. It is dosed four times a day.

Ciprofloxacin (Cipro) is indicated for the treatment of uncomplicated UTIs.

Do not take with
ANTACIDS

Quinolones such as ciprofloxacin should not be taken with antacids, calcium, magnesium, theophylline, or warfarin. It should be administered at least two hours before or six hours after antacids containing magnesium or aluminum, or other products containing metal cations. The tablet should not be split, crushed, or chewed. Because this drug increases sensitivity to the sun, it is important that patients be told to use sunscreen to protect the skin, even if sun exposure is minimal.

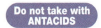

Methenamine (Cystex, Hiprex, Urex) has a local anesthetic effect on urinary tract mucosa in addition to its antimicrobial effect. It is classified as a miscellaneous antibiotic. Methenamine should be taken with food to minimize GI effects, and with sufficient fluids to ensure adequate urine flow. Alkaline foods, antacids, and other alkalinizing medication (e.g., bicarbonate) should be avoided. Skin rash, painful urination, or excessive abdominal pain should be reported to the physician. Administration with sulfonamides is contraindicated. If a dye is used in the formulation of Hiprex, it can turn urine blue and can cause allergic reactions.

Nitrofurantoin (Macrobid, Macrodantin) should be taken with food or milk. It may turn urine brown or dark yellow, and alcohol should be avoided. This drug has side effects resembling those of disulfiram (Antabuse), discussed in Chapter 7.

Sulfamethoxazole-trimethoprim (Bactrim, Bactrim DS, Cotrim, Cotrim DS, Septra, Septra DS, Sulfatrim) should be taken with plenty of water. A sunscreen should be used, because this drug increases sensitivity to the sun.

Phenazopyridine (Azo-Standard, Pyridium, Uristat) is an over-the-counter (OTC) agent that has a local anesthetic effect on urinary tract mucosa. It colors the urine orange and stains anything it contacts. It should not be used for more than two days and should be taken with an antibiotic because phenazopyridine by itself does not have antimicrobial activity. It is used for the symptomatic relief of urinary burning, itching, frequency, and urgency in association with UTIs or following urologic procedures. Antibiotics are discussed in greater detail in Chapter 4.

Benign Prostatic Hyperplasia

Benign prostatic hyperplasia (BPH) is one of the most common **prostatic diseases** that occur in older men. This abnormal enlargement of the prostate gland appears to occur with aging in combination with certain pathophysiologic influences. An enlarged prostate becomes a problem when it obstructs urine outflow from the bladder.

FIGURE 11.7
Male Urinary System

The prostate gland surrounds the neck of the bladder and releases prostatic fluid.

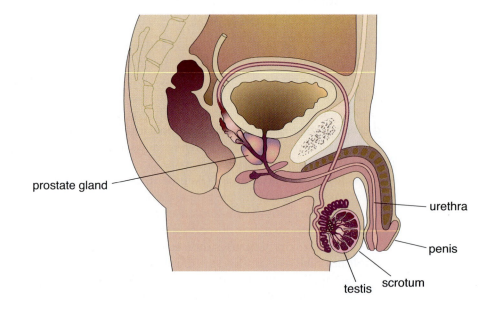

prostate gland

urethra

penis

testis   scrotum

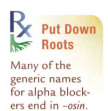

Put Down Roots

Many of the generic names for alpha blockers end in -*osin*.

Increasing evidence shows that nonsurgical interventions, especially drug therapy, may be effective as a primary treatment for selected patients with BPH. Alpha blockers and 5-alpha-reductase inhibitors represent promising and innovative approaches to pharmacologic management of BPH. Some drug therapies cause urinary retention and should not be used by patients with BPH. Potential alternative drugs are listed in Table 11.6.

Alpha Blockers

Alpha blockers are used to treat patients who have BPH, especially in those individuals who also have high blood pressure. These two conditions are a common combination in older men. These medications work by inhibiting the alpha-1 receptors in the prostate gland and bladder. This relaxes them as well as the blood vessels in the rest of the body. Commonly used alpha blockers for BPH appear in Table 11.7.

TABLE 11.6 Drugs to Avoid in BPH and Potential Substitutions

Drugs to Avoid	Potential Substitutions
Anticholinergics	Antacids, proton pump inhibitors (PPIs), sucralfate
Antihistamines	Nasal corticosteroids
Calcium channel blockers	Alpha blockers
Disopyramide	Quinidine
Oral bronchodilators	Inhaled bronchodilators
Tricyclic antidepressants (TCAs)	Selective serotonin reuptake inhibitors (SSRIs)

TABLE 11.7 Most Commonly Used Agents for BPH

Generic (Brand)	Pronunciation	Dosage Form	Dispensing Status
Alpha Blockers			
alfuzosin (Uroxatral)	al-FYOO-zoe-sin	Tablet	Rx
doxazosin (Cardura)	dox-AY-zoe-sin	Tablet	Rx
prazosin (Minipress)	PRAZ-oh-sin	Capsule	Rx
tamsulosin (Flomax)	tam-SOO-loe-sin	Capsule	Rx
terazosin (Hytrin)	ter-AY-zoe-sin	Capsule	Rx
5-Alpha-Reductase Inhibitors			
dutasteride (Avodart)	du-TAS-tur-ide	Capsule	Rx
dutasteride-tamsulosin (Jalyn)	du-TAS-tur-ide tam-SOO-loe-sin	Capsule	Rx
finasteride (Propecia, Proscar)	fin-AS-tur-ide	Tablet	Rx

In the urinary system, alpha blockers reduce urinary resistance and improve urine flow. They are sometimes used to help pass kidney stones that have become lodged in the ureters.

Common side effects of alpha blockers include dizziness, drowsiness, fatigue, headache, fainting, and **orthostatic hypotension**, which is a drop in blood pressure that causes dizziness when transitioning from sitting or lying down to standing up. Rising slowly from a seated or lying position can alleviate this effect.

Alpha blockers also have sexual side effects that are very rare but serious. One such effect is **priapism**, a prolonged and painful erection. If this condition occurs, patients should seek medical attention immediately to prevent permanent damage and impotence.

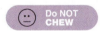

Alfuzosin (Uroxatral) may have fewer side effects than other alpha blockers and may be better tolerated. It does not require titration. The primary side effects are hypotension and dizziness. Alfuzosin helps relax the muscles in the prostate gland and the opening of the bladder, which improves the passage of urine. It should be taken with the same meal each day, and never on an empty stomach. Because it is a long-acting tablet, alfuzosin is dosed once a day. Therefore, the coating of the tablet must remain intact, and patients should not split, chew, or crush the tablets.

Doxazosin (Cardura) is an alpha blocker that prevents the constriction of blood vessels. It lowers blood pressure in this way. It was also found to relax the muscles around the prostate gland, making urination easier. First doses can cause excessive lowering of blood pressure, so it is often recommended that these doses be taken at bedtime to prevent dizziness and fainting. The drug may cause swelling of the ankles as well as fatigue.

Prazosin (Minipress) is a selective alpha blocker, approved for treating hypertension. Several studies have shown benefits in patients who have BPH, and the number of patients using this drug is increasing. Orthostatic hypotension is common, but this effect can sometimes be minimized by initiating the therapy at bedtime.

Tamsulosin (Flomax) is an alpha blocker, but it is more selective than other alpha blockers. It has little effect on blood pressure but works well for BPH. Fasting increases tamsulosin's bioavailability. It is recommended that doses be administered 30 minutes after the same meal each day.

Terazosin (Hytrin) is a long-acting, selective alpha blocker approved for use as an antihypertensive agent. It produces significant improvement in obstructive symptoms and urinary flow rates. Its primary advantage over prazosin is a

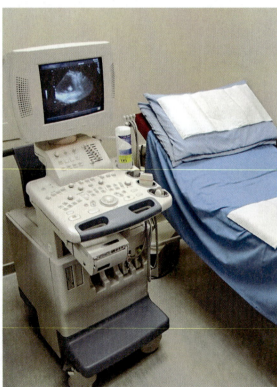

Along with digital rectal examinations and various body fluid tests, medical ultrasonography is often used to confirm a diagnosis of BPH.

longer half-life that allows for once-daily dosing and, presumably, better rates of patient adherence. The side effects of tiredness, dizziness, and orthostatic hypotension can be minimized by taking the drug at bedtime. Headache has also been reported. Prophylactic administration of acetaminophen, 650–675 mg a half hour before the terazosin dose, may lessen the severity of headache, which usually subsides after several weeks of treatment.

Contraindications Alfuzosin is contraindicated in patients with moderate-to-severe liver insufficiency and with medications that may increase its blood levels, such as itraconazole, ketoconazole, and ritonavir. Doxazosin and prazosin should be avoided in patients with a hypersensitivity to quinazolines. Tamsulosin and terazosin do not have any contraindications.

Cautions and Considerations Alpha blockers can have a first-dose effect, whereby blood pressure drops dramatically and causes dizziness or fainting. Patients are often observed closely during the first dose to monitor for this effect. Repeated blood pressure measurements may be required for four to six hours after taking the first dose. Consequently, patients should be careful about driving or operating machinery until they know how the medication affects them.

These agents must be used with caution in patients with GI disorders, liver disease, or kidney impairment. Alpha blockers can exacerbate GI motility disorders. Patients should inform their prescribers if they have any of these conditions before taking an alpha blocker. Healthcare practitioners should tell patients to take alpha blockers at night, before sleeping, and to avoid crushing or chewing alfuzosin, doxazosin, and tamsulosin. These medications should be swallowed whole.

Drug Interactions Alpha blockers may enhance the hypotensive effects of other drugs that lower blood pressure. For example, the hypotensive effects of beta blockers may be potentiated when used with alpha blockers. More than one alpha blocker should not be used at a time because of increased side effects. Cimetidine may exaggerate the hypotensive effects of tamsulosin.

5-Alpha-Reductase Inhibitors

The drug class known as **5-alpha-reductase inhibitors** is used to treat BPH, but these medications can also be used to treat male-pattern hair loss (see Table 11.7). The 5-alpha-reductase inhibitors work by inhibiting the conversion of testosterone into its active form, DHT in the prostate gland, hair follicles, and other androgen-sensitive tissues. Impeding this process reduces the size of the prostate because prostate tissue growth is testosterone dependent. Although blocking testosterone altogether would reduce prostate size, the side effects of reduced androgen production in the body are undesirable for most patients. With this class of drugs, only DHT production is blocked, thereby reducing prostate size while allowing adequate levels of testosterone to remain in the bloodstream.

Common side effects of 5-alpha-reductase inhibitors include decreased libido, erectile dysfunction, and ejaculation disorders. These medications can also cause **gynecomastia** (breast enlargement in men or boys). If these effects are bothersome, patients should speak with their prescribers to determine if drug therapy should be discontinued.

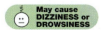

Dutasteride (Avodart) blocks both type 1 and type 2 5-alpha-reductase. It has been shown to shrink the prostate, keep it smaller, improve symptoms, and decrease the risk of long-term symptoms. It has also shown excellent results in the treatment and reversal of male pattern hair loss. Pregnant women should not handle this drug. It may take up to six months before urinary symptoms improve.

A combination drug, **dutasteride-tamsulosin (Jalyn)**, is used to treat an enlarged prostate in men with BPH. Dutasteride prevents the conversion of testosterone to dihydrotestosterone (DHT), which causes BPH. Tamsulosin relaxes the muscles in the prostate and bladder neck, making it easier to urinate. Because this combination medication causes birth defects, pregnant women should not handle it, and anyone taking it should not donate blood until at least six months after discontinuing the drug. Dizziness is the primary side effect. The pharmacy technician needs to be especially aware of interactions with this drug, and should inform the pharmacist if necessary.

Finasteride (Propecia, Proscar) blocks the enzyme that converts testosterone to DHT. The inhibition affects only DHT production and not testosterone, so the side effects of general androgen blockade are minimized. The drug results in an increase in intracellular testosterone levels, thereby minimizing sexual dysfunction, the primary drawback of hormonal therapy. The benefits of finasteride include:

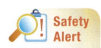
Safety Alert

Proscar (the brand name of finasteride), Prozac (the brand name of the antidepressant fluoxetine), and Prosom (the brand name of estazolam, a sleep inducer, now discontinued) could easily be confused.

- a reduction in prostate size, similar to the effect associated with other forms of androgen withdrawal;
- improved urine flow and symptom relief, similar to the effects associated with other forms of androgen withdrawal;
- minimal drug-related adverse effects, and
- a decrease in male pattern hair loss.

Finasteride is available as film-coated tablets. Crushed finasteride tablets or finasteride powder should not be handled by a woman who is or may become pregnant because it may present a risk to a male fetus.

Contraindications Dutasteride and finasteride are contraindicated in women of childbearing age.

Cautions and Considerations Because these agents block an active form of testosterone production, they could be harmful to a developing fetus in utero. Women of childbearing age must not handle these agents with bare skin. They should wear gloves to prevent measurable absorption of 5-alpha-reductase inhibitors, especially if handling broken tablets or opened capsules. They should also avoid contact with semen from a male partner exposed to 5-alpha-reductase inhibitors.

Drug Interactions Dutasteride levels may be increased by cimetidine, clarithromycin, erythromycin, isoniazid, itraconazole, ketoconazole, and nefazodone. Dutasteride levels may be decreased by carbamazepine, rifamycin derivatives, and St. John's wort. Finasteride does not have drug interactions.

Diuretics

A **diuretic** is a substance that increases the volume of urine output. The primary purpose of using diuretics is to rid the body of excess fluid and electrolytes. Diuretics are most often used as adjunct therapy to improve urine output in patients with kidney disease, to reduce blood volume in patients with high blood pressure, or to treat edema. In addition, the effectiveness of certain drugs may be enhanced by combination with a diuretic. Table 11.8 presents the most commonly used diuretics.

TABLE 11.8 Most Commonly Used Diuretics

Generic (Brand)	Pronunciation	Dosage Form	Dispensing Status
Carbonic Anhydrase Inhibitor			
acetazolamide (Diamox)	a-seet-a-ZOLE-a-mide	Capsule, injection, tablet	Rx
Loop Diuretics			
bumetanide (Bumex)	byoo-MET-a-nide	Injection, tablet	Rx
ethacrynic acid (Edecrin)	eth-a-KRIN-ik AS-id	Injection, tablet	Rx
furosemide (Lasix)	fur-OH-se-mide	Injection, oral liquid, tablet	Rx
torsemide (Demadex)	TORE-se-mide	Injection, tablet	Rx
Potassium-Sparing Diuretics			
amiloride (Midamor)	a-MIL-oh-ride	Tablet	Rx
eplerenone (Inspra)	ep-LAIR-a-none	Tablet	Rx
spironolactone (Aldactone)	speer-on-oh-LAK-tone	Tablet	Rx
triamterene (Dyrenium)	trye-AM-ter-een	Capsule	Rx
Thiazide and Thiazide-Related Diuretics			
atenolol-chlorthalidone (Tenoretic)	a-TEN-oh-lawl chlor-THAL-i-doan	Tablet	Rx
bisoprolol-hydrochlorothiazide (Ziac)	bis-OH-proe-lawl hye-droe-klor-oh-THYE-a-zide	Tablet	Rx
chlorthalidone (Hygroton)	klor-THAL-i-doan	Tablet	Rx
chlorothiazide (Diuril)	klor-oh-THYE-a-zide	Injection, oral liquid, tablet	Rx
hydrochlorothiazide, HCTZ (Microzide)	hye-droe-klor-oh-THYE-a-zide	Capsule, tablet	Rx
indapamide (Lozol)	in-DAP-a-mide	Tablet	Rx
lisinopril-hydrochlorothiazide (Prinzide, Zestoretic)	lyse-IN-oh-pril hye-droe-klor-oh-THYE-a-zide	Tablet	Rx
losartan-hydrochlorothiazide (Hyzaar)	loe-SAR-tan hye-droe-klor-oh-THYE-a-zide	Tablet	Rx
metolazone (Zaroxolyn)	me-TOLE-a-zone	Tablet	Rx
triamterene-hydrochlorothiazide (Dyazide, Maxide)	trye-AM-ter-een hye-droe-klor-oh-THYE-a-zide	Capsule, tablet	Rx

Classes of Diuretics

The various types of diuretics are discussed next in detail. Some diuretics, such as thiazide diuretics and potassium-sparing diuretics, tend to be used more for treating hypertension. Other diuretics, such as loop diuretics, are used more for treating kidney failure or reducing edema. Carbonic anhydrase inhibitors are usually used in patients with edema that have acid-base balance concerns. Combinations of these diuretic classes may be used in certain cases of kidney failure to maximize urine output.

Carbonic Anhydrase Inhibitor

Carbonic anhydrase inhibitors work in the nephrons by increasing excretion of bicarbonate ions, which carry sodium, potassium, and water into the urine. They increase urine volume and change the pH to alkaline. They are similar to sulfonamides in their chemical structure. These medications are used more frequently for open-angle glaucoma but are occasionally used for diuresis in congestive heart failure (CHF).

Common side effects of carbonic anhydrase inhibitors include **tinnitus** (ringing in the ears), tingling, nausea, vomiting, diarrhea, drowsiness, and changes in taste.

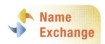

Acetazolamide (Diamox) is a commonly used carbonic anhydrase inhibitor. Acetazolamide has the unique indication of being used to prevent or treat symptoms associated with mountain sickness (or elevation change). Side effects include dizziness, drowsiness, and flushing. Oral acetazolamide may cause alteration in taste or leave a bitter flavor in the mouth.

Contraindications Acetazolamide should not be used in patients with a hypersensitivity to sulfonamides, liver disease or insufficiency, decreased sodium or potassium levels, adrenocortical insufficiency, cirrhosis, hyperchloremic acidosis, and severe kidney disease or dysfunction. Long-term use in narrow-angle glaucoma is contraindicated. It should also be avoided with concurrent aspirin use.

Cautions and Considerations Carbonic anhydrase inhibitors may have cross-reactivity in patients with a sulfa allergy. If patients experience a rash while taking one of these agents, they should notify their prescribers immediately.

Drug Interactions Use of more than one carbonic anhydrase inhibitor is not recommended. Salicylates may enhance the adverse effects of carbonic anhydrase inhibitors.

Loop Diuretics

Name Exchange

Even though the loop diuretic furosemide is widely available as a generic, it is often referred to in practice by its brand name, Lasix.

Loop diuretics work by inhibiting reabsorption of sodium, chloride, and water in the ascending loop of Henle. This unique site of action produces fast and profound diuresis (urine production). Sodium, chloride, magnesium, calcium, and potassium are all excreted quickly and efficiently with the use of a loop diuretic. For this reason, loop diuretics are used to pull fluid out of the body rapidly. Typically, these agents are used to treat swelling and fluid accumulation due to heart or kidney failure. Side effects of loop diuretics are similar to those of thiazide diuretics and include hypotension, dizziness, headache, rash, hair loss (alopecia), upset stomach, diarrhea, and constipation. Patients should be reminded to rise slowly from seated or lying positions to help with dizziness and decreases in blood pressure.

Bumetanide (Bumex) is a potent loop diuretic that can be administered orally or intravenously. Bumetanide has a black box warning for a risk of profound electrolyte depletion with excessive dosing. Careful medical supervision is required in patients using this drug. Patients may need to supplement potassium while using bumetanide.

Ethacrynic acid (Edecrin) is a loop diuretic that should not be used in patients who have a CrCl level that is <10 mL/min. It can be used orally or intravenously.

Furosemide (Lasix) is one of the most commonly used loop diuretics. It should be given in two doses per day at a six- to eight-hour interval. This dosage schedule produces more beneficial results, less toxicity, and fewer side effects. Also, if the first dose is given in morning and the next dose is given six hours later, the patient will not be up going to the bathroom all night.

Torsemide (Demadex) is a loop diuretic available in both oral and IV formulations. However, the IV form should be reserved for patients who require rapid diuresis. The IV and oral forms do not require dose conversion. Ototoxicity has been reported with oral and IV torsemide use.

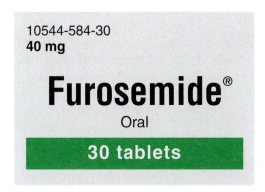

Contraindications Loop diuretics are contraindicated in patients with anuria (not producing urine). Bumetanide should not be used in patients with hepatic coma or severe electrolyte depletion. Ethacrynic acid should not be used in patients with a history of severe watery diarrhea with use and should not be used in infants.

Cautions and Considerations Loop diuretics deplete potassium levels in the body. Taking potassium supplements is often necessary with these diuretics to maintain proper electrolyte balance.

Drug Interactions Loop diuretics enhance the ability of other hypertensives to decrease blood pressure. Nonsteroidal anti-inflammatory drugs may decrease the efficacy of loop diuretics.

Potassium-Sparing Diuretics

Potassium-sparing diuretics work by blocking the exchange of potassium for sodium that takes place in the distal tubule. Therefore, more sodium is excreted while potassium is preserved in the body. Water follows sodium and, therefore, water is excreted along with sodium ions without depleting the body of potassium, which may happen with thiazide and loop diuretics. These drugs are used primarily to treat hypertension.

Aldosterone antagonists can be considered potassium-sparing, but these agents work by inhibiting a hormone that promotes fluid retention. Spironolactone, an older medication with this activity, works by inhibiting aldosterone, which promotes sodium and water reabsorption in the distal tubule and collecting duct of the nephron. Spironolactone is used primarily to treat hypertension and heart failure and sometimes may be used in **hyperaldosteronism** (a condition in which the body produces too much aldosterone).

Side effects of potassium-sparing diuretics can include gynecomastia. If bothersome, this effect may limit therapy because there is no treatment for it, other than to stop taking the drug. Other, less common side effects include upset stomach, headache, confusion, and drowsiness.

Spironolactone (Aldactone) is an antagonist of aldosterone, which in itself will promote potassium preservation. It may be used to treat edema, heart failure, primary hyperaldosteronism, and hypokalemia. Spironolactone is sometimes used to treat female hormonal acne.

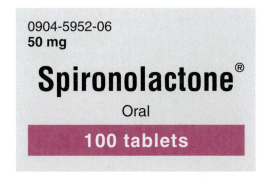

Amiloride (Midamor) is a potassium-sparing diuretic that is only available in an oral form. It should be administered with food to reduce upset stomach. Dose reduction is necessary in patients who have kidney dysfunction.

Eplerenone (Inspra) is a selective aldosterone blocker. It is 100 times more specific in its affinity for aldosterone than spironolactone, a first-generation aldosterone blocker. Eplerenone prevents sodium and water retention in the kidneys, thereby reducing blood volume and blood pressure. It is used for the treatment of hypertension alone or in combination with other drugs, and it is also indicated for the treatment of CHF after an acute myocardial infarction (MI). Potassium levels should be monitored when this drug is being taken. Patients should avoid foods containing salt substitutes and bananas. Hyperkalemia is the primary side effect.

Triamterene (Dyrenium) is a potassium-sparing diuretic. It is only available in an oral form and has a unique side effect. Triamterene can change the urine color to blue-green. Triamterene-hydrochlorothiazide (Dyazide, Maxzide) is a widely used combination diuretic. Even though this is a thiazide combination, it should not reduce potassium levels because triamterene is included.

Contraindications Potassium-sparing diuretics should not be used in the presence of elevated serum potassium, kidney insufficiency or impairment, or anuria. Amiloride should not be used if a patient is taking other potassium-conserving agents or supplements, or if that patient has diabetic nephropathy. Spironolactone is contraindicated in Addison's disease or other conditions associated with elevated potassium levels and with concomitant eplerenone use.

Contraindications to triamterene include severe liver disease and coadministration with other potassium-sparing agents.

Cautions and Considerations Potassium-sparing agents can cause hyperkalemia (high potassium levels) because they promote potassium retention. Periodic laboratory tests are needed to monitor for this effect.

Drug Interactions Potassium-sparing diuretics should be administered with caution in patients using drugs that increase potassium (such as ACE inhibitors).

Thiazide and Thiazide-Related Diuretics

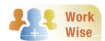
Work Wise

Hydrochlorothiazide is a commonly used thiazide diuretic. You may hear other healthcare practitioners refer to hydrochlorothiazide by its abbreviation, HCTZ.

A **thiazide diuretic** works by blocking a molecular pump that pulls sodium and chloride back into the blood from the distal tubule. Therefore, thiazides promote sodium and water excretion in the urine, lower the sodium level in the blood, and reduce vasoconstriction. These drugs have similar potencies but may differ in onset, peak, and duration of action. The increased sodium concentrations in the urine lead to an increased exchange of potassium for sodium, so potassium is lost too. Therefore, side effects of thiazide diuretics include hypokalemia, and patients should be told to ingest potassium (bananas, orange juice, citrus fruits) daily. Hypomagnesemia, hyperuricemia, hyperglycemia, and hypercalcemia are other side effects. A few patients become more sensitive to sunlight when taking a thiazide.

Chlorthalidone (Hygroton) inhibits sodium and chloride reabsorption in the cortical-diluting segment of the ascending loop of Henle. The primary side effect is hypokalemia. Chlorthalidone should be taken with food or milk early in the day; with multiple doses, the last dose should be taken no later than 6 p.m. to prevent **nocturia** (nighttime urination).

Atenolol-chlorthalidone (Tenoretic) is a cardioselective beta blocker combined with a diuretic, which is used to treat hypertension.

Hydrochlorothiazide (Microzide) is a thiazide diuretic that is only available in an oral form. Dosage forms include both capsules and tablets. Hydrochlorothiazide may be taken once or twice daily.

Bisoprolol-hydrochlorothiazide (Ziac) is a beta blocker combined with a diuretic. It can cause dizziness, headache, diarrhea, and fatigue.

Chlorothiazide (Diuril) is a thiazide diuretic that works by inhibiting sodium, chloride, and water reabsorption. This combined action leads to increased excretion of sodium, chloride, and water, which results in diuresis. Chlorothiazide is available in oral and injectable forms. The injection should only be given intravenously (never IM or SQ).

Indapamide (Lozol) enhances sodium, chloride, and water excretion by interfering with the transport of sodium ions across the renal tubular epithelium. The effect is localized at the proximal segment of the distal tubule of the nephron.

Lisinopril-hydrochlorothiazide (Prinzide, Zestoretic) is a combination ACE inhibitor and thiazide diuretic used for the treatment of hypertension, heart failure, and acute MI.

Losartan-hydrochlorothiazide (Hyzaar) is an ARB combined with a thiazide diuretic used for the treatment of hypertension and stroke risk reduction.

Metolazone (Zaroxolyn) inhibits sodium reabsorption in the distal tubules, causing an increased excretion of sodium, water, potassium, and hydrogen ions. It should be taken with food early in the day to prevent nocturia; the last dose should be taken no later than 6 p.m. It may increase a patient's sensitivity to sunlight.

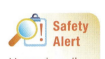

Safety Alert

Hyzaar is easily confused with Cozaar, which is simply losartan, the ARB component.

Contraindications Thiazide diuretics are related to sulfonamide drugs and therefore are contraindicated in patients with a hypersensitivity to sulfonamides. Thiazide diuretics are also contraindicated in patients with anuria. Metolazone has the additional contraindication of hepatic coma or precoma.

Cautions and Considerations Thiazide diuretics deplete potassium levels in the body. Taking potassium supplements with these diuretics is often necessary to maintain proper electrolyte balance. Patients should understand that taking these supplements is important because potassium is essential for effective cardiac function.

Drug Interactions Thiazide diuretics can interact with alcohol to contribute to drops in blood pressure. Patients should use caution when drinking alcohol while taking these medications. Thiazides also interact with drugs used to treat diabetes because they can raise blood glucose levels. However, this interaction is not a concern if a low-dose drug regimen is followed. In addition, thiazide diuretics interact with corticosteroids and lithium, so they are not usually used with them. Thiazide and thiazide-like diuretics may increase the QT-prolonging effects of dofetilide.

Complementary and Alternative Therapies

Saw palmetto is used to treat BPH symptoms, such as frequent or painful urination, as well as urinary hesitancy and urgency. Clinical studies have shown that this herbal treatment may have efficacy similar to that of finasteride in reducing these symptoms. Saw palmetto does not shrink overall prostate gland size; it works by reducing the thickness of the inner layer. It inhibits 5-alpha-reductase, which prevents conversion of testosterone to DHT. It has some anti-inflammatory effects but does not reduce prostate-specific antigen (PSA) levels. Side effects are mild and include dizziness,

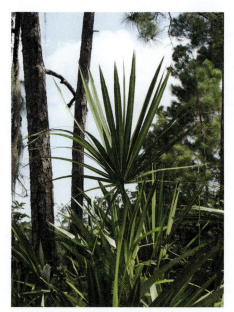

Saw palmetto may be used to treat patients with for BPH.

headache, nausea, vomiting, constipation, and diarrhea. Drug interactions with anticoagulants and some hormone therapies are possible. Patients should inform their physicians and pharmacists if they take saw palmetto. Typical doses are 160 mg twice a day or 320 mg once a day. Saw palmetto teas do not generally provide a high-enough dose to be effective.

Cranberry juice is used for the prevention of recurrent UTIs. Clinical trials have shown that daily ingestion of 16 ounces of cranberry juice is effective in preventing UTIs in elderly women, pregnant women, and inpatients. Oral capsules are not as effective. Although initially thought to acidify urine, cranberry juice is now thought to work by adhering to bacterial cells and preventing them from attaching to the inner walls of the bladder. Cranberry juice does not release bacteria that have already adhered to the bladder wall, so it does not treat an active UTI. Although side effects are few, cranberry juice, when consumed in large quantities, can cause stomach upset and diarrhea. Cranberry juice can interact with warfarin, so patients drinking it on a regular basis or in large amounts should let their healthcare practitioners know.

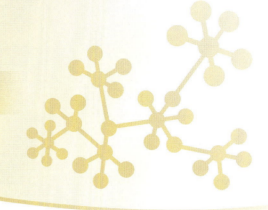

CHAPTER SUMMARY

Function of the Renal System

- The main function of the kidneys is to maintain the balance of water, electrolytes, and acids and bases in the body.

- The kidneys form urine, which is essential for normal body function.

- Acute renal failure is a rapid reduction in kidney function resulting in accumulation of nitrogen and other waste.

- Creatinine clearance is often used to assess renal function.

- Kidney disease is classified in stages (I–V).

Acute Kidney Injury and Chronic Kidney Disease

- Kidney disease treatment often involves therapy for hypertension.

- Most patients with renal failure show evidence of erythropoietin deficiency.

- Dialysis can be a lifesaving intervention for patients with kidney disease.

- If a renal transplant is necessary, the patient must take drugs to prevent the rejection of the new organ. Mycophenolic acid (Myfortic) is indicated specifically to prevent rejection of the kidney.

Drugs for Urinary Tract Disorders

- Urinary incontinence often affects older adults. Many medications are available for patients with urinary incontinence, including fesoterodine, flavoxate, oxybutynin, solifenacin, tolterodine, and trospium. Drugs for urinary incontinence have anticholinergic side effects such as dry mouth and constipation.

- BPH commonly affects older men.

- Alpha blockers, used to treat BPH, are associated with dizziness, fatigue, orthostatic hypotension, and priapism.

- Dutasteride (Avodart) and finasteride (Propecia, Proscar) are 5-alpha-reductase inhibitors used to treat BPH.

Diuretics

- The primary action of diuretics is to rid the body of excess fluid and electrolytes.

- Diuretics have different mechanisms of action. They are classified by where and how they work in the kidney: carbonic anhydrase inhibitors, loop diuretics, potassium sparing diuretics, and thiazide or thiazide-type diuretics.

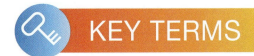

KEY TERMS

acute kidney injury a decrease in kidney function

acute renal failure a rapid reduction in kidney function resulting in the accumulation of nitrogen and other wastes

aldosterone antagonists agents that work by inhibiting a hormone that promotes fluid retention

alpha blockers drugs used to treat patients who have BPH; they block constriction of blood vessels, which may lead to vasodilation and hypotension

5-alpha-reductase inhibitors a class of drugs used to treat BPH and male-pattern hair loss

anemia a below-normal concentration of erythrocytes or hemoglobin in the blood

benign prostatic hyperplasia (BPH) an abnormal enlargement of the prostate gland, usually associated with aging

blood urea nitrogen (BUN) a blood test used to diagnose and monitor kidney function

carbonic anhydrase inhibitor a diuretic that acts in the proximal tubule to increase urine volume and change the pH from acidic to alkaline

chronic kidney disease (CKD) disease that involves progressive damage to the kidney tissue, resulting in the death of this tissue over time

Cockcroft and Gault equation a common formula used to calculate creatinine clearance (CrCl)

creatinine clearance (CrCl) a value used to determine kidney health; found from the amount of creatinine in urine and blood and also the amount of urine passed in 24 hours

detrusor muscles muscles that cause the bladder to contract and the external urinary sphincter to relax

dialysate a special fluid that draws toxins from the body into itself

dialysis an artificial method of filtering blood and correcting the electrolyte imbalances caused by kidney failure

diuretic a substance that rids the body of excess fluid and electrolytes by increasing the urine output

erythropoietin a hormone secreted by the kidneys that stimulates the production of red blood cells

external urinary sphincter a voluntary muscle that holds urine in the bladder before it exits the body

filtration the removal of substances from the blood as part of the formation of urine by the renal tubules

glomerular filtration rate (GFR) a value used to determine kidney health; an estimate of how much blood passes through glomeruli each minute

gynecomastia breast enlargement in men or boys

hemodialysis the process of diverting blood flow through a machine that mechanically filters blood and returns the blood to the body

hyperaldosteronism a condition in which the body produces too much aldosterone

hypercalcemia a condition in which the calcium level in the blood is above normal, with symptoms including weakened bones and kidney stones

hypocalcemia a condition in which the calcium level in the blood is below normal

incontinence an uncontrolled leaking of urine from the bladder

internal urinary sphincter an involuntary muscle that keeps urine from flowing back into the ureters once it enters the bladder

kidney a bean-shaped organ that filter excess minerals and water from the body to the bladder

kidney transplantation the process of surgically implanting a kidney from a living or deceased donor into a recipient

loop diuretic a drug that inhibits the reabsorption of sodium and chloride in the loop of Henle, thereby causing an increased urinary output

micturition the process in which detrusor muscles relax the external urinary sphincter, so urine is pushed out the body

national waiting list the list of candidates who are eligible for kidney transplant surgery; a person's place on the list depends on factors such as type of kidney problem, disease severity, and the likelihood of transplant success

nephron a glomerulotubular unit that is the working unit of the kidney

nocturia urinary frequency at night

orthostatic hypotension a drop in blood pressure upon positional change that causes dizziness

parenteral iron supplementation a process used in patients with CKD to replenish iron body stores in patients with iron deficiency

peritoneal dialysis a procedure that puts dialysate into the abdominal cavity and leaving it there for a certain period

potassium-sparing diuretic a drug that promotes excretion of water and sodium but inhibits the exchange of sodium for potassium

priapism a prolonged penile erection

prostatitis an inflammation of the prostate due to bacteria

reabsorption the process by which substances are pulled back into the blood after waste products have been removed during the formation of urine

renal artery a branch of the abdominal aorta that brings blood into the kidneys

renal cortex the outer layer of the kidneys; responsible for filtration

renal disease A disorder in which kidneys fail to filter waste products from the blood

renal medulla the structure that performs filtration in the kidneys

renal transplant drugs medications that assist the body in accepting a transplanted kidney

renal vein a vein that transfers filtered kidney blood back into the bloodstream

reticulocytes immature red blood cells

saw palmetto a plant that may provide treatment for BPH symptoms

secretion the release of cell products, including hydrogen and potassium ions, and acids and bases, into urine

serum creatinine (SCr) a blood test used to diagnose and monitor kidney function

thiazide diuretic a drug that blocks a pump that removes sodium and chloride together from the distal tubule

tinnitus ringing in the ears

uremia the clinical syndrome resulting from renal dysfunction in which excessive products of protein metabolism are retained in the blood

ureters paired muscular ducts that extend from the kidneys to the bladder

urinary analgesic a pain reliever used for treating UTIs

urinary bladder an organ that collects and holds urine until the fluid exits the body during urination

urinary incontinence the complaint of involuntary loss of urine

urinary retention A condition in which the kidneys when kidneys produce urine but the micturition process does not function properly, and urine accumulates in the bladder

urinary tract the group of organs that include the kidneys, ureters, bladder, and urethra; they are involved in the production and transportation of urine

urinary tract infection (UTI) an infection caused by bacteria, usually *E. coli*, that enter via the urethra and progress up the urinary tract; characterized by the presence of bacteria in the urine with localized symptoms

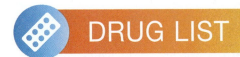

DRUG LIST

Renal Disease

Anemia Therapies
darbepoetin alfa (Aranesp)
epoetin alfa, erythropoietin (Epogen, Procrit)

Dialysis Therapies
cinacalcet (Sensipar)
sevelamer (Renagel, Renvela)

Supplemental Therapies
ergocalciferol, vitamin D (Deltalin, Drisdol)
ferumoxytol (Feraheme)
folic acid, vitamin B$_9$ (various brands)
iron dextran (INFeD)
iron sucrose (Venofer)
levocarnitine (Carnitor)
multiple vitamin complex (various brands)
pyridoxine, vitamin B$_6$ (various brands)
sodium ferric gluconate (Ferrlecit)

Renal Transplant Drugs
cyclosporine (Gengraf, Neoral Sandimmune)
mycophenolate (CellCept)
mycophenolic acid (Myfortic)
tacrolimus (Astagraf XL, Prograf)

Urinary Problems
darifenacin (Enablex)
fesoterodine (Toviaz)
flavoxate (Urispas)
oxybutynin (Ditropan, Oxytrol)
solifenacin (Vesicare)
tolterodine (Detrol)
trospium (Sanctura)

Medications to Treat UTIs

Antibiotics
amoxicillin (Amoxil)
amoxicillin-clavulanate (Augmentin)
ampicillin (Principen)
ciprofloxacin (Cipro)
methenamine (Cystex, Hiprex, Urex)
nitrofurantoin (Macrobid, Macrodantin)
sulfamethoxazole-trimethoprim (Bactrim, Bactrim DS, Cotrim, Cotrim DS, Septra, Septra DS, Sulfatrim)

Urinary Analgesic
phenazopyridine (Azo-Standard, Pyridium, Uristat)

BPH Agents

Alpha Blockers
alfuzosin (Uroxatral)
doxazosin (Cardura)
prazosin (Minipress)
tamsulosin (Flomax)
terazosin (Hytrin)

5-Alpha-Reductase Inhibitors
dutasteride (Avodart)
dutasteride-tamsulosin (Jalyn)
finasteride (Propecia, Proscar)

Diuretics

Carbonic Anhydrase Inhibitor
acetazolamide (Diamox)

Loop Diuretics
bumetanide (Bumex)
ethacrynic acid (Edecrin)
furosemide (Lasix)
torsemide (Demadex)

Potassium-Sparing Diuretics
amiloride (Midamor)
eplerenone (Inspra)
spironolactone (Aldactone)
triamterene (Dyrenium)

Thiazide and Thiazide-Related Diuretics
atenolol-chlorthalidone (Tenoretic)
bisoprolol-hydrochlorothiazide (Ziac)
chlorthalidone (Hygroton)
chlorothiazide (Diuril)
hydrochlorothiazide, HCTZ (Microzide)
indapamide (Lozol)
lisinopril-hydrochlorothiazide (Prinzide, Zestoretic)
losartan-hydrochlorothiazide (Hyzaar)
metolazone (Zaroxolyn)
triamterene-hydrochlorothiazide (Dyazide, Maxzide)

Black Box Warnings
amiloride (Midamor)
cyclosporine (Sandimmune)
epoetin alfa, erythopoietin (Epogen, Procrit)
iron dextran (Infed)
metolazone (Zaroxolyn)
mycophenolic acid (Myfortic)
mycophenolate mofetil (CellCept)
nilutamide (Nilandron)
tacrolimus (Astagraf XL, Prograf)
triamterene (Dyrenium)
spironolactone (Aldactone)

Medication Guides
ciprofloxacin (Cipro)
darbepoetin alfa (Aranesp)
epoetin alfa, erythropoietin (Epogen, Procrit)
mycophenolate mofetil (CellCept)
mycophenolic acid (Myfortic)

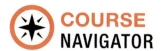

COURSE NAVIGATOR

Access interactive chapter review exercises, practice activities, flash cards, and study games.

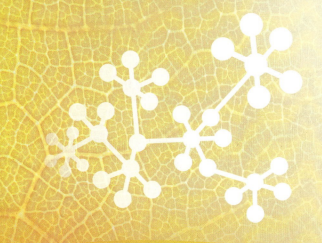

Drugs for Cardiovascular Diseases

12

Learning Objectives

1. Describe the anatomy and physiology of the cardiovascular system.

2. Describe the drugs and treatments for each type of cardiovascular disease.

3. Recognize anticoagulant and antiplatelet drugs, and describe their functions.

4. Explain a cerebrovascular accident (CVA) and the drugs used to treat it.

5. Identify drugs used to treat hyperlipidemia, and understand its role in heart disease and cerebrovascular accident treatment.

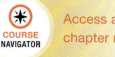

COURSE NAVIGATOR

Access additional chapter resources.

Cardiovascular diseases (those affecting the heart and blood vessels) account for a significant percentage of morbidity and mortality. Cardiovascular problems include arrhythmias, heart failure, myocardial infarction, angina, hypertension, coagulation, and excessive cholesterol in the blood. Many causative factors can be modified by lifestyle changes, and some are amenable to prophylaxis. Drugs have been developed to help manage these diseases. Drug therapy discussed in this chapter includes a large percentage of the most commonly prescribed drugs. Pharmacy technicians will encounter these drugs frequently on the job, and should commit them to memory.

The Cardiovascular System

The **cardiovascular system**, which includes the heart and blood vessels, circulates blood throughout the body, bringing needed oxygen and nutrients to tissues and carrying away carbon dioxide and toxic by-products. Without a properly functioning cardiovascular system, life is not sustainable. The heart pumps blood to the body through **arteries**, which carry blood away from the heart, and receives blood back from the tissues through **veins** (see Figure 12.1). In the **capillaries** (tiny blood vessels), critical fluids, gases, and nutrients are exchanged between the blood and body tissues. The heart also pumps blood through the lungs, where the blood is replenished with oxygen and releases carbon dioxide, which is then exhaled.

FIGURE 12.1
Blood Flow through the Cardiovascular System

Oxygenated blood is depicted in red, whereas blood returning from the body, in need of oxygen, is shown in blue.

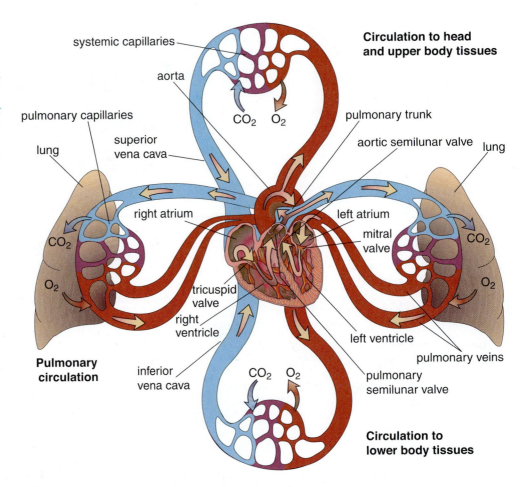

systemic capillaries

Circulation to head and upper body tissues

aorta

pulmonary capillaries

CO_2 O_2

pulmonary trunk

lung

superior vena cava

aortic semilunar valve lung

right atrium

left atrium

CO_2

mitral valve

CO_2

O_2

O_2

tricuspid valve

right ventricle

left ventricle

pulmonary veins

Pulmonary circulation

inferior vena cava

CO_2 O_2

pulmonary semilunar valve

Circulation to lower body tissues

The Heart

The heart has three functional parts: the cardiac muscle (myocardium), conducting system, and blood supply. Figure 12.2 shows the functional anatomy of the heart, and Figure 12.3 shows the internal heart structure and vessels leading to and exiting from the heart. **Cardiovascular (CV) disease**, also known as *heart disease*, can involve any or all of these functional parts.

A normal heartbeat is the result of a coordinated series of electrical events. It begins in the membranes of specialized cells in the **sinoatrial (SA) node**, often called the heart's natural pacemaker. Between beats, these membranes are polarized; that is, the inside of the cell is at a negative voltage relative to the outside. The beat originates when ion channels in the cell membrane open to allow positively charged sodium and calcium ions to flow into the cell, making the voltage positive instead of negative (**depolarization**). Other channels then open to allow positively charged potassium ions to flow out of the cell, making the voltage negative again (**repolarization**). The resulting **action potential** (electrical transmission developed in a muscle or nerve cell during activity) propagates through the conduction system to the muscle cells of the myocardium. When the action potential arrives at a myocardial cell, it depolarizes with a rapid inflow of sodium and a slower inflow of calcium (which releases intracellular calcium and triggers the muscle to contract), and it repolarizes with an outflow of potassium.

If the depolarizing and repolarizing flows were the only ion flows, the cell would run out of potassium and accumulate huge amounts of sodium and calcium. Other proteins in the cell membrane continually restore the balance by using energy to pump sodium and calcium out and potassium in simultaneously.

FIGURE 12.2
Functional Anatomy of the Heart

(a) Cardiac muscle
(b) Conducting system
(c) Blood supply

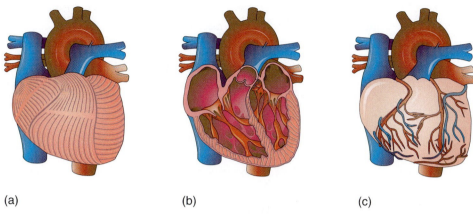

(a) (b) (c)

FIGURE 12.3
Internal Structures of the Heart

The heart is an organ with four chambers: the upper chambers are the right atrium and left atrium, and the lower chambers are the right ventricle and left ventricle.

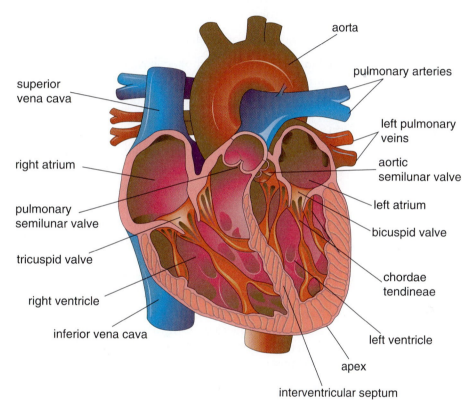

aorta

pulmonary arteries

superior vena cava

left pulmonary veins

aortic semilunar valve

right atrium

left atrium

pulmonary semilunar valve

bicuspid valve

tricuspid valve

chordae tendineae

right ventricle

left ventricle

inferior vena cava

apex

interventricular septum

The conduction system is arranged so that the action potential first arrives at the atria, which contract and pump blood received from veins into the ventricles, and then travels through the **atrioventricular (AV) node** to reach the ventricles, which pump blood out into the arteries. The first arteries to branch off from the aorta, which is the main artery from the left ventricle, are the coronary arteries, which carry oxygen and nutrients to the various parts of the heart itself. This conduction system is shown in Figure 12.4 on page 455.

Causative Factors of Cardiovascular Diseases

Various factors contribute to the development of CV diseases. Many cardiovascular problems develop because of poor health habits; however, some people are genetically predisposed to develop these problems. Even if a person has a genetic tendency toward a specific CV disease, proper diet, exercise, and rest can facilitate healthy heart function, prolong good health, and extend life span.

Predetermined factors include the following:

- **Heredity:** Children of parents with CV disease may have a higher risk of developing heart disease. Ethnicity may also play a role. For example, African Americans are two to three times more likely than other ethnic groups to have hypertension, or high blood pressure.
- **Gender:** Men face a greater risk of a myocardial infarction (MI), or heart attack, than women until age 55 years. At this age, a woman's risk increases tenfold and may surpass a man's if she smokes or has other conditions that cause CV disease.
- **Age:** More than half of all individuals who have had an MI are age 65 years or older. Of those who die from this condition, more than 80% are over age 65.

Other causative factors of CV disease can be influenced by lifestyle modification:

- **Cigarette smoking:** Smokers have more than twice the risk of an MI as nonsmokers. A smoker who has an MI is also more likely to die from it.
- **Hypertension:** High blood pressure stresses the heart over time and increases an individual's risk of a cerebrovascular accident (CVA), more commonly known as a *stroke*, or an MI. However, a nutritious diet, regular exercise, weight loss, reduction of salt intake, and drug therapy can lower blood pressure.
- **Hyperlipidemia:** Hyperlipidemia, a condition commonly referred to as *high cholesterol*, is associated with CV diseases. Too much cholesterol in the blood contributes to a buildup of plaque on the inner walls of the arteries that feed the heart and reduces blood flow to the heart. A diet low in saturated fats helps to lower blood cholesterol levels. Drugs can also lower blood cholesterol levels.
- **Obesity:** Obesity puts an added strain on the heart. This condition increases an individual's blood volume, blood pressure, and cholesterol levels. Obesity can also be a predisposing condition for diabetes.
- **Diabetes:** Individuals who have diabetes may have associated vascular problems. Consequently, they are prone to develop CV disease and are at an increased risk for an MI. Maintaining a healthy diet and weight, in conjunction with exercise and drugs, can help keep diabetes in check.

As this list indicates, lifestyle modification plays a critical role in reducing the risk of CV disease. The value of smoking cessation, dietary modifications, weight control, physical exercise, and adherence to a drug regimen should not be underestimated. The treatment of cardiovascular diseases requires permanent changes in lifestyle and may require drug therapy.

Angina

Angina pectoris (often referred to simply as *angina*) is chest pain due to an imbalance between oxygen supply and oxygen demand. Oxygen demand is directly related to heart rate, strength of contraction, and resistance to blood flow. **Ischemia** is an inadequate blood supply to an organ, especially the heart muscles. In angina, the inadequate blood supply does not cause the irreversible changes related to obstruction or narrowing of coronary arteries that occur in atherosclerosis, arterial spasm, pulmonary hypertension, and cardiac hypertrophy (enlargement of the heart).

Common types of angina include the following:

- **Stable angina** is characterized by effort-induced pain from physical activity or emotional stress. This pain is relieved by rest and is usually predictable and reproducible. Stable angina is the most common form.
- **Unstable angina** is characterized by pain that occurs with increasing frequency, diminishes the patient's ability to work, and has a decreasing response to treatment. It may signal an oncoming MI.
- **Variant angina** is characterized by pain due to a coronary artery spasm. This pain may occur at certain times of the day and is often induced by cold weather, stress, medications that constrict blood vessels, or smoking.

Symptoms and Risk Factors of Angina

The characteristic symptom of angina is severe chest discomfort, which may be described as heaviness, pressure, tightness, choking, a squeezing sensation, or a combination of these sensations. Other symptoms may include sweating, dizziness, and dyspnea (shortness of breath). Diagnosis is made from physical examination, electrocardiograms (ECGs), a coronary angiogram, and a radioisotope study. In angina, the ECG may be normal, but the T wave, discussed later in the chapter, is usually flat or inverted. Anginal pain is usually brief and predictable, often precipitated by exercise or emotional stress.

The risk factors for angina include the following:

- advanced age
- coronary artery disease (CAD)
- hypertension
- increased serum glucose levels (diabetes)
- increased serum lipoprotein levels
- obesity
- smoking
- type A personality

The following factors may initiate an anginal attack:

- cold weather (freezing air causes the body to constrict blood vessels)
- emotions (stressful situations can cause constriction)
- heavy meals (blood flow to the gut increases, resulting in decreased flow to the brain and heart)
- hypoglycemia (can lead to increased production of hormones associated with stress)
- pain (increases stress levels)
- smoking (nicotine causes arterial constriction and contributes to arteriosclerosis)

Antianginal Drugs

Angina may be relieved with rest. Treatment goals are to reduce symptoms and prevent heart attacks. Three major classes of drugs are used in the treatment of angina: beta blockers, calcium channel blockers, and nitrates. A fourth type of drug, ranolazine (Ranexa), is a metabolic modifier and is distinct from the drugs of the other three groups.

Beta Blockers

As described in Chapter 6, in response to increased anxiety, physical activity, or emotional stress, the sympathetic nervous system stimulates the release of catecholamines (the class of neurotransmitters that includes epinephrine and norepinephrine). The action of these neurotransmitters on the beta-1 receptors, in particular, increases heart rate and contractile force.

A **beta blocker** is a drug that is similar in molecular structure to a catecholamine and, therefore, competes for the same receptor sites. This action, in turn, inhibits neurotransmitter activity.

Beta blockers are designed to exert action on two types of beta receptors: beta-1 receptors and beta-2 receptors. Beta-1 receptors are found primarily in the heart and kidneys. Beta-2 receptors are found primarily in the lungs. In choosing a drug for the heart, a drug with more beta-1 blockage than beta-2 blockage may be preferred because beta-1 receptors are associated with cardiovascular function. Drugs that block beta-2 receptors can adversely affect respiration in patients with asthma, chronic obstructive pulmonary disease (COPD), or other respiratory problems. Beta blockers that are more selective for beta-1 receptors than beta-2 receptors are referred to as cardioselective beta blockers. Certain beta blockers also exhibit membrane-stabilizing and intrinsic sympathomimetic activity. More information on beta blockers can be found in Table 12.1.

Beta blockers are used to treat angina pectoris because of their effectiveness in slowing the heart rate, decreasing myocardial contractility, and lowering blood pressure, particularly during exercise. All of these actions reduce oxygen demand; thus, beta blockers reduce the frequency and severity of angina attacks. Beta blockers are also used to treat arrhythmias and hypertension and are most commonly used following an MI. They have been shown to improve morbidity and mortality rates. Though often the drug of choice in the early stages of heart failure (HF), beta blockers do not generally work well in decompensated heart failure (unstable patients). However, bisoprolol, carvedilol, and metoprolol have been approved to treat HF.

Most adverse reactions to beta blockers are mild and transient and rarely require withdrawal of therapy. The most common adverse reaction is fatigue. Beta blockers should not be withdrawn abruptly. Dosage should be reduced gradually over one to two weeks. The primary side effect of beta blockers is **bradycardia** (slowed heart rate). These drugs also mask symptoms of hyperthyroidism and hypoglycemia. For that reason, patients who have diabetes should avoid taking these medications. Beta blockers should also be used with caution in patients with bronchospastic disease because these drugs may inhibit the bronchodilating effects of endogenous catecholamines.

Acebutolol (Sectral) and **pindolol (Visken)** are beta blockers that have intrinsic sympathomimetic activity, so they reduce the heart rate less than other beta blockers. Side effects are bradycardia, increased airway resistance, fluid retention, masked signs of hypoglycemia, and depression.

Atenolol (Tenormin), **betaxolol (Kerlone)**, and **bisoprolol (Zebeta)** are beta-1 selective blockers. They are commonly used for hypertension, but they may also be used to treat angina and atrial fibrillation. Atenolol, betaxolol, and bisoprolol are available in oral formulations and may be taken without regard to meals.

Carvedilol (Coreg), the first beta blocker approved for the treatment of HF, is a nonselective beta blocker with vasodilating effects. The patient is started on a low dose, which is slowly increased. If the drug is taken with food, the risk of dizziness or **orthostatic hypotension** (a sudden rise in blood pressure upon standing) may be reduced. It can be used alone or in conjunction with other agents, especially thiazide diuretics, in the management of hypertension.

TABLE 12.1 Most Commonly Used Beta Blockers

Generic (Brand)	Pronunciation	Dosage Form	Dispensing Status
acebutolol (Sectral)	a-se-BYOO-toe-lawl	Capsule	Rx
atenolol (Tenormin)	a-TEN-oh-lawl	Tablet	Rx
betaxolol (Kerlone)	be-TAX-oh-lawl	Tablet	Rx
bisoprolol (Zebeta)	bis-OE-proe-lawl	Tablet	Rx
carvedilol (Coreg)	KAR-ve-dil-awl	Capsule, tablet	Rx
esmolol (Brevibloc)	ES-moe-lawl	Injection	Rx
labetalol (Normodyne, Trandate)	la-BET-a-lawl	Injection, tablet	Rx
metoprolol (Lopressor, Toprol-XL)	me-TOE-proe-lawl	Injection, tablet	Rx
nadolol (Corgard)	naye-DOE-lawl	Tablet	Rx
nebivolol (Bystolic)	neh-BIV-oe-lawl	Tablet	Rx
pindolol (Visken)	PIN-doe-lawl	Tablet	Rx
propranolol (Hemangeol, Inderal, InnoPran XL)	proe-PRAN-oh-lawl	Capsule, injection, oral liquid, tablet	Rx
sotalol (Betapace, Sorine, Sotylize)	SOE-ta-lawl	Injection, oral solution, tablet	Rx
timolol (Blocadren)	TYE-moe-lawl	Tablet	Rx

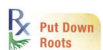

Put Down Roots

The generic names of beta blockers all end in *-lol*.

Practice Tip

Metoprolol, a commonly used beta blocker, comes in various oral dosage forms. The tartrate form is an immediate-release tablet that is best taken with food. The succinate salt form is an extended-release tablet to be taken with or without food. Be sure that your patients know which form they are taking.

Esmolol (Brevibloc) is a beta-1 selective blocker available in an intravenous (IV) dosage form only. As such, esmolol is usually reserved for emergency situations (such as arrhythmias and intraoperative tachycardia).

Labetalol (Normodyne, Trandate) is an alpha blocker and a nonspecific beta blocker. Pharmacy technicians should watch for a patient with prescriptions for both of these brands of labetalol. Prescribers often do not realize that the two brands are the same drug, so a patient could risk getting a double dose. Side effects are the same as for acebutolol and pindolol.

Metoprolol (Lopressor, Toprol-XL) is a beta-1 selective blocker that is available in oral and IV formulations. Metoprolol is used to treat angina, hypertension, and an MI. Oral metoprolol comes in immediate-release and extended-release forms. The extended-release tablets have an additional indication of heart failure. These tablets may be divided in half; however, they should not be crushed or chewed. Immediate-release tablets should be taken with meals. The IV dose of metoprolol is much smaller than the oral dose.

Nadolol (Corgard) and **timolol (Blocadren)** are nonselective beta blockers. They are both available as oral tablets.

Nebivolol (Bystolic) is a beta-1 selective blocker that causes vasodilation by increasing the production of nitric acid. In this way, it is different from other beta blockers. Nebivolol is approved only for the treatment of hypertension. It reduces vascular resistance and large-artery stiffness. The dosage should be reduced gradually when the patient stops taking the drug. Nebivolol cannot be discontinued abruptly.

Propranolol (Hemangeol, Inderal, InnoPran XL) is a nonselective beta blocker. Propranolol is used for multiple disorders including angina, cardiomyopathy, essential tremor, hypertension, arrhythmias, prevention of MI, and migraine headache.

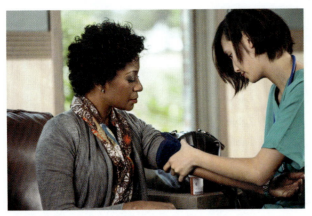
Beta blockers can be used to treat angina pectoris, arrhythmia, and hypertension.

Oral forms of propranolol include immediate-release and long-acting formulations. Immediate-release forms should be taken on an empty stomach; long-acting forms can be taken without regard to meals but should be taken consistently. Long-acting forms should not be crushed or chewed. Like metoprolol, the IV dose is much lower than the oral dose.

Sotalol (Betapace, Sorine, Sotylize) is indicated for the treatment of documented ventricular arrhythmia (e.g., sustained ventricular tachycardia, discussed later in this chapter) that, in the judgment of the physician, is life-threatening. The side effects are bradycardia, mental depression, and decreased sexual ability.

Contraindications Beta blockers are contraindicated in bradycardia (slow heart rate), cardiogenic shock, and heart block. Specific beta blockers may have additional contraindications. Atenolol should not be used in patients with pulmonary edema or in female patients who are pregnant. Carvedilol, labetalol, pindolol, propranolol, sotalol, and timolol are contraindicated in lung disorders such as asthma and COPD. Nebivolol should not be used in patients with liver impairment. Sotalol should be avoided in patients with long QT syndrome, kidney dysfunction, and low potassium levels.

Cautions and Considerations Atenolol, metoprolol, nadolol, propranolol, and timolol have black box warnings for increased cardiac symptoms (including worsening of angina and MI) with abrupt discontinuation. Gradual dose reduction is recommended over several weeks. Sotalol has a boxed warning for an increased risk of arrhythmia.

Blocking of beta-2 receptors constricts airways in the lungs in addition to lowering blood pressure. This effect can be harmful to patients with impaired respiratory function, for example, those with asthma or COPD. For these individuals, care must be taken to choose drugs that selectively block beta-1 receptors only. Beta blockers that can be used by patients with asthma or COPD include acebutolol, atenolol, betaxolol, bisoprolol, and metoprolol.

Abrupt withdrawal from a beta blocker can cause severe cardiac problems, such as an MI, angina, or arrhythmia. Thus, patients should not stop taking a beta blocker suddenly. If a change in medication is made, the dose will be decreased slowly until it is discontinued. Patients with diabetes should use beta blockers with caution. These drugs can inhibit the usual signs and symptoms of a reaction to low blood glucose. The only symptoms of low blood glucose that a patient taking a beta blocker may have are sweating and hunger. The pharmacist should counsel patients with diabetes who are taking beta blockers.

Drug Interactions Beta blockers may enhance the bradycardic effects of other drugs. Concurrent use with another drug that causes bradycardia is generally not recommended.

Beta blockers should not be used with beta agonists.

Over-the-counter (OTC) decongestants are vasoconstrictors that can raise blood pressure. Patients taking beta blockers to treat hypertension should avoid taking oral decongestants.

Sotalol should not be combined with other drugs that cause QT prolongation.

Nitrates

Nitrates relax vascular smooth muscle (venous more than arterial), which reduces venous return to the heart (**preload**) and cardiac filling and decreases tension in the heart walls. Nitrates dilate coronary vessels, allowing blood flow to redistribute to ischemic tissues. Because peripheral vasodilation decreases preload, nitroglycerin is also beneficial in the treatment of pulmonary edema in heart failure. Arterial vasodilation decreases arterial impedance (**afterload**), thereby lessening left ventricular work and aiding the failing heart. More information on nitrates can be found in Table 12.2.

Nitroglycerin (Minitran, Nitrolingual, Nitrostat, Nitro-Dur) is a common choice for acute anginal attacks. Nitroglycerin may be taken sublingually where the tablet is allowed to dissolve under the tongue. Nitroglycerin spray is applied under the tongue, one to two sprays every three to five minutes, with a maximum of three doses in a 15-minute period. If pain does not subside within five minutes after taking one dose of nitroglycerin, the patient should call 911. Both the tablets and the spray produce a stinging sensation under the tongue. Only the sublingual and translingual (absorption through the tongue into systemic circulation) routes should be used for acute attacks. Nitroglycerin may also be used as prophylaxis; in this case, the drug is taken a few minutes before the activity or stress that might cause an anginal attack.

Nitroglycerin patches (Nitro-Dur) should not be allowed to remain on the skin for 24 hours. There should be a patch-free time, usually when the patient is sleeping, or tolerance will develop. The label should instruct the patient in this procedure.

Nitroglycerin can cause severe headaches when first taken by a patient; aspirin or acetaminophen may provide relief. To prevent headaches, the dose of nitroglycerin can be reduced or, if administered as a patch or ointment, it can be placed lower on the body and gradually moved to the chest as the patient acclimates to the medication. Nitroglycerin can also cause orthostatic hypotension when first used, so patients should be advised to move slowly, especially when changing from a sitting or lying position. The drug can also cause flushing. When nitroglycerin must be discontinued, the drug should be tapered and not stopped abruptly.

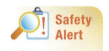

Safety Alert

Dilatrate-SR (a nitrate) and Dilacor XR (a calcium channel blocker) are often confused.

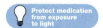

Protect medication from exposure to light

Nitroglycerin, whether in capsules or sublingual tablets, is sold in the original amber glass container. *Do not repackage this drug* because it adheres to soft plastic, which causes nitroglycerin to lose its effectiveness. The patient should replenish the sublingual tablets every six months, even if none have been taken, and the remaining tablets should be discarded.

Isosorbide dinitrate (Dilatrate-SR, Isordil) is used for the same purposes as nitroglycerin—the prevention of angina and HF. It is easily confused with Dilacor XR,

TABLE 12.2 Commonly Used Nitrates

Generic (Brand)	Pronunciation	Dosage Form	Dispensing Status
isosorbide dinitrate (Dilatrate-SR, Isordil)	eye-soe-SOR-bide dye-NYE-trate	Capsule, tablet	Rx
isosorbide mononitrate	eye-soe-SOR-bide mon-oh-NYE-trate	Tablet	Rx
nitroglycerin (Minitran, Nitrolingual, Nitrostat, Nitro-Dur)	nye-troe-GLISS-er-in	Capsule, injection, rectal ointment, sublingual tablet, transdermal ointment, transdermal patch, translingual solution, translingual spray	Rx

which is diltiazem, a calcium channel blocker. Pharmacy technicians should be careful, as they are very different drugs.

Isosorbide mononitrate is a nitrate used to treat angina. Isosorbide mononitrate is available as an immediate-release and extended-release tablet. Immediate-release isosorbide mononitrate is dosed twice a day, with each dose scheduled seven hours apart. Extended-release tablets are dosed once daily and are scored for splitting.

Contraindications Patients taking nitrates should not take erectile dysfunction drugs (such as sildenafil [Viagra], vardenafil [Levitra], and tadalafil [Cialis]). Erectile dysfunction agents also cause vasodilation, and additive effects between these drug classes could lower blood pressure to dangerous levels. Nitrates are contraindicated in patients with a hypersensitivity to organic nitrates. Nitroglycerin is contraindicated in patients with increased intracranial pressure and severe anemia.

Cautions and Considerations Because short-acting forms are designed for immediate absorption, sublingual and buccal (through the cheek) tablets should not be swallowed. Instead, they are placed in the mouth and allowed to dissolve. Long-acting oral forms are swallowed and should be taken on an empty stomach with a full glass of water.

If patients do not get relief from chest pain within 5 minutes of taking a dose of short-acting nitroglycerin they should call for emergency medical care (such as 911) and repeat their dose. If this second dose is needed, a patient could be experiencing a heart attack and should be medically evaluated immediately. A total of three doses can be used within a 15-minute time period.

Sublingual nitroglycerin tablets must be kept in their original amber-colored container and protected from light, heat, and moisture. These tablets lose their effectiveness easily in warm and moist conditions. Once the bottle is opened, the tablets are only good for six months, and the date on which it was opened should be written on the container. After six months have passed, the patient should throw away any remaining tablets.

Tolerance to the beneficial effects of nitrates is an additional concern. Tolerance occurs after constant exposure to the drug, resulting in reduced effectiveness of the medication for the patient. Therefore, a drug-free period of at least eight hours a day (usually overnight) is necessary. For example, the transdermal nitrate patch should be removed before bedtime and left off overnight. A new patch should be applied in the morning.

Drug Interactions Conivaptan, fusidic acid, and idelalisib may increase the concentrations of nitrates. Ergot derivatives may decrease the effects of nitrates. Nitrates should not be combined with nitric oxide because there is an increased risk of methemoglobinemia. Nitrates may enhance the adverse effects of riociguat.

Calcium Channel Blockers

A **calcium channel blocker** impedes the movement of calcium ions into cardiac muscle cells during depolarization by blocking the slow channels. Because the calcium is what triggers the contraction of the muscle, the calcium channel blocker reduces cell contractility and thus reduces the requirements of the cell for energy and oxygen. Moreover, calcium channel blockers also relax coronary vascular smooth muscle, allowing coronary arteries and arterioles to dilate, which in turn increases oxygen delivery. Thus, the oxygen demands of heart muscle tissue are reduced while the oxygen supply is increased.

Calcium channel blockers are commonly used to treat most supraventricular tachyarrhythmias (rapid, irregular atrial beats) and successfully convert most to normal (sinus) rhythm. Some calcium channel blockers slow conduction through the AV node, slow SA node action, and relax coronary artery smooth muscle. They are used to control fast ventricular rates in patients with atrial flutter and atrial fibrillation, two types of abnormal heart rhythms. Side effects include bradycardia, hypotension, heart block, cardiac failure, nausea, constipation, headache, dizziness, and fatigue, all of which lead to poor patient adherence. The patient sometimes does not understand that the drug is helping because he or she may feel worse after taking it. The most common side effect is constipation. Some patients experience drowsiness when they begin taking a calcium channel blocker. Some of these drugs should be taken with food, and caffeine should be limited. More information on calcium channel blockers can be found in Table 12.3.

Calcium channel blockers are also first-line therapy for hypertension. They reduce blood pressure by dilating the arterioles, which decreases peripheral vascular resistance to blood flow, energy consumption, and oxygen requirements. Diltiazem and verapamil also slow calcium movement into myocardial cells, thus reducing contraction ability and energy and oxygen requirements. Other calcium channel blockers act only on vascular smooth muscle and lack antiarrhythmic activity. Calcium channel blockers and diuretics are also used to treat isolated systolic hypertension.

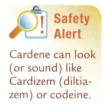

Safety Alert

Cardene can look (or sound) like Cardizem (diltiazem) or codeine.

Contraindications Contraindications to diltiazem include sick sinus syndrome, second- or third-degree AV block, severe hypotension, acute MI, and pulmonary congestion. Felodipine and nisoldipine should not be used in patients with a hypersensitivity to other calcium channel blockers. Nicardipine should not be used in patients with aortic stenosis. Nifedipine is contraindicated in patients with cardiogenic shock and acute heart attack. Contraindications to verapamil include severe left ventricular dysfunction, hypotension, cardiogenic shock, sick sinus syndrome, second- or third-degree AV block, Wolff-Parkinson-White syndrome, and Lown-Ganong-Levine syndrome. The IV form of verapamil is also contraindicated with concurrent use of beta blockers and in patients with ventricular tachycardia. Amlodipine and isradipine do not have contraindications.

TABLE 12.3 Commonly Used Calcium Channel Blockers

Generic (Brand)	Pronunciation	Dosage Form	Dispensing Status
amlodipine (Norvasc)	am-LOE-di-peen	Tablet	Rx
diltiazem (Cardizem, Dilacor XR)	dil-TYE-a-zem	Capsule, injection, tablet	Rx
felodipine (Plendil)	fe-LOE-di-peen	Tablet	Rx
isradipine (Dynacirc)	iz-RAD-i-peen	Capsule	Rx
nicardipine (Cardene)	nye-KAR-di-peen	Capsule, injection	Rx
nifedipine (Afeditab, Nifediac, Procardia)	nye-FED-i-peen	Capsule, tablet	Rx
nisoldipine (Sular)	nye-SOLE-di-peen	Tablet	Rx
verapamil (Calan, Verelan)	ver-AP-a-mil	Capsule, injection, tablet	Rx

Cautions and Considerations Some calcium channel blockers cause fluid retention (edema) and heart palpitations. To balance the positive and negative effects on the heart, healthcare practitioners closely monitor patients taking this class of drugs.

Select calcium channel blockers come in extended-release dosage forms that need to be taken just once a day. These products should be swallowed whole, not crushed or chewed. Crushing or chewing the medication ruins the release mechanism and could result in drastically lowered blood pressure because the entire large dose would be released at once.

Patients should be warned that some of the extended-release dosage forms (such as the oral form of verapamil) work by releasing the drug from a capsule or tablet called a *ghost pill* while in the digestive system. This ghost pill then moves through the gastrointestinal (GI) tract and appears in the patients' stool. Patients should be told they should not be alarmed by the appearance of this casing in their stool, and they should be reassured that the medication has been absorbed by the body.

Drug Interactions Additive or increased adverse effects occur when calcium channel blockers are used concurrently with beta blockers. Calcium channel blockers may increase digoxin levels.

Azole antifungals may increase concentrations of amlodipine, felodipine, isradipine, and nifedipine. Diltiazem and verapamil may result in altered drug levels and increased toxicity in lithium-using patients. Diltiazem, when used with amiodarone, may result in cardiotoxicity. Nafcillin decreases the effectiveness of nifedipine. Verapamil may increase tolvaptan concentrations.

Safety Alert

Cardura (doxazosin, an alpha blocker used to treat hypertension) and Cardene (nicardipine, a calcium channel blocker used to treat angina and hypertension) can also be misread for each other.

Metabolic Modifier

Ranolazine (Ranexa) is indicated for the treatment of chronic angina (see Table 12.4). Conventional angina drugs reduce cardiac oxygen demand, but ranolazine is a metabolic modifier that assists the heart to generate energy more efficiently by allowing the heart to function despite a decrease in oxygen. Ranolazine is used as an adjunct therapy for patients for whom other antianginal drugs do not work. It should be used concurrently with amlodipine, beta blockers, or nitrates. Ranolazine is produced as a light orange, oblong, extended-release tablet that cannot be cut or broken in half and must be swallowed whole. It may be taken without regard to meals.

Contraindications Patients who have liver cirrhosis should not use ranolazine.

Cautions and Considerations Ranolazine may prolong the QT interval. Acute kidney failure has occurred in patients who have kidney dysfunction and use ranolazine. Ranolazine should be used with caution in older adults because of increased risk of adverse events.

Drug Interactions Because ranolazine has many interactions, it is not used as first-line therapy. Ranolazine should not be given with simvastatin, because it can double the plasma concentration of the latter drug. Ranolazine may enhance the QT prolongation of other agents that prolong the QT interval.

TABLE 12.4 Metabolic Modifier for Angina

Generic (Brand)	Pronunciation	Dosage Form	Dispensing Status
ranolazine (Ranexa)	ra-NOE-la-zeen	Tablet	Rx

Arrhythmia

An **arrhythmia** is any variation from the normal rhythm of the heart. Heart rate and/or rhythm abnormalities occur when the heartbeat is too slow or too fast or when the contractions of the ventricles and atria are not synchronized.

Heart Rates and Rhythms

Normal cardiac rhythm is generated by the SA node at a rate of approximately 70 to 80 beats per minute. This rate exceeds the rate that can be produced by other potential pacemaking automatic (spontaneously depolarizing) cells, such as the AV node, the AV bundle (also called the bundle of His), and the Purkinje fibers (see Figure 12.4). An electrocardiogram (ECG) records and documents the signals sent through the conducting system of the heart, as shown in Figure 12.5. The QT interval, shown in the ECG recording in the figure, is a period in which the heart is refractory (nonresponsive) to all but the most powerful signals, if at all.

When the SA node works at less than optimal capacity, when conduction is interrupted, or when other areas become hyperexcitable, another discharging area may become the dominant pacemaker. A pacemaker other than the SA node is termed an **ectopic pacemaker**, also known as *ectopic focus*. Figure 12.6 shows a premature ventricular contraction (PVC), one example of an ectopic pacemaker. PVCs result in **tachycardia** (excessively high heart rate), flutter, or fibrillation.

Table 12.5 shows abnormal heart rhythms and rates and their ECG tracings. These conditions may be caused by ischemia, infarction, or alteration of body chemicals resulting in nonautomatic cells becoming automatic cells. Benign abnormalities have a low likelihood of sudden death. Potentially malignant abnormalities have a

FIGURE 12.4
Conduction System of the Heart

The conduction system of the heart is a group of specialized cardiac muscle cells that send signals to the heart muscle causing it to contract.

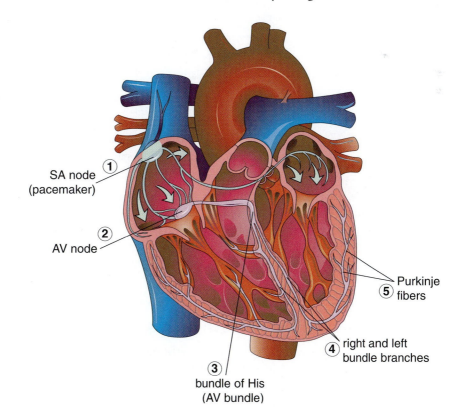

SA node (pacemaker) ①

AV node ②

Purkinje fibers ⑤

right and left bundle branches ④

bundle of His (AV bundle) ③

Typically, an ECG has five deflections (spikes and dips) named *P to T waves*. Each section of the ECG is labeled and corresponds to action in a particular part of the heart.

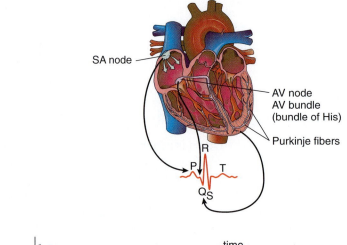

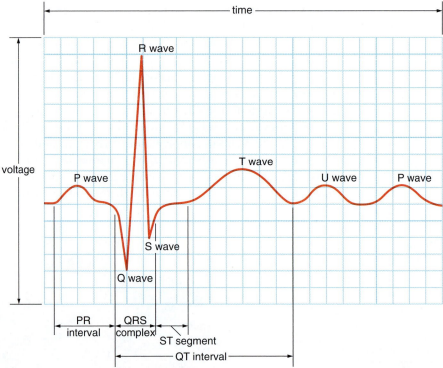

moderate risk of sudden death and indicate existing heart disease. Malignant abnormalities indicate an immediate risk of sudden death and serious heart disease. The symptoms of abnormal heart rhythms or rates include palpitations, syncope (loss of consciousness), light-headedness, visual disturbances, pallor (paleness), cyanosis (bluish skin discoloration), weakness, sweating, chest pain, and hypotension.

Pharmaceutical Treatment of Abnormal Heart Rates and Rhythms

Pharmaceutical treatment for arrhythmias is directed at preventing these life-threatening conditions by restoring sinus (normal) rhythm. The various classes of antiarrhythmic drugs have characteristic electrophysiologic effects on the myocardium

FIGURE 12.6
**Premature
Ventricular
Contraction**

When an area other than the SA node becomes the primary pacemaker, premature ventricular contractions can occur.

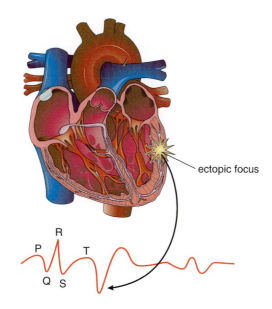

ectopic focus

TABLE 12.5 Abnormal Heart Rhythms

Arrhythmia	Beats per Minute	Electrocardiogram
tachycardia	150–250	
bradycardia	<60	
atrial flutter	200–350	
atrial fibrillation	>350	
premature atrial contraction	variable	
premature ventricular contraction	variable	
ventricular fibrillation	variable	

and the conducting system. Some drugs influence the heart rate directly or indirectly by affecting the movement of ions into or out of the cell. The excitability of the cells of the SA node is influenced by the permeability of the cell membrane to sodium and calcium ions. The sodium and calcium ions cross the cell membrane through openings called ion channels, which are actually protein molecules that are sensitive to specific electrical and chemical conditions. In effect, one can think of an ion channel as a gate or valve through which the ions pass (see Figure 12.7). Drugs may act to close the valve, allowing fewer ions to penetrate the membrane, or to open the valve, allowing more ions to penetrate. The objectives in managing atrial fibrillation are control of rate and rhythm and prevention of thromboembolism (obstruction of a blood vessel by a clot that has been dislodged from another site). Table 12.6 lists the most commonly used antiarrhythmic agents. Beta blockers and calcium channel blockers were discussed earlier in the section on angina.

Membrane-Stabilizing Agents (Class I)

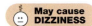
A **membrane-stabilizing agent** slows the movement of sodium ions into myocardial cells, thus requiring a stronger signal to trigger an action potential. The reduced ability to generate an action potential will dampen potential abnormal rhythms and heartbeats.

Disopyramide (Norpace) is used primarily in the treatment of ventricular arrhythmias but is avoided in patients with heart failure. Disopyramide is an anticholinergic, so dry mouth, urinary retention, constipation, and blurred vision are side effects.

Flecainide (Tambocor) prolongs refractory periods, action potential duration, and the QT interval. It is used for treating ventricular arrhythmias. The side effects are dizziness, blurred vision, tremors, nausea, and vomiting.

Lidocaine (Xylocaine), also used as a local anesthetic, reduces the ability of myocardial cells to respond to stimulation. Lidocaine is effective on the ventricles but has little effect on the atria. It must be given intravenously for PVCs associated with an MI. Common side effects of lidocaine are nausea, vomiting, constipation, and dizziness.

Mexiletine (Mexitil) has effects that are similar to lidocaine. It is used for the treatment of ventricular tachycardia but is more effective when used with another drug. Side effects include GI and neurologic symptoms and elevated liver enzyme levels. Mexiletine can also cause **leukopenia** (low white blood cell count) and **agranulocytosis** (a severe blood condition).

Propafenone (Rythmol) is used only for treating life-threatening arrhythmias because it may cause new arrhythmias or worsen existing ones. Propafenone may also worsen HF and interfere with pacemakers. Patients should be connected to a cardiac monitor at the beginning of therapy or with any increase in dosage.

Procainamide and **Quinidine** act to slow the SA node rate and AV conduction in atrial and ventricular arrhythmias. Side effects include **thrombocytopenia** (a decrease in the bone marrow production of blood platelets) and cinchonism (marked by headache, blurred vision, tinnitus, confusion, and nausea). Disopyramide and procainamide, discussed earlier, are similar to quinidine. Procainamide and quinidine are so similar that sometimes they may be used interchangeably.

Contraindications Disopyramide is contraindicated in patients with cardiogenic shock, preexisting second- or third-degree AV block, long QT syndrome, and sick sinus

FIGURE 12.7
The "Gatekeeper" Role of Cardiovascular Drugs

Drugs may act to close the ion channel, allowing fewer ions to penetrate the membrane, or to open the ion channel, allowing more ions to penetrate.

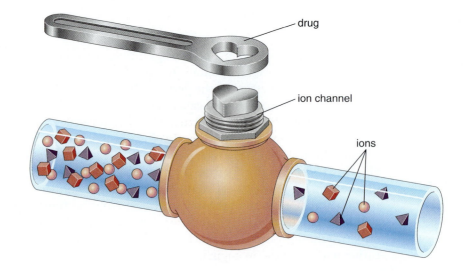

TABLE 12.6 Most Commonly Used Antiarrhythmic Agents

Generic (Brand)	Pronunciation	Dosage Form	Dispensing Status
Membrane-Stabilizing Agents (Class I)			
disopyramide (Norpace)	dye-soe-PEER-a-mide	Capsule	Rx
flecainide (Tambocor)	FLEK-a-nide	Tablet	Rx
lidocaine (Xylocaine)	LYE-doe-kane	Injection	Rx
mexiletine (Mexitil)	mex-IL-a-teen	Capsule	Rx
procainamide	proe-KANE-a-mide	Injection	Rx
propafenone (Rythmol)	proe-PAF-e-none	Capsule, tablet	Rx
quinidine	KWIN-i-deen	Injection, tablet	Rx
Beta Blockers (Class II), see Table 12.1			
Potassium Channel Blockers (Class III)			
amiodarone (Cordarone, Nexterone, Pacerone)	am-ee-OH-da-rone	Injection, tablet	Rx
dofetilide (Tikosyn)	doe-FET-il-ide	Capsule	Rx
dronedarone (Multaq)	droe-NE-da-rone	Tablet	Rx
Calcium Channel Blockers (Class IV), see Table 12.3			
Various Antiarrhythmic Agents			
atropine	AT-roe-peen	Injection, tablet	Rx
digoxin (Digitek, Digox, Lanoxin)	di-JOX-in	Injection, oral solution, tablet	Rx
isoproterenol (Isuprel)	eye-soe-proe-TER-e-nawl	Injection	Rx
Antidote for Digoxin Toxicity			
digoxin immune Fab (DigiFab)	di-JOX-in i-MYUN fab	Injection	Rx

syndrome. Contraindications to flecainide include preexisting second- or third-degree AV block, cardiogenic shock, CAD, and concurrent use of ritonavir or amprenavir. Systemic lidocaine should be avoided in patients with Adams-Stokes syndrome; Wolff-Parkinson-White syndrome; or severe degrees of SA, AV, or intraventricular heart block. Some commercially available forms of premixed lidocaine for injection may include corn-derived products and, therefore, should be avoided in patients with corn hypersensitivity. Mexiletine is contraindicated in patients with cardiogenic shock and second- or third-degree AV block. Procainamide should not be used in patients with complete heart block, second-degree AV block, and torsades de pointes. Contraindications to propafenone include SA, AV, and intraventricular disorders; Brugada syndrome; sinus bradycardia; cardiogenic shock; uncompensated cardiac failure; marked hypotension, bronchospastic disorders, or severe pulmonary disease; and uncorrected electrolyte abnormalities. Quinidine should not be used in patients with thrombocytopenia, thrombocytopenia purpura, myasthenia gravis, heart block greater than first degree, or idiopathic conduction delays, or with concurrent use of quinolone antibiotics, cisapride, amprenavir, or ritonavir.

Cautions and Considerations The use of membrane-stabilizing agents should be reserved for life-threatening arrhythmias. These agents should be used cautiously in patients with heart failure because of the potential to reduce heart rate too much.

Quinidine is available in gluconate, polyglyconate, and sulfate salts. Different salts of quinidine contain varying amounts of active drug and are not interchangeable.

Drug Interactions Membrane-stabilizing agents are associated with many drug interactions. Some major interactions are presented here. Quinidine may decrease the metabolism of codeine, digoxin, and tricyclic antidepressants (TCAs). Metabolism of quinidine may be decreased by cimetidine, and calcium channel blockers. Procainamide excretion may be inhibited by azole antifungals, cimetidine and trimethoprim. Other membrane-stabilizing agents may affect the disposition of TCAs, theophylline, and warfarin.

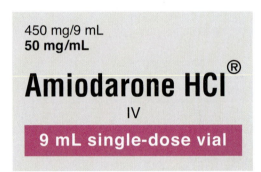

450 mg/9 mL
50 mg/mL

Amiodarone HCl®

IV

9 mL single-dose vial

Potassium Channel Blockers (Class III)

Potassium channel blockers delay repolarization of atrial and ventricular fibers by blocking the flow of potassium across cell membranes.

Amiodarone (Cordarone, Nexterone, Pacerone) is used to treat atrial and ventricular arrhythmias that do not respond to other medications. It is very effective, but it has a high incidence of significant and potentially fatal toxicities. Establishing control may take several days to several weeks with the IV form and up to one to four weeks with the oral dose. Many patients experience hypotension. Interactions can occur for several weeks or longer after cessation of amiodarone. Some patients will develop a slate blue rash from this drug. Because some of the side effects can be fatal, it is imperative that the prescriber carefully monitor the patient and order appropriate laboratory tests.

Dofetilide (Tikosyn) is used to maintain normal sinus rhythm in patients who have atrial fibrillation/atrial flutter lasting longer than one week and who have been converted to normal sinus rhythm. The drug itself can induce arrhythmias. Dofetilide must be initiated or reinitiated in a hospital setting. The patient must be placed in a facility that can provide monitoring and resuscitation for a period of three days. Dofetilide is available only to hospitals and to prescribers who have received training in the dosing and initiation of this drug. Dofetilide is part of the Risk Evaluation and Mitigation Strategies (REMS) program. Tikosyn in Pharmacy Systems (TIPS) is designed to allow retail pharmacies to dispense the drug, once the patient has been admitted to the hospital. Pharmacies must educate their staff, document that the prescriber is enrolled in the program, and document that the patient has been properly educated before dispensing the drug.

Dronedarone (Multaq) should be used for maintaining sinus rhythm in patients with no or minimal heart disease. It should be avoided in patients with heart failure. Dronedarone is better tolerated than amiodarone, which leads to better patient adherence, but it still has many serious side effects and interactions. Patients should watch for symptoms of liver disease and lung problems when taking dronedarone. Dronedarone is structurally related to amiodarone and is used to prevent hospitalization for patients who are in atrial fibrillation. It should be taken with the morning and evening meals. Grapefruit should be avoided.

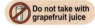
Do not take with grapefruit juice

Contraindications Amiodarone is contraindicated in patients with hypersensitivity to iodine, severe sinus-node dysfunction, second- or third-degree AV block, bradycardia, and cardiogenic shock.

Dofetilide is contraindicated in patients with long QT interval and severe kidney impairment. Concurrent use of cimetidine, dolutegravir, hydrochlorothiazide, itraconazole, ketoconazole, megestrol, prochlorperazine, trimethoprim, or verapamil contraindicates the administration of dofetilide.

Dronedarone should not be used in patients with permanent atrial fibrillation, symptomatic heart failure, liver or lung toxicity from amiodarone use, second- or third-degree AV block, bradycardia (heart rates below 60 beats per minute), severe liver impairment, pregnancy, and breast-feeding. Agents that prolong QT interval should not be used with dronedarone.

Cautions and Considerations Amiodarone has several black box warnings. Overall, there is a warning that amiodarone should only be used in patients who have life-threatening arrhythmias. Another warning is for the risk of severe liver toxicity. An additional warning cautions about amiodarone's potential to exacerbate arrhythmias. Pulmonary toxicity may occur with use, and amiodarone carries a black box warning for this adverse effect.

Dofetilide has a boxed warning saying that it must be initiated in a setting with clinical monitoring because there is a risk of arrhythmias. Dofetilide should be used cautiously in patients with renal impairment.

Dronedarone also has black box warnings. One warns that it should not be used in patients with symptomatic heart failure due to increased risk of death. When used in patients with permanent atrial fibrillation, dronedarone may also increase mortality.

Drug Interactions Potassium channel blockers are associated with many drug interactions. Several significant interactions are highlighted here. Amiodarone and dronedarone may decrease the metabolism of digoxin and warfarin. Amiodarone may also decrease the metabolism of theophylline. Dofetilide levels may be increased by azole antifungals, cimetidine, dolutegravir, lamotrigine, megestrol, prochlorperazine, thiazide diuretics, trimethoprim, and verapamil. Dofetilide may increase the QT prolonging effects of other drugs that prolong the QT interval.

Various Antiarrhythmic Agents

Other agents used to treat abnormal heart rates have different mechanisms of action.

Atropine is an anticholinergic agent that decreases the effect of vagal-mediated parasympathetic tone, allowing sympathetic action to take over. Atropine is used to treat bradycardia. Low doses may worsen the bradycardia, whereas high doses may cause cardioacceleration (a rate that is too high), which increases oxygen demand, resulting in ischemia and leading to arrhythmias. Atropine is also used as a preoperative medication to inhibit salivation and secretions during surgery.

Digoxin (Digitek, Digox, Lanoxin) may be used in the management of atrial flutter and fibrillation. Digoxin is also often used to treat HF. It has the following mechanisms of action:

- Increases the force of contraction.
- Increases the effective refractory period of the AV node (slows AV node stimulation).
- Increases the SA node, increasing automaticity due to ion imbalance (direct stimulation).

Digoxin is used to restore the force of myocardial contraction without increasing oxygen demands and to slow ventricular response to stimulation by slowing conduction in the AV node. It should be used with caution because of the possibility of systemic accumulation of the drug. Patients who take digoxin commonly experience digitalis toxicity, commonly referred to as *dig* (pronounced "didge") toxicity. This effect is especially common among older adults. The three primary signs of digitalis toxicity are nausea, vomiting, and arrhythmias. Patients become nauseated, have vertigo, experience general weakness, and may see yellow-green halos around objects. If these signs and symptoms occur, the drug should be withdrawn immediately. **Digoxin immune Fab (DigiFab)** is an antidote for digitalis toxicity. It is an antibody fragment that binds to digoxin, inactivating the drug, which is then excreted by the kidneys.

Isoproterenol (Isuprel) dilates coronary vessels. It is used parenterally to treat ventricular arrhythmias due to AV nodal block, and in bradyarrhythmias (slow, irregular heartbeats). It may be used temporarily to treat third-degree AV block until pacemaker insertion is performed. It increases heart rate and contractility.

Heart Failure

Heart failure (HF) is a chronic, progressive condition in which the heart is no longer able to pump enough oxygen-rich blood to meet the body's needs. In other words, the heart is unable to keep up with the demands of the body. Symptoms of heart failure include shortness of breath, fatigue, edema, and exercise intolerance. Figure 12.8 shows how blood regularly flows through the heart.

Treatment of Heart Failure

The goals of therapy are to prolong survival, relieve symptoms, improve quality of life, and prevent progression of disease. Most patients will be managed with a combination of drugs. Angiotensin-converting enzyme (ACE) inhibitors and beta blockers are commonly used. Diuretics are recommended for patients who retain fluid, and digoxin is recommended for patients who continue to experience symptoms after receiving optimal treatment with other drugs. The most commonly used agents for HF that have not been previously discussed in this text are listed in Table 12.7.

Vasodilators

Vasodilators are drugs that cause blood vessels to dilate. Vasodilators are used to treat HF because dilating the vessels reduces the resistance against which the heart must work. Some vasodilators are described here; others are discussed in the section on hypertension.

Isosorbide dinitrate-hydralazine (BiDil) is a combination drug used to supplement standard therapy and is also a reasonable alternative in patients who are unable to take an ACE inhibitor. Both components of this drug are vasodilators and enhance the relaxation of vessels using nitric oxide. Isosorbide dinitrate-hydralazine is dosed three times a day. It can cause headaches and dizziness. It is a film-coated tablet containing 20 mg of isosorbide dinitrate and 37.5 mg of hydralazine.

Contraindications Contraindications to the use of isosorbide dinitrate-hydralazine include hypersensitivity to organic nitrates and concomitant use of a phosphodiesterase-5 (PDE-5) inhibitor or riociguat.

FIGURE 12.8
Blood Flow through the Heart

Blood is prevented from flowing backward within the heart by the one-way valves between the atria and ventricles.

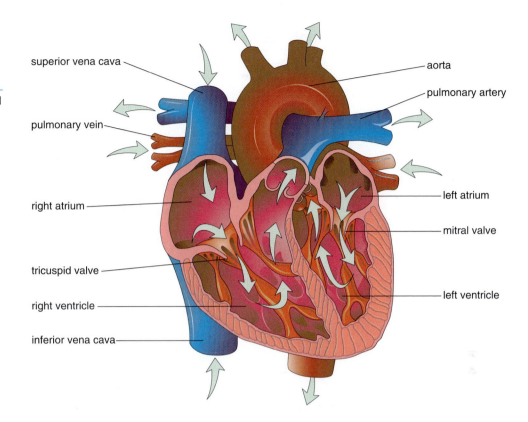

- superior vena cava
- pulmonary vein
- right atrium
- tricuspid valve
- right ventricle
- inferior vena cava
- aorta
- pulmonary artery
- left atrium
- mitral valve
- left ventricle

Cautions and Considerations The hydralazine component of isosorbide dinitrate-hydralazine may cause a lupus-like syndrome or fluid retention. Hydralazine is associated with peripheral neuritis (symptoms include numbness and tingling). Isosorbide dinitrate-hydralazine should be used with caution in patients who have CAD because it may worsen symptoms.

Drug Interactions Drugs with hypotensive effects should be used cautiously with isosorbide dinitrate-hydralazine. Conivaptan, fusidic acid, and idelalisib may increase concentrations of isosorbide dinitrate-hydralazine. PDE-5 inhibitors may enhance the vasodilatory effects of isosorbide dinitrate-hydralazine, and concurrent use should be avoided. Riociguat may enhance the hypotensive effects of isosorbide dinitrate-hydralazine.

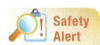

Safety Alert

Prinivil (lisinopril, an ACE inhibitor), Plendil (felodipine, a calcium channel blocker), Prevacid (lansoprazole, a gastric acid reducer), and Prilosec (omeprazole, a gastric acid reducer) look and sound alike.

Angiotensin-Converting Enzyme Inhibitors

An ACE inhibitor is a drug that competitively inhibits the conversion of angiotensin I to angiotensin II. (Angiotensin II is a potent vasoconstrictor that will be further discussed in the later section on hypertension.) The result is lower levels of angiotensin II and, therefore, less constriction of blood vessels, reducing resistance to blood flow. Lowering blood pressure puts less stress on the heart, allowing it to work more effectively. HF is especially responsive to ACE inhibitors. ACE inhibitors have been shown to decrease the risk of cardiovascular events for patients who have hypertension or HF and for patients post-MI.

A persistent cough seems to be the most troublesome side effect of ACE inhibitors. It is a dry, unproductive cough that can be extremely annoying. The cough may be the result of buildup of bradykinin, the breakdown of which is impeded by ACE inhibitors. As a result of the cough, patient adherence with ACE inhibitors may be poor. The most dangerous side effect is angioedema. It most commonly presents as swelling of

TABLE 12.7 Most Commonly Used Agents for Treating Heart Failure*

Generic (Brand)	Pronunciation	Dosage Form	Dispensing Status
ACE Inhibitors			
benazepril (Lotensin)	ben-AZ-eh-pril	Tablet	Rx
captopril (Capoten)	KAP-toe-pril	Tablet	Rx
enalapril (Epaned, Vasotec)	e-NAL-a-pril	Injection, tablet	Rx
fosinopril (Monopril)	foe-SIN-oh-pril	Tablet	Rx
lisinopril (Prinivil, Zestril)	lyse-IN-oh-pril	Tablet	Rx
moexipril (Univasc)	moe-EX-i-pril	Tablet	Rx
perindopril (Aceon)	per-IN-doe-pril	Tablet	Rx
quinapril (Accupril)	KWIN-a-pril	Tablet	Rx
ramipril (Altace)	RA-mi-pril	Capsule	Rx
trandolapril (Mavik)	tran-DOE-la-pril	Tablet	Rx
Vasodilators			
isosorbide dinitrate-hydralazine (BiDil)	eye-soe-SOR-bide hye-DRAL-a-zeen	Tablet	Rx
Human B-Type Natriuretic Peptide (hBNP)			
nesiritide (Natrecor)	ni-SIR-i-tide	Injection	Rx

* Not previously discussed in the text.

the face and tongue, which may begin a few hours after initiation of therapy or may not occur for several years into the treatment. The drug may cause dizziness, especially during the first few days. The patient should be told to stand up slowly to prevent orthostatic hypotension. Increased potassium levels occur with ACE inhibitor use, and patients are usually instructed to avoid salt substitutes, which often contain potassium. ACE inhibitors should be given with caution to patients taking lithium.

Contraindications ACE inhibitors should not be used in patients who have experienced angioedema with previous ACE inhibitor use. Other contraindications include idiopathic or hereditary angioedema and concomitant use with aliskiren in patients with diabetes mellitus.

Pregnant patients should not take ACE inhibitors because these agents can cause severe birth defects. Patients with a kidney condition called *bilateral renal artery stenosis* also should not take ACE inhibitors because the kidneys could shut down.

Cautions and Considerations In rare instances, hypotension, or low blood pressure, can occur. For ACE inhibitors, hypotension can happen dramatically, sometimes on the first dose. Careful monitoring is necessary when a patient starts taking an ACE inhibitor. In some cases, the first dose may be given in the physician's office, so the patient's blood pressure can be monitored for drastic drops.

Hyperkalemia, or an elevated potassium level, is another rare but serious side effect. It tends to occur when patients are also taking potassium-sparing diuretics such as spironolactone. Periodic blood tests for potassium levels will be conducted.

Patients who take diuretics along with an ACE inhibitor should be warned against taking potassium supplements.

Patients who have kidney problems (other than bilateral renal artery stenosis) can take ACE inhibitors, but doses are adjusted downward.

Drug Interactions Drugs with hypotensive effects should be used cautiously in patients taking ACE inhibitors. Other drugs that have hyperkalemic side effects (such as spironolactone) may enhance similar side effects from ACE inhibitors. ACE inhibitors should not be used with angiotensin II receptor blockers because of possible increased adverse effects.

Aldosterone Antagonists

Spironolactone, a potassium-sparing diuretic, is used to treat HF. Spironolactone was previously discussed in Chapter 11.

Beta Blockers

Beta blockers are commonly used to treat HF. Beta blockers were addressed earlier in the discussion of angina.

Antiarrhythmic Medications

Digoxin (Digitek, Digox, Lanoxin) is a drug used for treating HF as well as atrial fibrillation and flutter. It was previously described in the section discussing arrhythmias.

Human B-Type Natriuretic Peptide

Nesiritide (Natrecor) is one of a class of drugs that bind to guanylate cyclase–linked receptors on vascular smooth muscle, causing relaxation and thereby lowering blood pressure. It is a product of deoxyribonucleic acid (DNA) recombinant technology. Nesiritide improves circulation and relieves shortness of breath and fatigue in patients with acute HF. It should be used only in hospitalized patients with acute HF. Nesiritide is used as an alternative to IV nitroglycerin, milrinone, or nitroprusside. It is better tolerated than IV nitroglycerin and does not increase heart rate or cause arrhythmias. Side effects of nesiritide include urinating less than usual, fever, unusual tiredness, and light-headedness.

Contraindications Contraindications to nesiritide include cardiogenic shock and hypotension prior to starting therapy.

Cautions and Considerations Anaphylactic reactions have occurred with nesiritide use. It should be used with caution in patients who have kidney impairment.

Drug Interactions Drugs that have hypotensive effects should be used cautiously with nesiritide.

Hypertension

Blood pressure (BP) is defined as the product of cardiac output and total peripheral resistance. Cardiac output, which is the product of heart rate and stroke volume, is determined by three parameters: **preload**, **afterload**, and **contractility** (the capacity of the cardiac muscle for becoming shorter in response to a stimulus). Additional factors that affect blood pressure are blood viscosity, blood volume, and various nerve controls.

Blood pressure is expressed as the **systolic blood pressure** reading, which measures the pressure when the heart ejects blood, and the **diastolic blood pressure** reading, which measures the pressure when the heart relaxes and fills. Cardiac output is the major determinant of systolic pressure, which is the product of cardiac output and peripheral resistance. Diastolic pressure is related to the volume of venous blood return. Both readings are in millimeters of mercury (abbreviated "mm Hg"), that is, the height of a mercury column whose weight offsets the pressure. The reading is stated as systolic "over" diastolic pressure; measurements of 120 mm Hg systolic and 80 mm Hg diastolic are written "120/80" and read "120 over 80." This reading is often considered normal.

Hypertension is defined as elevated blood pressure. Blood pressure goals are determined by the patient and his or her prescriber. The "2014 Evidence-Based Guideline for the Management of High Blood Pressure in Adults," published in the *Journal of the American Medical Association*, offers recommendations for the management of hypertension. The article suggests treating high blood pressure when it exceeds 150/90 for people age 60 years and older and 140/90 for people younger than age 60 years. Patients with diabetes or kidney disease should begin treatment for high blood pressure when it exceeds 140/90 no matter what age they are.

The underlying basis of most cases of hypertension is unknown, although family history, cigarette smoking, and a high-fat diet are definite factors. Other factors include kidney disease, decreased pressure or delayed pulse in the lower extremities, obesity, adrenal tumor, and use of drugs such as oral contraceptives, corticosteroids, nonsteroidal anti-inflammatory drugs (NSAIDs), decongestants, and appetite suppressants.

Untreated Hypertension

Untreated hypertension can have devastating results, including the following:

- Cardiovascular disease can develop, characterized by enlargement of the heart (**cardiomegaly**), cardiac hypertrophy, the thickening of the cardiac wall, with loss of elasticity. Cardiac output is reduced, along with the ability of the heart to push blood through the body to perfuse tissue, leading to HF.
- HF results in inadequate perfusion, cold extremities (toes and fingers), pitting or whole-body edema (especially in the feet and legs), and accumulation of fluid in the lungs.
- Renal insufficiency can also result. The higher the blood pressure, the more the kidneys reduce renal blood flow and renal function.
- Accelerated cardiac and peripheral vascular disease can also result from hypertension.

In general, the higher the pressure, the greater the risk. Hypertension alters capillaries, venules, and arterioles. Blood cholesterol collects in arterial walls, reducing the size of the lumen and, therefore, the blood flow, leading to increased potential for infection, vascular problems (as in diabetes), and deterioration of nerves from diminished blood supply.

Hypertension Therapy

Hypertension control begins with detection and continued surveillance. Initial readings should be confirmed with subsequent readings for several weeks, unless the pressure is dangerously high at the first reading, in which case treatment begins immediately.

The goal of therapy is to prevent the morbidity and mortality associated with hypertension and to reduce blood pressure by the least intrusive means possible. A four-step regimen, presented in Table 12.8, is needed to reduce blood pressure.

Table 12.9 gives an overview of the main drug classes used in the treatment of hypertension, and Tables 12.10 and 12.11 list the most commonly prescribed agents for this disorder.

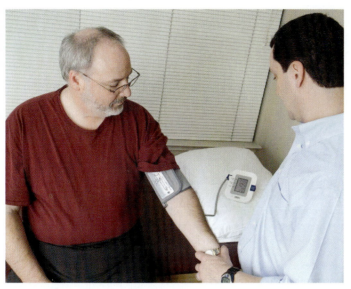
Monitoring blood pressure is an important component of managing hypertension.

Beta blockers, calcium channel blockers, and ACE inhibitors are important drugs used to treat hypertension. They have all been discussed previously in this chapter.

Diuretics

Diuretics are often used for treating hypertension. They reduce the cardiac output by increasing the elimination of urine and reducing the volume of fluid in the body, thereby reducing preload. Their ability to reduce the sodium load, however, is probably their most important effect on lowering blood pressure. Diuretics are discussed in Chapter 11.

TABLE 12.8   Regimen for Reducing Blood Pressure

Step 1	Modify lifestyle factors:		
	High sodium intake	to	moderate sodium intake
	Excess consumption of calories	to	weight reduction
	Physical inactivity	to	regular aerobic physical activity
	Excess alcohol consumption	to	moderate alcohol consumption
	Nicotine usage	to	cessation of nicotine usage
	High stress	to	control of stress
Step 2	Monotherapy: use a single drug, usually a diuretic, beta blocker, ACE inhibitor, angiotensin II receptor antagonist, or calcium channel blocker.		
Step 3	Add an additional drug (polytherapy).		
Step 4	Add a third agent that will act synergistically with the other two drugs in reducing blood pressure.		

TABLE 12.9 Pharmacologic Antihypertensive Therapies

Drug Class	Mechanism of Action
Alpha blockers	These drugs are peripheral-acting agents that block alpha receptor–induced constriction of blood vessels, leading indirectly to vasodilation and hypotension.
Angiotensin II receptor blockers (ARBs)	These drugs bind to the angiotensin II receptors, thereby blocking the vasoconstrictive effects of these receptors. Unlike ACE inhibitors, ARBs do not affect bradykinin-altered responses. Consequently, ARBs do not have the cough associated with ACE inhibitor use.
Angiotensin-converting enzyme (ACE) inhibitors	These drugs, addressed earlier in the section discussing heart failure, work by blocking the angiotensin-converting enzyme, thus preventing the conversion of angiotensin I to angiotensin II (a potent vasoconstrictor). The decrease in blood pressure is accompanied by a reduction in peripheral resistance and an increase in the elasticity of the large arteries, suggesting a direct effect on arterial smooth muscle.
Beta blockers	These drugs block beta-receptor response to adrenergic stimulation, thereby decreasing heart rate, myocardial contractility, blood pressure, and myocardial oxygen demand.
Calcium channel blockers	These drugs, addressed earlier in the section discussing angina, dilate the arterioles, thereby reducing peripheral resistance, energy consumption, and oxygen requirements.
Central nervous system agents	These drugs stimulate the alpha-2 adrenergic receptors in the brain and thereby reduce the sympathetic outflow from the vasomotor center in the brain. Thus, heart rate, cardiac output, and total peripheral resistance is decreased as a result of reduced stimulation of vascular muscle.
Combination drugs	Additive effects lower blood pressure.
Diuretics	These drugs, discussed in Chapter 11, reduce preload.
Selective aldosterone receptor antagonists	These drugs act as diuretics by binding to mineralocorticoid receptors, and blocking aldosterone action, thereby decreasing sodium retention and blood pressure.
Vasodilators	These drugs relax arterial smooth muscle and lower peripheral resistance via a direct mechanism.

Safety Alert

Many of the generic names of ARBs end in -sartan (e.g., losartan and valsartan), so pharmacy technicians must pay close attention to the first few letters of these drug names.

Angiotensin Receptor Blockers

Like ACE inhibitors, **angiotensin receptor blockers (ARBs)** are used to treat hypertension and heart failure. They are often an acceptable alternative for patients who cannot tolerate ACE inhibitors.

ARBs work by binding to the same receptors to which angiotensin II binds. Instead of stimulating vasoconstriction, as angiotensin II does, ARBs block these receptors, thereby preventing constriction and causing blood vessels to relax, which lowers blood pressure. ARBs do not cause bradykinin buildup as ACE inhibitors do, so coughing is not a typical side effect.

Azilsartan (Edarbi) lowers blood pressure slightly more than the other drugs in this class. It is only approved for hypertension. It is sensitive to moisture and light and must be dispensed and stored in the original bottle.

Candesartan (Atacand) is indicated for the treatment of hypertension and heart failure. While only available as a tablet, an oral suspension can be made for children or patients unable to swallow solids.

TABLE 12.10 Most Commonly Used Antihypertensive Therapeutic Agents

Generic (Brand)	Pronunciation	Dosage Form	Dispensing Status
ACE Inhibitors, see Table 12.7			
Angiotensin Receptor Blockers (ARBs)			
azilsartan (Edarbi)	ay-zil-SAR-tan	Tablet	Rx
candesartan (Atacand)	kan-de-SAR-tan	Tablet	Rx
eprosartan (Teveten)	ep-roe-SAR-tan	Tablet	Rx
irbesartan (Avapro)	ir-be-SAR-tan	Tablet	Rx
losartan (Cozaar)	loe-SAR-tan	Tablet	Rx
olmesartan (Benicar)	ohl-me-SAR-tan	Tablet	Rx
telmisartan (Micardis)	tel-me-SAR-tan	Tablet	Rx
valsartan (Diovan)	val-SAR-tan	Tablet	Rx
Beta Blockers, see Table 12.1			
Calcium Channel Blockers, see Table 12.3			
Central Nervous System Agents			
clonidine (Catapres, Catapres-TTS, Duraclon, Kapvay)	KLON-i-deen	Injection, tablet, transdermal patch	Rx
guanfacine (Tenex)	GWAHN-fa-seen	Tablet	Rx
methyldopa (Aldomet)	meth-il-DOE-pa	Injection, tablet	Rx
Direct Renin Inhibitor (DRI)			
aliskiren (Tekturna)	a-lis-KYE-ren	Tablet	Rx
Alpha Blockers			
alfuzosin (Uroxatral)	al-FYOO-zoe-sin	Tablet	Rx
doxazosin (Cardura)	dox-AY-zoe-sin	Tablet	Rx
prazosin (Minipress)	PRAY-zoe-sin	Capsule	Rx
terazosin (Hytrin)	ter-AYE-zoe-sin	Capsule	Rx

Eprosartan (Teveten) is indicated for the treatment of hypertension alone or in combination with other drugs. It is provided by the manufacturer in 400 mg oval, scored, pink tablets. Eprosartan tablets may be cut or broken in half. The 600 mg tablet is a white capsule and is dosed without regard to meals.

Irbesartan (Avapro) is approved for the treatment of hypertension and diabetic nephropathy in patients with type II diabetes. It slows the progression of kidney disease.

Losartan (Cozaar) is approved for the treatment of hypertension and diabetic nephropathy and for CVA prophylaxis. Research data show that twice-daily dosing may be more effective than once-daily dosing.

Olmesartan (Benicar) is a selective ARB. It is a prodrug that is converted to its active form during absorption in the GI tract. Olmesartan is indicated for the treatment of hypertension and may be used alone or with additional antihypertensive agents.

TABLE 12.11 Most Commonly Used Combination Antihypertensive Agents

Generic (Brand)	Pronunciation	Dosage Form	Dispensing Status
aliskiren-amlodipine-hydrochlorothiazide (Amturnide)	a-lis-KYE-ren am-LOE-di-peen hye-droe-klor-oh-THYE-a-zide	Tablet	Rx
aliskiren-valsartan (Valturna)	a-lis-KYE-ren val-SAR-tan	Tablet	Rx
amlodipine-benazepril (Lotrel)	am-LOE-di-peen ben-AYE-ze-pril	Capsule	Rx
amlodipine-valsartan (Exforge)	am-LOE-di-peen val-SAR-tan	Tablet	Rx
atenolol-chlorthalidone (Tenoretic)	a-TEN-oh-lawl klor-THAL-i-done	Tablet	Rx
benazepril-hydrochlorothiazide (Lotensin HCT)	ben-AZ-eh-pril hye-droe-klor-oh-THYE-a-zide	Tablet	Rx
bisoprolol-hydrochlorothiazide (Ziac)	bis-OE-proe-lawl hye-droe-klor-oh-THYE-a-zide	Tablet	Rx
enalapril-hydrochlorothiazide (Vaseretic)	e-NAL-a-pril hye-droe-klor-oh-THYE-a-zide	Tablet	Rx
irbesartan-hydrochlorothiazide (Avalide)	ir-be-SAR-tan hye-droe-klor-oh-THYE-a-zide	Tablet	Rx
lisinopril-hydrochlorothiazide (Prinzide, Zestoretic)	lyse-IN-oh-pril hye-droe-klor-oh-THYE-a-zide	Tablet	Rx
losartan-hydrochlorothiazide (Hyzaar)	loe-SAR-tan hye-droe-klor-oh-THYE-a-zide	Tablet	Rx
metoprolol-hydrochlorothiazide (Dutoprol, Lopressor HCT)	me-TOE-proe-lawl hye-droe-klor-oh-THYE-a-zide	Tablet	Rx
trandolapril-verapamil (Tarka)	tran-DOE-la-pril ver-AP-a-mil	Tablet	Rx
valsartan-hydrochlorothiazide (Diovan HCT)	val-SAR-tan hye-droe-klor-oh-THYE-a-zide	Tablet	Rx

Telmisartan (Micardis) may be used alone or in combination with other antihypertensive agents. It is specific and selective and maintains blood pressure reduction over a 24-hour period. Telmisartan has the longest half-life of all the ARBs. It is so sensitive to moisture that it is provided by the manufacturer in a foil blister pack. Because of this sensitivity to moisture, a telmisartan tablet cannot be cut in half. Pharmacy technicians should be aware that telmisartan will lose potency when the pack is opened.

Valsartan (Diovan) is approved for hypertension and heart failure. It may be dosed without regard for food.

Contraindications ARBs are contraindicated in patients with diabetes mellitus who are taking aliskiren.

Cautions and Considerations Patients taking diuretics along with ARBs may experience hypotension. Patients should be careful about getting up too quickly from a sitting or lying position until they know how these drugs affect them. Dizziness, fainting, and falling down may be signs of hypotension. Patients with kidney or liver impairment may need special dosing and monitoring if they are to take these medications.

Drug Interactions Drugs with hypotensive effects may enhance the hypotensive effects of ARBs. ARBs may enhance the adverse effects of ACE inhibitors. Pimozide concentrations may be increased by irbesartan and losartan. Telmisartan may enhance the adverse effects of ramipril.

Central Nervous System Agents

Central nervous system (CNS) agents stimulate the alpha-2 adrenergic receptors in the brain. This leads to a reduction in the sympathetic outflow from the vasomotor center in the brain and an associated increase in parasympathetic activity (vagal tone). As a consequence of these effects, heart rate, cardio output, total peripheral resistance, and plasma renin activity are decreased, and baroreceptor reflexes are blunted.

Clonidine (Catapres, Catapres-TTS, Duraclon, Kapvay) is the only antihypertensive supplied as a transdermal delivery system. The patch is worn for seven days. This delivery form seems to have fewer side effects than other formulations. Clonidine is also used to treat hypertension in patients experiencing withdrawal symptoms, especially alcoholics.

Guanfacine (Tenex) often has less of a sedative effect compared to clonidine. Its side effects are drowsiness, fatigue, dry mouth, depression, and fluid retention.

Contraindications Epidural clonidine administration is contraindicated with injection-site infection and concurrent anticoagulant therapy. Guanfacine does not have contraindications.

Cautions and Considerations Clonidine has a black box warning for epidural use. Epidural clonidine must be diluted prior to use. Clonidine may cause bradycardia, hypotension, and respiratory depression. It should be used with caution in patients who have cardiovascular disease or kidney impairment. Older adults may experience more intense side effects with the use of clonidine, consequently, this drug is not recommended for this patient population. Transdermal clonidine may contain metal that conducts electrical current. Therefore, transdermal patches should be removed prior to magnetic resonance imaging, cardioversion, or defibrillation. Discontinuation of therapy should be done gradually, over several days, to prevent rebound hypertension.

Guanfacine is available in immediate-release and extended-release formulations. These products are not interchangeable on a milligram-to-milligram basis. Guanfacine should be used cautiously in patients who have severe cardiac disease. Skin rash and skin exfoliation have occurred with use. It should be used with caution in patients with kidney or liver dysfunction. Use in older adults is not recommended because of the risk of CNS side effects. Discontinuation of guanfacine therapy should be tapered.

Drug Interactions Drugs that cause CNS depression (such as sleep aids) may enhance the CNS depressant effects of clonidine and guanfacine. Drugs that cause bradycardia (such as beta blockers) may enhance the bradycardic effects of clonidine and guanfacine. Mirtazapine may diminish the antihypertensive effects of clonidine.

Alpha Blockers

Alpha blockers are peripherally acting agents that reduce constriction of blood vessels by blocking alpha-adrenergic receptors. This action leads indirectly to vasodilation and hypotension. Alpha blockers are discussed in detail in Chapter 11.

Direct Renin Inhibitor

Aliskiren (Tekturna) inhibits renin, which controls the first rate-limiting step of the renin-angiotensin-aldosterone system (a hormone system is involved in the regulation of plasma sodium concentration and arterial blood pressure). It is indicated for the treatment of hypertension. The medication should not be taken with meals because a high-fat meal can reduce the absorption of this drug. Diarrhea appears to be the primary side effect.

Contraindications Aliskiren is contraindicated in patients with diabetes who are using an ACE inhibitor or ARB.

Cautions and Considerations Aliskiren has a black box that warns against use in pregnancy due to teratogenic effects. Hypersensitivity and angioedema have been reported with the use of aliskiren. Patients who have kidney impairment should use the drug cautiously.

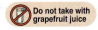 **Drug Interactions** Aliskiren may enhance the hyperkalemic effects of ACE inhibitors and ARBs, and the combination of these drugs should be avoided in most cases. Cyclosporine and itraconazole may increase the concentration of aliskiren. Grapefruit juice may decrease the concentration of aliskiren.

Combination Antihypertensives

Combination drugs have additive effects to relax blood vessels and lower blood pressure. Pharmacy technicians need to be aware that taking a combination drug may be more expensive than taking the two drugs separately, especially if two generic medications are available. Often the technician will pick up on this issue, call the prescriber, and explain how much can be saved if the patient takes two separate drugs in the same strength as the combination drug prescribed. If the prescriber will allow this, it is a great service to the patient. The pharmacist will need to make sure the patient is counseled to take the two drugs in place of the one drug.

Myocardial Infarction

Myocardial infarction (MI), commonly known as a heart attack, contributes greatly to CV disease, which is the leading cause of death in the United States according to the Centers for Disease Control and Prevention (CDC). An MI occurs when the flow of oxygenated blood to a section of the heart is blocked. This means that the heart is not receiving adequate oxygen, and if blood flow is not restored quickly, a section of the heart muscle begins to die (a process called **necrosis**). The damaged area is known as an *infarct*. Lesser infarcts undergo healing, in which muscle is replaced by scars made of connective tissue. The contractility of the heart is reduced around the scarring.

Causes of a Myocardial Infarction

An MI may occur when there is a prolonged decrease in oxygen delivery to a region of cardiac muscle. The likelihood of an MI increases substantially when the lumen (channel of a blood vessel) of one or more of the coronary arteries (the three major arteries that supply blood to the heart muscle) is narrowed by 70% or more. Factors that increase the risk of an MI include a history of angina, alcohol consumption, reduced pulmonary vital capacity, cigarette smoking, and atherosclerosis. Each year, more than 1 million individuals in the United States have an MI, and 50% of these individuals die from this event. For that reason, preventive measures are important.

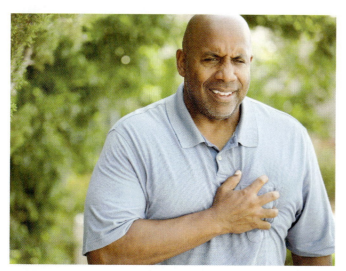

An MI can cause seemingly indirect symptoms such as anxiety and, most often, pain in the left arm.

Various lifestyle modifications may be recommended to reduce the risk of an MI:

- Eliminate smoking.
- Reduce hypertension by diet, medication, or both.
- Exercise moderately at least three times weekly.
- Adjust calories to achieve ideal body weight.
- Decrease alcohol consumption.
- Control diabetes.
- Use aspirin therapy in appropriate patients.
- Reduce dietary intake of cholesterol/triglycerides.

Symptoms of Myocardial Infarction

The most common symptoms of an MI include chest pain or discomfort, upper body discomfort, and shortness of breath. Pain and discomfort can range from mild to severe and may be experienced in the center or left side of the chest. It may feel like pressure or squeezing, or like heartburn or indigestion. Upper body discomfort may be in one or both arms, the back, shoulders, neck, jaw, or upper part of the stomach. Other common signs and symptoms include a cold sweat, unusual fatigue, nausea and vomiting, light-headedness, and dizziness. Men and women typically experience chest pain or discomfort. Women, however, are more likely to experience shortness of breath, nausea, and back or jaw pain.

Treatment of Myocardial Infarction

An MI is a medical emergency, and treatment is aimed at opening blocked arteries, controlling blood pressure, and regulating heart rhythm. In the acute phase, oxygen, nitroglycerin, and aspirin may be used. Chronic therapy may include the use of anticoagulants (discussed later in this chapter), beta blockers, ACE inhibitors, and medications to treat cholesterol. Beta blockers combined with low-dose (81 mg) aspirin are frequently prescribed to reduce the risk of death or recurrence following an MI. The beta blocker slows the action of the heart, thus reducing its workload. The aspirin prevents clot formation. Some prescribers may use an ACE inhibitor as adjunct therapy.

Clotting Disorders

Thrombin is an enzyme in blood plasma that causes the clotting of blood by reacting with fibrinogen to form fibrin. Blood clots transported in the blood, called thrombi (singular: **thrombus**), present a serious and potentially life-threatening problem. Thrombi develop from abnormalities in:

- blood coagulation, resulting in hypercoagulability;
- blood flow, leading to stasis;
- platelet adhesiveness, resulting in hypercoagulability; and
- vessel walls (from damage or surgery).

Venous thrombi usually form in areas of low-velocity blood flow, surgical or other vein injury, or large venous sinuses (pockets formed by valves in deep veins). Symptoms include swelling, discoloration, and pain. A piece of the clot may break off and travel to the lung, causing a **pulmonary embolism (PE)**, or sudden blocking of the pulmonary artery. Some patients have an undiagnosed deep vein thrombosis (DVT). A proximal (at or superior to the knee) DVT is the most serious and may be fatal.

Risk factors for DVT include the following:

- age over 40 years
- bed rest for more than four days
- estrogen combined with nicotine
- high-dose estrogen therapy
- major illness
- obesity
- pregnancy
- previous DVT
- surgery
- trauma
- varicose veins

Two classes of drugs—anticoagulants and antiplatelets—are used to reduce the risk of blood clots. An anticoagulant prevents clot formation by inhibiting clotting factors; an antiplatelet reduces the risk of clot formation by inhibiting platelet aggregation. Drugs in a third class, fibrinolytics, dissolve clots that have already formed.

Cell damage activates a pathway of coagulation, or **clotting cascade** (also referred to as *coagulation cascade*), as shown in Figure 12.9. If any factor along the path is missing, blood may not clot, as occurs in people with hemophilia. Each step involves the activation of a factor, which then triggers the next step, until finally the fibrin clot is formed. However, vessel blockage can occur as the result of fat, air, and debris gaining entry into circulation.

Anticoagulant Agents

An **anticoagulant** agent prevents clot formation by inhibiting clotting factors. Patients on anticoagulant drug therapy should be monitored to prevent future embolisms and minimize risk of hemorrhage. Patients taking anticoagulant agents must undergo frequent lab tests to monitor the drug's effectiveness.

FIGURE 12.9
**Clotting
Cascade**

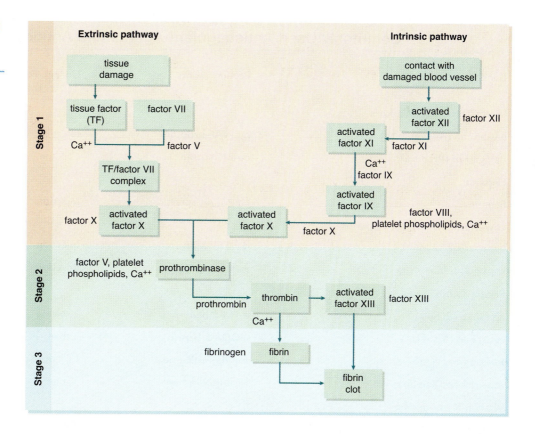

- **Partial thromboplastin time (PTT)** measures the function of the intrinsic and common pathways. (PTT is affected by heparin.)
- **Prothrombin time (PT)** assesses the function of the extrinsic and common pathways of the coagulation cascade; in particular, it measures the activity of the vitamin K–dependent factors. (PT is affected by warfarin.)
- The **international normalized ratio (INR)** standardizes the PT by comparing it to a standard index. This number will appear on the lab values. It is an important indicator because it compensates for differences in laboratories that do the blood samples. (INR is affected by warfarin.)
- **Hematocrit** is the proportion of the blood sample that is red blood cells.

Table 12.12 presents the most commonly used anticoagulant agents, as well as antidotes for them.

Direct Thrombin Inhibitors

Direct thrombin inhibitors bind directly to thrombin. They can inhibit circulating thrombin and thrombin that is bound to fibrin. Direct thrombin inhibitors may have a more predictable anticoagulant effect compared with heparins.

Bivalirudin (Angiomax) is used to treat patients with unstable angina who are undergoing angioplasty. It is a specific and reversible thrombin inhibitor.

Dabigatran (Pradaxa) is a direct thrombin inhibitor indicated for the treatment and prevention of venous thrombosis and PE and for the prevention of a CVA in non-valvular atrial fibrillation. It can be taken with or without food. The primary side effects are increased risk of bleeding, dyspepsia (upset stomach), and gastritis. Dabigatran is unique in that it must be stored and dispensed in the original container

Work Wise

Dispensing medications in the original containers may be advantageous. For one, it can save work and time for the pharmacy technician; more importantly, it can prevent drugs from being degraded by inappropriate storage.

TABLE 12.12   Commonly Used Anticoagulant Agents and Antidotes

Generic (Brand)	Pronunciation	Dosage Form	Dispensing Status
Direct Thrombin Inhibitors			
bivalirudin (Angiomax)	bye-VAL-i-roo-din	Injection	Rx
dabigatran (Pradaxa)	da-BIG-a-tran	Capsule	Rx
Heparin			
heparin	HEP-a-rin	Injection	Rx
Low-Molecular-Weight Heparins			
dalteparin (Fragmin)	dal-TEP-a-rin	Injection	Rx
enoxaparin (Lovenox)	ee-nox-a-PAIR-in	Injection	Rx
Factor Xa Inhibitors			
apixaban (Eliquis)	a-PIX-a-ban	Tablet	Rx
edoxaban (Savaysa)	e-DOX-a-ban	Tablet	Rx
fondaparinux (Arixtra)	fon-da-PAIR-i-nux	Injection	Rx
rivaroxaban (Xarelto)	ri-va-ROX-a-ban	Tablet	Rx
Vitamin K Antagonist			
warfarin (Coumadin)	WAR-far-in	Tablet	Rx
Antidote for Dabigatran			
idarucizumab (Praxbind)	EYE-da-roo-KIZ-ue-mab	Injection	Rx
Antidote for Heparin			
protamine sulfate	PROE-ta-meen SUL-fate	Injection	Rx
Antidote for Warfarin			
phytonadione or vitamin K (Mephyton)	fye-toe-na-DYE-own	Injection	Rx

(either a bottle or blister packs). Once a bottle of dabigatran is open, it must be used within four months.

More manufacturers are packaging drugs so they will not have to be repackaged in the pharmacy. There are several benefits of this practice:

1. It reduces the chance that the drug will be handled inappropriately or exposed to unclean or unsafe environments.

2. Some drugs are sensitive to light and/or moisture; leaving them in the original container protects them.

3. It may reduce confusion because the bottle appears different from others in the medicine cabinet.

4. It may be safer for the pharmacy technician and pharmacist who dispense the drugs, particularly in the case of teratogenic drugs, which should not be handled by pregnant women.

Contraindications Direct thrombin inhibitors are contraindicated in active bleeding. Dabigatran is also contraindicated in patients who have a mechanical prosthetic heart valve.

Cautions and Considerations Direct thrombin inhibitors increase the risk of bleeding that may potentially be fatal. These agents should be discontinued several days prior to surgery, if possible. Common side effects of direct thrombin inhibitors include nausea, headache, back pain, and bleeding due to excessive anticoagulation. Patients should report any signs of bleeding to their prescribers and follow instructions regarding laboratory tests.

Dabigatran carries black box warnings. One warning is for an increased risk of thrombotic events if it is discontinued prematurely. Another warning is for the risk of spinal or epidural hematoma. Older adults should use dabigatran with extreme caution, and other alternatives should be considered because of the increased risk of hemorrhage or stroke. Dabigatran should be used cautiously in patients who have kidney impairment; for these individuals, dose adjustment is necessary.

Drug Interactions Direct thrombin inhibitors may enhance the risk of bleeding with other anticoagulants. Concurrent use should be avoided if possible.

Urokinase may enhance the anticoagulant effects of dabigatran. P-glycoprotein inducers (such as carbamazepine, clotrimazole, phenytoin, and spironolactone) decrease concentrations of dabigatran; p-glycoprotein inhibitors (such as amiodarone, clarithromycin, dronedarone, itraconazole, ketoconazole, and verapamil) may increase dabigatran concentrations.

Heparin

Heparin is a naturally occurring circulatory anticoagulant produced in mast cells. It does not dissolve a clot that has already formed. Instead, heparin inhibits thrombin formation, thereby reducing the ability of blood to clot and preventing the formation of a new clot. Synthetic heparin is an IV anticoagulant medication. Heparin and low-molecular-weight heparins (LMWHs) are usually the anticoagulants of choice for pregnant patients because these drugs do not cross the placenta. Low-dose heparin may be used for prophylaxis of DVT or PE in postoperative patients, bedridden patients, obese patients, and patients with multiple bone fractures, hip prosthesis insertion, MI, or gynecologic or abdominothoracic surgery (for surgery when the limbs are not moving to assist blood flow). Heparin flushes are dilute solutions used to keep IV lines open. They should not be confused with therapeutic doses of heparin. Dosage of heparin is measured not in milligrams but in units based on biologic activity; the pharmacy technician must convert units to milliliters to determine the correct amount.

Common side effects of heparin include bruising, bleeding due to excessive anticoagulation, and **thrombocytopenia** (low platelet count). Heparin should be used with caution, however, because hemorrhaging may easily occur. **Heparin-induced thrombocytopenia (HIT)** is a rare but serious side effect that can be life-threatening. It can only be fully detected by laboratory tests but often is preceded by skin rash.

Contraindications Heparin should not be used in patients with severe thrombocytopenia or uncontrolled active bleeding (except when due to disseminated intravascular coagulation [DIC]). Full-dose heparin should also be avoided when proper coagulation tests cannot be obtained.

Cautions and Considerations To determine the presence of HIT, patients should report any signs of bleeding or skin rashes to their prescribers right away.

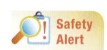

Safety Alert

Heparin can be given only intravenously or subcutaneously, usually in the abdomen. This drug must never be administered intramuscularly because an intramuscular (IM) injection will cause a hematoma (internal pooling of blood). Pharmacy technicians must be very careful to dispense the appropriate syringe and needle for subcutaneous heparin injections. If an IM syringe and needle is dispensed for heparin administration, serious damage could occur. Pharmacy personnel should know which drugs need which syringes.

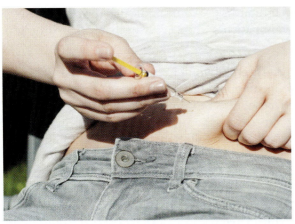

LMWHs are injected subcutaneously and come in prefilled syringes.

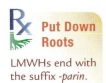

Put Down Roots

LMWHs end with the suffix *-parin*.

Drug Interactions Heparin may enhance the risk of serious bleeding of other anticoagulants. Concurrent use should be avoided, if possible.

Antidote for Heparin **Protamine sulfate** is the antidote for heparin; 1 mg neutralizes 90 to 120 units of heparin (approximately 1 mg per 100 units of heparin).

Low-Molecular-Weight Heparins

Low-molecular-weight heparins (LMWHs) are a class of anticoagulants derived from heparin. They may present a lower likelihood of bleeding compared with heparin. LMWHs are administered subcutaneously and are generally dosed once or twice daily.

LMWH products are available in vials and prefilled syringes with an attached needle intended for subcutaneous injection. Although doses are fixed by the manufacturer, prescribers will sometimes use a dose based on body weight. If a pharmacy technician receives a prescription for a fraction of a dose, or of a mixed dose, it is prudent to check with the prescriber to ensure accuracy.

Dalteparin (Fragmin) is an LMWH used to prevent thromboembolism. Unlike enoxaparin, dalteparin is dosed in units based on biologic activity.

Enoxaparin (Lovenox) is used to prevent thrombosis after surgery and to treat DVT with or without pulmonary embolism. It does not bind to heparin-binding proteins, and the half-life is two to four times that of heparin. The molecular weight of enoxaparin is approximately one-half that of heparin. At the recommended dose, single injections do not significantly influence platelet aggregation or affect clotting time. Platelet counts and the possibility of occult blood (blood that is present in small amounts only detected by laboratory tests) should be monitored, but it is not necessary to monitor PT or PTT. Side effects are hemorrhage and thrombocytopenia. In contrast to heparin and dalteparin, dosage strengths for enoxaparin are stated in milligrams rather than units based on biologic activity.

Contraindications LMWHs are contraindicated in patients who have a history of HIT, a hypersensitivity to heparin or pork products, and active major bleeding. Dalteparin is contraindicated in patients who have unstable angina, non–Q-wave MI, or prolonged venous thromboembolism prophylaxis undergoing epidural/neuraxial anesthesia.

Cautions and Considerations LMWHs require dose adjustment in patients who have impaired renal function and are contraindicated in some cases of severe kidney problems. Patients should inform their prescribers and pharmacists if they know they have kidney disease.

Drug Interactions Concurrent use of LMWHs with other anticoagulants should be avoided.

Factor Xa Inhibitors

Factor Xa is a clotting factor that is central to coagulation. Factor Xa inhibitors are anticoagulants that block the activity of factor Xa and prevent blood clots from developing or getting worse. These drugs can either directly or indirectly inhibit factor Xa.

Apixaban (Eliquis) is an oral factor Xa inhibitor that may be used for DVT prophylaxis and treatment, as well as thromboembolism prevention in nonvalvular atrial fibrillation.

Edoxaban (Savaysa) is used for the treatment of DVT and PE and for the prevention of thromboembolism in nonvalvular atrial fibrillation. Edoxaban should not be used in patients who have atrial fibrillation or a creatinine clearance greater than 95 mL/min because there is an increased risk of adverse effects.

Fondaparinux (Arixtra) is used to prevent or treat DVT. It cannot be used in patients who have kidney dysfunction or in patients weighing less than 50 kg (110 lb). A complete blood count (CBC), serum creatinine, and occult blood test are recommended periodically.

Rivaroxaban (Xarelto), a direct factor Xa inhibitor, prevents thrombosis (blood clots) in patients who have atrial fibrillation not associated with a heart valve problem. This condition places individuals at risk for a clot that forms in the heart and travels to the brain, causing a CVA. Rivaroxaban is also approved to prevent thrombosis after hip or knee replacement surgery and for patients with nonvalvular atrial fibrillation. It is the first factor Xa oral inhibitor and has a fast onset. It should be taken for 12 days after knee replacement and 35 days after hip replacement. Bleeding is the major side effect.

Contraindications Factor Xa inhibitors are contraindicated in active bleeding.

Fondaparinux is contraindicated in severe kidney impairment, bacterial endocarditis, and thrombocytopenia associated with a positive test for antiplatelet antibodies in the presence of fondaparinux.

Cautions and Considerations Factor Xa inhibitors have black box warnings. One warning is for a risk of spinal or epidural hematomas, which may result in long-term or permanent paralysis. Another warning is for thromboembolic events, which may result from premature discontinuation of these drugs.

Factor Xa inhibitors should be used with caution in patients who have kidney impairment; dose reduction is usually required.

Drug Interactions Drugs with anticoagulant properties should be avoided, if possible, with the use of factor Xa inhibitors because of a possible potentiated anticoagulant effect.

The concentrations of apixaban and rivaroxaban may be decreased by St. John's wort and increased by conivaptan and idelalisib. Edoxaban concentrations may be decreased by rifampin.

Vitamin K Antagonist

Warfarin (Coumadin) affects liver metabolism and prevents production of vitamin K–dependent clotting factors II, VII, IX, and X. The objective of warfarin therapy is to prevent future clots. As with heparin, warfarin has no effect on existing clots, but it can prevent clot formation, extension of formed clots, and secondary complications of thrombosis. Warfarin is rapidly and completely absorbed from the GI tract. Minor hemorrhaging (blood loss) may occur, but this is not an indication to stop warfarin therapy. At least three to five days are necessary for warfarin to achieve a therapeutic effect.

Contraindications Contraindications to warfarin include hemorrhagic tendencies, recent or potential surgery of the eye or CNS, major regional lumbar block anesthesia or traumatic surgery resulting in large open surfaces, blood dyscrasias, severe uncontrolled

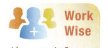
Work Wise

Always reinforce adherence to therapy and regular follow-up for patients who are receiving anticoagulation therapy. Patients who are taking warfarin initially require frequent blood tests, including an INR test every couple of days. Even after a patient has achieved a stable INR level, monthly or quarterly INR tests are generally required.

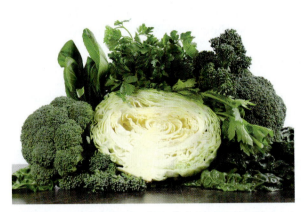

Patients who are taking oral warfarin must maintain a consistent diet of green vegetables such as kale, spinach, and broccoli to prevent a drug-food interaction.

hypertension, pericarditis or pericardial effusion, bacterial endocarditis, eclampsia or preeclampsia, threatened abortion, and pregnancy. Warfarin should also not be used in patients with a high potential of medication non-adherence.

Cautions and Considerations Patients who are prescribed warfarin are encouraged to take their warfarin at the same time each day to maintain steady drug levels in the body. Warfarin is also affected by certain foods. Because it inhibits vitamin K–dependent clotting factors, changes in the amount of vitamin K a patient ingests can affect warfarin activity. All patients, especially those just starting warfarin therapy, should learn about food and drug interactions. Foods high in vitamin K (such as green, leafy vegetables) do not have to be avoided entirely. Patients should simply avoid varying the amount of these foods that they typically eat, whether that be a little or a lot. Wide swings in the amount of vitamin K consumed will affect the activity of oral anticoagulants. Warfarin doses are adjusted according to each patient's typical daily food intake. Alcohol increases warfarin's effects. Patients taking anticoagulant drugs should not drink excessive amounts of alcohol or bleeding could occur. Moderate alcohol intake (one to two drinks a day) does not affect anticoagulation therapy.

Drug Interactions Warfarin is highly protein-bound and metabolized through the liver and therefore interacts with many alternative therapies, OTC drugs, and prescription drugs. The drug interactions with warfarin are too numerous to mention here, but some of the most common prescription drugs that interact with warfarin are listed in Table 12.13. Aspirin and NSAIDs affect clotting by changing platelet action, so they generally should not be taken with warfarin or other anticoagulants. (The risk is lower with some of the other anticoagulants, such as heparin and LMWHs.)

Interactions that affect warfarin activity can be serious. A decrease in effectiveness can cause unwanted clots; an increase in effectiveness can cause bleeding. Either way, the results of these interactions can be life-threatening. Patients should tell their prescribers and pharmacists about all medications they take so that potential interactions can be identified.

TABLE 12.13 Common Drugs that Interact with Warfarin

Amiodarone	Lovastatin
Carbamazepine	Metronidazole
Cimetidine	Phenytoin
Fenofibrate	Rifampin
Fluconazole	Rosuvastatin
Fluoxetine	Simvastatin
Fluvastatin	Sulfamethoxazole
Gemfibrozil	Tamoxifen
Levothyroxine	Voriconazole

Antidote for Warfarin Phytonadione or vitamin K (Mephyton), is an antagonist to warfarin. Charts are available to indicate the amount to administer based on the patient's INR. In severe hemorrhage, the patient is given fresh whole blood, which contains the clotting factors necessary to stop blood loss.

Antiplatelet Agents

Antiplatelet agents interfere with the chemical reactions that cause platelets to be sticky and aggregate. Table 12.14 presents the most commonly used antiplatelet agents.

General Antiplatelet Drugs

Safety Alert

Low-dose (81 mg) aspirin is often called *baby aspirin*. This designation does not mean it should be used for babies. In fact, aspirin should never be used in babies or children. Low-dose aspirin is formulated for adults and is enteric-coated to protect the lining of the stomach.

Aspirin and several other drugs are commonly used as antiplatelet medications.

Aspirin works as an antiplatelet agent by inhibiting cyclooxygenase, an enzyme that promotes clotting. This mechanism of action disrupts production of thromboxane, prostacyclin, and prostaglandin and is irreversible. In other words, clotting will be impaired until new platelets are circulating in the blood. Most patients who have had an MI, HF, CVA, or other CV conditions are instructed to take low-dose aspirin daily. It is extremely important to remember that uncoated aspirin is used when immediate absorption is needed, whereas enteric-coated aspirin is used to protect the lining of the stomach in nonemergency situations.

Aspirin has many side effects, especially GI symptoms. The labeled use of aspirin for the treatment of a CVA is only for the reduction of recurrent transient ischemic attacks (TIAs), discussed later in the chapter, or for the treatment of a CVA in patients who have had transient ischemia of the brain due to fibrin platelet emboli.

Cilostazol (Pletal) inhibits platelet phosphodiesterase. It increases a patient's ability to walk longer distances by decreasing shortness of breath. Cilostazol is used for symptomatic management of peripheral vascular disease. It is a reversible inhibitor of platelet aggregation.

Clopidogrel (Plavix) blocks adenosine diphosphate (ADP, a chemical involved in energy transmission in biologic systems) receptors and thus prevents fibrinogen binding and also reduces platelet adhesion and aggregation. Clopidogrel is approved to prevent the recurrence of atherosclerotic events such as an MI and a CVA. The major side effect of this drug is bleeding. Consequently, it should be discontinued seven days before surgery. Platelet transfusion may be appropriate if rapid reversal of the pharmacologic effects of the drug is warranted. Clopidogrel can be taken without regard to food.

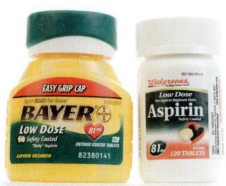

Aspirin, an antiplatelet drug, may be purchased over the counter as either a brand-name drug or a generic product.

Prasugrel (Effient) is taken with aspirin to reduce cardiovascular death, MI, and CVA. It is specifically for patients who have undergone angioplasty, which often involves the placement of a mechanical device to prevent thrombosis called a **stent**. When taken with aspirin, it reduces the risk of an MI. Prasugrel maintains the stent by keeping the platelets from sticking together and forming blood clots inside of it and the arteries of the heart. There is an increased risk of bleeding associated with the use of prasugrel. This drug must be dispensed and stored in the original container. This drug should be stopped at least seven days before surgery.

TABLE 12.14　Most Commonly Used Antiplatelet Agents

Generic (Brand)	Pronunciation	Dosage Form	Dispensing Status
General Antiplatelet Agents			
aspirin (various brands)	AS-pir-in	Caplet, capsule, rectal suppository, tablet	OTC
cilostazol (Pletal)	sil-OH-sta-zol	Tablet	Rx
clopidogrel (Plavix)	kloh-PID-oh-grel	Tablet	Rx
prasugrel (Effient)	PRA-soo-grel	Tablet	Rx
ticagrelor (Brilinta)	tye-KA-grel-or	Tablet	Rx
ticlopidine (Ticlid)	tye-KLOE-pi-deen	Tablet	Rx
Glycoprotein Antagonists			
abciximab (ReoPro)	ab-SIKS-ih-mab	Injection	Rx
eptifibatide (Integrilin)	ep-ti-FIB-a-tide	Injection	Rx
tirofiban (Aggrastat)	tye-roe-FYE-ban	Injection	Rx

Ticagrelor (Brilinta) blocks platelet aggregation. It should not be taken with aspirin that is more than 100 mg. It is used to decrease cardiovascular events in patients who have coronary syndromes. The primary side effect is bleeding. This drug is short acting; therefore, the best use of this medication may be for patients who need urgent surgery, although ticagrelor still needs to be stopped five days before surgery. It has a loading dose of 180 mg and then is taken twice daily with food. In contrast to the other drugs in this class, it may cause shortness of breath the first week, but this side effect seems to wear off.

Ticlopidine (Ticlid) is chemically related to clopidogrel. It is used to reduce the risk of thrombotic CVA (fatal or nonfatal), both for patients who have had such a CVA and for those who have experienced CVA precursors. Because ticlopidine carries a risk of neutropenia and/or agranulocytosis, the drug should be reserved for patients who cannot tolerate aspirin. Ticlopidine therapy may begin as soon as the diagnosis of TIA or thrombotic CVA has been made and cerebral hemorrhage has been ruled out. The drug may be used indefinitely. Adverse effects may include neutropenia, thrombocytopenia, diarrhea, nausea, and rash. The established protocol includes routine monitoring of CBCs and white blood cell (WBC) differentials during the first three months of therapy. After that, CBCs need to be obtained only when signs or symptoms suggest infection.

Contraindications　OTC aspirin labeling contraindicates use in patients who are allergic to other pain relievers or reducers. Aspirin should also not be taken for at least seven days after a tonsillectomy or oral surgery. Cilostazol is contraindicated in heart failure and active bleeding. Clopidogrel should not be used in active pathologic bleeding such as peptic ulcer or intracranial hemorrhage. Contraindications to prasugrel include active bleeding or prior stroke. Ticagrelor is contraindicated in active bleeding and in patients with history of intracranial hemorrhage and severe liver impairment. Contraindications to ticlopidine include active bleeding, intracranial hemorrhage, severe liver impairment, and hematopoietic disorders.

Aspirin should not be given to children. Reye's syndrome can develop in children who have been given aspirin after having been exposed to chickenpox or other viral infections. This syndrome includes a range of mental changes (mild amnesia, lethargy, disorientation, and agitation) that can culminate in coma and progressive unresponsiveness, seizures, relaxed muscles, dilated pupils, and respiratory failure. Pharmacy technicians must be mindful of combination preparations (e.g., Alka-Seltzer) that contain aspirin, if these preparations are intended for pediatric use.

Cautions and Considerations Aspirin is a salicylate and can cause salicylism, which is mild salicylate intoxication. Salicylism is characterized by tinnitus (ringing in the ears), dizziness, headache, and mental confusion. Severe intoxication is characterized by hyperpnea (abnormal increase in the depth of breathing), nausea, vomiting, acid-base disturbances, petechial hemorrhages, hyperthermia, delirium, convulsions, and coma. The lethal dose for aspirin is usually more than 10 g for an adult.

Cilostazol has a black box warning stating that it should not be used in patients with heart failure of any severity.

Clopidogrel and ticlopidine can cause thrombocytopenia (low platelet levels) and neutropenia (low WBC count).

Prasugrel has a black box warning for risk of significant or fatal bleeding. Another warning states that the use of prasugrel is generally not recommended in patients age 75 years or older. Prasugrel should not be used in patients likely to undergo coronary artery bypass surgery.

Ticagrelor has several black box warnings. One warning is for increased risk of bleeding (sometimes fatal). Another warning states that maintenance doses of aspirin should not be greater than 100 mg per day because it could decrease ticagrelor efficacy. Ticagrelor should be avoided in patients who require urgent coronary artery bypass surgery.

Drug Interactions All antiplatelet drugs can enhance the antiplatelet properties of other drugs. Combination use is not recommended. Concurrent anticoagulant use may increase risk of bleeding.

Using aspirin with other salicylates increases risk of salicylate toxicity. Aspirin increases the risk of bleeding when taken with anticoagulants.

Clopidogrel may increase concentrations of dasabuvir and enzalutamide. Esomeprazole, omeprazole, and pantoprazole may diminish the antiplatelet effects of clopidogrel.

Ticagrelor's activity may be diminished by dexamethasone. Pimozide and simvastatin concentrations may be increased by ticagrelor.

Ticlopidine may increase concentrations of pimozide and thioridazine.

Glycoprotein Antagonists

A **glycoprotein antagonist** binds to a receptor on platelets, preventing platelet aggregation as well as the binding of fibrinogen and other adhesive molecules. The action of these antagonists is reversible. Glycoprotein antagonists are indicated for acute coronary syndrome and are administered during invasive procedures to prevent artery closure.

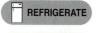

Abciximab (ReoPro) is a monoclonal antibody that is used to reduce acute cardiac complications in angioplasty patients at high risk for abrupt artery closure. The most common side effects are bleeding and thrombocytopenia. Abciximab should be refrigerated and protected from light; it should not be shaken.

Eptifibatide (Integrilin) mimics native protein sequences in the platelet receptors. It blocks binding of the platelet glycoprotein, thereby preventing platelet aggregation and thrombosis. It is reversible within two hours after infusion, which makes it a very attractive agent for invasive procedures, which are the primary use of this drug. It is also used for acute coronary syndrome to prevent the blood from clotting. The primary side effects are bleeding and thrombocytopenia. It should be refrigerated and protected from light until dispensed.

Tirofiban (Aggrastat) is used for prophylaxis or treatment of thrombosis in adults with HIT. It neutralizes clotting factor Xa and interrupts the blood coagulation cascade, thereby inhibiting thrombin formation. This drug must be protected from light.

Contraindications Hypersensitivity to murine proteins; active internal hemorrhage or recent GI or urogenital bleeding; a history of CVA within two years or with significant neurologic deficits; clotting abnormalities; administration of oral anticoagulants within seven days; thrombocytopenia; recent major surgery or trauma; intracranial tumor, arteriovenous malformation, or aneurysm; severe uncontrolled hypertension; history of vasculitis; use of dextran before percutaneous transluminal coronary angioplasty (PTCA) or intent to use dextran during PTCA; and concomitant use of another parenteral glycoprotein antagonist all contraindicate the use of abciximab.

Eptifibatide is contraindicated in active bleeding, a history of a CVA within the last month, a history of a hemorrhagic CVA, severe hypertension, recent major surgery, hemodialysis, and concurrent administration of another glycoprotein antagonist.

Tirofiban should not be used in patients who have a history of thrombocytopenia following tirofiban use, active internal bleeding, major surgical procedure, or severe recent physical trauma.

Cautions and Considerations The most common complication of glycoprotein antagonists is bleeding. Abciximab should be used with caution in older adults. Eptifibatide should be used with caution in patients who have kidney impairment. Tirofiban may cause thrombocytopenia. Tirofiban doses must be reduced in patients who have kidney impairment.

Drug Interactions Antiplatelet agents and anticoagulants increase the risk of bleeding with concurrent use of glycoprotein antagonists.

Fibrinolytic Agents

A **fibrinolytic agent** dissolves clots by binding to the clot protein formed by fibrin. Table 12.15 lists the most commonly used fibrinolytic agents. All of them are supplied in the form of a powder to be dissolved in sterile water for injection or the diluent supplied with the drug for IV use only. When reconstituting the drug from the powder, the vial should be gently swirled, never shaken, because shaking can disrupt the enzyme's molecular structure.

Alteplase (Activase) is a DNA recombinant technology product. It is a tissue plasminogen activator that dissolves clots. Side effects include bleeding, arrhythmias associated with reperfusion, allergy, nausea, vomiting, hypotension, and fever. Alteplase is most effective when administered within the first three hours after a CVA or an MI.

TABLE 12.15 Most Commonly Used Fibrinolytic Agents

Generic (Brand)	Pronunciation	Dosage Form	Dispensing Status
alteplase (Activase)	AL-te-plase	Injection	Rx
reteplase (Retavase)	REE-te-plase	Injection	Rx
tenecteplase (TNKase)	ten-EK-te-plase	Injection	Rx

Reteplase (Retavase) is given in two injections of 10 mL separated by an interval of 30 minutes. The powder must be refrigerated and must remain sealed to protect it from light until it is to be used. No other medication should be added to the IV solution line. Bleeding is the most pronounced side effect.

Tenecteplase (TNKase) is another DNA recombinant technology product that binds fibrin and converts plasminogen to plasmin. It is supplied as a powder to be dissolved in sterile water for injection, which is provided in an accompanying vial. This drug is incompatible with dextrose, so it should not be used in an IV line containing dextrose 5% in water; the line should be flushed with saline before and after injection. Tenecteplase should not be shaken before or after reconstitution. A light foaming is normal when the diluent is added to the powder. After reconstitution, tenecteplase should be allowed to sit for a few minutes to prevent denaturing (modifying the molecular structure) the solution.

Contraindications Fibrinolytics have many contraindications. They are all contraindicated in active internal bleeding. Alteplase is contraindicated in patients who have a history of a recent CVA, recent intracranial or intraspinal surgery or serious head trauma, and severe uncontrolled hypertension. Reteplase and tenecteplase should be avoided in patients with history of CVA, recent intracranial or intraspinal surgery or trauma, increased risk of intracranial bleeding, and severe uncontrolled hypertension.

Cautions and Considerations Fibrinolytics greatly increase the risk of bleeding and hemorrhage. Patients with conditions that increase the risk of bleeding should use fibrinolytics cautiously. They should be used with caution in older adults.

Drug Interactions Fibrinolytics may increase bleeding when used with other drugs that increase risk of bleeding.

Nitroglycerin may decrease the concentration of alteplase.

Cerebrovascular Accident

A **cerebrovascular accident (CVA)**, commonly known as a *stroke*, is the result of an event that interrupts the oxygen supply to a localized area of the brain. The brain is an oxygen-rich organ and requires a constant supply of oxygenated blood to keep brain tissue alive and functional. Consequently, a CVA is considered a medical emergency. Stroke can be considered as a finite event, an ongoing event, or a series of protracted occurrences. A stroke may evolve over several hours, days, or months. If the block in blood flow is brief, an individual may experience a **transient ischemic attack (TIA)**, or temporary neurologic changes during a brief period of time. TIAs may be important warning signs and predictors of imminent stroke.

Symptoms of a CVA include the following:

- sudden numbness or weakness of the face, arm, or leg (especially on one side of the body)
- sudden confusion and difficulty speaking or understanding speech
- sudden trouble seeing in one or both eyes
- sudden dizziness and loss of balance or coordination
- sudden severe headache with no known cause

Types of Cerebrovascular Accidents

There are two major types of CVA: ischemic and hemorrhagic. Each type is caused by different primary events: (1) an **ischemic stroke** or cerebral infarction, and (2) a hemorrhagic stroke or **cerebral hemorrhage**. Ischemic stroke and hemorrhagic stroke differ significantly. Ischemic stroke is the result of obstruction to blood flow, whereas a hemorrhage involves primary rupture of a blood vessel. Ischemic strokes are the most common type of strokes.

Ischemic Stroke

An **ischemic stroke**, which is the most common type of CVA, results from an obstruction of blood flow. This type of CVA may occur after a newly formed thrombus becomes lodged at its site of origin in a cerebral blood vessel. As the lumen of the vessel narrows and becomes obstructed, blood flow through the vessel slows, diminishes, and, in some cases, even ceases. The reduced blood supply to the brain results in cerebral ischemia, and infarction with tissue necrosis may follow. (see Figure 12.10)

Emboli that move from one cerebral vessel to another are known as *artery-to-artery emboli*. Both cardiogenic and artery-to-artery emboli can ultimately lodge in distal vessels, causing TIAs or infarction. Regardless of the source of the ischemia, the diminished blood flow results in less oxygen reaching the cerebral tissues.

FIGURE 12.10
Ischemic Stroke

An ischemic stroke occurs when a thrombus becomes lodged in a cerebral blood vessel.

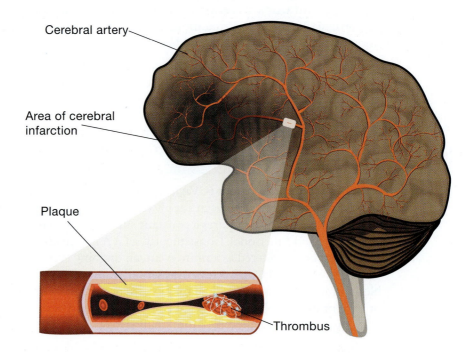

Cerebral artery

Area of cerebral infarction

Plaque

Thrombus

TABLE 12.16 CVA Risk Factors

Modifiable	Not Modifiable
Cigarette smoking	Age
Coronary artery disease	Gender
Diabetes	Genetic predisposition
Excessive alcohol intake	History of a cerebrovascular accident
Hyperlipidemia	Race
Hypertension	
Obesity	
Physical inactivity	

Hemorrhagic Stroke

A **hemorrhagic stroke** is a rupture in a blood vessel that supplies an area of the brain. This type of CVA may be marked by the sudden onset of severe headache, stiff neck, stupor, or a combination of these symptoms. Its effects are likely to be long-lasting and irreversible. A hemorrhagic stroke is most likely caused by hypertension, cerebral amyloid angiopathy, or arteriovenous malformation. Hypertensive hemorrhage and saccular (berry) aneurysms occur in separate parts of the brain with such predictability that the location itself is helpful in differential diagnosis of the stroke. Aneurysms are bulges in a blood vessel caused by weakening of the artery wall. They are usually found in the thalamus, pons, cerebellum, or putamen areas of the brain. Saccular aneurysms are thin-walled dilations that protrude off one of the arteries or proximate branches. When one of these weakened sacs ruptures, blood flows into the subarachnoid space. These aneurysms carry a high risk of death.

Risk Factors for Cerebrovascular Accident

Table 12.16 lists risk factors for a CVA. Note that some can be changed by lifestyle modifications, whereas others cannot. Important risk factors include advanced age, sex (24% higher risk for males than for females), hypertension, smoking, alcohol abuse, diabetes, and high cholesterol levels. In addition, oral contraceptive use by smokers, substance abuse, migraine headaches, and various cellular anomalies may contribute to ischemic strokes. Among the other important factors that contribute to the risk of a stroke are left ventricular hypertrophy and HF.

Several factors in a person's medical history are highly significant in the pathogenesis of cardiogenic embolic CVAs—strokes caused by heart disease. First is a history of atrial fibrillations. These very rapid, disorganized contractions of cardiac muscle lead to incomplete emptying of the atria. The blood that remains pooled in the atria has a propensity to clot. A portion of the clot may leave the heart and move into the vessels of the head and neck. Other factors that may predispose an individual to the occurrence of a CVA include rheumatic heart disease, acute MI, prosthetic heart valves, and left ventricular thrombi.

Management of a Cerebrovascular Accident

In managing a CVA, the emphasis is on prevention. There are six major categories of CVA management: antiplatelet therapy, anticoagulant therapy, fibrinolytic intervention, cerebrovascular surgery, nonpharmacologic therapy, and poststroke management.

Pharmacologic treatment options for TIAs and prevention of initial CVAs include antiplatelet and anticoagulant agents.

In the aftermath of a CVA, determination of the cause is critical for establishing optimal poststroke therapy. Antiplatelets, anticoagulants, and fibrinolytic agents play important but very different roles in CVA management. For example, treating a hemorrhage with anticoagulant or fibrinolytic agents would be detrimental. Treatment goals should confirm the diagnosis of the cause of the CVA, evaluate the cause, stabilize the event, and then establish a plan to prevent further loss to the brain. Antiplatelet agents, discussed previously, prevent platelet activation and formation of the platelet plug. Antiplatelet agents are often used to prevent recurrent thrombotic stroke and in high-risk patients, prevent initial episodes.

Treatment options for acute thrombotic CVA include anticoagulant agents and fibrinolytic agents. Anticoagulant agents interfere with the synthesis or activation of the coagulation factors in the blood. Formed clots have the potential to continue to expand and cause greater neurologic damage; anticoagulant agents may prevent existing clots from expanding. Anticoagulant agents have been routinely used to treat acute cardiogenic stroke and are used for the treatment of DVT and PE as well.

Fibrinolytic agents, also known as thrombolytic agents, differ from anticoagulant agents in one important aspect. Whereas anticoagulant agents can help prevent existing emboli and thrombi from expanding, fibrinolytic agents actually dissolve existing thrombi. Primary indications for fibrinolytic therapy include the following:

- DVT
- acute peripheral occlusion
- acute MI with embolization
- pulmonary thromboembolism
- coronary thromboembolism

Dissolution of the emboli and thrombi would appear to be preferable to simple containment. Nevertheless, adoption of fibrinolytic agents as the pharmaceutical therapy of choice has been slow, likely due to the side effects of these drugs. Additional information regarding fibrinolytics can be found in the section discussing blood clots.

Drug therapy for the prevention of CVAs and TIAs also includes several pharmaceutical products that do not fall into previously discussed drug classes. These are listed in Table 12.17 and are briefly described next.

May cause DIZZINESS

Dipyridamole (Persantine) inhibits platelet aggregation and may cause vasodilation. It maintains patency (ability to maintain open vessels) after surgical grafting procedures, including coronary artery bypass. It is used with warfarin to prevent other thromboembolic disorders. The primary side effect is dizziness. The pharmacy technician should notify the physician or pharmacist if the patient is taking other medications that affect bleeding, such as NSAIDs or warfarin. Dipyridamole is available in combination with aspirin. **Aspirin-dipyridamole (Aggrenox)** is approved to assist in preventing the recurrence of a TIA or CVA. Each dose contains 25 mg of aspirin and 200 mg of extended-release dipyridamole and is taken twice daily.

TABLE 12.17 **Preventive Drug Therapy for TIAs and CVAs**

Generic (Brand)	Pronunciation	Dosage Form	Dispensing Status
aspirin-dipyridamole (Aggrenox)	AS-pir-in dye-peer-ID-a-mole	Capsule	Rx
dipyridamole (Persantine)	dye-peer-ID-a-mole	Tablet	Rx

Contraindications Dipyridamole does not have contraindications. The combination product aspirin-dipyridamole is contraindicated in patients with hypersensitivity to aspirin or dipyridamole; an allergy to NSAIDs; and conditions such as asthma, rhinitis, and nasal polyps. Children or teenagers with viral infections should not use the combination product because aspirin may increase their risk of developing Reye's syndrome.

Cautions and Considerations Dipyridamole should be used with caution in patients with liver impairment. Older adults should be cautious of dipyridamole because it increases their risk of orthostatic hypotension.

Aspirin-dipyridamole contains salicylate, and patients are at risk for salicylate sensitivity. Tinnitus (or ringing in the ears) may occur with use. Aspirin-dipyridamole should be used with caution in patients with peptic ulcer disease or gastritis because it increases the risk of bleeding. Caution is also required in patients with kidney impairment.

Drug Interactions Increased bleeding may occur when these products are combined with other drugs that increase the risk of bleeding.

Aspirin-containing products may decrease the antihypertensive effect of ACE inhibitors. Live influenza virus and ketorolac may enhance the side effects of aspirin-containing products.

Cholesterol Abnormalities and Related Diseases

Cholesterol is an odorless, white, waxlike, powdery substance that is present in all foods of animal origin but not in foods of plant origin. Some cholesterol is essential for good health. It circulates continuously in the blood for use by all body cells. For example, lymphocytes, adrenal cortical cells, muscle cells, and renal cells use cholesterol to make cell membranes and steroid hormones, and the liver uses it to make bile acids. As mentioned earlier in the chapter, high blood cholesterol is an important risk factor for an MI or a CVA. Consequently, drugs that can lower blood cholesterol levels have come to play an important role in efforts to prevent cardiovascular disease. **Dyslipidemia** is a condition where levels of atherogenic lipoproteins are out of balance, and are either increased or decreased. An excessive amount of cholesterol in the blood is known as **hypercholesterolemia**. A related disease is **hyperlipidemia**, a condition in which the levels of one or more of the lipoproteins, discussed next, are elevated.

Causes of Dyslipidemia

Hypercholesterolemia can be an inherited disorder, or it can develop as a result of environmental factors, in particular, a diet that contains high levels of saturated fats. Food fats contain a mixture of three types of fatty acids: saturated, monounsaturated, and polyunsaturated. These terms refer to the chemical bonds that link carbon and hydrogen atoms in the fatty acid molecules. Saturated fatty acids contain as many hydrogen atoms as possible, and the molecules stick together densely.

In the body, the liver is responsible for making new cholesterol when needed and for processing cholesterol from food. The liver puts together packages containing triglycerides (the most common type of fat, in which a molecule of glycerin is bonded to three molecules of fatty acids), cholesterol, and carrier proteins, and then the liver releases these molecules into the bloodstream. Because they consist of lipids bound to proteins, these packages are called **lipoproteins**. They are spherical particles with a

FIGURE 12.11 Cross Section of Arteries

(a) Normal artery (b) Clogged artery

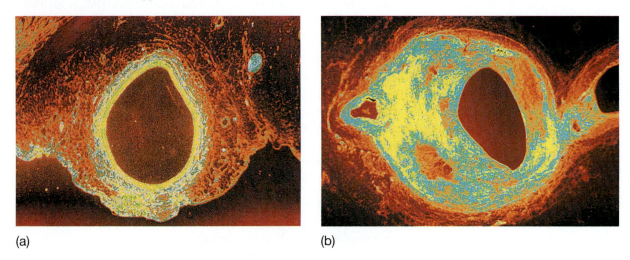

(a)   (b)

core of triglycerides and cholesterol, in varying proportions, surrounded by a surface coat of phospholipids. Most blood lipoproteins consist of two types:

- **High-density lipoproteins (HDLs)** absorb cholesterol and transport it back to the liver, where is can be excreted from the body. HDLs may be referred to as the "good cholesterol" because having elevated levels may reduce the risk for heart disease or a CVA.

- **Low-density lipoproteins (LDLs)** make up the majority of the body's cholesterol. LDLs may be referred to as the "bad cholesterol" because high levels may result in plaque buildup in the vasculature. This buildup can ultimately lead to heart disease or a CVA.

Triglycerides, a major component of lipoproteins, are neutral fats synthesized from carbohydrates for storage in adipose (fat) cells. They release free fatty acids in the blood. As the lipoproteins circulate, the triglycerides are drawn off for energy or storage.

Total cholesterol is a measure of the total amount of cholesterol in the body and is based on HDLs, LDLs, and triglycerides. In addition, in both men and women, total blood cholesterol increases throughout life. It enhances other risk factors for CAD. As described earlier, the LDLs that remain continue circulating to bring needed cholesterol to the cells of the body. LDLs not used by cells may be deposited in artery walls, eventually clogging them, as shown in Figure 12.11. The narrowing of the arteries due to deposits of cholesterol and fat on the inner surface of the vessel is known as **atherosclerosis**. Atherosclerosis can result in an MI or a CVA. Premature atherosclerosis is a common and significant consequence of dyslipidemia. Both disorders may be genetically determined but may be secondary to diabetes, obesity, alcoholism, hypothyroidism, liver disease, or kidney disease.

Lifestyle modifications are an important part of preventing and treating dyslipidemia. Most patients can achieve an average cholesterol reduction of 10%–15% through dietary interventions. The major dietary recommendations are to reduce the amount of saturated fats in the diet and increase dietary fiber intake. Physical activity is a lifestyle modification that can also be beneficial.

Drugs for Dyslipidemia

Cholesterol-lowering drugs are always used as an adjunct to proper diet control. Table 12.18 presents the most commonly used lipid-lowering agents. Some medications work better to decrease LDLs, some to decrease triglycerides, and others to increase HDLs. Drugs from different classifications are often prescribed together because they are synergistic. However, interactions between these and other drugs can cause serious muscle problems. Patients should report any symptom of myalgia (muscle pain) to their healthcare practitioners immediately.

TABLE 12.18 Most Commonly Used Lipid-Lowering Agents

Generic (Brand)	Pronunciation	Dosage Form	Dispensing Status
HMG-CoA Reductase Inhibitors			
atorvastatin (Lipitor)	a-tor-va-STAT-in	Tablet	Rx
fluvastatin (Lescol)	floo-va-STAT-in	Capsule	Rx
lovastatin (Altocor, Mevacor)	loe-va-STAT-in	Tablet	Rx
pitavastatin (Livalo)	pi-TA-va-sta-tin	Tablet	Rx
pravastatin (Pravachol)	prav-a-STAT-in	Tablet	Rx
rosuvastatin (Crestor)	roe-soo-va-STAT-in	Tablet	Rx
simvastatin (Zocor)	sim-va-STAT-in	Tablet	Rx
Fibric Acid Derivatives			
fenofibrate (TriCor)	fen-oh-FYE-brate	Tablet	Rx
fenofibric acid (Fibracor, Trilipix)	fen-oh-FYE-brik AS-id	Capsule	Rx
gemfibrozil (Lopid)	jem-FYE-broe-zil	Tablet	Rx
Bile Acid Sequestrants			
cholestyramine (Prevalite, Questran)	koe-les-TEER-a-meen	Packet, powder	Rx
colesevelam (Welchol)	koe-le-SEV-a-lam	Packet, tablet	Rx
colestipol (Colestid)	koe-LES-ti-pawl	Oral liquid, tablet	Rx
Other Cholesterol-Lowering Agents			
ezetimibe (Zetia)	ee-ZET-e-mib	Tablet	Rx
niacin (Niacor, Niaspan)	NYE-a-sin	Tablet	Rx
psyllium (Fiberall, Metamucil)	SIL-ee-um	Oral liquid	OTC
omega-3 fatty acid (Lovaza, Vascepa)	oh-MEG-ah-three FAT-ee as-id	Capsule	Rx
Combination Drugs			
amlodipine-atorvastatin (Caduet)	am-LOE-di-peen a-tor-va-STAT-in	Tablet	Rx
ezetimibe-simvastatin (Vytorin)	ee-ZET-e-mib sim-va-STAT-in	Tablet	Rx
pravastatin-buffered aspirin (Pravigard PAC)	prav-a-STAT-in BUF-erd AS-per-in	Tablet	Rx

TABLE 12.19 Drugs that May Adversely Impact Lipoproteins

Amiodarone	Estrogens
Anabolic steroids	Loop diuretics
Beta blockers	Progestins
Corticosteroids	Protease inhibitors
Cyclosporine	Thiazide diuretics

Some drugs increase cholesterol levels, and patients who have hyperlipidemia should avoid these medications. As in other situations, the advantages must be weighed against the disadvantages. See Table 12.19 for a listing of drugs that may adversely impact lipoprotein levels.

HMG-CoA Reductase Inhibitors

An **HMG-CoA reductase inhibitor**, also known as a *statin*, inhibits the enzyme that catalyzes the rate-limiting step in cholesterol biosynthesis. (HMG-CoA reductase is an abbreviated name for the enzyme.) Side effects include GI upset and headache, which may dissipate with time. Patients should report any unexplained muscle pain or weakness, especially with fever, to their healthcare practitioners immediately. Liver enzymes should also be monitored regularly. Studies have shown that fluvastatin, lovastatin, and simvastatin may have a greater cholesterol-lowering effect when taken at night because most cholesterol is produced at night. The most serious side effect of all statins is rhabdomyolysis (destruction of muscle accompanied by muscle pain).

Atorvastatin (Lipitor) is a potent lipid-lowering drug. It lowers LDLs significantly and may also lower triglycerides.

Fluvastatin (Lescol) and **lovastatin (Altocor, Mevacor)** are adjuncts to dietary therapy to decrease elevated serum total cholesterol and LDLs and may be used for primary and secondary prevention of cardiovascular disease.

Pitavastatin (Livalo) is a potent statin that can be taken any time during the day, not just in the evening like some other statins, with or without food.

Rosuvastatin (Crestor) is another potent statin. The most common side effect is muscle aches. It may be taken any time of the day with or without food.

Simvastatin (Zocor) should be taken at bedtime, and patients should report any muscle pain that is accompanied by fever. Simvastatin should be stored in well-sealed containers.

Contraindications Statins are contraindicated in patients with active liver disease or unexplained persistent elevations of liver enzymes. These medications are also contraindicated in patients who are pregnant or breast-feeding.

Lovastatin and simvastatin should not be used with boceprevir, clarithromycin, cobicistat, cyclosporine, erythromycin, gemfibrozil, human immunodeficiency (HIV) protease inhibitors, itraconazole, ketoconazole, nefazodone, posaconazole, telaprevir, telithromycin, and voriconazole. Simvastatin should not be used with danazol.

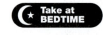

Put Down Roots

If you want to recognize the generic name of a HMG-CoA Reductase Inhibitor, just look at the ending. They all end in *-statin*.

Take at BEDTIME

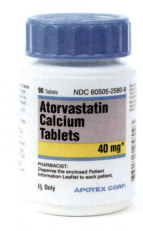

Atorvastatin is a commonly used HMG-CoA reductase inhibitor.

TABLE 12.20   Statin Equivalency Chart

Atorvastatin	Fluvastatin	Lovastatin	Pitavastatin	Pravastatin	Rosuvastatin	Simvastatin
—	40 mg	20 mg	1 mg	20 mg	—	10 mg
10 mg	80 mg	40 mg or 80 mg	2 mg	40 mg	—	20 mg
20 mg	—	80 mg	4 mg	80 mg	5 mg	40 mg
40 mg	—	—	—	—	10 mg	80 mg
80 mg	—	—	—	—	20 mg	—
—	—	—	—	—	40 mg	—

Work Wise

A prescriber may switch a patient from one statin to another. Table 12.20 lists the estimated equivalencies among HMG-CoA reductase inhibitors. For example, 10 mg of rosuvastatin is equivalent to 40 mg of atorvastatin.

Cautions and Considerations Statins are associated with rhabdomyolysis with acute kidney failure. Myopathy (a muscular disease marked by muscle pain, tenderness, or weakness) is also related to statin use. Older adults appear to be at increased risk of myopathy.

Liver function abnormalities are associated with statin use. Elevations in liver enzymes may occur and generally appear within the first year of treatment. Caution should be exercised in patients who consume substantial quantities of alcohol, have a history of liver disease, or show signs or symptoms of liver disease.

Increases in blood glucose levels may occur in patients using statins.

Dose adjustment may be necessary in patients with kidney dysfunction.

Drug Interactions Statins are associated with multiple drug interactions. Major interactions will be highlighted in this section.

Bile acid sequestrants may decrease the bioavailability of statins. Fibric acid derivatives and niacin may increase the risk of side effects of statins. Statins may increase the INR in patients using warfarin.

Amiodarone, dronedarone, macrolide antibiotics, nefazodone, protease inhibitors, and ranolazine may increase the levels and risk of myopathy of atorvastatin, lovastatin, and simvastatin. Azole antifungals and calcium channel blockers may increase the levels and risk of myopathy of atorvastatin, fluvastatin, lovastatin, and simvastatin. Colchicine may increase the risk of myopathy of atorvastatin, fluvastatin, lovastatin, pravastatin, and simvastatin. Grapefruit juice increases the risk of myopathy and decreases the metabolism of atorvastatin, lovastatin, and simvastatin. Avoidance of grapefruit juice with administration of these drugs is recommended.

Cimetidine may decrease the triglyceride-lowering effect of atorvastatin.

Atorvastatin and simvastatin may decrease levels of digoxin.

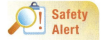

Safety Alert

High-dose (80 mg) simvastatin seems to increase patient risk of myopathy and rhabdomyolysis. Therefore, the 80-mg dose of simvastatin should only be used in patients who have been taking simvastatin long-tern without evidence of toxicity.

Fibric Acid Derivatives

Although the exact mechanism of action is unknown, **fibric acid derivatives** most likely increase the excretion of cholesterol in bile and therefore may increase the risk of gallstones. If an oral anticoagulant is being taken concurrently with a fibric acid derivative, the dose of the anticoagulant should be decreased to maintain a constant PT value. When a fibric acid derivative is used in combination with a statin, there is risk of a reaction that destroys skeletal muscle and damages the kidneys. As with statins, patients taking fibric acid derivatives should report any muscle pain to their healthcare practitioners.

Fenofibrate (TriCor) increases the catabolism (breakdown) of **very low-density lipoproteins (VLDLs)** by enhancing the synthesis of lipoprotein lipase. This drug is indicated as adjunctive therapy to dietary modification. If only marginal changes in total serum cholesterol and triglyceride concentrations are observed after six to eight weeks of therapy, fenofibrate should be discontinued. The primary side effects of fenofibrate are mild GI disturbances such as gas, diarrhea, or constipation. It should be taken with food.

Fenofibric acid (Fibricor, Trilipix) reduces cholesterol and triglycerides. It is the metabolite of fenofibrate (TriCor). Fenofibric acid should be taken either one hour after or four to six hours before other cholesterol medications. It should be discontinued if there is unexplained muscle pain, which, in rare cases, can be a result of a breakdown in skeletal muscle tissue, leading to kidney failure. Fenofibric acid is the only fibrate approved to be used with a statin. Side effects for fenofibric acid include GI symptoms, headache, and dizziness.

Gemfibrozil (Lopid) lowers triglyceride and VLDL levels while increasing HDL levels by reducing liver triglyceride production. Side effects are GI symptoms (abdominal pain, diarrhea, nausea, vomiting), CNS symptoms (vertigo, headache), alteration in taste, and skin rash.

Contraindications Fenofibrate and gemfibrozil are contraindicated in patients with active liver disease, severe kidney dysfunction, and gallbladder disease. Fenofibrate is contraindicated while breast-feeding. Gemfibrozil is contraindicated in patients using repaglinide.

Cautions and Considerations Patients with gallbladder problems usually should not use fibrates, and caution should be exercised when used in combination with statins because rhabdomyolysis can occur.

Drug Interactions Gemfibrozil may increase the risk of myopathy in patients using statins. It may also increase the adverse effects of ezetimibe.

Bile Acid Sequestrants

Bile acid sequestrants form a nonabsorbable complex with bile acids in the intestines. They block cholesterol absorption and decrease cholesterol synthesis. Constipation is the primary side effect.

Cholestyramine (Prevalite, Questran) stays in the intestines and combines with bile salts by binding with cholesterol and other fats, which are then removed in the feces. Side effects are nausea and vomiting because of the large doses required and pooling in the GI tract. Another effect is binding to medications and fat-soluble vitamins (A, D, E, K). For this reason, vitamin supplementation may be necessary.

Colesevelam (Welchol) binds bile acids in the intestines, impeding their reabsorption and increasing the fecal loss of LDLs. This drug should be taken with food.

Colestipol (Colestid) binds with bile acids to form an insoluble complex that is eliminated in the feces, thereby increasing fecal loss of LDLs. This drug should be taken with water or fruit juice or sprinkled on food. After taking the granular form, the patient should rinse the glass with a full amount of liquid and drink the contents to ensure that the full dose is taken. Other drugs should be taken at least one hour before or four hours afterward. Constipation is a side effect associated with the use of this drug.

Contraindications Cholestyramine is contraindicated in complete biliary obstruction. Colesevelam should not be used in patients with bowel obstruction, triglyceride levels greater than 500 mg/dL, or history of triglyceride-induced pancreatitis.

Cautions and Considerations Bile acid sequestrants should be used cautiously in patients with a triglyceride level greater than 300 mg/dL because these drugs may further elevate triglyceride levels.

Absorption of fat-soluble vitamins may be decreased in patients using bile acid sequestrants. They should be used with caution in patients with fat-soluble vitamin deficiencies.

Bile acid sequestrants may produce or exacerbate constipation and may cause fecal impaction.

Drug Interactions Bile acid sequestrants may decrease absorption of other drugs taken concurrently. Other drugs should be taken one hour before or six hours after other drugs.

Other Cholesterol-Lowering Agents

Ezetimibe (Zetia) lowers total cholesterol by inhibiting the absorption of cholesterol at the brush border of the small intestine (the lining of the small intestine covered by numerous folds called microvilli), leading to a decreased delivery of cholesterol to the liver. It has the additional benefit of increasing HDLs.

Niacin (Niacor) is vitamin B_3. It inhibits synthesis of VLDLs by the liver and lowers triglyceride and LDL cholesterol levels. When first taken, it induces a strange phenomenon of extreme skin flushing. This is avoidable with aspirin prophylaxis 30 minutes before taking the drug, by taking it with food, and by increasing the dose very slowly. Other side effects are nausea, vomiting, diarrhea, and an increase in uric acid levels, which can produce symptoms of gout.

Niacin (Niaspan) is a prescription form of vitamin B_3 and is an effective drug to increase HDL levels. Immediate-release forms of niacin may result in increased flushing; the extended-release prescription form decreases this side effect in many patients. Immediate-release and extended-release forms of this drug are not interchangeable. Niacin should be taken at bedtime. It should not be crushed or halved. It raises HDL cholesterol and lowers LDL cholesterol.

Psyllium (Fiberall, Metamucil) lowers cholesterol when used daily. It has the same effect as a high-fiber diet (as described in Chapter 10).

Contraindications Ezetimibe is contraindicated when used with a statin in patients with active liver disease.

Contraindications to niacin include active liver disease or persistent liver enzyme elevation, peptic ulcers, and arterial hemorrhage.

Cautions and Considerations Use ezetimibe with caution in patients with liver and kidney disease.

Niacin may increase blood glucose levels. Patients with diabetes or those individuals who are at risk for diabetes should use niacin with caution.

Drug Interactions Gemfibrozil may enhance the adverse effects of ezetimibe.

Alcohol may enhance the side effects of niacin. It may also increase the side effects of statins.

Omega-3 Fatty Acids

Omega-3 fatty acids in the form of fish oil supplements can be used as an alternative or adjunct therapy for lowering triglycerides. The omega-3 fatty acids in flaxseed and other products are different from the ones in fish. Diets high in these foods may decrease heart disease but not triglycerides.

Omega-3 fatty acids (Lovaza, Vescepa), derived from fish, interfere with the ability of the liver to synthesize triglycerides and are indicated as an adjunct to diet. Both products are available as a soft gelatin capsule.

Combination Drugs

The combination **amlodipine-atorvastatin (Caduet)** may be used to initiate treatment in patients with hyperlipidemia who have either hypertension or angina.

The combined ezetimibe-simvastatin product should not be used by patients who are pregnant or breastfeeding.

Varicose Veins

Veins are blood vessels that return blood from the organs to the heart. The organs release waste products into the blood to be transported to the heart and then to the lungs, where oxygen replaces the waste products. The blood is then transported back to the rest of the body by the arteries. The elasticity of veins allows these vessels to store unused blood while the body is at rest. In healthy veins, the valves help blood to travel toward the heart. Valves in **varicose veins** no longer function properly, thus allowing blood to travel back toward the extremities.

Treatment of Varicose Veins

Most varicose veins are relatively benign, but severe ones can lead to major complications from poor circulation through the affected limb. Inability to walk or stand, skin ulcers, skin conditions, and severe bleeding from minor trauma are a few of the complications of varicose veins. Support hose are the mainstay of treatment. When this treatment does not work, sclerotherapy, in which medication is injected into the veins to make them shrink, may be the answer. The medications used are called sclerosants (see Table 12.21). They scar and close the vein, forcing the blood to travel through healthier veins.

TABLE 12.21   Most Commonly Used Medication for Varicose Veins

Generic (Brand)	Pronunciation	Dosage Form	Dispensing Status
polidocanol (Asclera, Varithena)	pol-i-DOE-kuh-nol	Injection	Rx

Polidocanol (Asclera)

Polidocanol (Asclera, Varithena) is a sterile, colorless, sclerosing agent that is injected to treat varicose veins. It is important to prevent **extravasation** (leaking into the tissues) of this drug. Compression stockings should be worn immediately after the vein is sclerosed.

Contraindications Polidocanol is contraindicated in patients with acute thromboembolic disease.

Cautions and Considerations Severe allergic reactions are associated with polidocanol use.

Thrombosis may occur with use. Patients who have a history of thromboembolism or those individuals at risk for this condition should use this drug cautiously.

Drug Interactions There are no known significant interactions.

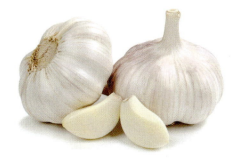

Garlic supplements may be effective in the prevention of certain cardiovascular disorders.

Complementary and Alternative Therapies

Plant sterol esters have been found to significantly lower LDL cholesterol and can be helpful adjuncts to diet and drug therapy for hyperlipidemia. Beta-sitosterol is a plant sterol similar in chemical structure to cholesterol. It is used in several food products (nutraceuticals), such as margarine and juice, for cardiovascular disease. The typical dosage of beta-sitosterol is 800 mg–6 g a day in divided doses with meals. It should not be taken with ezetimibe (Zetia) because this drug blocks sitosterol absorption and renders the dose ineffective.

Red yeast rice is a fermented rice product that is used in recipes and in medications to lower cholesterol and improve cardiovascular health. Red yeast rice is available in a capsule and tablet form and contains varying amounts of monacolins, agents with HMG-CoA reductase-inhibitor activity. There are other ingredients in red yeast rice that may lower cholesterol, such as sterols, isoflavones, and monounsaturated fatty acids. Red yeast rice supplements are usually taken at a dosage of 1,800 mg a day, divided in two doses.

Alpha tocopherol (vitamin E) supplements are used for a variety of conditions, such as cardiovascular disease, cancer, and diabetic neuropathy. The effectiveness of vitamin E for these uses has not been proven, and there is evidence to suggest vitamin E may increase the risk of heart failure. However, many individuals take this antioxidant for better health. A total dosage of 400 IU a day has been found to be safe and possibly effective for selected conditions, whereas higher dosages can cause side effects and are associated with poor outcomes.

Garlic contains organosulfur compounds that have antihyperlipidemic, antihypertensive, and antifungal effects. A variety of garlic products and supplements is available, and garlic has been found to be possibly effective in treating atherosclerosis, hypertension, some cancers, and skin fungal infections. The garlic product must contain allicin, the odorous, active ingredient produced upon crushing garlic cloves. A dosing regimen of 600–1,200 mg a day, divided into three doses, has been used in clinical trials. One clove of fresh garlic a day has also been used. Patients taking warfarin, saquinavir (a drug used to treat HIV), or other PIs should not take garlic.

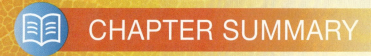

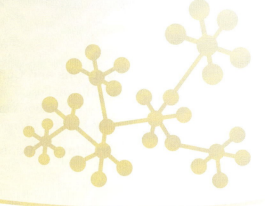

Cardiovascular System and Causative Factors of Cardiovascular Disease

- The heart is a complicated organ. Many factors contribute to the development of heart disease. Some factors, such as heredity, gender, and age, are predetermined, but others can be influenced by lifestyle modification.

- Proper diet, exercise, and rest can help to keep the heart functioning for a long time.

Angina

- Angina pectoris is an imbalance between oxygen supply to the heart and oxygen demand from the heart. The three main types are stable, unstable, and variant.

- Drugs used to treat angina include beta blockers, nitrates, calcium channel blockers, and a metabolic modifier.

- Beta blockers may mask symptoms of hypoglycemia; patients with diabetes should use these drugs cautiously.

- Carvedilol (Coreg) is a beta blocker used to treat hypertension and heart failure.

- Sotalol (Betapace) is a beta blocker indicated for the treatment of arrhythmias that are life-threatening.

- Nitrates are drugs commonly used to treat angina; they dilate coronary vessels, leading to redistribution of blood flow to ischemic tissues. Nitrates reduce preload on the heart, which reduces cardiac workload.

- A transdermal nitroglycerin patch should be removed at night to prevent development of tolerance to the drug. The label should instruct the patient in this procedure.

- Patients may experience a severe headache when initiating nitroglycerin therapy.

- Generic names of many beta blockers end in *-lol*.

- Generic names of many calcium channel blockers end in *-ipine*.

Arrhythmia

- Normal heart rhythm is generated by the sinoatrial (SA) node and propagated to the myocardium. In turn, the atria contract to fill the ventricles, and then the ventricles contract to eject blood into the arteries.

- Heart rate abnormalities can be caused by ischemia, infarction, or alteration of chemical balances that allow heart cells other than the SA node to fire automatically and become ectopic pacemakers.

- Various types of arrhythmias show specific patterns on the ECG and are associated with different degrees of danger.

- The various classes of antiarrhythmic drugs have characteristic electrophysiologic effects on the myocardium.

- The classes of drugs used to treat arrhythmias are grouped as class I (membrane-stabilizing agents), class II (beta blockers), class III (potassium channel blockers), class IV (calcium channel blockers), and others.

- Digoxin (Lanoxicaps, Lanoxin) may be used in managing atrial flutter, atrial fibrillation, and heart failure. It increases the force of contraction, the refractory period, and stimulation due to ion imbalance. The three primary signs of digitalis toxicity are nausea, vomiting, and arrhythmias.

- Atropine is used to treat bradycardia. It is also used preoperatively to inhibit salivation and secretions.

Heart Failure

- Heart failure occurs when the pumping ability of the heart can no longer sustain the blood flow required to meet the metabolic needs of the body.

- Medications to treat the effects of heart failure include vasodilators, angiotensin-converting enzyme (ACE) inhibitors, and human B-type natriuretic peptide.

- Generic names of most ACE inhibitors end in -pril.

Hypertension

- Cardiac output, which is the product of heart rate and stroke volume, is determined by preload, afterload, and contractility.

- Hypertension should be treated with salt restriction, weight control, regular exercise, reduction of alcohol consumption, cessation of smoking, stress control, and medication as prescribed.

- Drugs commonly used to treat hypertension include ACE inhibitors, angiotensin II receptor antagonists, beta blockers, calcium channel blockers, and diuretics.

- ACE inhibitors reduce blood pressure by competitive inhibition of the angiotensin-converting enzyme, preventing the conversion of angiotensin I to angiotensin II, a potent vasoconstrictor.

- Angiotensin receptor blockers (ARBs) reduce blood pressure by blocking angiotensin II at its receptors. Bound angiotensin II is not able to exert its effects. ARBs are less likely to cause coughing and angioedema than ACE inhibitors do because the angiotensin-converting enzyme, which also breaks down bradykinin, is not inhibited.

- Generic names of most ARBs end in *-artan*.

- Calcium channel blockers reduce blood pressure by arteriolar dilation, which leads to reduced peripheral resistance.

- Beta blockers, calcium channel blockers, and ACE inhibitors are all equally effective drugs used in the treatment of hypertension.

- Clonidine is an antihypertensive that has a transdermal delivery system.

Myocardial Infarction

- Myocardial infarction (MI) occurs when there is a prolonged decrease in oxygen delivery to a region of cardiac muscle; this hypoxia results in tissue death.

- MI is a leading cause of death in the United States.

- Symptoms of an MI include oppressive or burning tightness or squeezing in the chest; a feeling of choking and indigestion-like expansion; a sense of impending doom; and substernal pain, which may radiate to the neck, throat, jaw, shoulders, and one or both arms.

- Beta blockers and low-dose aspirin are prescribed for reducing the risk of death or recurrence following an MI.

Blood Clots

- Blood clots in the bloodstream (thrombi) can cause life-threatening pulmonary embolisms and other serious damage.

- Anticoagulants prevent clot formation by affecting clotting factors; antiplatelets reduce the risk of clot formation by inhibiting platelet aggregation.

- Partial thromboplastin time (PTT) measures the function of the intrinsic and common pathways; it is affected by heparin.

- Heparin inhibits thrombin formation, thereby reducing clot formation; it does not dissolve a clot that has already formed.

- Protamine sulfate is the antidote for heparin.

- Phytonadione or vitamin K₁ (Mephyton), is an antidote for warfarin.

- Aspirin may be prescribed to prevent a CVA or an MI.

- Glycoprotein antagonists are administered during invasive procedures to prevent artery closure.

- Fibrinolytic agents dissolve clots. They are used to treat a massive PE, an MI, and a CVA.

Cerebrovascular Accident

- A CVA may be caused by one of two primary events: a cerebral hemorrhage or a cerebral infarction.

- A TIA is a very strong predictor of an impending CVA.

- Risk factors for a CVA include advanced age, male sex, hypertension, smoking, alcohol abuse, diabetes, and high cholesterol levels.

- Emphasis should be on CVA prevention.

- Antiplatelet agents prevent platelet activation and formation of the platelet plug.

- Anticoagulant agents are used for deep vein thrombosis and pulmonary emboli and to prevent a CVA.

High Cholesterol and Related Diseases

- The liver packages triglycerides, cholesterol, and carrier proteins in spherical particles called *lipoproteins*, which circulate in the blood.

- Drugs are used as an adjunct to proper diet to prevent dyslipidemia.

- Some combinations of these drugs are synergistic; others can be dangerous. Any symptom of muscle pain should be reported to the physician immediately.

- Thiazide diuretics, loop diuretics, and glucocorticoids all increase the lipid profile unfavorably.

- Statins are HMG-CoA reductase inhibitors, and their generic names end in *-statin*.

action potential the electrical signal that causes a muscle to contract

afterload arterial impedance; it determines cardiac output

agranulocytosis a severe blood condition

angina pectoris spasmodic or suffocating chest pain caused by insufficient oxygen supply to meet oxygen demand

angiotensin receptor blockers (ARBs) drugs that block the action of angiotensin

anticoagulant a drug that prevents clot formation by affecting clotting factors

antiplatelet a drug that reduces the risk of clot formation by inhibiting platelet activation and aggregation

arrhythmia variation in heartbeat, irregular heartbeat

arteries vessels that carry blood from the heart

atherosclerosis accumulation of lipoproteins and fats on the inner surfaces of arteries, eventually clogging the arteries and leading to MI, stroke, or gangrene

atrioventricular (AV) node part of the conduction system of the heart that carries the action potential from the atria to the ventricles with a delay

beta-1 receptors receptors found primarily in the heart and kidneys

beta-2 receptors receptors found primarily in the lungs

beta blocker a class II antiarrhythmic drug that competitively blocks response to beta-adrenergic stimulation and therefore lowers heart rate, myocardial contractility, blood pressure, and myocardial oxygen demand; used to treat arrhythmias, MIs, hypertension, and angina

blood pressure (BP) the result of the heart forcing the blood through the capillaries; measured in millimeters of mercury, both when the heart is contracting and forcing the blood (systolic) and when the heart is relaxed and filling with blood (diastolic)

bradycardia abnormally slow heart rate

calcium channel blocker a class IV antiarrhythmic drug that prevents the movement of calcium ions through slow channels; used for most supraventricular tachyarrhythmias and in angina

capillaries tiny blood vessels

cardiogenic embolic CVAs strokes caused by heart disease

cardiomegaly enlargement of the heart due to overwork from overstimulation

cardiovascular (CV) disease pertaining to the heart and blood vessels

cardiovascular system the body system that includes the heart and blood vessels and circulates blood throughout the body

cerebral hemorrhage bleeding in the cerebrum

cerebrovascular accident (CVA) the result of an event that interrupts oxygen supply to an area of the brain; medical term for stroke

cholesterol an odorless, white, waxlike, powdery substance that is present in all foods of animal origin but not in foods of plant origin

clotting cascade a series of events that initiate blood clotting, or coagulation

contractility the cardiac muscle's capacity for becoming shorter in response to a stimulus; along with preload and afterload, it determines cardiac output

depolarization reversal of the negative voltage across a heart or nerve cell membrane, caused by an inflow of positive ions

diastolic blood pressure the blood pressure measurement that measures the pressure during the dilation of the heart

dyslipidemia an abnormal amount of lipids in the blood

ectopic pacemaker a pacemaker other than the SA node

extravasation leaking of fluid into the tissue

fibric acid derivatives drug that increases the excretion of cholesterol in bile and may increase the risk of gallstones

fibrinolytic an agent that dissolves clots

glycoprotein antagonist an antiplatelet agent that binds to receptors on platelets, preventing platelet aggregation as well as the binding of fibrinogen and other adhesive molecules

heart failure (HF) a condition in which the heart can no longer pump adequate blood to the body's tissues; results in engorgement of the pulmonary vessels

hematocrit a blood test that measures the percentage of the volume of whole blood that is made up of red blood cells

heparin-induced thrombocytopenia a potentially fatal immune-mediated adverse drug reaction caused by the emergence of antibodies that activate platelets in the presence of heparin

hemorrhagic stroke a rupture in a blood vessel that supplies an area of the brain

high-density lipoproteins (HDLs) lipoproteins containing 5% triglyceride, 25% cholesterol, and 50% protein; "good cholesterol"

HMG-CoA reductase inhibitor a drug that inhibits the rate-limiting step in cholesterol formation

hypercholesterolemia disorder characterized by excessive cholesterol

hyperkalemia an elevated potassium level

hyperlipidemia elevation of the levels of one or more of the lipoproteins in the blood

hypertension elevated blood pressure, in which systolic blood pressure is greater than 140 mm Hg and diastolic pressure is greater than 90 mm Hg

international normalized ratio (INR) a method of standardizing the prothrombin time (PT) by comparing it to a standard index

ischemia an inadequate blood supply to an organ, especially the heart muscles

ischemic stroke a cerebral infarction, in which a region of the brain is damaged by being deprived of oxygen

leukopenia low white blood cell count

lipoprotein a spherical particle containing a core of triglycerides and cholesterol, in varying proportions, surrounded by a surface coat of phospholipids that enables it to remain in solution

low-density lipoproteins (LDLs) lipoproteins containing 6% triglycerides and 65% cholesterol; "bad cholesterol"

low-molecular-weight heparin (LMWH) class of anticoagulants derived from heparin

membrane-stabilizing agent a class I antiarrhythmic drug that slows the movement of ions into cardiac cells, thus reducing the action potential and dampening abnormal rhythms and heartbeats

myocardial infarction (MI) a heart attack; occurs when a region of the heart muscle is deprived of oxygen

orthostatic hypotension a decrease in blood pressure within three minutes of standing when compared with blood pressure from sitting or lying down

partial thromboplastin time (PTT) a test that measures the function of the intrinsic and common pathways in blood clottin

preload the mechanical state of the heart at the end of diastole; along with afterload and contractility, it determines cardiac output

prothrombin time (PT) a test that assesses the function of the extrinsic pathways of the coagulation system; affected by warfarin

pulmonary embolism (PE) sudden blocking of the pulmonary artery by a blood clot

repolarization restoration of the negative voltage across a heart or nerve cell membrane, caused by an outflow of positive ions

sinoatrial (SA) node the pacemaker area of the heart

stable angina a type of angina characterized by effort-induced chest pain from physical activity or emotional stress; usually predictable and reproducible

stent a mechanical device placed to prevent thrombosis

systolic blood pressure a blood pressure measurement that measures the pressure during contraction of the heart

tachycardia excessively fast heart rate

thrombocytopenia a decrease in the bone marrow production of blood platelets

thrombin an enzyme in blood plasma that causes the clotting of blood by reacting with fibrinogen to form fibrin

thrombus blood clot

total cholesterol a measure of the total amount of cholesterol in the body and is based on HDL, LDL, and triglycerides

transient ischemic attack (TIA) temporary neurologic change that occurs when part of the brain lacks sufficient blood supply over a brief period of time; it may be a warning sign and predictor of imminent stroke

triglycerides a neutral fat stored in animal adipose tissue that releases free fatty acids into the blood

unstable angina a type of angina characterized by chest pain that occurs with increasing frequency, diminishes the patient's ability to work, and has a decreasing response to treatment; it may signal an oncoming MI

variant angina a type of angina characterized by chest pain due to coronary artery spasm; usually not stress induced

varicose vein a vein that has become enlarged or stressed because the valves no longer function properly, thus allowing blood to travel back toward the extremities

vasodilators drugs that cause blood vessels to dilate

vein a tube that carries oxygen-depleted blood toward the heart

very-low-density lipoproteins (VLDLs) lipoproteins containing 60% triglycerides and 12 % cholesterol

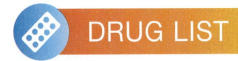

DRUG LIST

Antianginal Drugs

Beta Blockers

acebutolol (Sectral)
atenolol (Tenormin)
betaxolol (Kerlone)
bisoprolol (Zebeta)
carvedilol (Coreg)
esmolol (Brevibloc)
labetalol (Normodyne, Trandate)
metoprolol (Lopressor, Toprol-XL)
nadolol (Corgard)

nebivolol (Bystolic)
pindolol (Visken)
propranolol (Hemangeol, Inderal, InnoPran XL)
sotalol (Betapace)
timolol (Blocadren)

Nitrates

isosorbide dinitrate (Dilatrate-SR, Isordil)
isosorbide mononitrate (Imdur, Ismo)
nitroglycerin (Minitran, Nitrolingual, Nitrostat, Nitro-Dur)

Calcium Channel Blockers

amlodipine (Norvasc)
diltiazem (Cardizem, Dilacor XR)
felodipine (Plendil)
isradipine (Dynacirc)
nicardipine (Cardene)
nifedipine (Afeditab, Nifediac, Procardia)
nisoldipine (Sular)
verapamil (Calan, Verelan)

Metabolic Modifier

ranolazine (Ranexa)

Antiarrhythmic Agents

Membrane-Stabilizing Agents

disopyramide (Norpace)
flecainide (Tambocor)
lidocaine (Xylocaine)
mexiletine (Mexitil)
phenytoin (Dilantin)
procainamide (Procanbid, Pronestyl)
propafenone (Rythmol)
quinidine

Potassium Channel Blockers

amiodarone (Cordarone)
dofetilide (Tikosyn)
dronedarone (Multaq)

Other Antiarrhythmic Agents

atropine (none)
digoxin (Digitek, Digox, Lanoxicaps, Lanoxin)
isoproterenol (Isuprel)

Antidote for Digoxin Toxicity

digoxin immune Fab (Digibind, DigiFab)

ACE Inhibitors

benazepril (Lotensin)
captopril (Capoten)
enalapril (Epaned, Vasotec)
fosinopril (Monopril)
lisinopril (Prinivil, Zestril)
moexipril (Univasc)
perindopril (Aceon)
quinapril (Accupril)
ramipril (Altace)
trandolapril (Mavik)

Human B-type Natriuretic Peptide

nesiritide (Natrecor)

Vasodilators

hydralazine (Apresoline)
isoproterenol (Isuprel)
isosorbide dinitrate-hydralazine (BiDil)
milrinone (Primacor)
nitroprusside (Nitropress)

Drugs for Treating Hypertension

Angiotensin II Receptor Antagonists (ARBs)

azilsartan (Edarbi)
candesartan (Atacand)
eprosartan (Teveten)
irbesartan (Avapro)
losartan (Cozaar)
olmesartan (Benicar)
telmisartan (Micardis)
valsartan (Diovan)

CNS Agents

clonidine (Catapres, Catapres-TTS, Duraclon, Kapvay)
guanfacine (Tenex)
methyldopa (Aldomet)

Peripheral Acting Agents (Alpha Blockers)

alfuzosin (Uroxatral)
doxazosin (Cardura)
phentolamine (Regitine)
prazosin (Minipress)
terazosin (Hytrin)

Direct Renin Inhibitors

aliskiren (Tekturna)

Combinations

aliskiren-amlodipine-hydrochlorothiazide (Amturnide)
aliskiren-valsartan (Valturna)
amlodipine-benazepril (Lotrel)
amlodipine-telmisartan (Twynsta)
amlodipine-valsartan (Exforge)
atenolol-chlorthalidone (Tenoretic)
benazepril-hydrochlorothiazide (Lotensin HCT)
bisoprolol-hydrochlorothiazide (Ziac)

enalapril-hydrochlorothiazide (Vaseretic)
irbesartan-hydrochlorothiazide (Avalide)
lisinopril-hydrochlorothiazide (Prinzide,
   Zestoretic)
losartan-hydrochlorothiazide (Hyzaar)
trandolapril-verapamil (Tarka)
valsartan-hydrochlorothiazide
   (Diovan HCT)

Factor Xa Inhibitors

Apixaban (Eliquis)
Edoxaban (Savaysa)
Fondaparinux (Arixtra)
Rivaroxaban (Xarelto)

Anticoagulants

bivalirudin (Angiomax)
dabigatran (Pradaxa)
fondaparinux (Arixtra)
heparin
lepirudin (Refludan)
rivaroxaban (Xarelto)
warfarin (Coumadin)

Low-Molecular-Weight Heparins

dalteparin (Fragmin)
enoxaparin (Lovenox)

Antidote for Heparin

protamine sulfate

Antidote for Warfarin

phytonadione (Mephyton, Vitamin K$_1$)

Antiplatelet Agents

aspirin
cilostazol (Pletal)
clopidogrel (Plavix)
prasugrel (Effient)
ticagrelor (Brilinta)
ticlopidine (Ticlid)

Glycoprotein Antagonists

abciximab (ReoPro)
eptifibatide (Integrilin)
tirofiban (Aggrastat)

Fibrinolytic Agents

alteplase (Activase)
reteplase (Retavase)
tenecteplase (TNKase)

Stroke Prevention

aspirin-dipyridamole (Aggrenox)
dipyridamole (Persantine)

Lipid-Lowering Agents

HMG-CoA Reductase Inhibitors (Statins)

atorvastatin (Lipitor)
fluvastatin (Lescol)
lovastatin (Altocor, Mevacor)
pitavastatin (Livalo)
pravastatin (Pravachol)
rosuvastatin (Crestor)
simvastatin (Zocor)

Fibric Acid Derivatives

fenofibrate (TriCor)
fenofibric acid (Trilipix)
gemfibrozil (Lopid)

Bile Acid Sequestrants

cholestyramine (Questran, Prevalite)
colesevelam (WelChol)
colestipol (Colestid)

Miscellaneous Cholesterol-Lowering Drugs

ezetimibe (Zetia)
niacin (Niacor, Niapsan)
omega-3 fatty acid (Lovaza, Vescepa)
psyllium (Fiberall, Metamucil)

Combinations

amlodipine-atorvastatin (Caduet)
ezetimibe-simvastatin (Vytorin)
pravastatin-buffered aspirin (Pravigard PAC)

Sclerosing Agent

polidocanol (Asclera, Varithena)

Black Box Warnings

Note that, as a class, all beta blockers
   have Black Box warnings.

acebutolol (Sectral)
aliskiren (Tekturna)
aliskiren-valsartan (Valturna)
amiodarone (Cordarone)
aspirin (Many)
atenolol (Tenormin)
betaxolol (Kerlone)
bisoprolol (Zebeta)

carvedilol (Coreg)
cilostazol (Pletal)
clopidogrel (Plavix)
disopyramide (Norpace)
dofetilide (Tikosyn)
dronedarone (Multaq)
esmolol (Brevibloc)
flecainide (Tambocor)
fondaparinux (Arixta)
labetalol (Normodyne, Trandate)
metoprolol (Lopressor, Toprol-XL)
mexiletine (Mexitil)
minoxidil (Loniten, Rogaine)
moracizine (Ethmozine)
nadolol (Corgard)
nebivolol (Bystolic)
nitroprusside (Nitropress)
phenytoin (Dilantin)
pindolol (Visken)
procainamide (Procanbid, Pronestyl)
propafenone (Rythmol)
propranolol (Hemangeol, Inderal,
    InnoPran XL)
phytonadione (Mephyton, Vitamin K_1)
prasugrel (Effient)
protamine sulfate
quinidine
sotalol (Betapace)
ticagrelor (Brilinta)
ticlopidine (Ticlid)
timolol (Blocadren)
warfarin (Coumadin)

Medication Guides

amiodarone (Cordarone)
clopidogrel (Plavix)
dabigatran (Pradaxa)
dofetilide (Tikosyn)
dronedarone (Multaq)
fenofibric acid (Fibricor, Trilipix)
prasagral (Effient)
rivaroxaban (Xarelto)
ticagrelor (Brilinta)
warfarin (Coumadin)

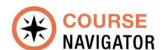

COURSE NAVIGATOR

Access interactive chapter review exercises, practice activities, flash cards, and study games.

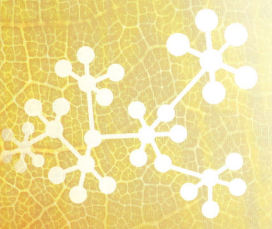

13

Drugs for Muscle and Joint Disease

Learning Objectives

1 Define the role of muscle relaxants.

2 Identify muscle relaxants and their various mechanisms of action.

3 Identify the nonnarcotic analgesics, and describe their uses and mechanisms of action.

4 Identify agents used to treat osteoarthritis, and gout and discuss their usage and side effects.

5 Define autoimmune diseases.

6 Describe treatments for autoimmune disorders including rheumatoid arthritis and systemic lupus erythematosus.

COURSE NAVIGATOR

Access additional chapter resources.

Conditions of the muscles and joints are quite common. Muscle relaxants are used to reduce spasticity associated with multiple sclerosis, cerebral palsy, skeletal muscle injuries, orthopedic surgery, postoperative recovery, and spinal cord injury. Other problems that involve muscles and joints are treated with nonsteroidal anti-inflammatory drugs (NSAIDs). Many NSAIDs are achieving over-the-counter (OTC) status, which means that more NSAIDs will be used by patients for self-medication. Osteoarthritis, rheumatoid arthritis, and gout are other ailments of the joints. These conditions are treated with various agents. The pharmacy technician must be aware of the side effects and proper use of these drugs.

Muscles and Joints

Bones of the skeletal system, which provides the framework of the human body, are connected at **joints**. A joint is the place of union or junction between two or more bones of the skeleton, which increases its flexibility. The work of movement at joints is performed by skeletal muscles, which are contractile tissues. That is, joints and muscles work together to allow the body to move. Any injury or illness that seriously affects a joint or muscle impedes movement of that part of the body and can have a devastating effect on the quality of life. Even relatively minor injuries, stiffness, or minor but persistent pain can be annoying.

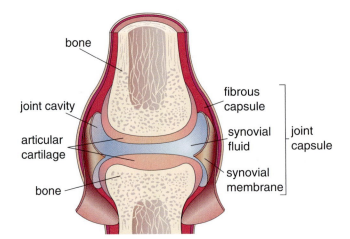

The human body contains a wide variety of joints. The anatomy of a typical joint is shown in Figure 13.1. In addition to the components shown in Figure 13.1, **ligaments** (noncontractile connective tissue that ties one bone to another bone) are essential for keeping bones aligned and forming the fibrous capsule that encloses the moving parts. Joints can be classified in a number of ways. One method of classification is joint structure according to the following categories:

- **Cartilaginous**—articulating bone surfaces are covered with cartilage
- **Fibrous**—articulating bone surfaces are attached by fibrous connective tissue
- **Synovial**—articulating surface is covered by a fluid-filled, fibrous sac

Furthermore, joints can be classified based on whether they permit no movement, a slight degree of movement, or a variety of types of movement. Figure 13.2 presents a variety of joint types.

A **muscle** is an organ that produces movement by contracting (shortening itself). Muscles are connected to bones by tough, cordlike tissues called tendons. Figure 13.3 shows the involvement of the bones, muscles, and tendons to produce movement at the elbow joint. In addition to creating skeletal movement, muscle contraction pumps blood, facilitates motility in the gastrointestinal tract, and produces uterine contractions during birth among other involuntary movements. Muscles are typically grouped into the following three types:

- **Skeletal**—striated muscle in which contraction is voluntary; contraction is used for locomotion and maintaining posture
- **Smooth**—muscle in which contraction is involuntary; occurs in the lining of various organs such as the stomach, esophagus, uterus, and bladder
- **Cardiac**—heart muscle; involuntary, but the texture of the muscle is striated

These three types of muscles are illustrated in Figure 13.4.

Muscles

Skeletal muscles are voluntarily controlled by impulses originating in the central nervous system (CNS). Electrical impulses are conducted through the spinal cord by somatic neurons that eventually communicate with the muscle at the neuromuscular junction. The neurotransmitter **acetylcholine (ACh)** is released to bind with nicotinic receptors on the muscle cell membrane. When the neurotransmitter binds to the

FIGURE 13.2   The Human Skeleton and Examples of Joints and Their Functions

Joints function in many different ways, such as ball-and-socket, hinge, pivot, glide, and others.

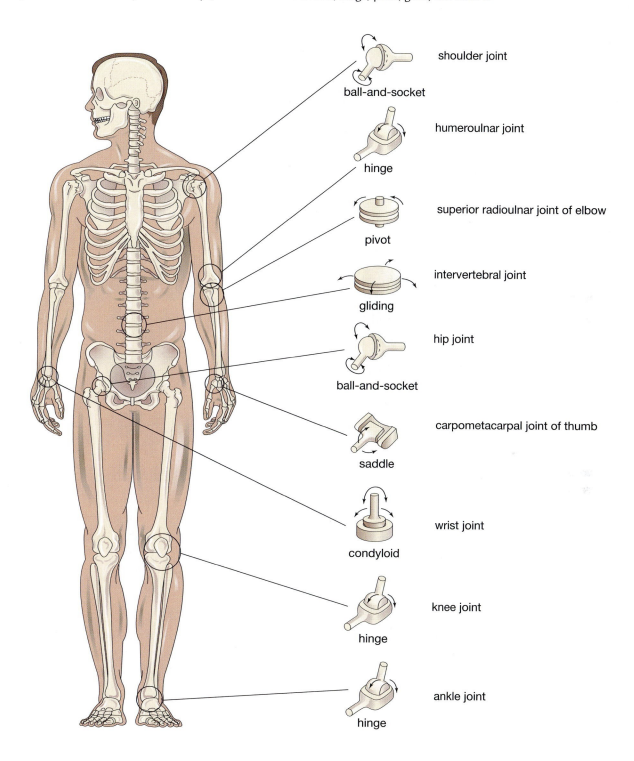

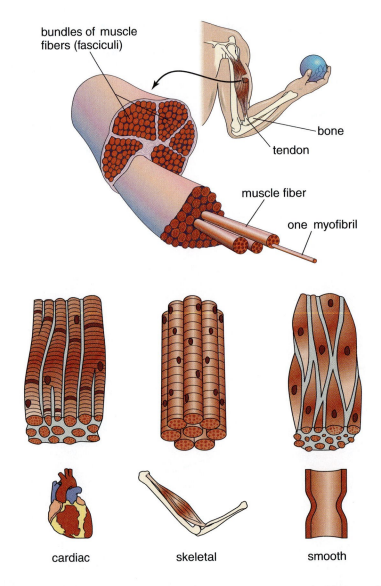

FIGURE 13.3
Bones, Muscles, and Tendons

In this figure, the involvement of bones, muscles, and tendons produce movement at the elbow joint.

bundles of muscle fibers (fasciculi)

bone

tendon

muscle fiber

one myofibril

FIGURE 13.4
Types of Muscle Tissue

There are different types of muscle tissue, such as cardiac, skeletal, and smooth.

cardiac   skeletal   smooth

receptor, calcium is released, causing a contraction in the muscle fibers. Relaxation occurs when ACh is broken down by acetylcholinesterase. Skeletal muscle contractions can be either voluntary (movement) or involuntary (tone, posture).

Muscle Relaxants

A **muscle relaxant** is an agent used specifically to reduce muscle tension. These substances act on motor neurons or at the neuromuscular junction. These agents block normal muscle function by one of the following mechanisms:

- blocking release of ACh
- preventing destruction of ACh at nicotinic receptors (continuous depolarization leads to paralysis by fatigue)
- preventing ACh from reaching nicotinic receptors (competitive nondepolarizing inhibitors)

Agents that continuously bind to ACh nicotinic receptors can also block normal muscle function; like the compounds that prevent destruction of ACh, these depolarize

TABLE 13.1 Most Commonly Used Muscle Relaxants

Generic (Brand)	Pronunciation	Dosage Form	Dispensing Status	Controlled-Substance Schedule
baclofen (Baclofen, EnovaRX-Equipto-Baclofen, Gablofen, Lioresal)	BAK-loe-fen	Injection, tablet, topical cream	Rx	
carisoprodol (Soma)	kar-eye-soe-PROE-dawl	Tablet	Rx	C-IV*
chlorzoxazone (Lorzone, Parafon Forte DSC)	klor-ZOX-a-zone	Tablet	Rx	
cyclobenzaprine (Amrix, Flexeril, Fexmid)	sye-kloe-BEN-za-preen	Tablet	Rx	
dantrolene (Dantrium, Revonto, Ryanodex)	DAN-troe-leen	Capsule, injection	Rx	
diazepam (Valium)	dye-AZ-e-pam	Injection, tablet, oral solution, rectal gel	Rx	C-IV
metaxalone (Metaxall, Skelaxin)	me-TAX-a-lone	Tablet	Rx	
methocarbamol (Robaxin)	meth-oh-KAR-ba-mawl	Injection, tablet	Rx	
orphenadrine (Norflex)	or-FEN-a-dreen	Injection, tablet	Rx	

*in some states

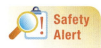

Safety Alert

The Institute for Safe Medication Practices (ISMP) includes baclofen on its list of drugs that have a heightened risk of causing significant patient harm when used in error.

muscle fibers, causing paralysis by fatigue. Centrally acting muscle relaxants do not directly relax muscles. Instead, they depress the CNS and thereby reduce the anxiety that increases muscle tone or the reflex signals that result in spasms. Table 13.1 presents the most commonly used muscle relaxants.

Muscle relaxants are used to reduce spasticity in multiple sclerosis, cerebral palsy, skeletal muscle injuries, orthopedic surgery, postoperative recovery, and spinal cord injury. Some dispensing issues are common among the muscle relaxants. To prevent possible drug interactions, a drug history should be completed for a patient before administering any of these drugs. The pharmacy technician will often obtain this history from the healthcare practitioner and update it as necessary. The sedative properties of these drugs cause the patient to relax, which in turn reduces reflex impulse conduction. Side effects of the muscle relaxants are sedation, reduced mental alertness, reduced motor abilities, and gastrointestinal (GI) upset. Patients taking these drugs should avoid alcohol.

Baclofen

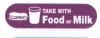

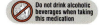

Baclofen (EnovaRX-Baclofen, Equipto-Baclofen, Gablofen, Lioresal) is a **centrally acting** muscle relaxant. That is, it does not directly act on the muscle or neuromuscular junction, but it inhibits transmission of monosynaptic and polysynaptic reflexes at the spinal cord level to relieve **muscle spasticity**, a condition whereby muscle fibers are in a state of continuous, involuntary contraction as a result of reflex impulses. Baclofen is used for treating reversible spasticity resulting from spinal cord lesions or multiple sclerosis. Its mode of action may be hyperpolarization of the terminals of the fibers that carry the initial stimulus signal that triggers the reflex. It also has a number of unlabeled uses, including hiccups and bladder spasticity. Baclofen should be taken with food or milk, can cause drowsiness, and may impair coordination and judgment. Concurrent alcohol use may potentiate these effects. Abrupt withdrawal after prolonged use may cause hallucinations, tachycardia, or spasticity.

Contraindications Topical and oral baclofen do not have contraindications. The intrathecal formula should not be given intravenously, intramuscularly, subcutaneously, or via epidural.

Cautions and Considerations Intrathecal baclofen carries a black box warning against abrupt discontinuation. Abrupt withdrawal has resulted in severe reactions that led to organ failure and death in some cases.
    Use with caution in older adults as they may be more sensitive to CNS side effects.

Drug Interactions The use of CNS depressants may exacerbate the CNS side effects of baclofen.

Carisoprodol

Carisoprodol (Soma) is a centrally acting skeletal muscle relaxant that is sometimes subject to abuse. Once carisoprodol is ingested, the molecules are cleaved to an active metabolite: meprobamate, which is a Schedule IV controlled substance that relieves anxiety leading to muscle tension. Because of the abuse potential, carisoprodol is a scheduled substance in many states. It causes drowsiness and dizziness.

Contraindications Contraindications include hypersensitivity to carbamates (such as meprobamate) and acute intermittent porphyria.

Cautions and Considerations Carisoprodol is on the Beers List as a drug that may be potentially inappropriate for use in older adults.
    Use with alcohol and other CNS depressants increases the risk of toxicity.

Drug Interactions Carisoprodol interacts with clindamycin, phenothiazines, and monoamine oxidase inhibitors (MAOIs).
    The use of CNS depressants may exacerbate the CNS side effects of carisoprodol.

Chlorzoxazone

Chlorzoxazone (Lorzone, Parafon Forte DSC) is indicated for symptomatic treatment of muscle spasms and pain associated with acute musculoskeletal conditions. It does not directly affect the muscle or the neuromuscular junction but is believed to act, like baclofen, on the spinal cord by depressing polysynaptic reflexes. Chlorzoxazone may cause drowsiness and dizziness. Alcohol consumption should be avoided while taking this medication.

Contraindications There are no contraindications for chlorzoxazone.

Cautions and Considerations Chlorzoxazone is on the Beers List as a drug that may be potentially inappropriate for use in older adults.
    Liver toxicity has occurred with use. Discontinue if elevated liver enzymes develop.

Drug Interactions The use of CNS depressants may exacerbate the CNS side effects of chlorzoxazone.

Cyclobenzaprine

Cyclobenzaprine (Amrix, Fexmid, Flexeril) is indicated for treating muscle spasms associated with acute painful musculoskeletal conditions and for supportive therapy in tetanus. It is a centrally acting skeletal muscle relaxant that is pharmacologically related to tricyclic antidepressants. It reduces tonic somatic motor activity influencing both alpha and gamma motor neurons. Onset of action is usually within one hour. Cyclobenzaprine should not be used for more than two to three weeks.

Contraindications Contraindications include use with or within 14 days of MAOIs, hyperthyroidism, congestive heart failure, heart block, and during the acute recovery phase of heart attacks.

Cautions and Considerations Cyclobenzaprine is on the Beers List as a drug that may be potentially inappropriate for use in older adults.

Cyclobenzaprine may impair the ability to perform hazardous activities requiring physical coordination.

Drug Interactions The use of CNS depressants may exacerbate the CNS side effects of cyclobenzaprine.

Anticholinergic medications may decrease the therapeutic effects of cyclobenzaprine.

Dantrolene

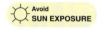

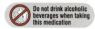

Dantrolene (Dantrium, Revonto, Ryanodex) acts on skeletal muscle beyond the neuromuscular junctions. It is considered to be a directly acting muscle relaxant and reduces muscle responsiveness to stimulation and decreases the force of contraction by reducing the amount of calcium released from the T tubules. It is used in treating spasticity related to spinal cord injuries, stroke, cerebral palsy, and multiple sclerosis. The side effects are malaise, weakness, fatigue, possible liver toxicity, and photosensitivity. Alcohol and other CNS depressants should be avoided.

Contraindications Dantrolene contraindications include active hepatic disease, such as hepatitis and cirrhosis; where spasticity is used to sustain upright posture and balance in locomotion; or whenever spasticity is used to obtain or maintain increased function.

Cautions and Considerations Dantrolene has a black box warning for hepatotoxicity. Patients using dantrolene should have their liver function monitored.

Drug Interactions Estrogen may increase the risk of liver toxicity.

The use of CNS depressants may exacerbate the CNS side effects of dantrolene. Dantrolene is also given before surgery to patients susceptible to malignant hyperthermia; this use is discussed in greater detail in Chapter 6.

Diazepam

Diazepam (Valium), a benzodiazepine, relieves anxiety causing muscle contraction. Some authorities consider it to be the best muscle relaxant, but it has significant abuse potential. It should not be discontinued abruptly after prolonged use. Commonly reported side effects include drowsiness, fatigue, and loss of body control.

Contraindications Contraindications to diazepam include children less than six months of age and in patients with acute narrow-angle glaucoma.

Cautions and Considerations Patients with hypersensitivity to other benzodiazepines may also react to diazepam. Diazepam should be used with caution in these patients.

Benzodiazepines are on the Beers List as being potentially inappropriate for use in older adults.

Drug Interactions Cimetidine and protease inhibitors may decrease clearance of benzodiazepines. Coadministration with disulfiram may produce alcohol intolerance.

The use of CNS depressants may exacerbate the CNS side effects of diazepam.

Metaxalone

Metaxalone (Metaxall, Skelaxin) is available in 400 mg and 800 mg scored tablets. The drug has no direct action on muscle, end plate, or fiber. It probably relaxes muscles through general CNS depression and may cause drowsiness. The patient should notify the physician if a skin rash or yellowish discoloration of the skin, eyes, or both occurs.

Contraindications Contraindications to metaxalone include significantly impaired hepatic or renal function, history of drug-induced hemolytic anemias, and other anemias.

Cautions and Considerations Metaxalone may cause CNS depression, and patients should be warned about decreased ability to perform tasks that require mental alertness.

Metaxalone should be used with caution in patients with liver or kidney impairment.

Caution must be exercised when used by older adults because of the increased risk of CNS and anticholinergic side effects.

Drug Interactions Metaxalone may enhance the effects of alcohol, barbiturates, and other CNS depressants.

Methocarbamol

Methocarbamol (Robaxin) is used to treat muscle spasms associated with acute painful musculoskeletal conditions and as supportive therapy in tetanus. It causes skeletal muscle relaxation by reducing the transmission of impulses from the spinal cord to skeletal muscles. Methocarbamol may cause drowsiness or impair judgment or coordination. Patients should avoid alcohol or other CNS depressants and should notify the physician of rash, itching, or nasal congestion. The drug may turn urine brown, black, or green.

Contraindications The injectable form of methocarbamol is contraindicated in renal impairment.

Cautions and Considerations Methocarbamol may cause CNS depression and patients should be warned about decreased ability to perform tasks that require mental alertness.

Methocarbamol is on the Beers List as a drug that may be potentially inappropriate for use in older adults.

Drug Interactions The use of CNS depressants may exacerbate the CNS side effects of methocarbamol.

Orphenadrine

Orphenadrine (Norflex) is indicated to treat muscle spasms and to provide supportive therapy in tetanus. It is an indirect skeletal muscle relaxant thought to work by central atropine-like effects; it has some euphorigenic (induces a state of euphoria) and analgesic properties. Orphenadrine may cause drowsiness. The tablet should be swallowed whole, not crushed or chewed. The patient should avoid alcohol, because orphenadrine also may impair coordination and judgment.

Contraindications Orphenadrine is contraindicated in patients with glaucoma, GI obstruction, peptic ulcer, prostatic hypertrophy, neck obstruction, cardiospasm, and myasthenia gravis.

Cautions and Considerations Orphenadrine may cause CNS depression, and patients should be warned about decreased ability to perform tasks that require mental alertness.

The injectable form of orphenadrine contains sulfites, which may cause allergic reaction in certain patients.

Orphenadrine is on the Beers List as a drug that may be potentially inappropriate for use in older adults.

Drug Interactions Anticholinergic medications may enhance the anticholinergic side effects of orphenadrine.

The use of CNS depressants may exacerbate the CNS side effects of orphenadrine.

Inflammation and Swelling

Recall from Chapter 6 that an analgesic is any medication taken to relieve pain. A **nonnarcotic analgesic** is used for mild-to-moderate pain, inflammation, and fever. Pain may be either dull, throbbing **somatic pain** from skin, muscle, and bone or sharp, stabbing **visceral pain** from organs. Figure 13.5 shows the pathway by which inflammation, pain, and fever develop when a tissue is injured. The nonnarcotic analgesics are believed to relieve pain by interrupting this pathway. They inhibit the enzyme cyclooxygenase and thereby decrease the conversion of arachidonic acid to prostaglandins (PGs), thromboxane A_2, and prostacyclin. Because the body cannot store PGs, they must be newly synthesized to be released during inflammation. Thus, the inhibition of cyclooxygenase reduces the synthesis of PGs and thereby reduces their influence at sites of inflammation and tissue damage.

Similarly, decreasing the synthesis of PGs can reduce a fever. Fever is a response by the body's temperature-regulating center, the hypothalamus, to substances called *endogenous pyrogens*, which are produced in response to bacterial or viral infections. The subsequent release of PGs from the brain causes the body "thermostat" to reset at a higher temperature—a fever. The higher temperature is meant to harm antigens and support the immune system.

Although nonnarcotic analgesics offer benefits, adverse gastrointestinal (GI) effects may limit their use because PGs promote mucosal production in the stomach, protecting the gastric lining from autodigestion by acids. By preventing the production of PGs, nonnarcotic analgesics risk exposing the stomach to ulceration. These products also elevate serum concentrations of hepatic enzymes, promote water and electrolyte retention, and can cause acute renal insufficiency. In addition, some nonnarcotic analgesics can displace oral anticoagulants, sulfonylureas, phenytoin, and

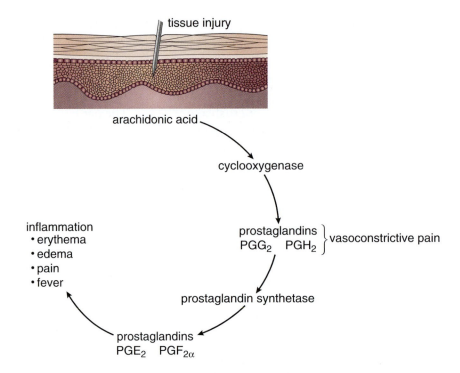

FIGURE 13.5
Pain Pathway in Tissue Injury

In addition to promoting inflammation and triggering the pain response, prostaglandins stimulate fever in the central nervous system.

sulfonamides from binding sites on plasma proteins. Nonsteroidal anti-inflammatory drugs (NSAIDs) are a class of drugs that are analgesic, **antipyretic** (fever reducing), and anti-inflammatory. The prototype NSAID is aspirin (salicylate). Acetaminophen, which is both analgesic and antipyretic, is not an NSAID, because it has little if any effect on inflammation.

Salicylates

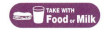

Salicylates were initially discovered and isolated from the bark of the white willow tree and were first used for rheumatic fever. Table 13.2 lists commonly used salicylates. They have analgesic, antipyretic, and anti-inflammatory properties. The primary analgesic action is peripheral rather than central. In contrast, the primary antipyretic action is central, presumably in the hypothalamus. Salicylates reduce fever by increasing blood flow to the skin and inhibiting PG synthesis. As a class, they must be taken with food and dispensed with a medication guide.

Salicylates are indicated for the following symptoms and conditions:

- arthritis
- inflammation of arthritis and rheumatism
- menstrual cramps
- muscular aches and pains
- pain and fever of influenza or other infections
- simple headache (headache other than migraine)

Low dosages (300–900 mg per day) of a salicylate can usually be taken safely. More than 4 g per day can cause problems; 10 g per day can be lethal. It is not uncommon, however, for a patient with rheumatoid arthritis to take 3–6 g per day under a physician's supervision.

Salicylates should be avoided after surgery or tooth extraction in patients with hemophilia (because they can interfere with normal clotting); in patients with asthma, nasal polyps, chronic sinusitis (because salicylates may trigger an allergic-like hypersensitivity reaction); and in patients with bleeding ulcers (due to bleeding risk).

If used during pregnancy, salicylates may result in anemia, prolonged pregnancy and labor, and excessive bleeding before, during, and after delivery. They can also contribute to birth defects. Use of salicylates in the last trimester may result in prematurity, stillbirth, newborn death, low birth weight, and bleeding into the fetal brain. Salicylates can also cause closure of the ductus arteriosus, causing premature distribution of blood to the lungs. Moreover, the gastric irritation caused by salicylates and other NSAIDs must not be treated with misoprostol (Cytotec), a PG analog, in pregnant patients, because PGs stimulate uterine contraction. Pharmacy technicians who are pregnant should wear gloves when dispensing misoprostol.

Patients taking probenecid should not take a salicylate, which can prevent the excretion of uric acid and precipitate an attack of gout. Salicylates should not be taken with methotrexate, because they can increase methotrexate levels to a life-threatening toxic range. If a patient taking warfarin (Coumadin) is also taking aspirin, the pharmacy technician should alert the pharmacist. Some prescribers use the two drugs in combination, but this increases bleeding times.

TABLE 13.2 Most Commonly Used Salicylates

Generic (Brand)	Pronunciation	Dosage Form	Common Dosage	Dispensing Status
aspirin (acetylsalicylic acid)	AS-pir-in	Caplet, capsule, gum, suppository	325–650 mg every 4–6 hours, not to exceed 4 g/day	OTC
buffered aspirin (Ascriptin, Bufferin)	BUF-erd AS-pir-in	Tablet	325–650 mg every 4–6 hours, not to exceed 4 g/day	OTC
choline magnesium trisalicylate (Trilisate)	KOE-leen mag-NEE-zhum trye-sa-LIS-il-ate	Liquid, tablet	Individualize based on patient response	Rx
salsalate (Amigesic)	SAL-sa-late	Tablet	3 g per day in 2–3 divided doses	Rx

TABLE 13.3 Acetaminophen and Acetylcysteine

Generic (Brand)	Pronunciation	Dosage Form	Common Dosage	Dispensing Status
Antipyretic Analgesic				
acetaminophen (Tylenol)	a-seat-a-MIN-oh-fen	Injection, oral liquid, suppository, tablet	325 mg–1000 mg every 4–6 hours, not to exceed 4 g/day from all sources	OTC
Acetaminophen Antidote				
acetylcysteine (Mucomyst, Acetadote)	a-set-il-SIS-teen	Injection, oral solution, solution for inhalation	varies based on weight and regimen	Rx

The side effects of salicylates include GI upset, tinnitus (ringing in the ears), and platelet changes. The nonionized portion of the acetylsalicylic acid is lipid soluble and is easily absorbed into the gastric mucosal cells, which in turn causes further damage that can disrupt the integrity of the gastric mucosal barrier. This is why pharmacy databases provide the pharmacy technician with warnings when these drugs are dispensed and also why the US Food and Drug Administration (FDA) stipulates that they be accompanied by a medication guide.

Aspirin

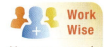

Work Wise

You may see aspirin abbreviated as ASA. This stands for it's chemical name, acetylsalicylic acid.

Aspirin is a commonly used OTC salicylate. Low-dose (81–325 mg) aspirin taken daily has been shown to reduce the risk of heart attacks and strokes in patients with a prior history of cardiovascular disease (heart attack, stroke, bypass surgery). At low doses, aspirin appears to irreversibly inhibit the formation of thromboxane A_2, a prostaglandin molecule that facilitates platelet aggregation in blood vessels. Although aspirin taken for a myocardial infarction (MI) must be plain so that it can more quickly enter the bloodstream, if a prescriber writes for aspirin to be taken daily, it should be for the enteric-coated (EC) form. This will protect the lining of the patient's stomach. To minimize interactions, aspirin should be taken at least one hour before any other NSAID. If a patient is on both aspirin and an NSAID and you get the warning of an interaction, remind the pharmacist to counsel the patient regarding this time interval.

Cautions and Considerations Salicylism, mild salicylate intoxication, is characterized by tinnitus (ringing in the ears), dizziness, headache, and mental confusion. Severe intoxication is characterized by hyperpnea (abnormal increase in the depth of breathing), nausea, vomiting, acid-base disturbances, petechial hemorrhages, hyperthermia, delirium, convulsions, and coma.

The lethal dose for aspirin is usually over 10 g for an adult. The advent of childproof caps for medicine has reduced the incidence of pediatric intoxication.

Aspirin should not be given to children. Reye's syndrome can develop in children who have been given aspirin after having been exposed to chickenpox or other viral infections. This syndrome includes a range of mental changes (mild amnesia, lethargy, disorientation, and agitation) that can culminate in coma and progressive unresponsiveness, seizures, relaxed muscles, dilated pupils, and respiratory failure. Pharmacy technicians must be mindful of combination preparations (e.g., Alka-Seltzer) that contain aspirin, if these preparations are intended for pediatric use.

Drug Interactions Using aspirin with other salicylates increases risk of toxicity. Aspirin increases the risk of bleeding when taken with anticoagulants.

Choline Magnesium Trisalicylate

Choline magnesium trisalicylate (Trilisate) is approved for the treatment of arthritis. It must be taken with food, but it does not cause as many stomach problems as other drugs in this class. It acts on the hypothalamus to reduce fever and block pain impulses. A much lower dose of choline magnesium trisalicylate is necessary to have an antipyretic effect than is needed to inhibit pain. The liquid form may be mixed with fruit juices, but one needs to remain in an upright position for 30 minutes after taking it.

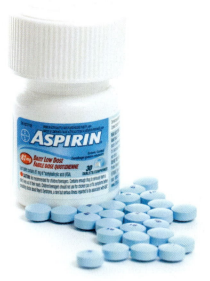

Aspirin is an OTC salicylate.

Contraindications Hypersensitivity to other nonacetylated salicylates contraindicates use.

Cautions and Considerations Choline magnesium trisalicylate should be used with caution in patients with asthma or liver or kidney dysfunction.

Because of the increased risk of salicylate-related toxicities, older adults should use the lowest possible effective dose.

Drug Interactions Choline magnesium trisalicylate may enhance adverse reactions of corticosteroids. Other salicylates my enhance side effects. Warfarin's anticoagulant effect may be increased with concurrent use.

Salsalate

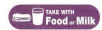

Salsalate (Amigesic) is approved for minor pain or fever and arthritis. It does not inhibit platelet aggregation as much as other drugs in this class and tends to cause fewer gastrointestinal side effects. Salsalate should be taken with food. The fact that it will not "thin" the blood makes it a very important member of this drug class.

Contraindications Contraindications of salsalate include asthma, urticaria, or allergic reaction.

Cautions and Considerations Salsalate has two boxed warnings. One is for increased risk of adverse cardiovascular thrombotic events (such as heart attack or stroke). The other warning is for gastrointestinal events such as ulceration, bleeding, and perforation.

Drug Interactions Salsalate may enhance the adverse effects of corticosteroids. NSAIDs may increase the toxic side effects of salsalate.

Mixed Analgesics

A mixed analgesic is a drug containing both a narcotic and an NSAID or acetaminophen. Chronic use of mixed analgesics can lead to kidney failure, because these drugs have additive toxic effects on the kidneys. Furthermore, many of the OTC analgesics can cause problems for persons who drink alcohol daily. The FDA wants manufacturers to put an alcohol warning on the labels of all OTC analgesics. For acetaminophen, the problem is liver toxicity; for ibuprofen, an NSAID, it is increased GI bleeding.

Mixed analgesics containing a narcotic combined with aspirin, ibuprofen, or acetaminophen are often prescribed with more concern for the narcotic than for the nonnarcotic dose. The pharmacy technician can play a critical role here. When a prescription for any of these drugs is received, it would be prudent to calculate the dose of the nonnarcotic to see whether it exceeds the toxicity dosage.

Osteoarthritis

The word **arthritis** is derived from the Greek word for joint, *arthron*, and it literally means "joint inflammation." Arthritis can take many forms, but the most common complaint of arthritis patients is persistent pain. This pain is caused by functional problems of the joints.

Osteoarthritis (OA) is a degenerative joint disease in which cartilage in joints becomes thinner and less elastic, eventually causing bone to wear and become deformed (see Figure 13.6). It is a common age-related condition of synovial joints. The most commonly affected joints are the sternoclavicular joint, spine, hips, knees, fingers, and big toes. Joints carrying large loads (knees) and those under stress (fingers) are especially likely to be affected. Osteoarthritis generally appears after age 40. The disease is characterized by progressive pain, stiffness, limitation of motion, and deformed joints. Stiffness in the morning is the most prevalent complaint; it is also common after inactivity such as sitting. Drug therapy for OA is aimed at the reduction of symptoms and the prevention of disability. If OA is severe enough, surgery or joint replacement is performed.

FIGURE 13.6
Osteoarthritis

Osteoarthritis, which commonly affects the knee joint, may result in a total knee replacement if pain or stiffness does not improve with other treatments such as medication or physical therapy.

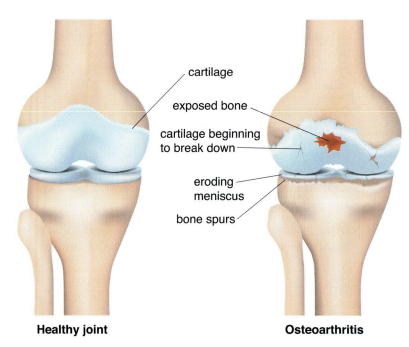

cartilage

exposed bone

cartilage beginning to break down

eroding meniscus

bone spurs

Healthy joint　　　　**Osteoarthritis**

Safety Alert

Acetaminophen is a component of hundreds of medications. When used correctly, acetaminophen is remarkably safe. However, when taken at doses above recommended levels, acetaminophen may cause serious liver damage. Acetaminophen poisoning has become the most common cause of acute liver failure in the United States.

Acetaminophen

Acetaminophen (Tylenol) is an **antipyretic analgesic** and has a limited side effect profile (see Table 13.3). Furthermore, acetaminophen may be taken during pregnancy. However, if over-ingested it can be lethal, and because it is in so many pain medications, an overdose can happen without prescribers realizing it. Pharmacy technicians need to be aware of the maximum acetaminophen dose when dispensing combination narcotics. Most prescribers do not take this into consideration. If the prescription allows the patient to take more than 4 g per day, the prescriber must be notified. Acetaminophen is still a first-line medication for mild-to-moderate pain.

It can be especially useful in patients who:

- have a peptic ulcer,
- take a uricosuric agent for gout,
- take an oral anticoagulant,
- have a clotting disorder,
- are at risk for Reye's syndrome,
- are intolerant to aspirin (still a 6% chance of cross-intolerance), or
- have post-surgical pain.

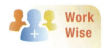

Acetaminophen does not cause GI irritation, bleeding, alteration of platelet adhesiveness, or potentiation of oral anticoagulants. There are few interactions; indeed, it is even safe to take during pregnancy. However, it should be taken with caution and under medical supervision if a patient has severe liver disease or alcoholism. At a dosage of more than 4 g per day, liver damage can occur. This risk increases if the patient is fasting or is ingesting alcohol.

Acetaminophen is a popular choice for OA, particularly the noninflammatory type. Many patients do not take acetaminophen for arthritis, because it must be taken multiple times a day to maintain pain control. Arthritis can become so severe that acetaminophen no longer manages the pain.

Contraindications Patients who have severe liver impairment or severe active liver disease should avoid acetaminophen use.

Cautions and Considerations Acetaminophen should be used cautiously in patients with alcoholic liver disease or patients who consume three or more alcoholic drinks each day.

An acute overdose of acetaminophen or doses greater than 4,000 mg a day may cause liver toxicity. Long-term daily use of this medication may lead to liver damage in some patients. Use caution with concomitant acetaminophen and alcohol use.

Acetylcysteine (Mucomyst, Acetadote) is the only antidote for an acetaminophen overdose; it is also approved for some bronchial diseases. It acts as an alternate substrate and conjugates with the acetaminophen, detoxifying the active metabolite.

Acetylcysteine has a strong, rotten egg-like smell, which limits its use. The IV form is primarily used because of the convenience. For bronchial conditions, it comes in a form that can be inhaled, through a vaporizer, and an oral dose form. Acetylcysteine when used for acetaminophen poisoning can be administered orally or intravenously. Each has a different dosing regimen (72-hours when administered orally and 21-hours when intravenous) and vary based on patient-specific factors. Both regimens include a loading dose and are followed by maintenance doses. Administration may vary depending upon acetaminophen levels. Acetylcysteine should be administered as soon as possible, preferably within 4 hours of ingestion, but it can be effective in patients treated up to 8 to 10 hours after ingestion.

Drug Interactions Probenecid may increase the serum concentration of acetaminophen.

Nonsteroidal Anti-Inflammatory Drugs

Nonsteroidal anti-inflammatory drugs (NSAIDs) are often used as first-line therapy in patients with inflammatory OA. In noninflammatory OA, NSAIDs are used when patients experience inadequate pain reduction with acetaminophen. Other indications for the use of NSAIDs include inflammation associated with injury, dysmenorrhea (painful menstrual cycle), and fever. They relieve inflammation, swelling, and pain. NSAIDs may take longer to reduce fever than other agents, but the effects last longer, and they do not cause euphoria.

NSAIDs work by inhibiting prostaglandin (PG) synthesis in tissues, thereby preventing the sensitization of pain receptors to other mediators of inflammation. Thus, they generally act in the affected tissues, rather than centrally as opiates do. Any central actions that NSAIDs do exhibit are usually unwanted side effects, with the exception of lowered body temperature. It is unlikely, though, that all NSAIDs act only on PGs and by only one mechanism. The following cautions and considerations, contraindications, and drug interactions apply to all of the following drugs unless otherwise elaborated upon in the description of the specific drug.

Contraindications All NSAIDs that appear in Table 13.4 are contraindicated for peri-operative pain during coronary artery bypass graft (CABG) surgery. NSAID use is also contraindicated if an individual has asthma, hives, or other allergic reactions after taking aspirin or other NSAIDs. For example, if an individual experienced hives and an asthma exacerbation with ibuprofen use, all other NSAIDs would also be contraindicated, because of concerns about cross-sensitivity.

Cautions and Considerations The action of NSAIDs in inhibiting PG synthesis explains their primary side effect: GI upset. PGs perform three protective functions in the GI tract: increasing mucosal blood flow, increasing mucus production, and decreasing free acid production. Thus, by inhibiting PG synthesis, NSAIDs also inhibit the protective effect of PGs on the gastric mucosa, so it is no surprise that one in five chronic NSAID users develops some type of GI gastropathy. This drug class should always be taken with food, be administered at the lowest dose for the shortest period of time possible, and be dispensed with a medication guide. Nausea, abdominal cramps, heartburn, ulcers, and indigestion are all associated with NSAID use. For this reason, a proton pump inhibitor, misoprostol, or an H_2 blocker will be prescribed with these agents in some patients. Because they upset the balance of vasoconstricting and vasodilating chemicals in the body, NSAIDs can also increase heart or circulation problems, and this effect must be considered.

The next most common side effect of NSAID use is kidney damage. Acute renal failure, fluid retention, hypertension, hyperkalemia, interstitial nephritis, and papillary necrosis can all be attributed to NSAID use. Other side effects include liver abnormalities, blood clotting irregularities, bone marrow depression, tinnitus, jaundice, dizziness, drowsiness, rash, and dry mouth.

Drug Interactions NSAIDs can interact with the following drugs:

• other NSAIDs, including aspirin
• beta blockers
• cyclosporine
• digoxin
• diuretics
• methotrexate
• oral hypoglycemics
• warfarin

Because NSAIDs are protein-bound, concentrations can be altered by other drugs such as aspirin. Consequently, concurrent use of the two should be discouraged, as the combination may lead to additive or synergistic toxicity rather than increased efficacy. Also, other NSAIDs may interfere with the cardioprotective effects of low-dose (81–325 mg) aspirin.

Table 13.4 presents the most commonly used NSAIDs. Many NSAIDs are OTC, or OTC status has been requested. This means they will be used to self-medicate. It is most important to realize that, although all NSAIDs have similar mechanisms of action, patient response to these drugs varies widely. Clinical trials have not shown any of these agents to be superior to the others for managing osteoarthritis. Given the wide variation in patients' reactions, inadequate response or loss of response to one NSAID does not imply inefficacy of others. If one drug does not achieve the desired

TABLE 13.4   Most Commonly Used Drugs for Arthritis and Related Disorders

Generic (Brand)	Pronunciation	Dosage Form	Common Dosage	Dispensing Status
Conventional NSAIDs				
diclofenac (Cambia, Cataflam, Flector, Pennsaid, Rexaphenac, Solaraze, Voltaren, Zipsor, Zorvolex)	dye-KLOE-fen-ak	Capsule, injection, oral packet, ophthalmic, patch, tablet, transdermal gel, transdermal solution, topical solution	PO: 100–200 mg a day Topical: 2–4 g every 6 hr	Rx
etodolac (Lodine)	ee-TOE-doe-lak	Capsule, tablet	600–1,000 mg a day	Rx
ibuprofen (Advil, Motrin)	eye-byoo-PROE-fen	Capsule, cream, injection, oral liquid, tablet	OTC: 200 mg taken 3 or 4 times a day; Rx: 400–800 mg taken 3 or 4 times a day	OTC, Rx
indomethacin (Indocin)	in-doe-METH-a-sin	Capsule, injection, oral liquid, suppository	PO: 50–200 mg a day Rectal: 50–200 mg a day	Rx
ketoprofen (Orudis, Oruvail)	kee-toe-PROE-fen	Capsule, cream	200–300 mg a day	Rx
ketorolac (Toradol)	kee-toe-ROLE-ak	Injection, tablet, ophthalmic	IM/IV: 30–60 mg every 4–6 hr PO: 10–20 mg every 4–6 hr but not to exceed 40 mg in 24 hr	Rx
meloxicam (Mobic)	mel-OX-i-kam	Capsule, oral liquid, tablet	7.5–15 mg a day	Rx
nabumetone (Relafen)	na-BYOO-me-tone	Tablet	1,000–2,000 mg a day	Rx
naproxen (Aleve, Anaprox, Naprosyn)	na-PROX-en	Capsule, cream, oral suspension, tablet	250–550 mg twice a day	OTC Rx
oxaprozin (Daypro)	ox-a-PROE-zin	Tablet	600–1,200 mg a day	Rx
piroxicam (Feldene)	peer-OX-i-kam	Capsule	20 mg a day	Rx
sulindac (Clinoril)	sul-IN-dak	Tablet	150–200 mg a day	Rx
COX-2 Inhibitor				
celecoxib (Celebrex)	sel-a-KOX-ib	Capsule	200 mg once a day	Rx
Combination Drugs				
diclofenac-misoprostol (Arthrotec)	dye-KLOE-fen-ak mye-soe-PROST-awl	Tablet	diclofenac sodium 50 mg and misoprostol 200 mcg 3 times a day	Rx
esomeprazole-naproxen (Vimovo)	ee-soe-MEP-ra-zole na-PROX-en	Tablet	naproxen 375–500 mg and esomeprazole 20 mg twice a day	Rx
ibuprofen-famotidine (Duexis)	eye-byoo-PROE-fen fa-MOE-ti-deen	Tablet	800 mg ibuprofen and 26.6 mg famotidine 3 times a day	Rx
Other				
tramadol (Active-Tramadol, ConZip, EnovaRX-Tramadol, Synapryn FusePaq, Ultram, Ultram ER)	TRA-ma-dawl	Capsule, cream, oral liquid, tablet	Immediate-release/oral disintegrating tablets: 50–100 mg every 4–6 hours, not to exceed 400 mg/day; Extended-release: 100–300 mg a day	Rx

results, treatment with another NSAID is appropriate before considering adding other agents. Rotating these agents is common, and patients seem to get better results when this is done; although it is important to allow two to three weeks with one agent before switching to another.

The only NSAIDs with parenteral forms are indomethacin and ketorolac, and these are for short-term use only.

Diclofenac

Diclofenac (Cambia, Cataflam, Flector, Pennsaid, Rexaphenac, Solaraze, Voltaren, Zipsor, Zorvolex) can induce signs and symptoms of hepatotoxicity: nausea, fatigue, pruritus, jaundice, upper-right-quadrant tenderness, and flu-like symptoms. Therefore, regular liver function tests are important. The patient should report any blood in the stool to the prescriber. Cataflam has a more rapid onset of action than does the sodium salt, Voltaren, because it is absorbed in the stomach rather than the duodenum. Topical forms are Solaraze and Voltaren Topical. These forms are dispensed with dosing cards, which patients should use to measure the amount to be applied. The prescribed amount should be massaged into the area that is painful, and the area where the drug is applied should not be washed for at least an hour. Flector is the patch form. It should be applied to the most painful area and changed every 12 hours. It must be kept dry. Arthrotec is diclofenac combined with misoprostol; it protects the stomach from NSAID-induced ulcers.

Etodolac

Etodolac (Lodine) dosage should not exceed 1,200 mg per day. Patients should be told not to crush the tablets and to report any blood in the stool to the prescriber. Black or tarry stools usually indicate blood of gastric origin. Bright red blood in the stool is usually from rectal origin and indicates hemorrhoids.

Ibuprofen

Ibuprofen (Advil, Motrin) comes in liquid dosage forms and is the first OTC analgesic for children since acetaminophen was approved. It controls fever well and can be alternated with acetaminophen. Ibuprofen has a slower onset of action than acetaminophen but a longer duration. Consequently, alternating ibuprofen and acetaminophen works well. The adult formulations are also available OTC in strengths of 200 mg per tablet, caplet, or capsule. However, the patient can easily take more than one tablet at a time and attain the 400 mg, 600 mg, or 800 mg prescription formulation. Unless recommended by the physician, this could be very dangerous. If the patient is taking OTC agents, the physician should be notified if a fever lasts more than three days or pain lasts longer than 10 days.

Ibuprofen-famotidine (Duexis) has been shown to reduce NSAID-induced ulcers. It is dosed three times daily and is often used in patients who cannot tolerate a proton pump inhibitor. It is meant for patients with low cardiovascular risk who need GI protection. However, depending on the patient's insurance, it may be more affordable to separate these two drugs. If so, this is a much-appreciated service the pharmacy technician can provide for the patient.

Indomethacin

Indomethacin (Indocin) is a potent NSAID, and its effects are believed to be mediated by PGs. However, it has more adverse effects than the newer agents. Because of its side effect profile, indomethacin is not used as frequently as the other NSAIDs for arthritis. Indomethacin is the only NSAID available as a suppository. Intravenously administered indomethacin is used in neonates to promote closure of the patent ductus arteriosus and to alleviate the associated symptoms of cardiac failure. It should be administered over 20 to 30 minutes at a concentration of 0.5 to 1.0 mg/mL in preservative-free sterile water for injection. The IV formula should be reconstituted just before administration and any unused portion discarded. The latter is especially important in a neonatal unit.

Contraindications Indomethacin suppositories should not be used in people with inflammation of the rectal lining or recent rectal bleeding.

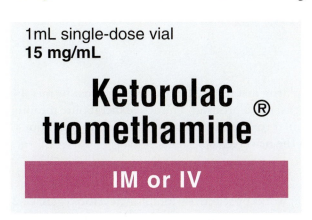

1mL single-dose vial
15 mg/mL

Ketorolac tromethamine ®

IM or IV

A ketorolac injection is an NSAID commonly used to treat the moderate-to-severe pain associated with OA. Labels for injectable products and oral products often look different.

Ketorolac

Ketorolac (Toradol) is indicated for short-term use (less than five days) in moderate-to-severe pain. It acts peripherally to inhibit PG synthesis. It is useful in patients who cannot tolerate narcotics. When injected, a dose of 30 mg provides pain relief comparable to 12 mg of morphine or 100 mg of meperidine. Side effects include nausea, dyspepsia (abdominal discomfort, heartburn), GI pain, and drowsiness.

Contraindications Ketorolac use is contraindicated in patients with peptic ulcer disease, a history of GI bleeding or perforation, advanced kidney disease or risk of kidney failure, suspected or confirmed cerebral bleeding, or a high risk of bleeding. Ketorolac should not be used in combination with aspirin or other NSAIDs, probenecid, or pentoxifylline. In addition, ketorolac should not be given by epidural or intrathecal administration and should not be used during labor and delivery.

Meloxicam

Meloxicam (Mobic) appears to cause less GI toxicity than other NSAIDs. For that reason, it has become a very popular drug for arthritis. It can be dosed once or twice daily.

Nabumetone

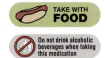

Nabumetone (Relafen) should be taken in the morning with food. The lowest effective dose should be used for chronic treatment. As with other NSAIDs, alcohol should be avoided because it may add to the irritant action of the drug in the stomach.

Naproxen

Naproxen (Aleve, Anaprox, Naprosyn) is an NSAID that should be used in the lowest effective dose for the least amount of time possible. Aleve is available as an OTC product.

Esomeprazole-naproxen (Vimovo) is an NSAID and a proton pump inhibitor. The NSAID reduces substances in the body that cause inflammation, pain, and fever. The proton pump inhibitor decreases the amount of acid produced in the stomach. This drug is approved to treat osteoarthritis, rheumatoid arthritis, and ankylosing spondylitis, and to decrease the risk of gastric ulcers in patients at risk of developing these from treatment with NSAIDs. It is enteric coated, so it should not be halved or crushed. The tablet should be taken 30 minutes before a meal. The drug should be used at the lowest effective dose for the shortest amount of time, and should not be used for a period longer than six months.

Piroxicam

Piroxicam (Feldene) has the advantage of once-a-day dosing. It is for acute or long-term therapy of arthritis. Therapeutic effects are evident early in treatment, and the response increases over several weeks. As with other NSAIDs, the patient needs to take the drug for at least two weeks to allow the drug sufficient time to reach its therapeutic effectiveness.

Sulindac

Sulindac (Clinoril) is a renal-sparing drug metabolized in the liver. It must be metabolized to the active form. In other words, it is a prodrug. The active metabolite inhibits cyclooxygenase and is structurally similar to indomethacin. Both sulindac and indomethacin have more side effects than the newer agents.

Celecoxib

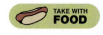

Celebrex is easily confused with Cerebyx (fosphenytoin, an anticonvulsant).

Celecoxib (Celebrex) is an NSAID that works by selectively inhibiting **cyclooxygenase-2 (COX-2)**, an enzyme that promotes production of the prostaglandins that cause pain and inflammation but not those prostaglandins that protect the GI lining. It is the only COX-2 inhibitor available in the United States. NSAIDs and salicylates block both **cyclooxygenase-1 (COX-1)** and COX-2, which arrests prostaglandins in the GI lining. Celecoxib is taken for arthritis pain and other pain in patients with a history of ulcers or GI bleeding. It can be taken on a short-term or long-term basis. Although GI upset is less than with the older NSAIDs, it remains the primary side effect. Fluid retention is another significant side effect with this drug. Celecoxib has the potential for cross-reactivity in patients who are allergic to sulfonamides, and it may increase cardiovascular risk. A label should be attached when dispensing this drug to instruct patients to take it with food. At the time of this writing, celecoxib is the only COX-2 inhibitor still on the market, because all of the others have been recalled by the FDA.

Contraindications As with the NSAIDs discussed previously, celecoxib should not be used for treatment of perioperative pain related to CABG surgery. Allergy to sulfonamides, aspirin, or other NSAIDs contraindicates celecoxib use.

Cautions and Considerations Other COX-2 inhibitors were removed from the market in the United States because of adverse effects involving heart problems and death from cardiac complications. Some patients recall the news coverage of this event and are hesitant to take a COX-2 inhibitor. Celecoxib has not been associated with such effects, but patients should work with their prescribers to monitor health conditions.

Drug Interactions Nephrotoxic agents (angiotensin-converting enzyme inhibitors, other NSAIDs) will increase the nephrotoxic effects of celecoxib. Anticoagulants may increase bleeding risk.

Rheumatoid Arthritis

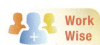
Rheumatoid arthritis (RA) is an entirely different disease from OA because it is an autoimmune disorder. RA involves an abnormal process in which the immune system destroys the synovial membrane of the joint, producing inflammation. The synovium (see Figure 13.1) swells and thickens. Fingerlike projections grow from the synovium into cartilage, bone, tendon, and joint spaces, causing reabsorption of bone and cartilage. As the disease progresses, bone to bone contact occurs, with eventual joint fusion. Most destruction occurs close to the inflamed synovial membrane. Because cartilage has no nerves, pain originates from the surrounding joint structures, such as bones, tendons, ligaments, and muscles. The same joints on both sides are affected approximately 70% of the time. The small joints of the hand are usually affected first, followed by the feet, ankles, knees, wrists, elbows, shoulders, temporomandibular joints, and vertebral column.

Signs of RA are morning pain and stiffness, are usually symmetrical, last longer than an hour, and are not relieved by activity. Patients are prone to cold temperatures and feel changes in barometric pressure. Four main laboratory tests are used to help diagnose RA: rheumatoid factor (RF), anti-cyclic citrullinated peptide (anti-CCP) antibodies, erythrocyte sedimentation rate (ESR), and C-reactive protein (CRP). The disease is not curable but can be slowed with medication.

The goal of drug therapy in RA is to maintain mobility and delay disability for as long as possible. Medication cannot cure RA, but it can improve pain symptoms, increase function, and slow the disease progression that eventually erodes and distorts joints. Some of the drugs used to treat RA, such as NSAIDs, are used to treat symptoms, whereas other drugs can modify the course and progression of the disease.

To treat rheumatoid arthritis, drugs must be administered that turn off the immune system. This makes the body very susceptible to infections, cancer, and other diseases. That is why infection and malignancies are the primary side effects of the drugs.

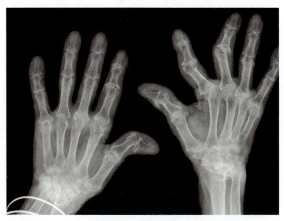

X-ray images of wrists and hands affected by rheumatoid arthritis.

Disease-Modifying Antirheumatic Drugs

The existing treatments for rheumatoid arthritis are divided into two categories:

1. agents that provide only symptomatic relief
2. agents that can potentially modify disease progression

The former category includes NSAIDs, discussed earlier, and corticosteroids, discussed in other chapters. The latter category includes a variety of agents that are collectively referred to as **disease-modifying antirheumatic drugs (DMARDs)**. The latest evidence shows that early, mild RA should be treated with more than NSAIDs, because joint damage occurs earlier than previously thought. The newer therapeutic approaches to the treatment of RA focus on the use of new **biologic response modifiers** with the ability to inhibit lymphocytes and cytokine activity. Table 13.5 gives an overview of the most commonly used DMARDs. DMARDs are taken regularly to maintain disease and symptom control. If one agent does not generate a response, others are tried or combinations of multiple DMARDs are used. They work best when started within the first three months after RA diagnosis. Disease remission can sometimes be achieved. At a minimum, early therapy slows the joint destruction that creates disability. Azathioprine (Imuran) and cyclosporine (Neoral, Sandimmune) have two approved uses according to the FDA: as immunosuppressants after organ transplantation and as DMARDs for RA. The injectable biologic response modifiers, including etanercept (Enbrel), infliximab (Remicade), adalimumab (Humira), and anakinra (Kineret), are made through recombinant DNA technology and work by inhibiting either interleukin-1 (IL-1) or tumor necrosis factors (TNFs), two substances that cause inflammation and joint damage.

TABLE 13.5 Most Commonly Used DMARDs

Generic (Brand)	Pronunciation	Dosage Form	Common Dosage	Dispensing Status
adalimumab (Humira)	a-da-LIM-yoo-mab	Injection	40 mg every 2 weeks	Rx
anakinra (Kineret)	an-a-KIN-ra	Injection	100 mg a day	Rx
auranofin (Ridaura)	aw-RAN-noh-fin	Capsule	6–9 mg/kg/day, divided 2–3 times a day	Rx
azathioprine (Imuran)	az-a-THYE-oh-preen	Tablet	3–5 mg/kg/day initially, then 1–3 mg/kg/day	Rx
cyclophosphamide (Cytoxan)	sye-kloe-FOSS-fa-mide	Injection, tablet	1.5–2.5 mg/kg/day	Rx
cyclosporine (Neoral, Sandimmune)	sye-kloe-SPOR-een	Capsule, injection	2.5 mg/kg, divided twice a day	Rx
etanercept (Enbrel)	ee-TAN-er-sept	Injection	25 mg twice a week or 50 mg once a week	Rx
golimumab (Simponi)	goe-LIM-ue-mab	Injection	50 mg once a month	Rx
hydroxychloroquine (Plaquenil)	hye-drox-ee-KLOR-oh-kwin	Tablet	200–300 mg a day	Rx
infliximab (Remicade)	in-FLIX-i-mab	Injection	3 mg/kg at 0, 2, and 6 weeks, then every 8 weeks	Rx
leflunomide (Arava)	le-FLOO-noe-mide	Tablet	100 mg a day for 3 days, then 10–20 mg once a week	Rx
methotrexate (Rheumatrex)	meth-oh-TREX-ate	Injection, tablet	7.5–15 mg a week	Rx
sulfasalazine (Azulfidine)	sul-fa-SAL-a-zeen	Tablet	500 mg twice a day, then increase to 1 g twice a day	Rx

Adalimumab

Adalimumab (Humira) is a biologic response modifier that blocks TNF. Adalimumab increases the risk of infections and cancer. It is approved for RA, but also for ankylosing spondylitis, Crohn's disease, juvenile idiopathic arthritis, plaque psoriasis, psoriatic arthritis, rheumatoid arthritis, and ulcerative colitis. Adalimumab is available as a prefilled syringe or a pen injector. It is administered every other week as a subcutaneous injection. Adalimumab is stored in the refrigerator. Side effects include headache, nausea, vomiting, flu-like symptoms, rash, itching, heart problems, anemia and blood disorders, secondary malignancy, nephrotic syndrome, confusion, tremor, and reactivation of hepatitis B.

Contraindications Adalimumab does not have any contraindications.

Cautions and Considerations Adalimumab has several black box warnings. The first is an increased risk of serious infection that may result in hospitalization and death. Patients at risk for infection should use the medication with caution. Adalimumab has a boxed warning for lymphoma and other malignancies in children. The third boxed warning is for hepatosplenic T-cell lymphoma, a rare disease reported primarily in patients using adalimumab for Crohn's disease or ulcerative colitis. The last warning deals with tuberculosis (TB) reactivation with use. Patients should be evaluated for latent TB prior to therapy initiation.

Drug Interactions Adalimumab may enhance the adverse effects of abatacept, anakinra, belimumab, canakinumab, certolizumab, infliximab, natalizumab, pimecrolimus, rilonacept, tacrolimus, tocilizumab, tofacitinib, and vedolizumab.

Live vaccines should be avoided while patients are using immunosuppressant therapy.

Adalimumab may decrease serum concentration of warfarin.

Anakinra

Anakinra (Kineret) is an interleukin receptor antagonist used for arthritis. Anakinra is available as an injection. The primary side effects include headache, nausea, vomiting, diarrhea, redness and pain at injection site, flu-like symptoms, and blood disorders.

Contraindications Anakinra is contraindicated in patients with a hypersensitivity to proteins derived from *Escherichia coli*.

Cautions and Considerations Hypersensitivity reactions may occur with use, including anaphylaxis.

Anakinra should be used with caution by patients with asthma, because of an increased risk of infection.

The needle cover of anakinra contains latex. Patients with latex sensitivity should not use this product. The product also contains polysorbate 80.

Drug Interactions Anakinra may enhance the adverse effects of abatacept, natalizumab, pimecrolimus, tacrolimus, and tofacitinib.

Live vaccines should not be used concurrently because of an increased risk of infection.

Auranofin

Auranofin (Ridaura) is used for RA and is administered orally. It comes as a capsule and is taken once or twice a day. Side effects include diarrhea, nausea, vomiting, abdominal pain, anorexia, indigestion, gas, constipation, itching, rash, hair loss, photosensitivity, blood disorders, kidney and liver damage, and lung problems (serious but rare).

Contraindications Auranofin is contraindicated in patients with a history of severe toxicity to gold compounds.

Cautions and Considerations Auranofin has several black box warnings, all relating to gold toxicity. The first is for general signs of gold toxicity (rash, stomatitis, pruritis), as auranofin contains gold. Another boxed warning is for gastrointestinal effects such as persistent diarrhea, nausea, vomiting, or ulcerative colitis. The next warning is for hematologic effects such as decreased hemoglobin, white blood cells, and platelets. The last warning is for proteinuria and hematuria.

Drug Interactions There are no known drug interactions for auranofin.

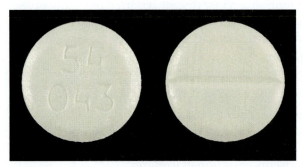

Azathioprine is available in tablet dosage form as pictured.

Azathioprine

Azathioprine (Imuran) depresses bone marrow function, thereby increasing the potential for infection. Response in RA may not occur for up to three months. Side effects include malaise, nausea, vomiting, leukopenia, neoplasia, thrombocytopenia, liver toxicity, myalgia, and fever.

Contraindications Contraindications include pregnancy (in patients with RA) and patients with RA who have a history of use of alkylating agents.

Cautions and Considerations Azathioprine has a black box warning for increased risk of development of malignancy (such as lymphoma). Patients should be informed of risk before use. Another boxed warning advises that only experienced prescribers should prescribe azathioprine.

Severe gastrointestinal toxicity may occur with use. This includes nausea, vomiting, diarrhea, myalgia, hypotension, and liver enzyme abnormalities.

Drug Interactions Adverse effects of other immunosuppressants may be enhanced by azathioprine.

Febuxostat may increase serum concentrations of azathioprine.

Azathioprine may increase the risk of infection with live vaccines. Concurrent use should be avoided.

Cyclophosphamide

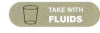

Cyclophosphamide (Cytoxan) depresses bone marrow function, increasing the potential for infection. Patients must remain well hydrated during use of this drug. Without proper hydration, the drug can cause irreparable damage to the urinary bladder. Fluid ingestion should increase by at least several cups a day when cyclophosphamide therapy commences. Side effects include anorexia, nausea, vomiting, hair loss, blood disorders, kidney damage, infertility, fluid imbalance, secondary malignancy (cancer), heart problems, and lung problems (serious but rare).

Contraindications Cyclophosphamide should not be used in patients with urinary flow obstruction.

Cautions and Considerations The ISMP includes cyclophosphamide among its list of drugs with increased risk of harm when used in error.

Cyclophosphamide is considered a hazardous agent, and appropriate handling precautions must be taken.

Cardiotoxicity has been associated with cyclophosphamide use.

Drug Interactions Belimumab, etanercept, pimecrolimus, and tacrolimus may enhance the toxicities of cyclophosphamide.

Cyclophosphamide may increase adverse effects of clozapine, natalizumab, and tofacitinib.

Live vaccines may cause infection and concurrent use is not recommended.

Etanercept

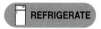

Etanercept (Enbrel) is a biologically engineered protein that inhibits the action of tumor necrosis factor (TNF). (Growing evidence suggests that TNF plays a key role in the pathogenesis of RA.) Etanercept was the first biologically engineered product approved for the treatment of RA. This drug is indicated in the treatment of moderate-to-severe RA in patients who have experienced an inadequate response to one or more of the other arthritis drugs. Etanercept can be used in combination with methotrexate in patients who do not respond adequately to methotrexate alone. Etanercept must be stored in the refrigerator. Injection site reactions are the primary side effect. Other side effects include headache, nausea, vomiting, hair loss, cough, dizziness, abdominal pain, rash, indigestion, swelling, mouth sores, blood disorders, secondary lymphoma, Stevens-Johnson syndrome, seizures, heart problems, pancreatitis, and difficulty breathing.

Contraindications Sepsis contraindicates etanercept use.

Cautions and Considerations Etanercept has three boxed warnings. The first is for increased risk of serious infection that may lead to hospitalization or even death. The second is for lymphoma and other malignancies in children. The last is for TB reactivation with etanercept use. Patients starting etanercept should be evaluated for TB.

Drug Interactions Etanercept may increase the adverse effects of abatacept, anakinra, belimumab, canakinumab, certolizumab, cyclophosphamide, infliximab, natalizumab, rilonacept, tacrolimus, tofacitinib, and vedolizumab.

Pimecrolimus and tocilizumab may enhance the adverse effects of etanercept.

Live vaccines may cause infection, and concurrent use is not recommended.

Golimumab

Golimumab (Simponi) is a TNF inhibitor used to treat RA, psoriatic arthritis, and ankylosing sponodylitis. It is injected subcutaneously once a month. Golimumab should be used with methotrexate for RA, with or without methotrexate for psoriatic arthritis, and alone for ankylosing spondylitis. All three are chronic disorders in which the immune system attacks joints. Side effects include upper respiratory tract infections, runny nose, fever/chills, dizziness, and redness at injection site.

Contraindications Golimumab does not have contraindications.

Cautions and Considerations Golimumab has three boxed warnings. The first is for increased risk of serious infection that may lead to hospitalization or even death. The second is for lymphoma and other malignancies in children. The last is for TB reactivation with golimumab use. Patients starting golimumab should be evaluated for TB.

Drug Interactions Golimumab may increase the adverse effects of abatacept, anakinra, belimumab, canakinumab, certolizumab, cyclophosphamide, infliximab, natalizumab, rilonacept, tacrolimus, tofacitinib, and vedolizumab.

Pimecrolimus and tocilizumab may enhance the adverse effects of golimumab. Live vaccines may cause infection, and concurrent use is not recommended.

Hydroxychloroquine

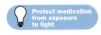

Hydroxychloroquine (Plaquenil) is used to suppress acute attacks of malaria and to treat systemic lupus and RA. It can cause corneal deposits, retinal changes, GI upset, and skin rash. Patients should wear sunglasses in sunlight and watch for vision changes, ringing in the ears, and hearing loss. Side effects include nausea, vomiting, abdominal pain, diarrhea, anorexia, headache, dizziness, confusion, seizures, blurred vision or vision changes, allergy, skin rash, muscle weakness/pain, anemia, blood disorders, hearing loss, and heart problems.

Contraindications Hydroxychloroquine is contraindicated in individuals with hypersensitivities to 4-aminoquinoline derivatives or retinal or visual field changes attributable to 4-aminoquinolines. Hydroxychloroquine also should not be used on a long-term basis in children.

Cautions and Considerations Hydroxychloroquine has a boxed warning advising that only an experienced prescriber should be prescribing this medication.

Drug Interactions Artemether may enhance the adverse effects of hydroxychloroquine. Hydroxychloroquine may enhance the toxicities of lumefantrine and mefloquine.

Infliximab

Infliximab (Remicade) was initially approved for Crohn's disease, but it is now approved for RA, ankylosing spondylitis, plaque psoriasis, psoriatic arthritis, and ulcerative colitis. It is given intravenously with an induction regimen of 5 mg at weeks 0, 2, and 6, followed by a maintenance regimen every 8 weeks. Side effects include nausea, vomiting, headache, diarrhea, abdominal pain, cough, indigestion, fatigue, back pain, fever/chills, chest pain, flushing, dizziness, heart failure, nerve problems, seizures, and Stevens-Johnson syndrome.

Contraindications Infliximab should be avoided in patients with a hypersensitivity to murine (mouse family) proteins.

Cautions and Considerations Infliximab has three boxed warnings. The first is for increased risk of serious infection that may lead to hospitalization or even death. The second is for lymphoma and other malignancies in children. The last is for TB reactivation with infliximab use. Patients starting infliximab should be evaluated for TB.

Drug Interactions Infliximab may increase the toxicities of abatacept, anakinra, belimumab, canakinumab, certolizumab, natalizumab, pimecrolimus, rilonacept, tacrolimus, tofacitinib, and vedolizumab.

Adalimumab, etanercept, golimumab, tocilizumab, and ustekinumab may enhance infliximab's toxicities.

Live vaccines may cause infection, and concurrent use is not recommended.

Leflunomide

Leflunomide (Arava) is a pyrimidine synthesis inhibitor that interferes with the proliferation of lymphocytes. Leflunomide slows the progression of rheumatoid arthritis, reduces pain and joint swelling, and improves functional ability. Evidence suggests that this drug exhibits an additive effect when combined with methotrexate. In the event of overdose or toxicity, cholestyramine should be administered. Leflunomide tablets should be protected from light. Side effects include headache, dizziness, diarrhea, abdominal pain, indigestion, weight loss, liver problems, peripheral neuropathy (nerve pain), hair loss, high blood pressure, anemia, blood disorders, and lung disease.

Contraindications Leflunomide is contraindicated in pregnancy.

Cautions and Considerations Leflunomide has a boxed warning for reports of hepatotoxicity. Liver function should be monitored in patients using leflunomide. The other black box warning is for women of childbearing potential. They should not receive therapy until pregnancy has been ruled out and they receive counseling concerning the fetal risk.

Leflunomide use may increase risk of serious infection. It is considered a hazardous agent, and special handling precautions should be taken.

Drug Interactions Bile acid sequestrants may decrease serum concentrations of the active metabolite. In fact, cholestyramine can be used if too much leflunomide has been ingested. Activated charcoal may also decrease serum concentrations.

The adverse effects of natalizumab, teriflunomide, and tofacitinib may be enhanced by leflunomide.

Pimecrolimus and tacrolimus may enhance the adverse effects of leflunomide.

Live vaccines should be used concurrently with leflunomide.

Methotrexate

Methotrexate (Rheumatrex) is an antineoplastic agent used to treat cancers, arthritic conditions, and psoriasis. It should be taken on an empty stomach. Exposure to sunlight should be avoided. Side effects include mouth sores, nausea, vomiting, abdominal distress, anemia and blood disorders, liver and kidney damage, Stevens-Johnson syndrome, eye irritation, and heart problems.

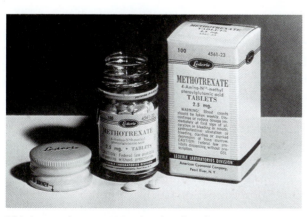

This image shows a 1950s bottle of methotrexate.

Contraindications Methotrexate is contraindicated in breastfeeding, pregnancy, alcoholism, alcoholic liver disease or other chronic liver disease, immunosuppressed states, and preexisting blood diseases.

Cautions and Considerations Methotrexate has many boxed warnings. It may cause kidney damage; bone marrow suppression (that may be fatal); severe and potentially fatal dermatologic reactions; gastrointestinal toxicity; liver damage (acute and fatal); immune suppression (leading to potentially fatal infections); pneumonitis; malignant lymphomas; tumor lysis syndrome; and decreased elimination in patients with ascites or reduced kidney impairment. There is also a boxed warning for severe bone marrow suppression with concurrent NSAID use. Methotrexate may cause fetal death or congenital abnormalities in pregnant patients. Concurrent methotrexate and radiotherapy may increase the risk of soft tissue necrosis and osteonecrosis. The methotrexate products that contain preservatives should not be used for intrathecal administration.

Drug Interactions Acitretin, foscarnet, pimecrolimus, and tacrolimus may enhance the toxic effects of methotrexate.

Methotrexate may increase the toxic effects of clozapine, dipyrone, and natalizumab.

Live vaccines should not be used concurrently.

Sulfasalazine

Sulfasalazine is used to treat ulcerative colitis and rheumatoid arthritis. Sulfasalazine helps to reduce joint pain, swelling, and stiffness. Tablets should be administered in evenly divided doses, preferably after meals. Enteric-coated tablets should be swallowed whole. Side effects include anorexia, diarrhea, abdominal pain, indigestion, headache, nausea/vomiting, colitis, blood disorders, rash, Stevens-Johnson syndrome, liver and kidney problems, hair loss, and male infertility.

Contraindications Sulfasalazine should be avoided in patients with a hypersensitivity to sulfa drugs or salicylates and in patients who have an intestinal or urinary obstruction or porphyria.

Cautions and Considerations Sulfasalazine may have cross-reactivity in patients with sulfa allergy.

Blood diseases have occurred with sulfasalazine use. Use with extreme caution in patients with diseases.

Severe skin reactions, including fatal ones, have occurred with sulfasalazine use.

Enteric-coated tablets may not be fully absorbed in some patients. If tablets pass in stool, discontinue this formulation.

Drug Interactions Sulfasalazine interacts with ketorolac and methotrexate. Live vaccines should be avoided in patients using sulfasalazine.

Systemic Lupus Erythematosus

Systemic lupus erythematosus (SLE or lupus) is a chronic **autoimmune disease** that can affect the skin, joints, kidneys, lungs, nervous system, membranes, and other organs. SLE is characterized by periods of acute relapses and of remission. Common symptoms of SLE include fatigue, fever, and weight gain. Symptoms that patients may experience depend on the areas that are affected. Some of these symptoms include arthritis, skin lesions, Raynaud's phenomenon (a disorder characterized by cold-induced color changes of the hands and feet), kidney dysfunction, GI problems (such as gastritis), pulmonary dysfunction, cardiovascular dysfunction, neurologic complications, ophthalmic issues, and hematologic dysfunction (such as thromboembolism). Treatment of SLE is based on a myriad of factors, including patient preference, disease activity, and comorbidities.

TABLE 13.6 Common Treatments for SLE

Generic (Brand)	Pronunciation	Dosage Form	Common Dosage	Dispensing Status
Antimalarials				
chloroquine (Aralen)	KLOR-oh-kwin	Tablet	250 mg a day	Rx
hydroxychloroquine (Plaquenil)	hye-drox-ee-KLOR-oh-kwin	Tablet	200–400 mg a day	Rx
Immunosuppressants				
azathioprine (Imuran)	az-a-THYE-oh-preen	Tablet	2 mg/kg a day	Rx
methotrexate (Rheumatrex)	meth-oh-TREX-ate	Injection, tablet	7.5–15 mg a week	Rx

Most patients with SLE are treated with hydroxychloroquine (discussed with rheumatoid arthritis) or chloroquine, which are traditionally drugs used for malaria. Oral corticosteroids (such as prednisone) or injectable corticosteroids (such as methylprednisolone) may also be used. Corticosteroids are covered more thoroughly in Chapter 14. Immunosuppressants such as azathioprine or methotrexate may also be used; both were discussed earlier in this chapter. Typical doses of SLE treatments are included in Table 13.6.

Chloroquine

Chloroquine (Aralen) is an **antimalarial**, a class of medications traditionally used to treat malaria. However, antimalarials can improve SLE by decreasing autoantibody production, protecting the skin, and improving skin lesions. Hydroxychloroquine (discussed earlier in this chapter) and chloroquine are the most frequently used antimalarials for the treatment of SLE. Side effects of chloroquine include upset stomach, skin discoloration, agitation, and anxiety.

Contraindications Contraindications to chloroquine include previous retinal and visual field changes.

Cautions and Considerations Chloroquine has been associated with cardiovascular effects, including QT prolongation. Use should be avoided in patients with QT prolongation. Ophthalmic effects (such as macular degeneration and irreversible retinal damage) have occurred with use of chloroquine. Patients should be monitored for ophthalmic effects, and treatment should be discontinued immediately if signs or symptoms of visual changes occur.

Drug Interactions Abiraterone, conivaptan, fusidic acid, and idelalisib may increase serum concentrations of chloroquine.

Chloroquine may decrease the effects of agalsidase alfa, agalsidase beta, and ampicillin.

Artemether may increase the toxic effects of chloroquine.

The adverse reactions of mefloquine and thioridazine may be enhanced by chloroquine.

QT-prolonging agents, ivabradine, and mifepristone may increase the QT-prolonging effects of chloroquine.

Gouty Arthritis

Gouty arthritis, often referred to merely as gout, usually affects single joints, causing a **tophus** (a deposit of sodium urate) to form around the joint. Tophi may form in tissues, joint cartilage, ear lobes, and metatarsals. Typically, the first joint affected is the big toe; it becomes painful, swollen, and red. The disease is related to the patient's metabolism of uric acid, which is normally excreted by the kidneys. The affected patient overproduces or has improper excretion of uric acid, so aspirin is contraindicated because it competes with uric acid for kidney excretion. The condition is usually inherited. Persons prone to gout should avoid the following drugs, which could precipitate an attack:

- cytotoxic agents
- diuretics
- ethanol
- nicotinic acid
- salicylates

Acute Gout Treatment

A gout attack is a severe and debilitating pain episode, with the worst pain occurring in the first 24 hours. Most attacks usually resolve within 3 to 10 days with proper medication. Potent and fast-acting NSAIDs (indomethacin, naproxen) are often used. NSAIDs may help with pain and swelling.

Colchicine

Colchicine (Colcrys, Mitigare) can be used to treat an acute gout attack and to reduce the frequency of recurrent episodes of gouty arthritis. When used for preventive gout treatment, therapy is often short term because of its potentially toxic side effects. Colchicine's exact mechanism of action is not completely known, but it is thought to work as an anti-inflammatory and may decrease uric acid deposition. Side effects include diarrhea, nausea, and vomiting.

Contraindications Colchicine use is contraindicated in patients with kidney or liver impairment. Colchicine should not be used in combination with drugs that may slow the drug's clearance from the body, such as P-glycoprotein inhibitors or strong cytochrome P-450 (CYP) 3A4 inhibitors.

Cautions and Considerations Colchicine should be used with caution in older adults, and dosage adjustments should be considered. Clearance of colchicine is decreased in patients with liver or kidney impairment.

Drug Interactions Conivaptan, fusidic acid, and idelalisib may increase serum concentrations of colchicine.

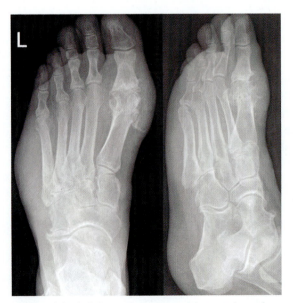

X-rays of the left foot of a person with gout show the characteristic swelling of the joint of the big toe and the side of the foot.

Preventive Gout Treatment

Chronic preventive therapy of gout is indicated in certain patients. There are various agents used to prevent gout. Allopurinol, colchicine (discussed earlier), febuxostat, and probenecid are all common preventive gout options.

Allopurinol

Allopurinol (Zyloprim) is often used for preventive gout treatment and is usually one of the top 200 drugs dispensed in pharmacies. Allopurinol works by inhibiting the production of uric acid. It is classified as a xanthine oxidase inhibitor. Side effects include skin rash, nausea, and diarrhea.

Contraindications Allopurinol does not have any reported contraindications.

Cautions and Considerations Allopurinol use has been associated with severe hypersensitivity reactions and should be discontinued if signs are present. Allopurinol should be used with caution in patients with kidney impairment because of the increased risk of hypersensitivity reactions.

Drug Interactions Allopurinol may increase concentrations of didanosine.
Allopurinol may enhance toxic effects of pegloticase.
The anticoagulant effects of warfarin may be enhanced by allopurinol use.

Febuxostat

Febuxostat (Uloric) works by inhibiting uric acid production. Like allopurinol, it is classified as a xanthine oxidase inhibitor. Febuxostat is used for chronic management of high uric acid levels in patients with gout. Side effects include diarrhea, headache, and angioedema.

TABLE 13.7 Most Commonly Used Drugs for Gouty Arthritis

Generic (Brand)	Pronunciation	Dosage Form	Common Dosage	Dispensing Status
Acute Attack Therapy				
colchicine (Colcrys, Mitigare)	KOL-chi-seen	Injection, tablet	1.2 mg initially, followed in 1 hr with 0.6 mg. Maximum dose of 1.8 mg within 1 hr	Rx
Preventive Gout Therapy				
allopurinol (Zyloprim)	al-oh-PURE-i-nawl	Tablet	200–600 mg a day	Rx
colchicine (Colcrys, Mitigare)	KOL-chi-seen	Capsule, tablet	0.6 mg twice a day	Rx
febuxostat (Uloric)	feb-UX-oh-stat	Tablet	80–120 mg a day	Rx
probenecid	proe-BEN-e-sid	Tablet	250 mg twice a day for 1 week, then 500 mg twice a day for 2 weeks; increase 500 mg/day every other week until at 3,000 mg a day	Rx

Contraindications Febuxostat should not be used concurrently with azathioprine or mercaptopurine.

Cautions and Considerations Febuxostat use has been associated with severe hypersensitivity reactions and should be discontinued if signs are present. Liver failure has been reported with febuxostat use. Febuxostat should also be used with caution in patients with severe hypersensitivity reactions to allopurinol.

Drug Interactions Febuxostat may increase the serum concentrations of azathioprine, didanosine, mercaptopurine, and pegloticase.

Probenecid

Probenecid is used for preventive gout treatment in patients with relatively low kidney uric acid excretion. It works by inhibiting the renal reabsorption of uric acid and therefore promotes uric acid excretion. Side effects include nausea, vomiting, and anorexia.

Contraindications Probenecid should not be used in children less than two years of age, and therapy should not be initiated during an acute gout attack.

Cautions and Considerations Probenecid use has been associated with severe hypersensitivity reactions and should be discontinued if signs are present.

Drug Interactions Probenecid may increase the concentrations of avibactam, doripenem, ketorolac, meropenem, and penicillins.

Adverse reactions of pegloticase may be enhanced by probenecid.

Complementary and Alternative Therapies

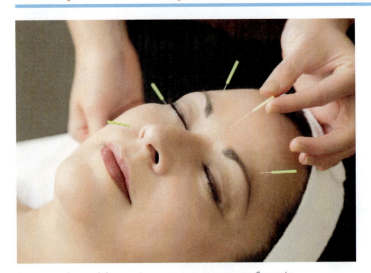

A woman is receiving an acupuncture treatment for pain.

Acupuncture, a process that involves penetrating the skin with thin needles in specific areas, is used for pain. Acupuncture has been used for thousands of years in Chinese medicine. There are several studies that show acupuncture to be beneficial for acute and chronic pain. In fact, some insurance plans cover acupuncture as a benefit.

Chondroitin is taken by some individuals in combination with glucosamine for hip and knee OA. However, studies do not clearly show that chondroitin taken with glucosamine is effective for OA. Chondroitin is derived from shark cartilage and bovine (cow) sources and is thought to work by inhibiting an enzyme that promotes inflammation. If patients want to take chondroitin, typical dosing is 200–400 mg two or three times a day. Common side effects tend to be mild and include nausea, heartburn, diarrhea, and constipation. Rare side effects include eyelid swelling, lower limb swelling, hair loss, and allergic reaction. If patients experience any of these effects, they should stop taking chondroitin.

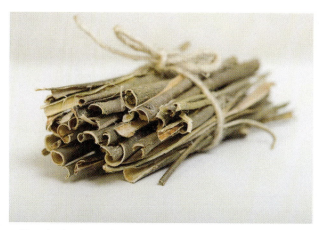
Willow bark contains salicin and is used for pain.

Glucosamine is used by some individuals to improve pain and stiffness from OA. This supplement is derived from the exoskeleton of shellfish and is thought to slow joint degeneration. If patients want to take glucosamine, typical dosing is 1,500 mg a day (given in divided doses, 500 mg 3 times a day). Side effects are usually mild and include nausea, heartburn, diarrhea, and constipation. Taking glucosamine with food can decrease these effects. Although glucosamine has not proven to be harmful in studies, it is recommended that patients with shellfish allergies avoid taking it.

Willow bark (*Salix alba*), which is a bark that contains salicin, has been used to treat many different kinds of pain. Willow bark is a traditional analgesic (pain relieving) therapy for osteoarthritis. Several studies have confirmed this finding. Additional studies comparing willow bark to conventional medicinal agents for safety and effectiveness are warranted.

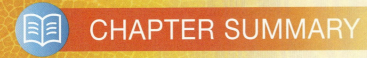
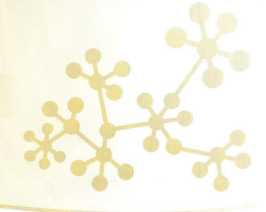

CHAPTER SUMMARY

Muscle Relaxants

- The side effects of muscle relaxants are sedation, reduced mental alertness, reduced motor abilities, and GI upset. Patients taking these drugs should avoid alcohol.

- Methocarbamol (Robaxin) causes skeletal muscle relaxation by reducing the transmission of impulses from the spinal cord to skeletal muscles.

- Orphenadrine (Norflex) is an indirect skeletal muscle relaxant thought to work by central atropine-like effects. The tablet should be swallowed whole, not crushed or chewed.

- Carisoprodol (Soma) is subject to abuse. Once the drug is ingested, the molecules are cleaved to the major metabolite, meprobamate, which is a controlled substance. Carisoprodol is a controlled substance in many states.

- Cyclobenzaprine (Flexeril) is a centrally acting skeletal muscle relaxant that is pharmacologically related to tricyclic antidepressants. Onset of action is usually within one hour, and the drug should not be used for more than two to three weeks.

- Baclofen (Lioresal) is used for treating reversible spasticity, spinal cord lesions, and multiple sclerosis and is sometimes used for hiccups. It should be taken with food or milk.

Inflammation and Swelling

- Analgesics are used for mild-to-moderate pain, inflammation, and fever. A widely accepted mechanism for many of their actions is their ability to inhibit the enzyme cyclooxygenase and thereby decrease the conversion of arachidonic acid to prostaglandins (PGs), thromboxane A_2, or prostacyclin.

- Somatic pain (from injury to skin, muscle, and bone) is dull and throbbing, whereas visceral pain (from the organs) is sharp and stabbing.

- Fever is a response by the body's temperature-regulating center (the hypothalamus) to substances called endogenous pyrogens produced as a result of bacterial or viral infections. The subsequent release of PGs from the brain causes the body "thermostat" to reset at a higher temperature.

- Adverse GI effects may limit the use of nonnarcotic analgesics.

- Salicylates have analgesic (pain-relieving), anti-inflammatory, and antipyretic (fever-reducing) properties.

- The primary analgesic actions of salicylates are peripheral rather than central. Their primary antipyretic action is central and presumed to be in the hypothalamus.

- Salicylates are indicated for simple headache, arthritis, pain and fever with influenza, muscular aches and pains, menstrual cramps, and inflammation.

- Salicylates cause gastrointestinal ulceration. They should be avoided by patients with asthma, nasal polyps, chronic sinusitis, bleeding ulcers, and hemophilia. They should not be taken after surgery or tooth extraction.

- More than 4 g of aspirin per day can cause problems; 10 g can be lethal.

- Mild salicylate intoxication is characterized by ringing in the ears (tinnitus), dizziness, headache, and mental confusion.

Osteoarthritis

- The most common complaint from arthritis patients is persistent pain. Because cartilage has no nerves, pain originates from surrounding joint structures, such as bones, tendons, ligaments, and muscles.

- Therapy for arthritis is aimed at relieving pain, maintaining or improving mobility, and minimizing disability. It may include medication, physical therapy, and patient education.

- Acetaminophen acts centrally to cause antipyresis. It is an effective analgesic and antipyretic without the anti-inflammatory, antirheumatic, or uric acid excretory effects of aspirin. A patient with severe liver disease or alcoholism should not take acetaminophen.

- At a dose of above 4 g of acetaminophen per day, liver damage can occur.

- Alcohol can cause a problem with OTC analgesics, according to the FDA. For acetaminophen, the problem is liver toxicity; for NSAIDs, it is increased GI bleeding.

- NSAIDs take longer to reduce fever than other products, but the effect may last longer.

- NSAIDs are used for headache, menstrual cramps, backache, muscle aches, flu, fever, and the pain and inflammation of arthritis, rheumatism, and gouty arthritis.

- NSAIDs inhibit PG synthesis in inflamed tissues, thereby preventing the sensitization of pain receptors to mediators of inflammation. Thus, they generally act peripherally rather than centrally as other pain killers do.

- PGs perform three protective functions in the GI tract: increase mucosal blood flow, increase mucus production, and decrease free acid production.

- Side effects of NSAIDs are GI upset, nausea, abdominal cramps, heartburn, indigestion, ringing in the ears, ulcers, jaundice, dizziness, and rash. Gastropathy develops in one in five chronic NSAID users.

- Many patients will need to take a proton pump inhibitor with NSAIDs.

- Concurrent use of multiple NSAIDs (including aspirin) should be discouraged, because the combination may lead to additive or synergistic toxicity rather than increased efficacy.

- Clinical trials have not shown the superiority of any single NSAID over the others for the management of osteoarthritis.

- All NSAIDs should be administered with food and dispensed with a medication guide.

- When injected, ketorolac (Toradol) has shown pain relief equal to narcotics. It is for short-term use only.

- Sulindac (Clinoril) is a renal-sparing drug that is metabolized in the liver.

- Nabumetone (Relafen) should be taken in the morning with food.

Rheumatoid Arthritis, Systemic Lupus Erythematosus, Gouty Arthritis

- DMARDs are disease-modifying antirheumatic drugs that may slow the progression of the disease, but the side effects limit their use.

- Methotrexate (Rheumatrex) should be taken on an empty stomach, and exposure to the sun should be avoided. Methotrexate is an antineoplastic agent commonly used to treat RA.

- Hydroxychloroquine (Plaquenil) is an antimalarial drug also used to treat RA and lupus.

- Lupus (SLE) is an autoimmune disease for which there is no cure. It affects multiple systems of the body. Drugs used to treat it are NSAIDs, antimalarials, corticosteroids, and immunosuppressants.

- Aspirin should not be given to a patient with gout; it competes with uric acid for kidney excretion.

- Cytotoxic agents, diuretics, ethanol, nicotinic acid, and salicylates can precipitate a gout attack.

- Colchicine and NSAIDs are used for acute gout attacks.

- Colchicine, indomethacin, and allopurinol are all used as chronic preventative therapies for gout.

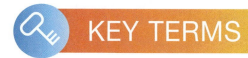

KEY TERMS

acetylcholine (ACh) a neurotransmitter that binds to ACh receptors on the membranes of muscle cells, beginning a process that ultimately results in muscle contraction

acupuncture a process that involves penetrating the skin with thin needles in specific areas to manage pain

antimalarial medication used to treat malaria

antipyretic fever reducing

antipyretic analgesic drug that reduces both fever and pain

arthritis joint inflammation; persistent pain due to functional problems of the joints

autoimmune disease illness in which the immune system attacks and destroys healthy tissue within the body

biologic response modifiers drugs that work by inhibiting substances that cause inflammation and joint damage

cardiac heart muscle

cartilaginous articulating bone surfaces are covered with cartilage

centrally acting drug that does not act directly on the muscle

cyclooxygenase-1 (COX-1) an enzyme that is present in most body tissues and produces protective prostaglandins to regulate physiological processes such as GI mucosal integrity

cyclooxygenase-2 (COX-2) an enzyme that is present in the synovial fluid of arthritis patients and is associated with the pain and inflammation of arthritis

disease-modifying antirheumatic drugs (DMARDs) agents that can modify the progression of rheumatoid arthritis

fibrous articulating bone surfaces are attached by fibrous connective tissue

gouty arthritis a disease resulting from the improper excretion of uric acid; also called *gout*

joints parts of the human body where bone meets bone

ligaments noncontractile connective tissue that ties one bone to another bone

lupus see systemic lupus erythematosus

muscle an organ that produces movement by contracting

muscle relaxant a drug that reduces or prevents skeletal muscle contraction

muscle spasticity a condition whereby muscle fibers are in a state of involuntary, continuous contraction that causes pain

nonnarcotic analgesic a drug used for pain, inflammation, and fever that is not a controlled substance

nonsteroidal anti-inflammatory drugs (NSAIDs) a class of drugs that provide pain, swelling, and fever reduction

osteoarthritis (OA) a degenerative joint disease resulting in loss of cartilage, elasticity, and bone thickness

salicylates a class of nonnarcotic analgesics that have both pain-relieving and antipyretic (fever-reducing) properties

skeletal striated muscle in which contraction is voluntary

smooth muscle in which contraction is involuntary

somatic pain dull, throbbing pain from skin, muscle, and bone

synovial articulating surface that is covered by a fluid-filled, fibrous sac

systemic lupus erythematosus (SLE) an autoimmune disease that affects multiple systems of the body, leading to painful inflammation; the underlying cause is not known

tophus a deposit of sodium urate around a joint, symptom of gout

visceral pain sharp, stabbing pain from the organs

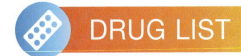

DRUG LIST

Muscle Relaxants

baclofen (Lioresal, EnovaRX-Baclofen, Equipto-Baclofen, Gablofen)
carisoprodol (Soma)
chlorzoxazone (Lorzone, Parafon Forte DSC)
cyclobenzaprine (Flexeril, Amrix, Fexmid)
dantrolene (Dantrium, Revonto, Ryanodex)
diazepam (Valium)
metaxalone (Metaxall, Skelaxin)
methocarbamol (Robaxin)
orphenadrine (Norflex)

Salicylates

aspirin
buffered aspirin (Ascriptin, Bufferin)
choline magnesium trisalicylate (Trilisate)
salsalate (Amigesic)
willow bark (*Salix alba*)

Antipyretic Analgesic

acetaminophen (Tylenol)

Antidote to Acetaminophen

Acetylcysteine (Mucomyst, Acetadote)

Nonsteroidal Anti-Inflammatory Drugs (NSAIDs)

diclofenac (Cambia, Cataflam, Flector, Pennsaid, Rexaphenac, Solaraze, Voltaren, Zipsor, Zorvolex)
diclofenac-misoprostol (Arthrotec)
esomeprazole-naproxen (Vimovo)
etodolac (Lodine)
ibuprofen (Advil, Motrin)
indomethacin (Indocin)
ketoprofen (Orudis, Oruvail)
ketorolac (Toradol)
meloxicam (Mobic)
nabumetone (Relafen)
naproxen (Aleve, Anaprox, Naprosyn)
oxaprozin (Daypro)
piroxicam (Feldene)
sulindac (Clinoril)

COX-2 Inhibitors

celecoxib (Celebrex)

Other

ibuprofen-famotidine (Duexis)
tramadol (Active-Tramadol, ConZip, EnovaRX-Tramadol, Synapryn FusePaq, Ultram, Ultram ER)

Disease-Modifying Antirheumatic Drugs (DMARDs)

adalimumab (Humira)
anakinra (Kineret)
auranofin (Ridaura)
azathioprine (Imuran)
cyclophosphamide (Cytoxan)
cyclosporine (Neoral, Sandimmune)
etanercept (Enbrel)
golimumab (Simponi)
hydroxychloroquine (Plaquenil)
infliximab (Remicade)
leflunomide (Arava)
methotrexate (Rheumatrex)
sulfasalazine (Azulfidine)

Drug to Treat Lupus

azathioprine (Imuran)
chloroquine (Aralen)
hydroxychloroquine (Plaquenil)
methotrexate (Rheumatrex)

Drugs to Treat Gout

allopurinol (Zyloprim)
colchicine (Colcrys, Mitigare)
febuxostat (Uloric)
indomethacin (Indocin)
probenecid

Black Box Warnings

acetylcysteine (Mucomyst, Acetadote)
adalimumab (Humira)
aspirin (Ascriptin, Bufferin)
azathioprine (Imuran)
celecoxib (Celebrex)
dantrolene (Dantrium)
diclofenac (Cambia, Cataflam, Flector,
    Pennsaid, Rexaphenac, Solaraze,
    Voltaren, Zipsor, Zorvolex)
diclofenac-misoprostol (Arthrotec)
esomeprazole-naproxen (Vimovo)
etanercept (Enbrel)
etodolac (Lodine)

golimumab (Simponi)
hydroxychloroquine (Plaquenil)
ibuprofen (Advil, Motrin)
ibuprofen-famotidine (Duexis)
indomethacin (Indocin)
infliximab (Remicade)
ketoprofen (Orudis, Oruvail)
ketorolac (Toradol)
leflunomide (Arava)
meloxicam (Mobic)
methotrexate (Rheumatrex)
nabumetone (Relafen)
naproxen (Aleve, Anaprox, Naprosyn)
oxaprozin (Daypro)
piroxicam (Feldene)
salsalate (Amigesic)
sulindac (Clinoril)
tocilizumab (Actemra)
tramadol (Active-Tramadol, ConZip,
    EnovaRX-Tramadol, Synapryn FusePaq,
    Ultram, Ultram ER)

Medication Guides

aspirin
belimumab (Benlysta)
celecoxib (Celebrex)
colchicine (Colcrys)
diclofenac (Cataflam, Flector, Solaraze,
    Voltaren)
diclofenac-misoprostol (Arthrotec)
esomeprazole-naproxen (Vimovo)
etodolac (Lodine)
golimumab (Simponi)
ibuprofen (Advil, Motrin)
ibuprofen-famotidine (Duexis)
indomethacin (Indocin)
ketoprofen (Orudis, Oruvail)
ketorolac (Toradol)
meloxicam (Mobic)
nabumetone (Relafen)
naproxen (Aleve, Anaprox, Nparosyn)
oxaprozin (Daypro)
pegloticase (Krystexxa)
piroxicam (Feldene)
sulindac (Clinoril)
tocilizumab (Actemra)

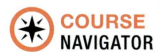
COURSE NAVIGATOR

Access interactive chapter review exercises, practice activities, flash cards, and study games.

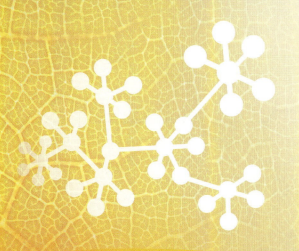

14

Hormonal Disorders and Their Treatment

Learning Objectives

1. Summarize the concept of hormones and how they regulate the body.

2. Explain the treatments for disorders of the thyroid.

3. Discuss adrenal sex hormones and male erectile dysfunction.

4. Outline the concept of hormone replacement therapy.

5. Distinguish the various formulations of oral contraceptives.

6. Outline the drugs used urgently during labor and at delivery.

7. Describe the diseases of the genital systems and how to avoid them.

8. List commonly used corticosteroids.

9. Summarize diabetes and the proper treatment and care of patients.

10. State the applications for growth hormone.

COURSE NAVIGATOR

Access additional chapter resources.

The endocrine system regulates a number of functions to keep the body in balance as well as to control complicated processes such as those involved in reproduction. The same hormones that trigger activity may also be used in treatment. The pharmacologic agents used in these treatments include thyroid preparations, calcium, oral contraceptives, drugs used during labor and delivery, corticosteroids, drugs used in treatment of diabetes, and growth hormones.

The Endocrine System

The **endocrine system**, illustrated in Figure 14.1, consists of glands and other structures produce secretions called **hormones** and release them directly into the circulatory system. The various hormones are responsible for specific regulatory effects on organs and other tissues of the body. The tissue affected by a hormone is called its **target**. Through the work of hormones, the endocrine system maintains homeostasis of the body by regulating the physiologic functions involved in normal daily living and in times of stress.

FIGURE 14.1
Endocrine System

Endocrine glands release hormones directly into the bloodstream, where they travel throughout the body to trigger responses in specific target tissues.

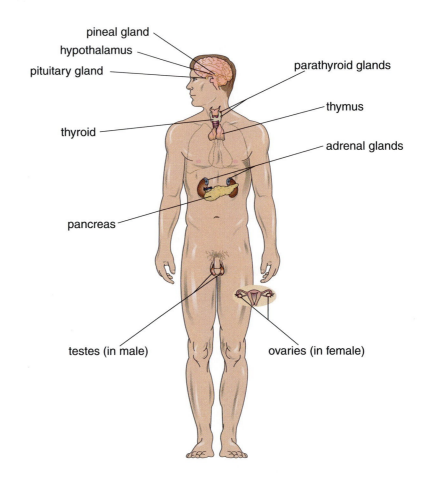

pineal gland
hypothalamus
pituitary gland
parathyroid glands
thymus
thyroid
adrenal glands
pancreas
testes (in male)
ovaries (in female)

Within the endocrine system, the pituitary gland plays a leading role because its hormones regulate several other endocrine glands, as well as a number of body activities, as shown in Figure 14.2. Regulation of hormone synthesis by a particular gland is achieved via an intricate negative feedback mechanism involving that gland, the hypothalamic-pituitary axis, and autoregulation. In a **feedback mechanism**, some of the output signals of a system return as input to exert some control over the process. Physiologic factors such as dopamine and stress can also influence the hypothalamic-pituitary axis and autoregulation.

Thyroid Disorders

The **thyroid gland**, shown in Figure 14.3, produces hormones that stimulate various body tissues to increase their metabolic activity. These hormones, **triiodothyronine (T_3)** and **thyroxine (T_4)**, are both stored as thyroglobulin, which the thyroid cells must break down before they can be released into the bloodstream. Both T_3 and T_4 are generally bound to protein molecules. Activity occurs when the hormones are not bound. T_3 is more physiologically active than T_4. The feedback mechanism that controls the thyroid is the hypothalamic-pituitary axis, which produces thyroid-stimulating hormone (TSH), which in turn stimulates the thyroid to produce T_3 and T_4 (see Figure 14.4). These hormones build up in circulating blood and slow the pituitary gland's production and release of TSH. For a patient with signs of hormonal imbalance,

FIGURE 14.2
Pituitary Hormones

The pituitary gland plays a key role in growth, onset of puberty, and reproductive cycles.

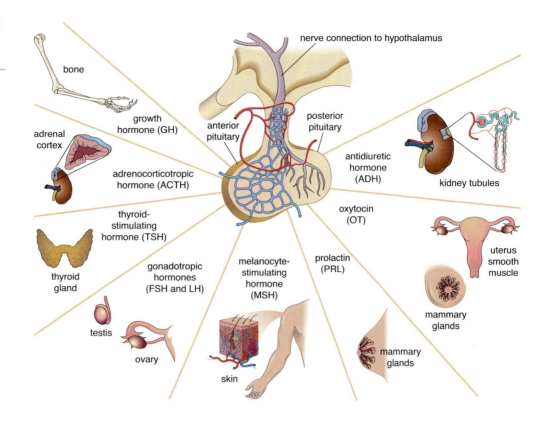

FIGURE 14.3
Thyroid Gland

The thyroid gland is located in the neck surrounding the trachea.

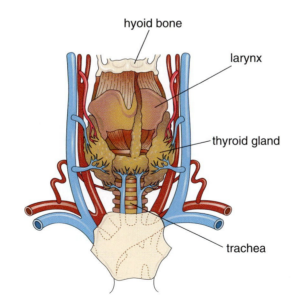

FIGURE 14.4

FIGURE 14.4
The Hypothalamic-Pituitary Axis

A high TSH test result means that T_3 and T_4 levels are low (hypothyroidism).

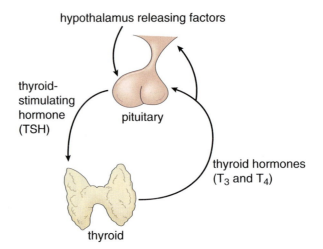

hypothalamus releasing factors

thyroid-stimulating hormone (TSH)

pituitary

thyroid hormones (T_3 and T_4)

thyroid

measuring the amount of serum TSH can determine whether the thyroid is functioning normally; in some instances, other tests for T_4 and T_3 may be needed. It is also important to note, though, that some peripheral conversion of T_4 to T_3 occurs in the tissues.

Safety Alert

Levothyroxine and levofloxacin (an antibiotic) can be misread for each other.

Hypothyroidism

Hypothyroidism refers to conditions in which the production of thyroid hormones is below normal. Congenital (at birth) hypothyroidism may arise in infants and is often caused by an iodine deficiency in the mother's diet during pregnancy. It can cause severe impairment of mental growth and is marked by a thick tongue, lethargy, lack of response to commands, and short stature. It can be corrected if treated within the first 6 to 12 months of life.

The causes of hypothyroidism include a defect in the function of the thyroid due to autoimmune destruction of the gland, radioactive iodine therapy, or surgical removal of the thyroid. Pituitary dysfunction or an abnormality in the hypothalamus can also cause thyroid failure.

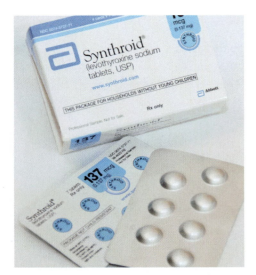

Levothyroxine is available as a generic drug or as the brand product Synthroid.

Treatment of Hypothyroidism

Thyroid replacement therapy is indicated for hypothyroid states and thyroid cancer. In the absence of natural hormones, thyroid hormone replacement is required. Although thyroid hormone increases metabolism, replacement therapy should not be used to treat obesity. Drugs commonly used to treat hypothyroidism are listed in Table 14.1. Hypothyroidism causes increased sensitivity to numerous drugs. Correction may increase requirements for other drugs because of increases in their metabolism and conversion.

Levothyroxine (Levothroid, Levoxyl, Synthroid) is synthetic T_4. It is recommended for chronic therapy. Levothyroxine can have cardiovascular side effects, so patients should immediately report any chest pain, increased pulse, palpitations, heat intolerance, or excessive sweating. In overdose, it can cause "too rapid" a correction and, therefore, a risk of cardiotoxicity and hyperthyroidism. Levothyroxine

| 25 mcg orange | 50 mcg white | 75 mcg violet | 88 mcg olive | 100 mcg yellow | 112 mcg rose |

| 125 mcg brown | 137 mcg turquoise | 150 mcg blue | 175 mcg lilac | 200 mcg pink | 300 mcg green |

Levothyroxine is available in multiple strengths, each with different colors.

may alter the protein binding of other drugs, so the technician should check the patient profile for drugs currently being taken.

Generic levothyroxine products and Synthroid are therapeutically equivalent, and they are now **AB rated** according to the US Food and Drug Administration (FDA) (that is, shown by studies to be bioequivalent, as a generic should be to the corresponding brand name drug). One clinical study showed that switching products does not cause problems, but it is usually undesirable to switch brands once a patient has become stable. Some prescribers are concerned that the small FDA-allowable compositional differences between Synthroid and generic levothyroxine brands could affect blood levels. All patients taking thyroid hormones should undergo TSH tests periodically, as well as approximately six weeks after changes in dosage or brands. Once the patient is stable on a brand, the prescriber will typically write **Dispense as Written (DAW)** and write the prescription for that brand name only. Most pharmacy computer programs automatically switch all drugs to a generic; when the switch happens with this drug, the technician may frequently need to switch the drug back to the brand if indicated by the prescriber.

Liothyronine (Cytomel, Triostat) is synthetic T_3. It may be used for hypothyroidism and management of goiter. Liothyronine is available in oral and injectable forms.

Contraindications Levothyroxine and liothyronine use is contraindicated in the presence of an acute heart attack, untreated hyperthyroidism, and uncorrected adrenal insufficiency. Thyroid extract (Armour Thyroid), which contains beef and pork products, should not be used in patients with a hypersensitivity to beef or pork.

The capsule form of levothyroxine should not be used in individuals who cannot swallow capsules. The injection form of liothyronine should not be used in patients who are undergoing artificial rewarming.

Cautions and Considerations Thyroid hormones have a black box warning saying they should not be used for the treatment of obesity or for weight loss.

Serious and potentially life-threatening toxic effects can occur with higher doses, especially in patients with normal levels of thyroid hormones. Patients should be reminded to get regular blood tests to check thyroid hormone levels. Various brands of thyroid hormone may contain slightly different amounts, enough for changes in

TABLE 14.1 Most Commonly Used Agents for Hypothyroidism

Generic (Brand)	Pronunciation	Dosage Form	Dispensing Status
levothyroxine, T_4 (Levoxyl, Synthroid, Tirosint, Unithroid)	lee-voe-thye-ROX-een	Capsule, injection, tablet	Rx
liothyronine (Cytomel, Triostat)	lye-oh-THYE-roe-neen	Injection, tablet	Rx
thyroid extract (Armour Thyroid)	THYE-roid EX-trakt	Tablet	Rx

therapy to be experienced by individual patients. Once one brand of thyroid hormone is chosen, the patient should continue receiving that brand at each refill.

Drug Interactions Aluminum-containing products may decrease concentrations of levothyroxine when taken within four hours of each other.

Bile acid sequestrants, calcium-containing products, magnesium-containing products, and multivitamins may decrease the concentrations or all thyroid replacement therapies. Thyroid products should not be taken at the same time as bile acid sequestrants.

Carbamazepine, ciprofloxacin, estrogen products, fosphenytoin, iron salts, phenytoin, rifampin, and selective serotonin reuptake inhibitors (SSRIs) may decrease the efficacy of thyroid hormones. Tricyclic antidepressants may enhance the cardiotoxic effects of thyroid agents.

Orlistat, raloxifene, and sevelamer may decrease the concentrations of levothyroxine.

Thyroid products may increase the metabolism of theophylline.

Warfarin's anticoagulant effect may be enhanced by thyroid products.

Hyperthyroidism

Hyperthyroidism, also called thyrotoxicosis, is due to excessive levels of thyroid hormone. This condition is less common than hypothyroidism. Common causes of hyperthyroidism include **Graves' disease**, thyroid nodules or tumors, and pituitary nodules or tumors.

Symptoms of hyperthyroidism are varied, with the most prominent being weight loss and hair loss. Another prominent symptom is **exophthalmos**, a condition in which fat collects behind the eyeball, causing the eyeball to protrude and making it difficult to close the eye. This condition can cause corneal ulceration. Adults with hyperthyroidism may have heart problems due to prolonged hyperactivity caused by the excessive hormone levels.

For children, hyperthyroidism is managed with surgery and hormone replacement therapy. In adults, surgery is indicated for malignant lesions, esophageal obstruction, failure of thyroid therapy, or large multinodular goiters.

Thyroid storm presents with clinical features similar to thyrotoxicosis, but the features are more exaggerated. It is a life-threatening medical emergency. Thyroid storm commonly lasts approximately three days, although symptoms may persist for an additional eight days. Treatment includes IV fluids, antipyretics, cooling blankets, and sedation. Antithyroid drugs are given in large doses. Table 14.2 presents the most commonly used agents for hyperthyroidism.

TABLE 14.2 Most Commonly Used Agents for Hyperthyroidism

Generic (Brand)	Pronunciation	Dosage Form	Dispensing Status
methimazole (Tapazole)	meth-IM-a-zole	Tablet	Rx
propylthiouracil (PTU)	proe-pil-thye-oh-YOOR-a-sil	Tablet	Rx

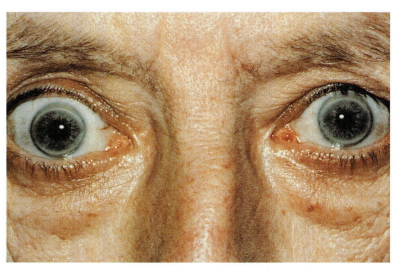

Protrusion of the eyeballs, known as exophthalmos, is a symptom of hyperthyroidism.

Treatment of Hyperthyroidism

Treatment for hyperthyroidism usually involves surgery, which removes or reduces the malfunctioning gland, or **ablation**, which destroys the thyroid gland via radioactive iodine. Afterward, **oral thyroid supplementation** is given to artificially provide adequate hormone levels. Propylthiouracil and methimazole are sometimes used for short-term suppression of thyroid hormones.

Methimazole (Tapazole) is used for the treatment of hyperthyroidism in patients where surgery or radioactive iodine therapy is not appropriate. It may also be used to treat hyperthyroid symptoms in patients awaiting thyroidectomy or radioactive iodine therapy. The patient should be monitored for hypothyroidism, T_3 and T_4 levels, complete blood count (CBC) with differential, and liver function (baseline and as needed).

Propylthiouracil (PTU) blocks the synthesis of T_3 and T_4 and the conversion of T_4 to T_3. This drug is used for palliative treatment of hyperthyroidism, as adjunctive therapy to improve hyperthyroidism in preparation for surgical treatment, and management of thyroid storm. The recommended dose should not be exceeded. Patients should notify the prescriber or pharmacist in the event of fever, sore throat, unusual bleeding or bruising, headache, or general malaise. If the patient is taking chronic therapy, the following parameters should be monitored: CBC with differential, prothrombin time (PT), liver function tests, thyroid function tests (T_4, T_3, and TSH), and periodic blood cell counts. Administration of propylthiouracil is preferred over methimazole in thyroid storm.

Both propylthiouracil and methimazole cause altered taste and mild **alopecia** (hair loss). Bone marrow depression with fever, sore throat, and malaise can occur and can be serious. An autoimmune reaction and a warfarin-like anticoagulant reaction can also occur.

Contraindications Methimazole and propylthiouracil do not have contraindications.

Cautions and Considerations Propylthiouracil carries a boxed warning for liver toxicity, which may be fatal in some cases.

Methimazole use is also associated with liver toxicity. In addition, it is associated with increased bleeding, bone marrow suppression, and dermatitis.

Drug Interactions Methimazole and propylthiouracil may decrease the anticoagulant effects of warfarin.

The adverse effects of clozapine may be exacerbated by methimazole and propylthiouracil.

Male Hormones and Sexual Dysfunction

The sex hormones are controlled by pituitary hormones, particularly follicle-stimulating hormone (FSH) and luteinizing hormone (LH).

An **androgen** is a hormone that promotes development and maintenance of male physical characteristics. In males, androgens are produced by the testes. They are also produced by the ovaries in females, but they are largely converted into female hormones (discussed in the following section). In both males and females, they are also produced in the adrenal glands and the peripheral fat tissue. An important androgen is **testosterone**, which is produced by the testes. The pituitary hormones travel in the bloodstream to the testes, where they stimulate the Leydig cells to produce testosterone and release it into the blood. Through a feedback mechanism, the increased testosterone levels then slow the secretion of the releasing factors by the hypothalamus.

Testosterone is responsible for initiating sperm production and for behavioral characteristics (e.g., aggressiveness), libido, and sexual potency. It is required during adulthood for the maintenance of libido, sexual potency, fertility (sperm production), muscle mass and strength, fat distribution, bone mass, erythropoiesis (red blood cell production), and prevention of baldness.

Disorders of Male Hormones

Hypogonadism is a condition where the body's sex glands produce little or no hormones. In male hypogonadism the testes are not secreting sufficient hormones and usual development of muscle, facial hair, genitals, and voice is altered. Symptoms include breast enlargement, muscle loss, and decreased libido. If hypogonadism is secondary to brain tumors, additional symptoms may include headache, visual disturbances, and breast discharge. Hypogonadism in men is usually treated with androgens.

Androgens can cause **hirsutism** (abnormal hairiness) and acne. Hepatoxicity and abnormally high levels of red blood cells are also side effects. Other adverse effects from androgen therapy include oily skin, ankle edema, priapism (frequent or prolonged, painful penile erections), and **gynecomastia** (breast enlargement in males, with or without tenderness). Use of a low initial dosage in **nonvirilized** men (i.e., those lacking male secondary sex characteristics) mimics the natural increase in serum testosterone concentration during puberty. It produces **virilization** gradually, which minimizes adverse effects of androgens, especially priapism. Gynecomastia is the result of the conversion of testosterone to estradiol (E_2) through peripheral pathways. Men with hepatic cirrhosis are predisposed to gynecomastia.

When administered orally, testosterone undergoes extensive first-pass metabolism in the gastrointestinal tract and liver. To overcome this problem, various testosterone derivatives (e.g., fluoxymesterone and methyltestosterone) have been developed for oral administration. In the past, most men with hypogonadism received biweekly, deep intramuscular injections of testosterone.

Scrotal, transdermal dosage forms overcome some of the drawbacks associated with oral and intramuscular administration. Applying a transdermal testosterone patch to the scrotal skin in the morning provides a serum testosterone concentration that mimics the natural **circadian** (on a 24-hour cycle) secretion of the hormone in young, healthy men. Because scrotal skin is at least five times more permeable than skin at other sites, an inadequate serum testosterone concentration results if a scrotal patch is applied to other areas of the body. To optimize contact, the scrotal skin should be dry-shaved before the patch is applied. Many men prefer scrotal, transdermal formulations to intramuscular testosterone injections because the patch is easy to apply, and the pain and discomfort of the injections can be avoided. Other patients find it embarrassing to explain the transdermal patch to their sex partners. Testosterone patches, like other testosterone dosage forms, are classified as Schedule III-controlled substances because of the abuse potential as an anabolic steroid.

Erectile dysfunction (ED) (failure to initiate or to maintain an erection until ejaculation) may have many causes, including testosterone deficiency, alcoholism, cigarette smoking, psychological factors, and medications. ED may also be referred to as *male impotence* or *male dysfunction*. Table 14.3 lists drugs that may cause ED. Alcohol is a primary reason for ED.

Treatment of Male Hormonal Disorders

Table 14.4 lists common ED medications. The drugs most frequently used to treat ED are the **phosphodiesterase-5 (PDE-5) inhibitors**. In fact, they are usually listed in the top 50 drugs dispensed in pharmacies today. Even though much of the media attention is paid to PDE-5 inhibitors, there are other treatment options for patients to consider. However, the routes of administration for these products are not as convenient as the oral route of PDE-5 inhibitors. One of these alternative treatment options is alprostadil. Considered a second-line choice of therapy for ED, alprostadil is a prostaglandin that works by relaxing smooth muscle in the vasculature of the penis. Alprostadil is injected into the base of the penis or inserted as a pellet into the urethra.

Testosterone (Androderm, AndroGel, Striant, Testoderm) is delivered through transdermal systems or patches. Androderm and AndroGel are applied to a fleshy area of the back, abdomen, upper arm, or thigh, whereas Testoderm is applied to the scrotum. The usual starting dosage for Androderm is two patches applied every evening (approximately every 24 hours). Patients should be cautioned not to use the same site more than once every seven days. The system may be worn while taking a shower or bath. Virilization of a female sex partner is unlikely, because the occlusive outer film prevents the partner from coming in contact with the drug. The application site should be allowed to dry before dressing. Patients should wash their hands with soap and water after handling this drug. AndroGel should be applied once daily, preferably in the morning, to clean, dry, intact skin. Striant, another brand name for testosterone, is a buccal (under the tongue) system. These drugs increase libido and sexual potency within weeks or months and also improve the patient's sense of well-being.

Alprostadil (Caverject, Edex, Muse, Prostin) is available under various brand names to treat ED. Caverject and Edex are penile injections, and Muse (Medicated Urethral System for Erection) is a urethral suppository. Muse comes with a small plastic applicator that inserts a micropellet of alprostadil into the urethra. Muse works quickly, usually within 10 minutes. The side effects are penile pain and urethral burning.

TABLE 14.3 Drugs That May Cause Erectile Dysfunction

Alcohol	H$_2$ blockers
Amphetamines	Haloperidol
Antihypertensives	Lithium
Corticosteroids	Opiates
Estrogens	Some antidepressants

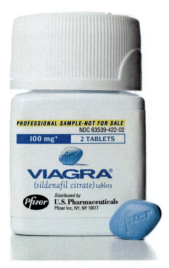

Sildenafil is sold under the brand name Viagra.

 May cause BLURRED VISION

High doses can cause hypotension and dizziness. Muse can also affect the female partner, causing vaginal burning and itching. It should be refrigerated unless it is going to be used within 14 days. Caverject is administered as an injection into the corpora cavernosa on the sides of the penis (hence the name). The manufacturer provides Caverject as a kit that contains six syringes and single-dose vials of freeze-dried powder for reconstitution and administration. The vials should be refrigerated until dispensed, but they may be kept at room temperature for up to three months. In Caverject Impulse, the powder and the water are stored in separate chambers in the prefilled syringe. Turning the plunger before injection mixes the powder and water and dials the specified dose.

PDE-5 inhibitors, have replaced other drugs used for male ED. These drugs produce smooth muscle relaxation and inflow of blood into the penis in response to sexual stimulation. They have many interactions with other drugs, most notably a potentially lethal interaction with nitrates (nitroglycerin, isosorbide dinitrate, and isosorbide mononitrate) used to treat ischemic heart disease, as described in Chapter 12.

Sildenafil (Viagra), enhances the relaxant effect of nitric oxide released in response to sexual stimulation. This allows an erection to occur naturally. It should be taken at least one hour before sexual activity. Pharmacy technicians must watch the interaction profile carefully, because sildenafil has several interactions. Its interaction with nitrates is potentially lethal. Other interactions to watch for are erythromycin and antifungal medications. Sildenafil can cause temporary vision disturbances, headache, and indigestion. It will decrease blood pressure for several hours.

Vardenafil (Levitra) has the same side effect profile as sildenafil, but is often prescribed when sildenafil proves ineffective. Patients should be discouraged from smoking or drinking alcohol for a few hours before sexual activity.

TABLE 14.4 Most Commonly Used Agents for Erectile Dysfunction

Generic (Brand)	Pronunciation	Dosage Form	Dispensing Status	Control Schedule
alprostadil (Caverject, Edex, Muse)	al-PROS-ta-dil	Injection, urethral pellet	Rx	
testosterone (Androderm [nonscrotal], AndroGel, Striant, Testoderm [scrotal])	tes-TOS-te-rone	Cream, injection, ointment, pellet for implant, transdermal patch, transdermal solution	Rx	C-III
Phosphodiesterase-5 Inhibitors				
avanafil (Stendra)	av-AN-a-fil	Tablet	Rx	
sildenafil (Viagra)	sil-DEN-a-fil	Tablet	Rx	
tadalafil (Cialis)	tah-DAL-a-fil	Tablet	Rx	
vardenafil (Levitra)	var-DEN-a-fil	Tablet	Rx	

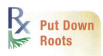
Tadalafil (Cialis) is sometimes called the "weekender" because it is effective for 36 hours. Peak plasma levels of the drug are obtained in two hours. It has a faster onset and longer duration than the other PDE-5 inhibitors. Tadalafil has the same interactions with nitrates and other drugs as sildenafil and vardenafil, but it has a significantly different chemical structure.

Avanafil (Stendra) is the newest PDE-5 inhibitor. It appears to have enhanced PDE-5 selectivity compared to the other PDE-5 inhibitors, a more rapid onset of action, and its absorption is not significantly impacted by food.

Contraindications PDE-5 inhibitors are contraindicated in patients who take nitrates or alpha blockers. The combination of PDE-5 inhibitors and these other medications can cause a dangerous drop in blood pressure. Alprostadil is an alternative when PDE-5 inhibitors are contraindicated. Patients must be appropriately instructed in the preparation and administration of alprostadil.

Cautions and Considerations Patients taking other medications for blood pressure should first discuss the use of PDE-5 inhibitors with their prescribers. Drinking alcohol while taking a PDE-5 inhibitor can worsen these blood pressure effects. Patients may also experience increased heart rate, dizziness, and headache.

Drug Interactions PDE-5 inhibitors interact with several other medications, most notably a potentially lethal interaction with nitrates (nitroglycerin, isosorbide dinitrate, and isosorbide mononitrate) used to treat ischemic heart disease. The patient should be sure that his pharmacist and prescriber know all the medications and over-the-counter (OTC) dietary supplements he takes to avoid any dangerous interactions. You can help by obtaining thorough medication histories for patients who bring in prescriptions for PDE-5 inhibitors.

Female Hormones and Sexual Dysfunction

Exogenously administered female hormones can prevent conception, ease the symptoms of menopause, and help prevent osteoporosis. Two of the most important female hormones are estrogen and progesterone. Estrogen stimulates the development of female secondary sex characteristics and promotes the growth and maintenance of the female reproductive system. Progesterone is responsible for controlling the preparation of the uterus for a fertilized ovum.

Estrogen

Estrogen is a group of hormones that are formed in the ovaries from androgenic precursors. When the hypothalamic-pituitary axis releases FSH to the ovaries, it stimulates estrogen production for 1 to 14 days and progesterone production for 14 to 28 days. As both hormones build up in the bloodstream, a feedback mechanism reduces the activity of the hypothalamus in producing and releasing the gonadotropin-releasing hormone (GnRH).

Estrogen compounds are the growth hormones of reproductive tissue in females. In addition, they share some actions of androgens on the skeleton and other tissues. Estrogen produces endometrial growth, increased cervical mucus, cornification (thickening and maturing) of vaginal mucosa, growth of breast tissue (ducts and fat deposits), increased epiphyseal closure, sodium retention, carbohydrate metabolism, and calcium utilization.

Estrogen is used for contraceptive formulations (discussed at length later in this chapter), relief of menopausal symptoms, reduction of osteoporosis in combination with other drugs (e.g., **bisphosphonates**), gonadal failure, and prostatic cancer. Symptoms of estrogen deficiency include irregular bleeding and irregular menstrual cycles. **Vasomotor** symptoms, which affect the blood vessels, may also appear. Commonly known as hot flashes, vasomotor instability starts in the face and moves down over the body; the severity is related to the rate of estrogen decline. Other symptoms of estrogen deficiency may include atrophic vulvovaginitis, characterized by excessive vaginal dryness; **dyspareunia** (painful intercourse); and infections (due to a dryness-related reduction in the number of lactobacilli that produce protective acids). Estrogen depletion also leads to a reduction in the amount of glycogen to be metabolized, an increase in pH of the vaginal area, and loss of lubrication, causing urethral and bladder atrophy. **Hormone therapy (HT)** relieves the symptoms of estrogen deficiency.

The rate of estrogen production declines with the onset of menopause, which is defined as the cessation of menses for one year; it is accompanied by a change in the site, amount, and pattern of estrogen production. The **climacteric** (the syndrome of endocrine, somatic, and psychological changes that occur at the end of the female reproductive period) is characterized by gradual loss of ovarian function and irregular bleeding before the termination of menses. With decreased estrogen production at menopause, estrogen-responsive tissues atrophy. Menopausal symptoms may include vasomotor instability (hot flashes), drying and atrophy of the vaginal mucosa, insomnia, irritability, and other mood changes, including a certain amount of depression.

As ovarian function declines with age, androstenedione, produced in the adrenal cortex, becomes the primary source of estrogen, and estrone becomes the dominant circulating estrogen. Because the naturally occurring concentration of androstenedione and the efficiency of its conversion may vary considerably among women, HT is often provided to ease the transition into menopause. A small amount of estrogen continues to be produced through the metabolism of adrenal steroids to estradiol in peripheral fat tissue. Depending on body fat, some women may not need estrogen replacement. Estrogen is also effective in preventing bone loss, lowering cholesterol levels, and improving the color and turgor of skin. Table 14.5 lists more information about estrogens.

Progestins

Progestins are a group of synthetic forms of **progesterone**. Both progesterone and estrogen prevent ovulation. Progesterone achieves this by inhibiting the secretion of LH, whereas estrogen suppresses the secretion of FSH, thereby blocking follicular development and ovulation.

Progestin is used primarily in oral contraceptive pills and to prevent uterine cancer in postmenopausal women who take hormone replacement therapy. Types of progestin include levonorgestrel, medroxyprogesterone, norethindrone, and norgestimate. Generally, progestin is offered in combination with estrogen. Another important use is to treat menstrual dysfunction, such as irregular cycles, protracted uterine bleeding, dysmenorrhea, amenorrhea, and endometriosis. It is believed that poorly cycling estrogens may promote enlargement of the **endometrium** (the inner membrane of the uterus). Treatment with a progestin lowers the incidence of endometrial enlargement. Progestin alone does not promote menstrual bleeding, but in patients who either have endogenous estrogen or are treated first with estrogen, cyclic treatment with progestin helps to restore normal cycling. Table 14.5 lists the most commonly used types of progestin.

Hormone Therapy

Table 14.5 presents the most commonly used supplements for hormone therapy for the symptoms of menopause. It is important for the technician to know that, even if these medications have the exact same ingredients, they cannot be interchanged. The doses will differ slightly in each.

Patients taking any form of estrogen, whether it is in contraceptives or hormone therapy, should be aware that smoking is associated with greater morbidity, especially in patients over 35 years of age. Estrogen therapy and smoking increase the risk of blood clots, which increases the risk of deep vein thrombosis (discussed in Chapter 12).

Research is continually revealing new information about hormone therapy's risks and benefits. Some studies recommend that it be used only to manage the vasomotor symptoms of menopause and that use should be limited to the shortest duration possible. Hormone therapy is also associated with some risk of breast cancer. For this reason, some practitioners do not prescribe estrogen to patients who have had breast cancer or who have a family history of breast cancer. Depending on the patient, the benefits of HT in reducing the symptoms of menopause and especially decreasing bone loss may outweigh the risk of breast cancer.

TABLE 14.5   Most Commonly Used Progestin and Estrogen Supplements

Generic (Brand)	Pronunciation	Dosage Form	Dispensing Status
Estrogen Only			
conjugated estrogen (Cenestin, Enjuvia, Premarin)	CON-ju-gate-ed ES-troe-jen	Cream, injection, tablet	Rx
estradiol (Alora, Climara, Divigel, Elestrin, Estrogel, Estring, Evamist, Femring, Menostar, Minivelle, Vagifem, Vivelle-Dot)	es-tra-DYE-awl	Cream, emulsion, gel, injection, patch, tablet, transdermal solution, vaginal ring	Rx
Progestin Only			
progesterone (Crinone, Endometrin, First-Progesterone, Prometrium)	pro-JES-te-rone	Capsule, cream, gel, injection, vaginal suppository	Rx
Estrogen-Progestin			
conjugated estrogen-medroxyprogesterone (Premphase, Prempro)	CON-ju-gate-ed ES-troe-jen me-DROX-ee-pro-JES-te-rone	Tablet	Rx
estradiol-drospirenone (Angeliq)	es-tra-DYE-awl droe-SPY-re-nown	Tablet	Rx
estradiol-levonorgestrel (Climara Pro)	es-tra-DYE-awl lee-voe-nor-JES-trel	Patch	Rx
estradiol-norethindrone (Activella, CombiPatch)	es-tra-DYE-awl nor-eth-IN-drone	Patch, tablet	Rx
estradiol-norgestimate (Prefest)	es-tra-DYE-awl nor-JES-ti-mate	Tablet	Rx
ethinyl estradiol-norethindrone (femhrt)	ETH-in-il es-tra-DYE-awl nor-eth-IN-drone	Tablet	Rx

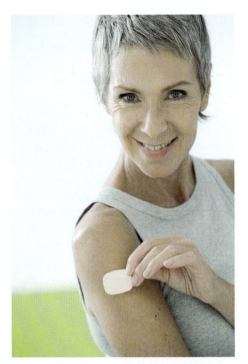

Hormone therapy can be administered via different dosage forms. Patches, as pictured, are one such dosage form.

Whether or not to use HT is a decision for a woman and her physician. The advantages and disadvantages will be different for each woman depending on her family history and her physical condition. If a woman who has been on HT for a long time chooses not to continue, however, hormones should be tapered off.

Estrogen-Only Hormone Therapy Products

Conjugated estrogens (Premarin) are estrogens of equine origin. In fact the brand name comes from the source which is pregnant mares' urine.

Estradiol (Alora, Climara, Divigel, Elestrin, Estrogel, Estring, Evamist, Femring, Menostar, Minivelle, Vagifem, Vivelle-Dot) is bioidentical to human hormones. It is produced in many shapes and forms, none of which are interchangeable. Topical estrogen may be safer than pills because it avoids first pass metabolism through the liver. Vivelle-Dot, a small patch, is placed on the abdomen for three and a half days. Elestrin is a gel that is contained in a pump and should be applied over the entire upper arm and shoulder area.

Estring and Femring contain the medication in a ring that is inserted in the vagina. The ring releases an initial burst of estradiol, followed by a tapered, low dose for a 90-day period. Insertion of the ring is similar to using a diaphragm. If removed, the ring should be rinsed in lukewarm water before reinsertion. This drug relieves symptoms of weak pelvic muscles without releasing significant systemic concentrations of estradiol. Therefore, it is not used for vasomotor symptoms or for the prevention of osteoporosis. If the patient has an intact uterus, she will also need a progestin product so as to prevent endometrial hyperplasia.

Evamist is a topical estrogen spray in a metered-dose pump. The initial dose is one spray per day, which is titrated to relief of symptoms not to exceed two or three sprays. It is applied to the inside of the forearm at the same time each day. The spray should be allowed to dry for a few minutes. Sunscreen should be applied before the spray; if applied after, it decreases the effectiveness of the spray.

Common side effects of estrogen hormone therapy include dizziness, abdominal pain or bloating, diarrhea, nausea, headache, breast tenderness, vaginal discharge, fluid retention, hair loss, and depression. The other effects may subside with continued therapy. Sometimes, hormone replacement therapy can cause dark skin patches on the face, called **melasma**. Patients should inform their prescribers about these effects so that necessary dose changes can be made. Some women find that specialty and extemporaneous, compounded forms of estrogen, with or without progesterone, produce fewer side effects.

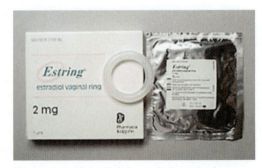

Estrogen can be administered via vaginal rings, such as the product pictured.

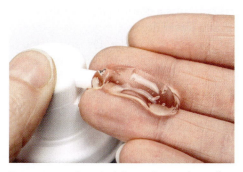
Estrogen can be administered transdermally. The product pictured is a gel that is applied topically.

Contraindications Contraindications to estrogens include known or suspected history of breast cancer; estrogen-dependent malignancy; undiagnosed abnormal genital bleeding; active deep vein thrombosis, pulmonary embolism (PE), or a history of these conditions; active arterial thromboembolic disease or a history of these conditions; liver impairment or disease; and pregnancy.

Cautions and Considerations Estrogen-only hormone replacement has several boxed warnings. They may increase the risk of endometrial cancer in women with an intact uterus using these products. Estrogen-only therapy is also associated with cardiovascular disorders and dementia.

Drug Interactions Estrogen derivatives may diminish the therapeutic effect of anastrozole, anticoagulants, and somatotropin. Estrogen may decrease the serum concentration of simeprevir.

Progestin Hormone Therapy Products

Progesterone (Crinone, Endometrin, First-Progesterone, Prometrium) is used for amenorrhea (absence of menstruation) and for the prevention of endometrial hyperplasia in women with an intact uterus using estrogen therapy. Progesterone products come in a wide variety of dosage forms to suit patient needs. Headache, dizziness, and depression are commonly reported side effects.

Contraindications Contraindications to progesterone include undiagnosed abnormal vaginal bleeding; active deep vein thrombosis, PE, or a history of these conditions; active or history of arterial thromboembolic disease; history of or suspected malignancy of the breast or genitals; liver dysfunction or disease; ectopic pregnancy; and pregnancy.

Cautions and Considerations Progesterone has several black box warnings. There is a warning about the increased risk of breast cancer and a second warning regarding the risk of dementia. A third black box warning indicates HT should be used for the shortest duration at the lowest effective dose possible.

Drug Interactions Progesterone may diminish the therapeutic effects of anticoagulants and diabetes agents. Colchicine, doxorubicin, pazopanib, rivaroxaban, silodosin, topotecan, and vincristine concentrations may be increased by progesterone. Ulipristal may diminish the effects of progesterone.

Estrogen-Progestin Hormone Therapy Products

Combination therapy with an estrogen product and a progestin is used if a patient has an intact uterus. In the normal cycle, high levels of estrogen before ovulation cause cells in the uterine lining to multiply. Estrogen can cause the same effect when given for HT, leading to endometrial hyperplasia, which may progress to uterine cancer. A progestin counteracts these effects. Therefore, women with an intact uterus should receive both an estrogen and a progestin. If progestin therapy can be avoided, however, the risk of side effects from HT medication decreases tremendously.

Conjugated estrogen-medroxyprogesterone (Premphase, Prempro) contains the same estrogens as Premarin with the addition of a progestin. Each Prempro tablet contains both estrogen and progestin. The contents of Premphase depends on the day of therapy. The first 14 days contain estrogen only (tablets are maroon) and the subsequent 14 tablets contain both estrogen and progestin (tablets are blue).

Ethinyl estradiol–norethindrone (femhrt) contains a combination of hormones commonly used in oral contraceptives, but at a lower dosage.

Estradiol-drospirenone (Angeliq) is available in an oral tablet. Drospirenone is a progestin with antiandrogen activity. For this reason, estradiol-drospirenone may result in decreased acne.

Estradiol-levonorgestrel (Climara Pro) is provided by the manufacturer as a patch. It may decrease the intensity and number of hot flashes, night sweats, and vaginal dryness associated with menopause. The patch is stored at room temperature and is applied once weekly.

Estradiol-norethindrone (CombiPatch) is a matrix transdermal in which the drugs are incorporated within the adhesive matrix layer and released continuously. The patch should be applied twice weekly to a smooth, fold-free area of dry skin on the abdomen and should be worn continuously. It should be stored in the refrigerator before dispensing. **Estradiol-norethindrone (Activella)** is the tablet form of this drug combination. Activella is indicated for symptoms of menopause, vulvar atrophy, and the prevention of osteoporosis. It also decreases total cholesterol but at the expense of decreased high density lipoprotein (HDL) levels. It is derived from soy and a synthetic progestin. Activella is used to control moderate-to-severe vasomotor symptoms of menopause.

Contraindications Contraindications to estrogen-progestin products include unusual genital bleeding; history of breast cancer; known or suspected estrogen-dependent tumor; active thrombosis; liver impairment or disease; known or suspected pregnancy; and kidney insufficiency.

Cautions and Considerations Estrogen plus progestin therapy is associated with cardiovascular disease and dementia. Breast cancer risk may be increased in patients using these products.

Drug Interactions Estrogen derivatives may diminish the therapeutic effect of anastrozole, anticoagulants, and somatotropin. Estrogen may decrease the serum concentration of simeprevir.

Progesterone-containing agents may diminish the therapeutic effects of anticoagulants and diabetes agents. Colchicine, doxorubicin, pazopanib, rivaroxaban, silodosin, topotecan, and vincristine concentrations may be increased by progesterone-containing products. Ulipristal may diminish the effects of progesterone-containing products.

Female Sexual Dysfunction

Female sexual dysfunction is marked by persistent, recurrent problems with sexual response. Many women experience sexual dysfunction at some point in their lives. Female sexual dysfunction can take different forms, including decreased desire, reduced arousal, anorgasmia (or inability to achieve orgasm), and pain.

Treatment should be directed at the causes of sexual dysfunction, which are often multifactorial. Nonpharmacological options such as counseling, lifestyle changes, and the use of vaginal lubricants and moisturizers may provide relief. Androgen therapy (discussed previously) and antidepressants (see Chapter 7) may also improve sexual function.

Drug Treatment for Female Sexual Dysfunction

There is only one FDA-approved drug used to treat female sexual dysfunction in premenopausal women, **flibanserin (Addyi)**. Flibanserin works by modulating the neurotransmitters serotonin, dopamine, and norepinephrine and has been shown to increase sexual desire. Like other drugs that effect neurotransmitters, it may take six to eight weeks before improvement is noticed. Flibanserin is available as a 100-mg tablet that is taken once a day before sleep to mitigate certain side effects. The most serious side effects of flibanserin are hypotension and fainting. Other common effects associated with flibanserin include fatigue, dizziness, headache, nausea, and sedation.

Contraindications Contraindications to flibanserin include concomitant alcohol use, liver impairment, and concomitant use of drugs that strongly inhibit its metabolism.

Cautions and Considerations Flibanserin has black box warnings for increased risk of severe hypotension and loss of consciousness in patients with liver impairment and those using alcohol concurrently. Due to these adverse effects, flibanserin has an FDA-required Risk Evaluation and Mitigation Strategy program for prescribers and pharmacies.

CNS depression may result from flibanserin. Patients should be cautioned about performing tasks that require them to be mentally alert.

Little is known about adverse effects on women who take flibanserin while pregnant or breastfeeding, and is not recommended to treat these populations.

Drug Interactions Flibanserin has multiple drug interactions. The following drugs should not be used with flibanserin: alcohol, azelastine, bosutinib, conivaptan, fusidic acid, idelalisib, orphenadrine, paraldehyde, pazopanib, silodosin, thalidomide, topotecan, and vincristine.

Hormones in Gender Reassignment

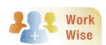

Work Wise

Those seeking hormone therapy for gender reassignment sometimes self-medicate for fear of rejection by healthcare providers and the cost of treatment. Maintaining a professional and nonjudgmental work environment helps all your patients feel comfortable seeking care.

Transgender people experience a gender identity that is inconsistent with their somatic sexual differentiation. Gender identity is a complex psychological concept, but it may be outwardly marked by expressions through clothing, hairstyle, or manner. A transgender person may desire to permanently transition to the gender they identify with, through a process called **gender reassignment**. Those who choose to go through this process are **transsexual**. Gender reassignment can include hormonal, anatomical, and psychosocial change. Following psychological counseling, patients may also eventually choose surgical means of gender reassignment. Generally, hormone therapy is a precursor to that final step. Hormone therapy in gender reassignment usually has two main goals. The first is to suppress the hormones of the individual's natal sex. The second is to introduce characteristics of the reassigned sex.

Female-to-male (FTM) gender reassignment involves terminating menstruation and inducing the development of a traditionally male appearance. Testosterone is traditionally used, either through injections; transdermal patches, creams, or gels; subcutaneous pellets; or sublingual lozenges. Using testosterone typically produces oily skin, facial and body hair growth, balding, increased muscle mass, redistribution of body fat, loss of menses, enlargement of the clitoris, vaginal atrophy, and a deepened voice. Side effects include polycythemia (the production of too many red blood cells), weight gain, acne, and sleep apnea. These hormones may also lead to elevated liver enzymes and high blood cholesterol levels. The transdermal treatments can cause skin irritation, and women who are pregnant should not come in contact with patients receiving such treatments. The lozenges may cause gum irritation, taste changes, and headaches, which usually diminish after a few weeks.

Male-to-female (MTF) transgender patients usually require reduction in the effects of androgens. This may be achieved by the use of estrogen, progesterone, progestins, and antiandrogens. Use of these hormones may result in changes in body fat distribution, decreased muscle mass, softening of the skin and decreased oiliness, declines in libido and erections, breast growth, shrinking of the testes and decreased sperm production, thinning and slowed growth of facial and body hair, and male pattern baldness. Side effects include venous thromboembolic disease, gallstones, elevated liver enzymes, weight gain, hypertriglyceridemia (high levels of triglycerides in the blood), cardiovascular disease, and hypertension.

Contraception, Pregnancy, and Childbirth

Pharmacology plays an important role in family planning today. Medications can factor into women's decisions to have or not have children, help them successfully carry a child to term, and even ease the pain of childbirth.

Contraception

Contraception is any practice that serves to prevent pregnancy during sexual activity. These practices can be either nonpharmacologic or pharmacologic. Contraceptive methods that are nonpharmacologic include abstinence and natural birth control. Contraceptive methods that are pharmacologic include oral contraceptives; various barrier products, such as male and female condoms; transdermal and vaginal contraceptives; and various injections, implants, and intrauterine devices. Because of the pharmacology foundation of this textbook, the pharmacologic methods of contraception are discussed in depth in this section.

Choosing a method of contraception is a personal decision, and individuals must consider several factors, including rates of effectiveness, ease of use, and adherence requirements. Patients should understand that rates of effectiveness for preventing pregnancy reported in product labeling refer to "perfect use." These rates are only achieved when the patient follows instructions exactly. If a product is difficult to use or undesirable for a particular patient, adherence and effectiveness of the product will not be ideal. Perfect use is not representative of actual use in many cases, and all products have some failures, even if such failures are rare.

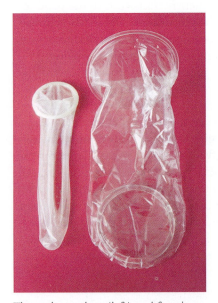

The male condom (left) and female condom (right) are barrier methods of contraception. Both devices are OTC products that prevent sperm from entering a woman's vagina.

Contraceptive Products for the Male Reproductive System

Contraceptive products on the market that work for the male reproductive system generally use physical barriers that prevent sperm and ova from coming into contact. Drug therapy that alters sperm production and thus affects male fertility has been researched, but no effective products have yet been brought to market.

Barrier Products

Barrier birth control products are used when intercourse is anticipated. These products form a physical barrier that prevents sperm from entering the uterus through the cervix. To be effective, the products are put in place prior to intercourse, left there for a specific amount of time, and then removed.

The **male condom** is placed over the erect penis before entering the vagina. Condoms collect the ejaculate (semen and sperm) and prevent it from coming into contact with the vagina or cervix. Ejaculate material is removed along with the condom. Condoms are the only birth control method that also prevent or lower the risk of transmission of sexually transmitted infections (STIs), also referred to as sexually transmitted diseases (STDs). Latex and polyurethane condoms provide the best protection because they are impermeable. Other than latex allergy and skin irritation, no apparent side effects are typically associated with condom use.

Contraindications Latex allergy is a contraindication to latex condom use. Men and women who have a latex allergy should use polyurethane condoms.

Cautions and Considerations Getting the proper fit, keeping the condom on during the entire sexual activity, and maintaining an erection while wearing a condom have been reported as problems that decrease the ease of use and effectiveness of condoms. Concurrent use of male and female condoms is not recommended because friction between the condoms can cause them to break.

Water-based lubricants such as K-Y Jelly and Astroglide can be used with latex condoms. However, oil-based lubricants can can cause the condom to break and are not recommended for use with condoms. Some other vaginal products and medications can contain oil-based ingredients such as butoconazole and mineral oil. Therefore, patients using these therapies should abstain from intercourse or use polyurethane condoms until this therapy is completed.

Contraceptive Products for the Female Reproductive System

Contraceptive products on the market today that affect the female reproductive system generally apply one or more of the following contraception approaches:

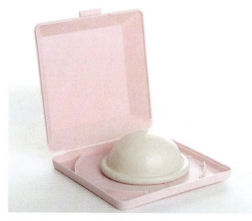

A diaphragm, as pictured, is a barrier device that fits over the cervix.

- physical or pharmacologic barriers that prevent sperm and ova from coming into contact
- drug therapy that prevents ovulation from occurring
- drug therapy that prevents implantation of a fertilized ovum in the uterus

As mentioned earlier, patients should understand that rates of effectiveness for contraception methods are only achieved when the patient follows instructions exactly. However, there are circumstances that may hinder the effectiveness of certain contraceptive products, despite perfect adherence by the patient. For example, specific drugs and conditions may adversely affect the efficacy of the oral contraceptive pill.

Barrier Products

As mentioned earlier, barrier birth control products are used when intercourse is anticipated. These products form a physical barrier that prevents sperm from entering the uterus through the cervix. To be effective, the products are put in place prior to intercourse, left there for a specific period, and then removed. Barrier products do not alter normal ovulation, cervical mucus, or endometrial lining formation.

The **female condom** is worn by a woman and forms a physical barrier between the penis and the vagina. The female condom is made of nitrile material instead of latex, and it is inserted up to eight hours before sexual activity. When used properly, the condom holding the ejaculate material is removed after intercourse. As mentioned earlier, condoms are the only contraception method that also prevent or lower the risk of STI transmission. Few if any side effects are typically associated with the use of female condoms.

The **diaphragm** and the **cervical cap** are made of rubber, latex, or silicone and are bordered by a rounded ring that fits over the cervix inside the vagina. They form a barrier that covers the cervical opening and prevents sperm from entering the uterus and traveling to the fallopian tubes. A diaphragm is larger than a cervical cap and covers a larger area over the cervix. These products work best when used with a **spermicide** that kills sperm cells on contact. Diaphragms and cervical caps are prescription items that must be fitted or sized to a woman's internal anatomy by her prescriber. They are self-inserted prior to sexual intercourse and left in place for at least six hours after sexual intercourse. Some women experience more frequent urinary tract infections when using diaphragms or cervical caps. This effect is thought to be related to changes in the normal vaginal flora from exposure to the spermicide that is used along with these devices. Use of a diaphragm without a spermicide, however, will diminish its effectiveness at preventing pregnancy. Therefore, to reduce the incidence of urinary tract infections, it is recommended that women urinate before insertion of these devices and right after intercourse.

Diaphragms and cervical caps used with spermicide may cause irritation, burning, or itching of mucous membranes. If irritation, burning, or rash from the spermicide continues, an alternative form of contraceptive should be considered.

Contraindications The female condom is not contraindicated in any specific patient population. This type of condom can be used as an alternative barrier method when one of the partners has a latex allergy.

The diaphragm should not be used by women who have an allergy to latex or spermicide, frequent urinary tract infections, or a history of toxic shock syndrome. Some anatomic differences (such as uterine prolapse) can make it difficult to get a proper fit for a diaphragm and preclude some patients from being able to use one. Diaphragms and cervical caps that include spermicide contain the ingredient nonoxynol-9. Patients with hypersensitivity to nonoxynol-9 should avoid products with spermicide.

Cautions and Considerations To ensure effectiveness of a female condom, partners must be sure that the penis does not slip between the vagina and the outer surface of the condom or that the outer ring does not get pushed inside of the vagina. Although the female condom can be removed at any time after intercourse, it is most effective when removed before the woman stands up to avoid spilling semen. To remove the condom, the outer ring is twisted to seal it and then pulled out.

As mentioned earlier, patients should also be aware that concurrent use of male and female condoms is not recommended, as friction between the condoms can cause them to break. Finally, patients should understand that the female condom is more expensive than the male condom and has a slightly lower rate of effectiveness at preventing pregnancy.

Diaphragms and cervical caps do not protect against transmission of STIs. These contraceptives are meant to be reused, but they must be thoroughly cleaned with mild soap and water and properly stored after each use. In addition, women should be refitted for a diaphragm or cervical cap after pregnancy, miscarriage, abortion, pelvic surgery, or significant weight loss or gain because the shape of the uterus and vagina changes.

Oral Contraceptives

Pharmacologic contraception involves manipulating hormones to prevent ovulation and change the texture of cervical mucus. These drugs contain ethinyl estradiol, a synthetic estrogen, and/or one of several synthetic progestins. **Oral contraceptives (OCs)** that contain synthetic estrogens work by suppressing production of LH, the hormone that triggers ovulation. OCs that contain progestins suppress LH production and thicken cervical mucus, making movement difficult for sperm.

Typically, OCs are among the most frequently prescribed pharmaceutical agents in the United States. For these products to be optimally effective with the lowest frequency of side effects, patients should be well-informed as to their proper use.

OCs are taken daily at the same time to maintain a steady and elevated hormone level. Depending on the product chosen, patients begin therapy on the first day of their menstrual flow, the first Sunday after their menstrual flow, or whenever desired. In any case, backup contraception, such as a barrier method, must be used to prevent pregnancy for at least the first seven days of therapy, if not for the entire first cycle.

There are several OC products on the market. No matter the brand, all OC products have special packaging and dispensing regulations. These regulations state that all patients, upon receipt of their prescriptions, must receive a patient information leaflet that has been approved by the FDA.

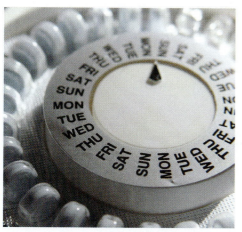

A variety of birth control pills are available.

Commonly Prescribed Oral Contraceptives

OCs contain either a combination of estrogen and progestin or progestins only (see Table 14.6). Combination OCs come in monophasic, biphasic, and triphasic dosing regimens. Monophasic regimens contain the same dose throughout the cycle, whereas biphasic and triphasic regimens increase the dosage once or twice during a menstrual cycle. The color of the tablet usually changes as the dose changes.

New approaches to oral contraception have brought about extended oral regimens. Such products involve taking a steady dose for 84 days before allowing a hormone-free week during which menstruation occurs. In effect, patients experience bleeding only once every three or four months. Although concern about endometrial thickening exists, such a regimen works well for patients who have menstrual cycle–related migraines, severe premenstrual symptoms, endometriosis, or polycystic ovarian syndrome (PCOS). Prescribers occasionally order a similar extended regimen of monophasic oral contraceptives.

Common side effects of OCs include weight gain, nausea, vomiting, bloating, increased appetite, fatigue, breast tenderness or enlargement, headaches, and edema (fluid retention). These effects tend to subside with continued use but can be a reason to stop or change therapy if bothersome. Patients should discuss these effects with their prescribers. Breakthrough bleeding (blood flow in the middle of a menstrual cycle) can occur, especially at the start of therapy. If it continues, the patient should talk with her prescriber. An increase in blood pressure can occur in the first few months of OC therapy. Patients with high blood pressure should be encouraged to use other methods of contraception, if possible. The most serious adverse effect of OCs is the development of cardiovascular complications, such as heart attack, stroke, or other forms of thromboembolic disease.

TABLE 14.6   Most Commonly Used Contraceptive Agents

Generic (Brand)	Pronunciation	Dosage Form	Dispensing Status
Combination Oral Contraceptives			
ethinyl estradiol-desogestrel (Apri, Azurette, Caziant, Cyclessa, Desogen, Emoquette, Enskyce, Kariva, Mircette, Ortho-Cept, Reclipsen, Solia, Velivet, Viorele)	ETH-in-il es-tra-DYE-awl des-oh-JES-trel	Tablet	Rx
ethinyl estradiol-drospirenone (Beyaz, Gianvi, Loryna, Nikki, Ocella, Syeda, Vestura, Yasmin, Yaz, Zarah)	ETH-in-il es-tra-DYE-awl droh-SPYE-re-none	Tablet	Rx
ethinyl estradiol-ethynodiol diacetate (Kelnor, Zovia)	ETH-in-il es-tra-DYE-awl e-thye-noe-DYE-awl dye-AS-e-tate	Tablet	Rx
ethinyl estradiol-levonorgestrel (Traditional: Altavera, Amethyst, Aviane, Enpresse, Falmina, Lessina, Levora, Lutera, Lybrel, Marlissa, Myzilra, Orsythia, Portia, Trivora; Extended combinations: Amethia, Camrese, Introvale, Jolessa, Quasense, Quartette, Seasonique)	ETH-in-il es-tra-DYE-awl LEE-voe-nor-jes-trel	Tablet	Rx
ethinyl estradiol-norethindrone (Alyacen, Aranelle, Brevicon, Cyclafem, Dasetta, Estrostep, femhrt, Leena, Junel, Loestrin, Lo Minastrin, Microgestin, Necon, Norinyl, Nortrel, Ortho-Novum, Ovcon, Tilia, Tri-Legest, Tri-Norinyl)	ETH-in-il es-tra-DYE-awl nor-ETH-in-drone	Tablet	Rx
ethinyl estradiol-norgestimate (MonoNessa, Ortho-Cyclen, Ortho Tri-Cyclen, Ortho Tri-Cyclen Lo, Previfem, Sprintec, TriNessa, Tri-Previfem, Tri-Sprintec)	ETH-in-il es-tra-DYE-awl nor-JES-ti-mate	Tablet	Rx
ethinyl estradiol-norgestrel (Cryselle 28, Elinest, Low-Ogestrel, Norgestrel, Ogestrel, Ovral)	ETH-in-il es-tra-DYE-awl nor-JES-trel	Tablet	Rx
Progestin-Only Contraceptives			
norethindrone (Camila, Errin, Heather, Jolivette, Lyza, Micronor, Nora-Be, Nor-QD)	nor-ETH-in-drone	Tablet	Rx
Emergency Contraceptives			
levonorgestrel (Plan B, Plan B One-Step, Next Choice, Next Choice One Dose, Take Action)	LEE-voe-nor-jes-trel	Tablet	OTC or Rx
ulipristal (ella)	yoo-li-PRISS-tal	Tablet	OTC or Rx
Other Hormonal Contraceptives			
ethinyl estradiol-etonogestrel (NuvaRing)	ETH-in-il es-tra-DYE-awle ee-toe-noe-JES-trel	Vaginal ring	Rx
ethinyl estradiol-norelgestromin (Ortho Evra)	ETH-in-il es-tra-DYE-awl nor-el-JES-troe-min	Patch	Rx

Ethinyl estradiol-desogestrel (Apri, Azurette, Caziant, Cyclessa, Desogen, Emoquette, Enskyce, Kariva, Mircette, Orth-Cept, Reclipsen, Solia, Velivet, Viorele) contains a type of progestin classified as third generation. Third-generation progestins are thought to have less androgen activity.

Ethinyl estradiol-drospirenone (Beyaz, Gianvi, Loryna, Nikki, Ocella, Syeda, Vestura, Yasmin, Yaz, Zarah) contains a progestin that is known as a spironolactone analog. Drospirenone has mineralocorticoid activity as well as progestin activity, so it works as a potassium-sparing diuretic, thereby potentially reducing the risk of sodium and fluid retention and weight gain.

Ethinyl estradiol-ethynodiol diacetate (Kelnor, Zovia) contains a first generation progestin. Ethynodiol diacetate may exhibit estrogen-like activity.

Ethinyl estradiol-levonorgestrel (Altavera, Amethyst, Aviane, Enpresse, Falmina, Lessina, Levora, Lutera, Lybrel, Marlissa, Myzilra, Nordette, Orsythia, Portia, Trivora, Amethia, Camrese, Introvale, Jolessa, Quasense, Quartette, Seasonique) contains a second-generation progestin. Levonorgestrel has androgen-like properties. This may result in adverse effects such as lowering high density lipoprotein concentrations.

Ethinyl estradiol-norethindrone (Alyacen, Aranelle, Brevicon, Cyclafem, Dasetta, Estrostep, Femhrt, Leena, Junel, Loestrin, Lo Minastrin, Microgestin, Necon, Norinyl, Nortrel, Ortho-Novum, Ovcon, Tilia, Tri-Legest, Tri-Norinyl) contains a first-generation progestin and is a commonly prescribed OC.

Norethindrone (Camila, Errin, Heather, Jolivette, Lyza, Micronor, Nora-Be, Nor-QD) is a progestin-only contraceptive. This means it does not contain an estrogen component. Progestins act to prevent pregnancy by inhibiting the secretion of LH, which causes egg release; causing thickening of the cervical mucus to impede the entry of sperm; and altering the uterine lining to prevent implantation of a fertilized egg. Therefore, progestins can be used as contraceptives by themselves without additional estrogens.

Contraindications Patients with clotting disorders should not take OCs because these agents can increase the formation of blood clots. Blood clots, depending on their location and severity, may be fatal. Patients who have disorders that affect potassium levels, such as kidney disease, liver dysfunction, or adrenal insufficiency, should not take ethinyl estradiol-drosperinone. Patients with heart or cerebrovascular disease should not take OCs. Drospirenone has actions similar to the diuretic spironolactone and can adversely affect potassium levels.

Cautions and Considerations Patients with a history of breast, endometrial, ovarian, or cervical cancer should discuss the risks and benefits of OCs with their healthcare practitioners. Some controversy exists about whether OCs increase a woman's risk of cancer in these organs, so patients should make informed decisions about their own care.

The advantage of products containing only progestin is that the lower hormone dose reduces side effects, such as headaches and elevated blood pressure. These products are commonly used in patients for whom OCs are typically not appropriate (i.e., women who have high blood pressure or heart disease, women older than 35 years, and women with blood clotting disorders, especially those who smoke). Smoking in conjunction with hormone therapy increases the risk of heart attack, blood clots, and stroke.

The disadvantage of products containing only progestin is that missed doses affect failure rate more quickly than contraceptives containing estrogen. If a dose of a progestin-only pill is missed by more than three hours, the patient should take it as soon as she remembers and use a backup birth control method, such as condoms, for at least 48 hours.

Technicians should remind patients that oral contraceptives do not prevent transmission of STIs. To avoid transmission, patients must use a barrier method.

Drug Interactions Other medications, herbal preparations, and supplements can interact with oral contraceptives and reduce their effectiveness. Table 14.7 describes various drug interactions. Patients may need to use additional or alternative methods of contraception to prevent pregnancy while taking interacting medications.

TABLE 14.7 Oral Contraceptive Interactions

Class	Drug(s)	Type of Interaction
Antibiotics	erythromycin, griseofulvin, penicillins, rifampin, tetracyclines	May decrease OC effectiveness; interfere with enterohepatic cycling and recycling of estrogen, which can cause a fluctuation in hormone levels
Anticonvulsants	carbamazepine, felbamate, phenobarbital, phenytoin, primidone	Decrease OC action through increased metabolism of hormones
Antifungals	fluconazole, itraconazole, ketoconazole	May decrease OC action (see *antibiotics*)
Benzodiazepines	alprazolam, chlordiazepoxide, diazepam, flurazepam, triazolam	Metabolism of benzodiazepines that undergo oxidation may be decreased, increasing central nervous system (CNS) effects
Bronchodilators	theophylline	Theophylline metabolism may be decreased, increasing side effects
Corticosteroids	hydrocortisone, methylprednisolone, prednisolone, prednisone	Effects may be increased owing to inhibition of metabolism by OC
Lipid-lowering agents	clofibrate	Metabolism of clofibrate may be increased, decreasing OC effect
Tricyclic antidepressants (TCAs)	amitriptyline, imipramine	TCA metabolism may be decreased, increasing the side effects

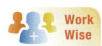

Work Wise

Emergency contraceptives may be colloquially referred to as the "morning-after pill."

Emergency Contraceptives

In the event of unprotected sex, administration of an **emergency contraceptive** may prevent pregnancy if medications are taken quickly, up to 120 hours after unprotected sex. These medications cannot interfere with a pregnancy after implantation; that is why timing is so important. Emergency contraception is not intended to be used as a primary method of contraception.

There are different options for emergency contraception. Products containing levonorgestrel, ulipristal, and estradiol plus levonorgestrel are used. Levonorgestrel products include Plan B, Plan B One-Step, Next Choice, Next Choice One Dose, and Take Action. One-pill products including Plan B One-Step, Next Choice One Dose, and Take Action are OTC products with no age restrictions for purchase. Ulipristal (ella) is available by prescription only. Two-pill products such as Plan B and Next Choice are available by prescription. Estradiol plus levonorgestrel is not sold in a form specific to emergency contraception. This method uses commercially available oral contraceptives at increased doses.

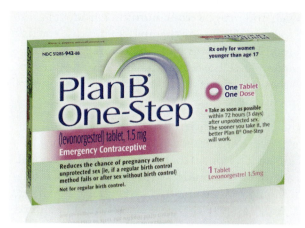

PlanB One-Step is an example of emergency contraception.

Nausea and vomiting are the most common side effects of emergency contraceptives. Antiemetic medication (meclizine or metoclopramide) can be given prior to the emergency contraceptive to reduce these side effects. If a patient vomits within three hours of taking emergency contraception, the medication should be taken again along with an antiemetic medication to reach its full effectiveness. Headache, dizziness, and abdominal pain are also possible.

Contraindications Levonorgestrel and ulipristal are contraindicated in pregnant women. There are no other contraindications for the use of emergency contraception. Even conditions that would typically make long-term oral contraception use dangerous (clotting disorders and cardiovascular or liver disease) are not contraindicated in the short-term use of emergency contraception.

Cautions and Considerations Some medications that affect liver function can alter the effectiveness of emergency contraception. These medications may include antiseizure and antiretroviral (human immunodeficiency virus [HIV]) agents.

Drug Interactions Oral contraceptive drug interactions can be found in Table 14.7, and they refer to emergency contraceptives as well.

Ulipristal levels may be decreased by barbiturates, bosentan, efavirenz, felbamate, griseofulvin, oxcarbazepine, St. John's wort, and topiramate.

Other Hormonal Contraceptives

Hormonal contraceptives may be administered by routes other than oral. For example, transdermal contraceptives deliver the drug systemically through the skin and vaginal contraceptives deliver the drug locally in the vagina. They provide alternatives for patients who do not want or cannot remember to take a daily oral medication. Patients who experience unwanted side effects of oral contraceptives often find these alternatives an attractive choice.

Transdermal Contraceptives

Transdermal contraceptives use a stick-on patch to deliver a combination of estrogen and progesterone in a steady supply through the skin (see Table 14.6). As is true for oral contraceptives, the hormones that are delivered alter the menstrual cycle and prevent follicle maturation and ovulation. They also thicken cervical mucus, making it difficult for sperm to pass through the cervix. One patch is applied each week for three weeks and then left off for one week while menstruation occurs. The patch should be replaced the same day of the week. It is placed on a clean, dry, intact area of skin on the buttock, abdomen, upper outer arm, or upper torso (not the breasts). The area of the patch application should be rotated.

Common side effects of transdermal contraceptives are similar to those of oral contraceptives and include breast tenderness, headache, irritation at the application site, nausea, menstrual cramps, and abdominal pain. These effects tend to subside with continued use. If these effects remain bothersome, an alternative contraceptive agent should be tried.

Contraindications As with all estrogen and progesterone hormone products, benefits and risks of therapy must be weighed. Hormone therapy can increase the risk of cardiovascular events, stroke, and blood clots. Risk of blood clots is especially high for patients 35 years and older who smoke. These hormones can exacerbate depression and migraine headaches. Patients with these conditions should discuss use of hormone contraception with their healthcare practitioners.

Cautions and Considerations If the patch detaches (fully or partially) from the skin, it should be reapplied if possible. If detachment lasts for less than a day, no backup birth control is needed. If detachment lasts longer than a day, then nonhormonal methods of birth control such as a barrier method should be used for seven days. If the patch cannot be reapplied, a new patch should be used and backup contraception used for seven days. A new cycle then begins, and the day to change the patch must be altered.

Drug Interactions See Table 14.7 for drug interactions.

Vaginal Contraceptives

The **vaginal ring** is a combination contraceptive that contains synthetic estrogen and progesterone: **ethinyl estradiol-etonogestrel (NuvaRing)**. The ring is inserted into the vagina where the hormones are absorbed through the vaginal mucosa. This device is left in place for three weeks and then removed for a week while menstruation occurs.

Common side effects of the vaginal ring include headache, nausea, vaginal secretion, vaginitis, bloating, cramps, and weight gain. Use of the vaginal ring may be associated with fewer side effects than experienced with oral contraceptives, presumably because the ring delivers a lower hormonal dose to a localized area. Side effects may subside with continued use. If the effects continue to be bothersome, patients should discontinue therapy and talk with their prescribers.

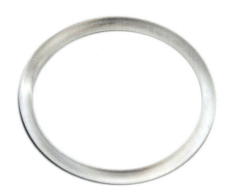

The soft, flexible vaginal ring is compressed and inserted into the vagina to prevent ovulation.

Contraindications The vaginal ring should not be used in patients with breast cancer or other estrogen- or progestin-dependent tumors, liver tumors or disease, pregnancy, or undiagnosed uterine bleeding. Women at high risk for aterial or venous thrombosis (such as cerebrovascular disease, coronary artery disease, diabetes mellitus with vascular disease, deep vein thrombosis [DVT] or pulmonary embolism defined earlier, migraine, uncontrolled hypertension, women over the age of 35 years old who smoke, or with inherited coagulopathies) should not use the vaginal ring.

Cautions and Considerations When stored in a pharmacy, vaginal rings such as the NuvaRing must be kept in the refrigerator to maintain their potency until patients pick up their prescribed products. Patients should be directed to keep their vaginal rings in the refrigerator until they plan to use them.

Drug Interactions See Table 14.7 for drug interactions.

Injections

Medroxyprogesterone (Depo-Provera) is an intramuscular injection given in the deltoid or gluteus maximus every three months. It is administered by a healthcare practitioner and works by inhibiting ovulation, thickening the cervical mucus, and changing the endometrium to inhibit implantation.

150 mg per mL

Depo-Provera
Contraceptive Injection ®
IM

1 mL prefilled syringe (single dose)

Common side effects of medroxyprogesterone injection include menstrual irregularity, abdominal pain, weight changes, dizziness, headache, weakness, fatigue, and nervousness. Also possible are decreased libido, inability to achieve orgasm, pelvic pain, backache, breast pain, leg cramps, hair loss, depression, bloating, nausea, rash, insomnia, edema, hot flashes, acne, sore joints, and vaginitis. Patients should understand the risks of these potential side effects along with the benefits when choosing this long-term contraception option. Because the drug is long-acting, these effects are unavoidable once they occur and will probably continue for three months.

Contraindications Patients with clotting disorders should not take medroxyprogesterone because it can increase the formation of blood clots. In addition, patients with heart or cerebral vascular disease should not take systemic contraceptive medications. A clot in either a coronary artery or cerebral artery could be fatal.

Cautions and Considerations Medroxyprogesterone should not be used if conception has already occurred. For this reason, the patient may be required to take a pregnancy test before administration. It can take weeks for a normal menstrual cycle to resume after using medroxyprogesterone.

Drug Interactions Medroxyprogesterone may diminish the effectiveness of anticoagulants, diabetes medications, and aripiprazole.

Medroxyprogesterone's effectiveness may be decreased by acitretin, aprepitant, atazanavir, barbiturates, bile acid sequestrants, carbamazepine, darunavir, efavirenz, fosphenytoin, griseofulvin, lamotrigine, mifepristone, mycophenolate, phenytoin, and ulipristal.

Medroxyprogesterone may increase the blood clotting effects of tranexamic acid.

Implants

Etonogestrel (Implanon) is an implant placed just under the skin on the inner upper arm and replaced every three years to prevent pregnancy. This product must be inserted by a healthcare practitioner. It works by inhibiting ovulation, thickening the cervical mucus, and changing the endometrium to inhibit implantation.

Common side effects of etonogestrel include changes in menstrual bleeding, weight gain, and mood swings. Other potential side effects include upper respiratory tract infection, vaginitis, breast pain, acne, and abdominal pain. These effects, if particularly bothersome, can be sufficient reason to have the implant removed.

Contraindications Etonogestrel should not be used if conception has already occurred. For this reason, the patient may be required to take a pregnancy test before insertion of the implant. Patients with clotting disorders should not take etonogestrel because it can increase the formation of blood clots. In addition, patients with heart or cerebrovascular disease should not take systemic contraceptive medications. A clot in either a coronary artery or cerebral artery could be fatal.

Cautions and Considerations Because this product is a long-term option for contraception, patients should understand the risks and potential complications of using this drug. It can take three to four weeks for ovulation to resume after removing this implant.

Drug Interactions Etonogestrel may diminish the effectiveness of anticoagulants and diabetes medications.

The effectiveness of etonogestrel may be decreased by acitretin, aprepitant, atazanavir, barbiturates, bile acid sequestrants, carbamazepine, darunavir, efavirenz, fosphenytoin, griseofulvin, lamotrigine, mifepristone, mycophenolate, phenytoin, and uliprista.

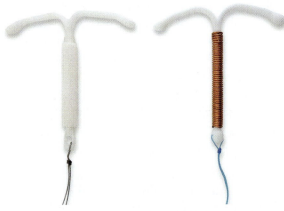

IUDs can contain hormones (pictured left) and others contain copper (pictured right).

Intrauterine Devices

An **intrauterine device (IUD)** is placed into the uterus by a healthcare practitioner and may stay in place for up to 10 years, depending on the product. There are several types of IUDs on the market. Some IUDs contain **levonorgestrel (Liletta, Mirena, Skyla)**, a hormone that alters the endometrium to prevent implantation; other IUDs contain copper **(ParaGard)**.

Although the exact mechanism of action is not well understood, IUDs primarily prevent pregnancy by impeding fertilization. The presence of the IUD device in the uterus causes an inflammatory response that is toxic to sperm and ova and impairs implantation.

Common side effects of IUDs can include spontaneous abortion, septicemia, pelvic infection, perforation of the uterus, vaginitis, abnormal menstrual bleeding, anemia, pain, cramping, backaches, and tubal damage. These effects can be serious and should be fully discussed and understood before patients choose this contraception method.

Contraindications Women with an abnormal or distorted uterine shape, active pelvic inflammatory disease (PID), endometriosis, Wilson's disease, allergy to copper, or unexplained uterine bleeding should not use IUDs. Women with breast cancer should not use an IUD that contains an active hormone (levonorgestrel).

Cautions and Considerations IUDs should not be used if conception has already occurred. For this reason, the patient may be required to take a pregnancy test before administration. An IUD is a long-term but reversible option for contraception.

Drug Interactions Copper IUDs do not contain drugs and are not associated with interactions.

Hormonal IUDs may decrease the effectiveness of other drugs, such as anticoagulants and medications that lower blood glucose.

Heavy Menstrual Bleeding

If a woman's period involves a blood loss greater than 80 mL, it may be considered heavy menstrual bleeding. Many prescribers treat this with nonsteroidal anti-inflammatory drugs (NSAIDs) or an oral contraceptive to decrease cramps and bleeding. Heavy menstrual bleeding is usually caused by too little progesterone. Drugs to treat heavy menstrual bleeding are described in Table 14.8.

Estradiol-dienogest (Natazia) reduces blood loss by about 50%, and is the first OC approved to treat this problem. It has antiandrogenic effects. The drug requires a four-phase regimen. Estradiol is decreased as dienogest is increased during the cycle to prevent breakthrough bleeding. It has four estrogen-only tablets instead of the hormone-free period of other oral contraceptives.

TABLE 14.8 Drugs to Treat Heavy Menstrual Bleeding

Generic (Brand)	Pronunciation	Dosage Form	Dispensing Status
estradiol-dienogest (Natazia)	es-tra-DYE-ole dye-EN-oh-jest	Tablet	Rx
tranexamic acid (Lysteda)	tran-eks-AM-ik AS-id	Injection, tablet	Rx

Tranexamic acid (Lysteda) is a synthetic antifibrinolytic drug. It prevents the binding of fibrin and plasmin in a reversible manner. This drug should be taken for five days during menstruation. Any vision changes should be reported immediately because such symptoms could signal clotting within the retina.

Contraindications Estradiol-dienogest is contraindicated in breast cancer or other estrogen- or progestin-dependent tumors, liver disease, pregnancy, undiagnosed abnormal uterine bleeding, and women at high risk of arterial or venous thrombotic disease.

Tranexamic acid injection is contraindicated in patients with acquired defective color vision, active blood clotting, and subarachnoid hemorrhage. Oral tranexamic acid should not be used in patients with active thromboembolic disease or risk of thrombosis, and concurrent use of combination OCs.

Cautions and Considerations Patients with a history of breast, endometrial, ovarian, or cervical cancer should discuss the risks and benefits of estradiol-dienogest with their healthcare practitioners. Some controversy exists about whether estradiol-dienogest increases a woman's risk for these types of cancer, so patients should make informed decisions about their own care.

Tranexamic acid is associated with visual defects. If visual changes are noted, patients should discontinue use. Clotting has been reported with tranexamic acid use.

Drug Interactions Estradiol-dienogest interactions are the same as those for OCs and can be found in Table 14.7.

OCs and tretinoin may increase the thrombotic effects of tranexamic acid.

Pregnancy Tests and Pregnancy

Detecting a pregnancy early allows a woman to make informed lifestyle decisions and seek appropriate healthcare resources for an optimal outcome. Critical organ systems develop during the first month of embryogenesis; these systems are affected by the mother's diet (e.g., vitamins, caffeine), environment (e.g., smoking), and medications. Early confirmation of pregnancy allows for earlier prenatal care, earlier detection of an ectopic pregnancy (a potentially life-threatening condition), and more time for counseling and consideration of alternatives.

Pregnancy tests are based on detecting the hormone **human chorionic gonadotropin (hCG)**, a glycoprotein produced by trophoblastic cells (the outer cells of the blastocyst) and their descendants in the placenta. Because hCG levels can be measured as early as six to eight days after conception, a woman can test for pregnancy after the first day of a missed menstrual period (depending on the test used). All currently marketed tests detect hCG with monoclonal antibodies (MCAs) specific for the hormone. A chromogen-reactive enzyme linked to one of the antibodies changes color in the presence of hCG, indicating pregnancy. MCA tests provide

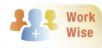

results in one to five minutes. These tests differ in the time and number of steps required to complete the test, the clarity of instructions, and the ease with which the test results can be determined. Consumers generally achieve better than 95% accuracy with home pregnancy tests. Brand names of pregnancy tests include First Response, e.p.t., and Clearblue.

To use a kit properly, patients should:

1. Check the expiration date.
2. Read the instructions twice.
3. Wait the recommended number of days after the first day of menstrual period.
4. Collect the sample from the first morning urine.
5. Collect the urine in a clean container; do not use a plastic cup.
6. If the test cannot be done immediately, refrigerate the urine. Patients should be sure to set out the container with the urine 20 to 30 minutes before the test is performed.
7. If the test is positive, patients would make an appointment to see a doctor.
8. If the test is negative, patients should wait three to five days. If menstruation does not begin, perform the test again. If the second test is negative and menstruation has not started, patients should see a doctor.

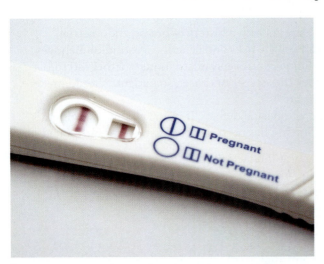

Pregnancy tests can be purchased over the counter for home use.

False-negative test results can be due to chilled urine, chilled test reagents, diluted urine, or high-dose pancreatic enzyme replacement. False-positive results can be due to collecting the urine in a waxed paper cup, an undetected miscarriage or recent abortion, or elevated levels of hCG (e.g., due to a tumor).

Sexually active women should make sure they get the daily requirements of folic acid, iron, and calcium. Pregnancy commonly occurs without the mother even being aware that she is pregnant, and these three substances are very important in the formation of the fetus. Folic acid prevents tubular defects; iron prevents anemia, preterm delivery, and low birth weight in infants; and calcium is important for bone development.

Drugs Used During Childbirth

Childbirth poses dangers to both the mother and child, and death or serious injury is not uncommon. Even during relatively uncomplicated deliveries, childbirth is extremely painful for the mother. With the advent of modern medicine and pharmaceutical products, women and their healthcare providers have numerous tools at their disposal. For uncomplicated deliveries, women may choose not to use drugs, though they are available to control pain. For emergency situations, however, drugs are necessary. If labor ceases, use of a drug that induces labor could prevent the need for a caesarean section (C-section). If a C-section is performed, then other drugs are involved. If uncontrolled bleeding occurs, drugs are usually indicated. Table 14.9 lists the drugs most commonly used during childbirth.

Drugs Used to Induce Labor

Labor induction is the process of stimulating uterine contractions to speed the onset of labor. Inducing labor may be indicated in pregnancies that last longer than 39 weeks, prelabor rupture of membranes, fetal demise, maternal diabetes, and delivery of twins. Both pharmacologic and nonpharmacologic strategies may be used.

Dinoprostone (Cervidil, Prepidil, Prostin E2) promotes cervical ripening (softening to permit delivery) in patients when there is medical or obstetrical indication for the induction of labor. Prepidil is a gel that is packaged in a syringe. Prostin E is a suppository in a foil wrapper. Cervidil is a vaginal insert with a string attached so that it can be removed at the appropriate time.

Misoprostol (Cytotec) is also used for cervical ripening. It is a prostaglandin E analog and is also used for labor induction. The tablets are usually cut into halves or quarters and inserted into the vagina. Pregnant women should not touch misoprostol because it can induce premature labor.

Oxytocin (Pitocin) is a synthetic duplicate of a natural hormone secreted by the posterior lobe of the pituitary gland. The hormone stimulates the contraction of uterine smooth muscle at term, when uterine muscle is most sensitive to the hormone. Such a drug is called an **oxytocic agent**. Side effects for the mother may include vomiting, irregular heart rate, tachycardia, and postpartum bleeding. The child may experience bradycardia, arrhythmias, and jaundice. This drug should be used as a last resort.

Contraindications Dinoprostone is contraindicated in cases where vaginal delivery is contraindicated.

Misoprostol should not be given to patients with hypersensitivity to prostaglandins.

Oxytocin is contraindicated in pregnant patients with unfavorable fetal positions, fetal distress, hypertonic or hyperactive uterus, contraindications to vaginal delivery, emergencies where surgical intervention is preferred, and where adequate uterine activity fails to achieve progress.

Cautions and Considerations Dinoprostone has boxed warnings to be used only by an experienced physician and to adhere strictly to dosage recommendations.

Misoprostol also carries boxed warnings. It can result in abortion, premature birth, or birth defects. It should not be used to reduce the risk of NSAID-induced ulcers in women of childbearing potential.

Oxytocin has a boxed warning that it should not be used for elective induction of labor.

TABLE 14.9 Most Commonly Used Drugs during Childbirth

Generic (Brand)	Pronunciation	Dosage Form	Dispensing Status
dinoprostone (Cervidil, Prepidil, Prostin E2)	dye-noe-PROST-oan	Gel, vaginal insert, suppository	Rx
magnesium sulfate (none)	mag-NEE-zhum-SUL-fate	Injection	Rx
misoprostol (Cytotec)	mye-soe-PROS-tawl	Tablet	Rx
nifedipine (Procardia)	nye-FED-i-peen	Capsule	Rx
oxytocin (Pitocin)	ox-i-TOE-sin	Injection	Rx

Drug Interactions Dinoprostone may enhance the adverse effects of carbetocin and oxytocin.

Antacids may enhance the adverse effects of misoprostol.

Misoprostol may enhance the adverse effects of oxytocin agents. Oxytocin may cause QT prolongation and should be used cautiously with other agents that may prolong the QT interval.

Drugs Used for Premature Labor

A drug used to slow labor is called a **tocolytic agent**. Very few tocolytic agents are available.

Magnesium sulfate is used to prevent seizures in preeclampsia or eclampsia (caused by hypertension) during pregnancy. This drug has severe consequences when used in error. It is a high-alert drug, so special care needs to be taken when dispensing this intravenous drug. It has a tocolytic effect (slows uterine contraction) and is also used frequently for this purpose.

Nifedipine (Procardia) is a calcium channel blocker (see Chapter 12) used as a tocolytic agent. It relaxes smooth muscle. The soft capsule contains 10 or 20 mg of nifedipine. The capsule is punctured and placed under the tongue so that it will be absorbed more quickly.

Osteoporosis

Bone is a living tissue that is continuously being replaced as a result of the balance between **osteoclast** (a cell that resorbs bone) and **osteoblast** (a cell that forms bone) activity. In normal, healthy bone (see Figure 14.5), the opposing activities of osteoclasts and osteoblasts are balanced. As adults age, however, resorption of bone tissue exceeds the deposit of new bone. Furthermore, newly formed bone is less dense and more fragile than original bone. Reduction or weakening of bone mass increases the risk of bone fracture. For adults over 50 years old, these processes occur at a faster rate for women than for men. The condition of reduced bone mineral density, disrupted microarchitecture of bone structure, and increased likelihood of fracture is known as **osteoporosis**. Osteoporosis occurs as a result of deficiency in estrogen, calcium, and vitamin D. The reduction in bone mass is accelerated and more severe in women who have had an early hysterectomy because without a uterus a woman's body produces less estrogen. With less estrogen, lower amounts of calcium are used by bony tissue. Daily calcium intake with vitamin D is essential to the prevention of bone loss.

Osteoporosis can cause fractures in the hips, spine, and wrists, which are painful and debilitating. **Hip fractures** can be life-threatening because the subsequent hip replacement surgery, recovery, and potential complications are often dramatic. Older patients may never return to normal function after a hip fracture.

Risk Factors

Individuals at risk for developing osteoporosis typically have one or more of these characteristics:

- female gender (90% of patients)
- white or Asian race
- family history of osteoporosis

- small body frame
- history of smoking
- heavy caffeine intake
- suboptimal nutrition (e.g., low calcium intake)

The risk for osteoporosis can be assessed using a **bone mineral density (BMD)** machine. This machine uses X-ray and ultrasound technology to determine bone density measurements. Typically, the heel bone is measured because it is a good estimate of hip and spine bone density. The result of a BMD screening yields a **T-score**, which is an estimate of risk, not a diagnosis. Armed with such information, patients can make changes in their lives, such as performing weight-bearing exercises, eating foods high in calcium, quitting smoking, and decreasing caffeine intake, which are all ways to increase bone density. If a diagnosis of osteoporosis is made by a healthcare practitioner, drug therapy may be prescribed.

FIGURE 14.5
Microscopic View of Bone

Osteoclasts and osteoblasts provide bone remodeling, a continual process that grows and repairs bone.

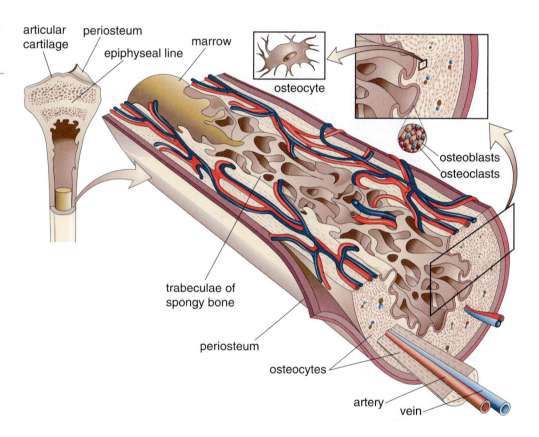

Drugs for Osteoporosis

It makes sense that supplementing estrogen in women whose levels are declining would stave off drastic drops in bone mineral density. However, the increased risk of heart disease, cancer, and stroke associated with estrogen replacement products has been found to outweigh this benefit. Consequently, hormone replacement therapy (HRT) with estrogen has fallen out of favor as a treatment for osteoporosis but is taken at the lowest dose for the shortest time possible with the sole goal of alleviating menopausal symptoms. The most common drugs to treat osteoporosis include the bisphosphonates. These drugs work by inhibiting bone resorption. Other treatments aim to mimic the beneficial effects of estrogen without the deleterious effects. Some osteoporosis therapies suppress osteoclasts or regulate calcium and phosphate metabolism.

Table 14.10 lists the most commonly used agents for the prevention and treatment of osteoporosis.

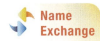

Name Exchange

You may hear the generic drug alendronate, a commonly used bisphosphonate, called by its brand name, Fosamax.

Bisphosphonates

Bisphosphonates inhibit osteoclasts from removing calcium from bone tissue. These medications prevent bone breakdown so that stronger bones are maintained. Over time, bone density can be maintained, and hopefully, fractures can be prevented. Bisphosphonates are used primarily for osteoporosis but can be used to treat Paget's disease (a chronic disorder that results in weakened bones, fractures, and arthritis). Sometimes, bisphosphonates are used in bone and spinal injury cases to promote bone regrowth and strengthening. Depending on the product chosen, bisphosphonates can be taken orally on a daily, weekly, or monthly basis. They can even be administered intravenously (IV) every month, every three months, or annually. The variety of dosage regimens allows prescribers to individualize drug therapy.

Side effects of bisphosphonates can include headache, nausea, vomiting, diarrhea, constipation, abdominal pain, indigestion, and esophagitis. Taking oral dosage forms with a full glass of water and remaining upright afterward can reduce side effects such as reflux and esophageal issues. Other side effects include insomnia and anemia, for which patients must seek medical advice to manage. A less common yet severe side effect is osteonecrosis (bone tissue death) of the jaw. The IV dosage forms can cause fever, so acetaminophen is given simultaneously.

TABLE 14.10 Most Commonly Used Agents for Osteoporosis

Generic (Brand)	Pronunciation	Dosage Form	Dispensing Status
Bisphosphonates			
alendronate (Fosamax, Fosamax Plus D)	a-LEN-droe-nate	Tablet	Rx
ibandronate (Boniva)	eye-BAN-droh-nate	Tablet, injection	Rx
pamidronate (Aredia)	pa-MID-roe-nate	Injection	Rx
risedronate (Actonel)	ris-ED-roe-nate	Tablet	Rx
zoledronic acid (Reclast)	zo-le-DROE-nik AS-id	Injection	Rx
Selective Estrogen Receptor Modulators (SERM)			
raloxifene (Evista)	ra-LOX-i-feen	Tablet	Rx
Other Drugs for Osteoporosis			
calcitonin (Miacalcin)	kal-si-TOE-nin	Injection, nasal spray	Rx
denosumab (Prolia, Xgeva)	den-OH-sue-mab	Injection	Rx
teriparatide (Forteo)	ter-i-PAR-a-tide	Injection	Rx

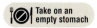

Take on an empty stomach

Put Down Roots

Almost all of the bisphosphonate agents used to treat osteoporosis end with the suffix *-ate*. The exception to this rule is zoledronic acid, which is a bisphosphonate derivative.

Alendronate (Fosamax) is a bisphosphonate compound approved by the FDA for treating osteoporosis. In addition, alendronate is used for hypercalcemia of malignancy and in Paget's bone disease, a disorder of unknown cause that affects middle-aged and older adults and results in excess bone destruction and unorganized bone repair.

To enhance absorption, alendronate must be taken at least 30 minutes before the first food, beverage, or medication of the day. In order to prevent esophageal damage, the patient should drink six to eight ounces of water while swallowing the alendronate tablet and should not lie down for at least 30 minutes afterward. Alendronate is dosed once daily or once weekly, depending on the dosage.

Ibandronate (Boniva) is also a bisphosphonate approved for the treatment of osteoporosis. It is manufactured in a once-a-month tablet or an IV formulation that is administerd every three months. The IV form is associated with more side effects than the oral form. Oral ibandronate must be taken with care; it must be taken 60 minutes before the first food or drink of the day, with six to eight ounces of plain water, and the patient must remain upright for 60 minutes. These requirements may lead to nonadherence.

Pamidronate (Aredia) is a bisphosphonate that is not FDA approved for osteoporosis. It is approved for hypercalcemia of malignancy, osteolytic bone metastases and lesions, and Paget's disease. It is available only as an injection and is administered once a month.

Risedronate (Actonel) is a bisphosphonate that inhibits bone resorption by acting on osteoclasts or osteoclast precursors. It is indicated for the treatment and prevention of osteoporosis in postmenopausal women and of Paget's disease for both men and women. Risedronate is taken either once weekly or twice monthly.

Zoledronic acid (Reclast) is a bisphosphonate for IV infusion. The usual dose is 5 mg and must be administered over no less than 15 minutes. It may have a quicker onset and a longer duration of action than other drugs used to treat hypercalcemia.

Contraindications Bisphosphonates are contraindicated in the case of hypersensitivity to other bisphosphonates. For example, if a patient has a hypersensitivity to alendronate, the use of all other bisphosphonates is contraindicated.

Specific bisphosphonates have unique contraindications. Alendronate, ibandronate, and risedronate are contraindicated in patients with hypocalcemia, abnormalities of the esophagus, and an inability to stand or sit upright for at least 30 minutes. The effervescent tablets and oral solution of alendronate are contraindicated in patients at increased risk for aspiration. Zoledronic acid should not be used in patients with hypocalcemia and kidney dysfunction.

Cautions and Considerations Oral bisphosphonates are poorly absorbed from the GI tract and are adversely affected by food. Therefore, they must be taken on an empty stomach (preferably first thing in the morning) with water. After taking a bisphosphonate, patients should wait at least 30 minutes before eating. Bisphosphonates are also highly irritating to the GI tract, so they must be taken with a full glass of water to ensure that they do not become lodged in the esophagus. Patients must remain upright for at least 30 minutes after medication administration to prevent reflux. In most cases, bisphosphonate infusions are administered in a physician's office or clinic.

Drug Interactions Antacids, calcium, iron, magnesium, and multivitamins may decrease the concentration of oral bisphosphonates. Antacids should be taken two hours before or one hour after bisphosphonates. Proton pump inhibitors may decrease the effectiveness of bisphosphonates.

Selective Estrogen Receptor Modulators

Selective estrogen receptor modulators (SERMs) work as estrogen receptors by mimicking the beneficial effects of estrogen on bone mineral density. However, they do not increase the risk of breast or uterine cancer the way regular estrogen can. In fact, they can improve cholesterol levels, although they are not used for hyperlipidemia. While there are multiple SERMs on the market, **raloxifene (Evista)** is the one indicated to treat osteoporosis.

Common side effects of SERMs are hot flashes, headache, diarrhea, joint pain, leg cramps, and flu-like symptoms. The most serious side effect is deep vein thrombosis or blood clots.

Contraindications Raloxifene is contraindicated in patients who have a history of or current venous thromboembolic disorders (including deep vein thrombosis and pulmonary embolism). This medication should not be taken by women who are pregnant or could become pregnant, or by women who are breastfeeding.

Cautions and Considerations Raloxifene should not be taken if prolonged immobility is anticipated because the drug carries an increased risk of thromboembolic events. If patients using SERMs experience pain, swelling, or bruising in one leg or difficulty breathing, they should seek medical care immediately.

Drug Interactions Cholestyramine may decrease absorption of raloxifene, and concurrent use should be avoided. Raloxifene may decrease the effectiveness of warfarin.

Other Osteoporosis Medications

There are several other medications used for osteoporosis in addition to those previously mentioned. These medications include calcitonin, denosumab, and teriparatide.

Calcitonin (Miacalcin) is a peptide hormone that suppresses the activity of osteoclasts. A synthetic replica of the calcitonin produced by salmon is used because this molecule is more potent than the calcitonin produced by the human thyroid gland. Calcitonin may be used at any time of day. Calcitonin nasal spray should be applied to a different nostril each day. The pump must be activated before the first dose. Most adverse effects of the intranasal product are local, such as runny nose. Flushing may occur with use of the injectable formulation.

Denosumab (Prolia, Xgeva) inhibits osteoclast formation, which decreases bone resorption and increases bone mass strength. It comes as a prefilled syringe and is administered by a healthcare professional subcutaneously every six months. Denosumab is indicated for patients who have failed other osteoporosis therapy and are at high risk for fracture. Patients should also take calcium and vitamin D with this drug. The solution may appear clear and colorless or it may look pale yellow. Denosumab is stored in the refrigerator and should be removed 15 to 30 minutes before administration. No other method should be used to warm the drug. Side effects such as dermatitis, eczema, and skin rash are reported with denosumab use.

Teriparatide (Forteo) is a human parathyroid hormone used for treating osteoporosis. It stimulates bone formation and resorption by regulating calcium and phosphate metabolism with bony tissue. Whereas other drugs only slow osteoporosis, teriparatide actually stimulates new bone growth. It is indicated for postmenopausal women with osteoporosis who are at high risk for fracture. Teriparatide is pen injected subcutaneously and must be stored in a refrigerator. Teriparatide use is associated with hypercalcemia and dizziness.

Contraindications There are no contraindications to calcitonin and teriparatide use. Denosumab is contraindicated in pregnancy and preexisting hypocalcemia.

Cautions and Considerations Calcitonin is derived from salmon; therefore, there is a risk for hypersensitivity reactions in patients with fish allergies. In addition, there is concern over an increased risk of cancer development with long-term use of calcitonin.

Bone fractures have been reported with denosumab use. Consider discontinuing use if severe dermatologic symptoms occur. Use teriparatide with caution in patients who have an increased risk for dizziness or falling.

Teriparatide has been associated with osteosarcoma, so patients with Paget's disease or with an increased risk for bone cancer should not use teriparatide. Teriparatide has a boxed warning for this.

Drug Interactions Calcitonin may decrease the serum concentrations of lithium. Denosumab may enhance the adverse effects of immunosuppressants. Teriparatide has no known drug interactions.

Adrenal Gland Disorders and Corticosteroid Therapy

The adrenal glands are located on the top of the kidneys. The medulla, or inner portion, functions like the sympathetic nervous system and produces catecholamines such as epinephrine (adrenaline). The cortex, or outer portion, produces several types of steroid hormones. Each such hormone, known as a **corticosteroid**, has its own combination of **glucocorticoid** (involved in cholesterol, fat, and protein metabolism) and **mineralocorticoid** (involved in regulating electrolyte and water balance) activity. The principal adrenal steroid hormone is cortisol. It is responsible for **gluconeogenesis** (conversion of fatty acids and proteins to glucose), protein catabolism, anti-inflammatory reactions, stimulation of fat deposition, and sodium and water retention (steroids are necessary for mineral retention). The adrenal cortex also produces various sex hormones.

As with the other hormones discussed earlier, the production of cortisol and other steroids begins in the hypothalamic-pituitary axis. The hypothalamus produces corticotropin-releasing factor (CRF), which stimulates the pituitary gland to produce adrenocorticotropic hormone (ACTH), which in turn enters the bloodstream and travels to the adrenal cortex, where it stimulates the release of cortisol into the blood. Through a feedback mechanism, the rising cortisol levels slow the action of the hypothalamus in producing and releasing CRF. Steroid production follows a circadian rhythm (regular recurrence in cycles of 24 hours). As Figure 14.6 shows, it peaks in the morning, and the low point occurs close to midnight.

When the corticosteroid cortisol **(hydrocortisone)** was isolated, a milestone in medicine was reached. Results of clinical trials in rheumatoid arthritis were dramatic, and soon cortisone, another corticosteroid, was found to improve symptoms in an amazing number of disease states. Further research led to the development of other corticosteroids—**prednisone**, **methylprednisolone**, **triamcinolone**, and **dexamethasone**—that had greater anti-inflammatory potency (glucocorticoid) and less effect on renal sodium resorption (mineralocorticoid). These drugs are used as anti-inflammatory or immunosuppressive agents in treating a variety of diseases, including those of hematologic, allergic, inflammatory, neoplastic, and autoimmune origin.

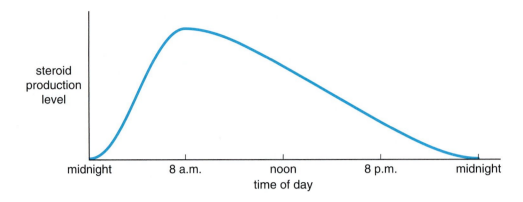

FIGURE 14.6
Steroid Production

Steroid production follows a circadian rhythm, with a peak in the morning and a low point around midnight.

steroid production level

midnight   8 a.m.   noon   8 p.m.   midnight

time of day

Addison's Disease

Addison's disease is a life-threatening deficiency of glucocorticoids and mineralocorticoids that is treated with daily administration of a corticosteroid. Commonly used corticosteroids are described in Table 14.11. The symptoms of Addison's disease include the following:

- debilitating weakness (may have respiratory failure)
- hyperkalemia
- bronze color of skin, produced by excessive melanin production, typically on the nipples, at creases, on the lips, and inside the mouth
- low levels of serum sodium and glucose
- reduced blood pressure
- weight loss

TABLE 14.11   Commonly Used Corticosteroids

Generic (Brand)	Pronunciation	Dosage Form	Dispensing Status
betamethasone (Celestone)	bay-ta-METH-a-sone	Injection, oral solution	Rx
budesonide (Entocort EC)	byoo-DES-oh-nide	Capsule, tablet	Rx
cortisone	KOR-ti-sone	Tablet	Rx
dexamethasone (Baycadron, Dexamethasone, DexPak)	dex-a-METH-a-sone	Elixir, injection, oral solution, tablet	Rx
hydrocortisone (A-Hydrocort, Cortef, Solu-Cortef)	hye-droe-KOR-ti-sone	Injection, tablet	Rx
methylprednisolone (A-MethaPred, Depo-Medrol, Medrol, Solu-Medrol)	meth-ill-pred-NISS-oh-lone	Injection, tablet	Rx
prednisolone (Flo-Pred, Orapred, Pediapred, Prelone)	pred-NISS-oh-lone	Oral solution, suspension, syrup, tablet	Rx
prednisone (Prednisone Intensol, Rayos)	PRED-ni-sone	Oral solution, tablet	Rx

Corticosteroid Therapy

Acute adrenal deficiency can be life-threatening and is treated with IV fluids and systemic corticosteroids. Systemic corticosteroids replace corticosteroids in a deficiency. They are also used for a variety of other conditions, particularly for their anti-inflammatory and immunosuppressant properties. Systemic corticosteroids may be used for asthma, autoimmune disorders, and hypersensitivity and allergic reactions.

Common side effects of corticosteroids include headache, dizziness, insomnia, and hunger. Taking corticosteroids in the morning may lessen these effects, especially insomnia. Long-term or excessive use can affect normal metabolism in the body and cause symptoms of steroid overproduction. Severe effects include high blood pressure, loss of bone mass (osteoporosis), electrolyte imbalance, cataracts or glaucoma, and insulin resistance (diabetes). Patients taking corticosteroids for long periods need special monitoring to prevent or treat these effects.

Corticosteroids are available in many dosage forms: tablets, syrups, injections, inhalants, eye drops, creams, ointments, lotions, suppositories, and others. They are commonly packed in dose packs. For example, the Medrol Dosepak contains 21 4 mg tablets. On the first day, the patient takes a loading dose; the dose decreases each day thereafter, as described on the package.

Contraindications Dexamethasone use is contraindicated in systemic fungal infections and cerebral malaria. Contraindications to hydrocortisone include serious infections (except septic shock or tuberculous meningitis) and skin lesions of viral, fungal, or tubercular origin. Injectable hydrocortisone should not be administered intramuscularly in patients with idiopathic thrombocytopenic purpura or via the intrathecal route.

Cautions and Considerations Patients should not stop taking corticosteroids abruptly. Untoward and life-threatening effects can occur if a patient who has been taking chronic corticosteroids discontinues them suddenly. Because these medications can suppress the immune system if taken in large doses, patients taking them may be at an increased risk for infection. Growth and development must be monitored closely in children taking corticosteroids for long periods because these drugs have the potential to stunt growth. Corticosteroids may cause gastrointestinal events, including gastritis, ulcer formation, and gastrointestinal bleeding.

Drug Interactions Corticosteroids may render anticoagulants less effective. Diabetes medications may be less effective when patients are using corticosteroids. Risk of infections with live vaccines increases with concurrent corticosteroid use.

Aprepitant, azole antifungals, and protease inhibitors may increase corticosteroid levels. Carbamazepine, phenytoin, and rifampin may decrease corticosteroid levels.

Adverse reactions of other immunosuppressants may increase the adverse effects of corticosteroids. The fluid-retaining side effects of androgens are enhanced by corticosteroids. Corticosteroids may diminish the therapeutic effects of diabetes agents. Quinolones used with corticosteroids increase the risk of tendon rupture.

Cushing's Syndrome

Cushing's syndrome is caused by an overproduction of cortisol; it can also result from excessive administration of corticosteroids over an extended period. Cushing's syndrome may also be caused by tumors in the adrenal glands. Patients have a protruding abdomen; a round, puffy face; and fat deposits above the shoulder blades. The fat distribution may not change even with cessation of corticosteroid therapy.

Surgery is used most often to remove tumors causing Cushing's syndrome. Sometimes cytotoxic or chemotherapy drugs are used to treat the tumor and suppress corticosteroid production. (See Chapter 16 for more information on chemotherapeutic agents.)

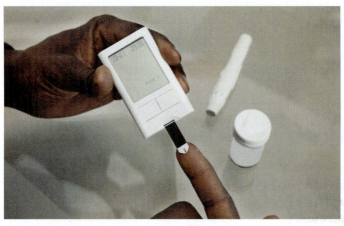

Since the mid-1960s, testing blood sugar levels has been a critical daily component of maintaining health while living with diabetes. Today's meters require less blood and are less painful than before.

Diabetes

Diabetes is a serious disease that affects millions of people. It is characterized by high blood glucose, which is due to insufficient levels of the critically important hormone insulin. If left untreated, diabetes can cause a range of serious conditions and, eventually, death.

The pancreas contains specialized cells, called the islets of Langerhans, that produce insulin. **Insulin** helps cells burn glucose for energy, combines with membrane receptors to allow glucose uptake, enhances transport and incorporation of amino acids into protein, increases ion transport into tissues, and inhibits fat breakdown. Thus, insulin is critical in maintaining blood glucose levels, as well as having other metabolic roles.

In persons with diabetes, either the secretion or the use of insulin is inadequate, which leads to excessive blood glucose levels. The normal blood glucose level is around 100 mg/dL. At elevated levels, the kidneys will not be able to reabsorb the excess, and glucose will spill into the urine. Levels consistently above 140 to 160 mg/dL are associated with long-term effects of diabetes. An elevated blood sugar level is known as **hyperglycemia**.

Diabetes is a devastating disorder that can damage all major organ systems. Over time, diabetes can destroy eyesight, kidneys, and peripheral circulation. The results are blindness, a need for dialysis, and amputation of limbs. Although approximately 20% of persons older than 60 years have diabetes, some estimates suggest that only half of those with diabetes in the United States are diagnosed. Furthermore, many patients with diabetes do not properly manage their disease.

Types of Diabetes

Type 1 diabetes occurs most commonly in children and young adults, but it may occur at any age. The average age of diagnosis is 11 or 12 years old. These patients are insulin dependent; that is, they have no ability to produce insulin. They may produce antibodies to islet cells in an autoimmune response. This group comprises 5%–10% of diabetes patients.

Type 2 diabetes comprises 80%–90% of diabetes cases. Most patients are over 40 years of age, with the majority being female. Patients with type 2 diabetes may have a relative insulin insufficiency (impaired insulin secretion); however, insulin receptor resistance on cells may be the primary culprit. The peripheral target tissues are resistant to insulin produced. Glucose is not absorbed because the cells do not respond to insulin. Most type 2 diabetes patients are overweight, and the best treatment is to lose weight.

Gestational diabetes occurs during pregnancy and increases the risk of fetal morbidity and death. The onset occurs during the second and third trimesters. Gestational diabetes can be treated with diet, exercise, and insulin. Usually, it disappears after the birth of the baby, but 30%–40% of women who have gestational diabetes will develop type 2 diabetes in 5 to 10 years. Oral contraceptives raise blood glucose levels, especially in women who had gestational diabetes, so whether they should use this type of contraception is debatable.

Secondary diabetes is caused by drugs. Among these drugs are oral contraceptives, beta blockers, diuretics, calcium channel blockers, glucocorticoids, and phenytoin. Secondary diabetes may cease when the drug is discontinued.

Symptoms and Complications of Diabetes

Symptoms of diabetes include the following:

- frequent infections
- glycosuria (presence of glucose in the urine)
- hunger
- increased urination (polyuria) and nocturia (excessive urination at night)
- numbness and tingling
- slow wound healing (hyperglycemia inhibits activity of neutrophils, a type of white blood cell)
- thirst
- visual changes
- nausea and vomiting
- weight loss, easy fatigability, irritability, and ketoacidosis

Although acute **hypoglycemia**, in which blood glucose levels fall below 70 mg/dL, is the more dangerous condition, chronic hyperglycemia, if unchecked, can result in long-term complications that can destroy the quality of life. If diabetes goes unchecked, there is risk of developing the following complications:

- **Retinopathy** is the leading cause of blindness in the United States. The vessels of the eyes become damaged, resulting in insufficient blood supply; rupture causes loss of sight.
- **Neuropathy** is the result of a lack of blood flow to nerves, leaving them unable to function. Symptoms are dull aching to sharp stabbing pains.
- Vascular problems lead to atherosclerosis of peripheral coronary and cerebrovascular vessels. The decreased blood flow causes neuropathy and slows healing, especially in the feet and legs. Wounds that fail to heal may need to be amputated.
- Dermatologic issues are often expressed as boils, acne, or fungal infections.
- Nephropathy, or kidney damage, occurs in 10%–21% of patients with diabetes and is the primary cause of end-stage renal disease.

Treatment of Diabetes

The goal of treatment of diabetes is to approximate nondiabetic physiology as closely as possible. The treatment consists of diet, exercise, and medications. Blood glucose monitoring is very important to prevent both acute and long-term complications and to guide treatment for reaching target fasting blood glucose goals. To prevent long-term complications, diabetes should be controlled to maintain fasting blood glucose levels between 80 and 130 mg/dL. Patients with type 1 diabetes must receive insulin. Patients with type 2 diabetes may be able to control the disease through diet and exercise alone, but commonly they have to add a drug therapy. Cases of diabetes that are difficult to control may be referred to as "brittle."

General treatment guidelines for a patient with any type of diabetes include the following:

- attention to diet
- blood pressure control
- adherence to the medication regimen
- control of hyperlipidemia
- daily foot inspections
- increased physical activity
- learning to recognize hypoglycemia
- monitoring progress at home through blood glucose testing
- monitoring progress at the doctor's office through measurement of **glycosylated hemoglobin (HbA1C)**
- patient education
- prompt treatment of all infections
- setting individual goals

Patients with diabetes must also take very good care of their feet, which are particularly vulnerable to infections. Diabetic ulcers (open wounds that are typically slow to heal) are the leading cause of foot and leg amputation and a leading reason for hospital admissions among patients with diabetes. Patients should be instructed to avoid the use of OTC foot products, unless otherwise directed by a physician. They should be instructed to moisturize their feet daily to prevent the skin from cracking. They should also keep nails trimmed to prevent ingrown toenails. It is common for patients with diabetes to have neuropathies of the legs. This sensation can be very painful, or the patient may feel total numbness in the extremities. With numbness, patients can injure their feet and not even be aware of it, which in turn can lead to serious infections.

Becaplermin gel (Regranex), listed in Table 14.12, is a recombinant human platelet-derived growth factor that speeds the healing of lower extremity diabetic ulcers. Some studies have shown that this drug, which acts locally and has very little systemic

TABLE 14.12   Most Commonly Used Drug for Lower-Extremity Diabetic Ulcers

Generic (Brand)	Pronunciation	Dosage Form	Dispensing Status
becaplermin gel (Regranex)	be-KAP-ler-min	Gel	Rx

FIGURE 14.7
Normal Glucose Production

The timing of bolus insulin released with meals is called prandial, which means "with meals."

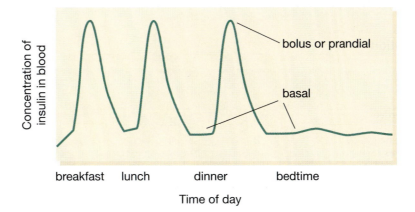

bolus or prandial

basal

breakfast   lunch   dinner   bedtime

Time of day

Concentration of insulin in blood

effect, can increase the incidence of complete healing of diabetic foot ulcers. If the wound does not decrease in size by 30% in 10 weeks or heal in 20 weeks, use of this drug should be reassessed.

Insulin

Safety Alert

It is very easy to grab the wrong type of insulin from the refrigerator. Always double-check insulins, because they look alike. All types of insulin are designated as high-alert medications by the Institute of Safe Medication Practices.

Insulin is normally produced in a combination of basal and bolus rates to maintain steady glucose concentrations in the blood (see Figure 14.7). **Basal insulin** is slowly released throughout the day and night to allow energy for basic cellular function. In contrast, **bolus insulin** is released at mealtimes to react with glucose entering the body from food intake. When insulin is given by injection, the goal is to mimic this natural physiologic insulin production. For patients with type 1 diabetes, multiple injections each day of combination basal and bolus insulins are necessary to achieve physiologic insulin dosing. Patients with type 2 diabetes may be given insulin using a similar physiologic dosing schedule or as one injection of long-acting insulin at bedtime in addition to oral medications.

Based on the duration of their pharmacological action, insulin products are classified as rapid-acting, short-acting, intermediate-acting, or long-acting. The differences are related to the molecular structure of insulin. **Rapid-acting insulin** begins to work in approximately 10 minutes and, for practical purposes, lasts as long as 2 hours. It is given just before meals to reduce **prandial** (mealtime) elevations in blood glucose. **Short-acting insulin** begins to work in around 30 minutes and lasts up to 4 hours in most cases. It is also taken prior to meals. **Intermediate-acting insulin** begins to be effective in 30 to 60 minutes and lasts 6 to 8 hours in most cases. It is used either once or twice a day. **Long-acting insulin** works for approximately 24 hours and is injected once a day.

Insulin is available in **vials** for use with **syringes** and in **self-injector pens**. **Insulin pumps** are also available; these deliver insulin through a tiny tube inserted just under the skin. These pumps can be programmed to deliver just the right amount of insulin each hour of the day for an individual patient. The tube must be reinserted every three days. Pumps eliminate the need for multiple injections a day but must be

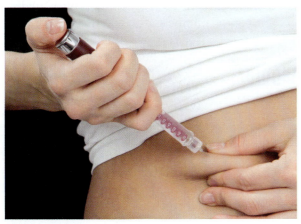

Patient injecting herself with insulin.

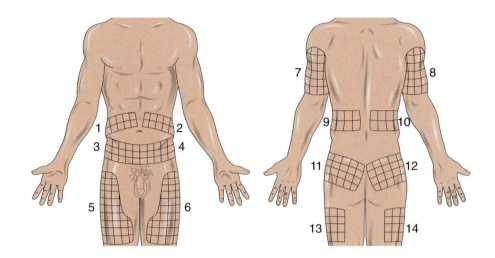

FIGURE 14.8
Rotation of Administration Sites for Insulin

The numbers indicate the order in which each region should be used. The boxes within the regions indicate a single injection site. After injecting all the first boxes in each region, the patient will inject the second box in each region, working sequentially through the entire series.

well understood and properly maintained to work effectively. Inhaled insulin is also available and does not require injection.

Insulin should not be injected into an area of the body that will receive a rigorous workout. The injection site should be rotated frequently because decreased subcutaneous fat can lead to lipoatrophy (loss of fat) at the injection site. Figure 14.8 illustrates the method of rotating insulin administration sites. Insulin enters the blood best from the abdomen, then the arms and legs, and last the buttocks.

The most common "side effect" of insulin is hypoglycemia. Although often listed as a side effect, hypoglycemia is, in fact, the intended effect of insulin. However, someone using insulin is an increased risk of developing serious hypoglycemia when doses are too high or meals are skipped. If blood glucose concentrations are lower than 40 mg/dL, loss of consciousness and brain damage can occur. Diabetic coma is life-threatening if not treated immediately. Symptoms of hypoglycemia include shakiness, headache, blurred vision, dizziness, confusion, irritability, hunger, and tiredness.

Other side effects are rare but can include lipodystrophy (fat accumulation or depletion at injection site). This effect can be largely avoided by rotating injection sites.

Table 14.13 lists the most commonly used types of insulin. Most insulin formulations are available by prescription only. Neutral protamine Hagedorn (NPH) insulin and the U-100 strength of regular insulin are available without a prescription. In an emergency situation, insulin does not require a prescription, but the person dispensing this drug will need documentation to make sure the correct insulin is dispensed.

Some states require a prescription for a syringe, and many states require proof of need. Regular and short-acting insulin solutions are clear; all others are cloudy. When two types of insulin are combined, a longer-acting insulin is paired with an insulin of rapid onset, causing the insulin to take effect quicker and last longer. When mixing two types of insulin, the regular type should be drawn up first.

10 mL
Humulin R Regular®
U-100
Injection
100 units/mL vial

20 mL (High Potency)
Humulin R Regular®
U-500
Injection
500 units/mL vial

Regular insulin is available in two concentrations, 100 units/mL and 500 units/mL. Pharmacy technicians should take extra caution to ensure they are dispensing the correct concentration. Errors can be potentially fatal.

TABLE 14.13 Profile of Common Insulin Products

Generic (Brand)	Pronunciation	Onset of Action	Maximum Peak and Duration	Appearance and Dispensing Status
Rapid-Acting				
inhaled regular insulin* (Afrezza)	in-hail-d RE-gyoo-lar IN-soo-lin	1–5 minutes	12–15 minutes; 3–4 hours	Colored cartridge; Rx only
insulin aspart (NovoLog)	IN-soo-lin AS-part	10–15 minutes	1–2 hours; 4 hours	Clear; Rx
insulin glulisine (Apidra)	IN-soo-lin-GLOO-lis-een	Few minutes	1 hour; 2 hours	Clear; Rx
insulin lispro (Humalog)	IN-soo-lin LYE-sproe	10–15 minutes	1–2 hours; 4 hours	Clear; Rx
Short-Acting				
regular insulin U-100 (Humulin R, Novolin R)	RE-gyoo-lar IN-soo-lin	30 minutes	4 hours; 8 hours	Clear; OTC
Intermediate-Acting				
neutral protamine Hagedorn (NPH) insulin (Humulin N, Novolin N)	NPH IN-soo-lin	1 hour	6–8 hours; 24 hours	Cloudy; OTC
regular insulin U-500 (Humulin R U-500)	RE-gyoo-lar IN-soo-lin	30 minutes	8 hours; 24 hours	Clear; Rx
Long-Acting				
insulin degludec (Tresiba)	IN-soo-lin DEG-lu-dek	1 hour	9 hours; 25 hours	Clear; Rx
insulin detemir (Levemir)	IN-soo-lin-DET-e-meer	1 hour	24–36 hours	Clear; Rx
insulin glargine (Lantus, Toujeo SoloStar)	IN-soo-lin GLAR-jeen	1 hour	None; 24–36 hours	Clear; Rx
Premixed				
insulin NPH/regular 70/30 (Humulin 70/30, Novolin 70/30, ReliOn Novolin 70/30)	IN-soo-lin NPH RE-gyoo-lar	30–60 minutes	2–10 hours; 18–24 hours	Cloudy; Rx
insulin lispro protamine/lispro 75/25 (Humalog 75/25)	IN-soo-lin LYE-sproe PRO-tah-meen LYE-sproe	10–30 minutes	1–6 hours; 14–24 hours	Cloudy; Rx
insulin aspart protamine/aspart 70/30 (Novolog 70/30)	IN-soo-lin AS-part PRO-tah-meen AS-part	10–30 minutes	1–6 hours; 14–24 hours	Cloudy; Rx
insulin lispro protamine/lispro 50/50 (Humalog 50/50)	IN-soo-lin LYE-sproe PRO-tah-meen LYE-sproe	10–30 minutes	1–6 hours; 14–24 hours	Cloudy; Rx

*This insulin is inhaled; all others listed in this table are injectable.

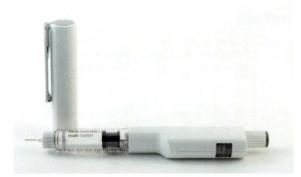

Insulin pens were developed to improve convenience.

Degludec (Tresiba), detemir (Levemir), glargine (Lantus), and regular insulin U-500 should not be mixed with any other type of insulin. All insulins are stored in the pharmacy refrigerator.

Manufacturers have developed pens for the easy administration of insulin. The pen consists of a disposable needle and a syringe of insulin. Insulin pens are available in various shapes and forms, and most are very easy to use.

Regular insulin U-100 (Humulin R, Novolin R) may be administered subcutaneously, intramuscularly, or intravenously. This is the only type of insulin that may be administered intravenously. Regular insulin U-500 (Humulin R U-500) should only be administered subcutaneously.

Inhaled regular insulin (Afrezza) is unique. It is administered by inhalation. It is available in different colored cartridges.

Insulin aspart (NovoLog) is a rapid-acting insulin analog. It is made by substituting aspartic acid for one of the amino acids in insulin. It is similar to Humalog, but Humalog contains the amino acid lysine. Insulin aspart may also be used with a pump. Each dose should be injected before meals. In order to maintain glucose levels, a longer-acting insulin may be needed.

Insulin glulisine (Apidra) is another rapid-acting insulin. Insulin glulisine is available in vials and in pens. It can be injected immediately before or after meals.

Insulin lispro (Humalog) is a rapid-onset insulin, so patients can inject it immediately before or after meals. In this way, the dose can be adjusted depending on the amounts and types of foods eaten. In addition, blood glucose can be tested, and then the drug can be dosed accordingly. It may be used with a pump to maintain proper blood glucose levels. Insulin lispro is available in two concentrations: 100 units/mL and 200 units/mL. The 100 units/mL formulation is available in vials and insulin pens; the 200 units/mL formulation is available in insulin pens only.

Neutral protamine Hagedorn (NPH) insulin (Humulin N, Novolin N) is an intermediate-acting insulin. NPH insulin can be used alone or in combination with other insulins, such as regular insulin. NPH insulin appears cloudy.

Insulin glargine (Lantus, Toujeo SoloStar) is a synthetic type of long-acting insulin. It differs from human insulin by three amino acids. Insulin glargine is associated with less nocturnal hypoglycemia and weight gain than conventional insulin. Because it precipitates when injected in subcutaneous tissue, insulin glargine may cause pain at the injection site. The precipitation causes the insulin to be absorbed slowly and to maintain a relatively constant blood level over 24 hours. There is no noticeable peak in action, and insulin glargine more closely approximates physiologic

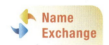

Name Exchange

You may hear other healthcare practitioners refer to insulin glargine more frequently by the brand name Lantus.

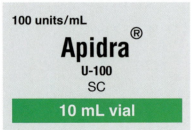

100 units/mL
Apidra®
U-100
SC
10 mL vial

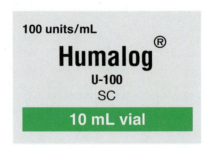

100 units/mL
Humalog®
U-100
SC
10 mL vial

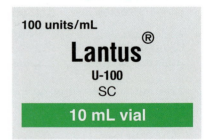

100 units/mL
Lantus®
U-100
SC
10 mL vial

Insulin is available in various types.

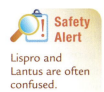

insulin release. It cannot be mixed with any other insulin. Insulin glargine is available in two concentrations: 100 units/mL and 300 units/mL. The 100 units/mL product is available under the brand name Lantus (in both vials and pens) and the 300 units/mL product is available as Toujeo SoloStar (only as a pen).

Insulin detemir (Levemir) is also classified as a long-acting insulin. Insulin detemir is used as a basal insulin. It may require twice daily administration. Insulin detemir is available in vials and insulin pens.

Insulin degludec (Tresiba FlexTouch) is the newest long-acting insulin available and is available in two concentrations: 100 units/mL and 200 units/mL. Technicians must be alert to select the proper concentration. Selecting the wrong concentration could result in serious adverse effects, including death.

Contraindications Insulin glulisine, insulin lispro, and regular insulin are contraindicated during episodes of hypoglycemia.

Inhaled regular insulin is contraindicated in patients with chronic lung disease, such as asthma or chronic obstructive pulmonary disease (COPD).

Cautions and Considerations Because most hospitalizations and emergency room visits for patients with type 1 diabetes result from hypoglycemic events, the risk of hypoglycemia cannot be overemphasized. Patients must be instructed to recognize and treat low blood glucose when it occurs. Family members of an individual who uses insulin should be taught how to administer glucagon. This medication is given when the patient is unconscious because of hypoglycemia and cannot self-treat by ingesting a food or beverage containing sugar.

The different types of insulin are packaged in similar appearing boxes in similar volumes, which can cause confusion.

For most insulin products there are 100 units of insulin per mL, which means one bottle of insulin has 1,000 units. Remember that insulin is dispensed in milliliters, but administered in units, and the pharmacy technician must determine how long the insulin will last for each patient. Furthermore, doses must be correct for insurance reimbursement.

More concentrated insulin products (200 units/mL, 300 units/mL, and 500 units/mL) are available—pharmacy technicians should make sure that these are not given to patients in place of the 100 units per mL dose, as this mistake could be fatal.

All insulin products must be stored in the refrigerator until dispensed or used by the patient. Once insulin warms to room temperature, the protein begins to degrade. Therefore, patients should keep insulin vials or pens in the refrigerator until they use them. Once opened, most insulin vials will expire in 28 to 30 days. Most insulin pens are also good for one month after opening, but a few expire in 14 days. It is not considered counseling to make the patient aware of these dates because drug storage does not require the judgment of the pharmacist. If exposed to extreme heat or cold, insulin can be degraded. Patients should protect insulin from heat (e.g., do not keep it in a car during the summer) or freezing temperatures. Patients who are traveling by plane should keep insulin with them in a carry-on bag because air cargo areas on planes are not climate-controlled. Finally, patients should discard any insulin package that contains clumps or appears frosty.

Inhaled regular insulin has a boxed warning for acute bronchospasm in patients with chronic lung disease.

Drug Interactions Insulin may enhance the hypoglycemic effects of other agents used for diabetes. Beta blockers and salicylates may enhance the hypoglycemic effects of insulin. Thiazide diuretics may decrease the efficacy of insulin.

Incretin Therapies

Incretin drugs either mimic endogenous incretin hormones or change their metabolism to increase their activity. **Glucagon-like peptide-1 (GLP-1)** and **glucose-dependent insulinotropic polypeptide** are endogenous incretin hormones, which are produced in response to glucose arriving from the intestines. They have multiple physiologic effects. First, incretins facilitate proper timing and function of phase I and phase II insulin response. **Phase I insulin response** refers to the immediate burst of insulin that occurs with, or even slightly before, the first bite of food. **Phase II insulin response** refers to the continued but somewhat slower release of insulin in the hours after eating. In type 2 diabetes, both phase I and phase II insulin responses are blunted. Second, incretins inhibit glucagon production in the pancreas that otherwise promotes an undesirable increase in blood glucose. Third, incretins have some effect on appetite by producing **satiety**, a sensation of fullness and satisfaction. Many patients experience significant and sustained weight loss on incretin mimetics. (Other medications to treat diabetes—such as insulin, sulfonylureas and thiazolidinediones—are associated with weight gain.) Incretin drug therapies are used most often in combination with other medications used to treat type 2 diabetes. Common incretin drugs are listed in Table 14.14.

Abiglutide (Tanzeum), dulaglutide (Trulicity), exenatide (Byetta), exenatide ER (Bydureon), and **liraglutide (Victoza)** are injectable products that mimic the action of GLP-1. Because GLP-1 is released only when glucose is introduced to the bloodstream, hypoglycemia between meals does not occur. Like GLP-1, then, these drugs do not carry a risk of causing low blood glucose levels.

Pramlintide (Symlin) mimics **amylin**, a hormone coproduced with insulin that reduces glucagon production, slows gastric emptying, and produces satiety. This incretin mimetic can be used by patients with type 1 diabetes to supplement insulin.

TABLE 14.14   Commonly Used Incretin Therapies

Generic (Brand)	Pronunciation	Dosage Form	Dispensing Status
GLP-1 Agonists			
albiglutide (Tanzeum)	al-bi-GLOO-tide	Injection	Rx
dulaglutide (Trulicity)	doo-la-GLOO-tide	Injection	Rx
exenatide (Byetta)	ex-EN-a-tide	Injection	Rx
exenatide ER (Bydureon)	ex-EN-a-tide ee-rr	Injection	Rx
liraglutide (Victoza)	lir-a-GLOO-tide	Injection	Rx
pramlintide (Symlin)	PRAM-lin-tide	Injection	Rx
DPP-4 Inhibitors			
alogliptin (Nesina)	al-oh-GLIP-tin	Tablet	Rx
linagliptin (Tradjenta)	lin-a-GLIP-tin	Tablet	Rx
saxagliptin (Onglyza)	sax-a-GLIP-tin	Tablet	Rx
sitagliptin (Januvia)	si-ta-GLIP-tin	Tablet	Rx

The addition of pramlintide to an insulin regimen can dramatically reduce the amount of insulin a patient has to take. Pramlintide is injected 30 minutes prior to each meal or snack containing at least 30 g of carbohydrate.

Common side effects of GLP-1 drugs include nausea, vomiting, diarrhea, dizziness, fatigue, and headache. Nausea is common at the beginning of therapy but diminishes over time. Side effects can be minimized by beginning treatment at a low dose and increasing the dose slowly. Timing injections immediately before eating can reduce nausea, vomiting, and upset stomach. Over a period of several weeks, the patient can move the time of injection further ahead of eating until reaching 30 to 60 minutes prior to a meal.

Alogliptin (Nesina), linagliptin (Tradjenta), saxagliptin (Onglyza), and **sitagliptin (Januvia),** are oral **dipeptidyl peptidase-4 (DPP-4) inhibitors** that slow inactivation of incretin hormones, thereby allowing them to persist longer and produce beneficial effects. Satiety does not seem to be as pronounced with these agents, and thus weight loss is not usually an added benefit. They are taken daily without regard to food.

Common side effects of DPP-4 inhibitors include headache, nasopharyngitis (runny nose and sore throat), and upper respiratory tract infection. The reason for these unusual side effects is not fully understood.

Contraindications Contraindications for exenatide ER and liraglutide include a patient or family history of medullary thyroid carcinoma and multiple endocrine neoplasia type 2. Pramlintide use is contraindicated in patients with gastroparesis and hypoglycemia unawareness.

DPP-4 inhibitors should not be used for patients with pancreatitis.

Cautions and Considerations Exenatide use has been associated with pancreatitis (inflammation of the pancreas). Patients should stop taking exenatide immediately and seek medical attention if they experience persistent or serious abdominal pain, especially if it is accompanied by vomiting.

If pramlintide is given with insulin, the patient can be at serious risk for low blood glucose levels, and those signs and symptoms can appear within three hours of taking the medications. Blood glucose levels should be checked before and after the injection. In addition, patients should be instructed on how to treat low blood glucose when it occurs.

Doses of DPP-4 inhibitors are cleared by the kidneys, so they must be adjusted for patients with kidney disease. Patients with kidney problems should alert their prescribers so that proper dosing is ordered.

Injectable incretin products must be stored in the refrigerator until dispensed. Once these products reach room temperature, they begin to degrade. Injectable incretin products are good at room temperature for only 30 days. Therefore, patients should keep these products in the refrigerator until they begin using them. Once opened, they can be kept at room temperature. Patients should protect these products from temperature extremes.

Drug Interactions Androgens and corticosteroids may increase the hypoglycemic effects of all diabetes medications. All diabetes medications may enhance the hypoglycemic effects of other diabetes medications.

Exenatide may decrease the effectiveness of oral contraceptives.

DPP-4 inhibitors may enhance the adverse effects of other diabetes medications and angiotensin converting enzyme (ACE) inhibitors.

Metformin

Initial drug therapy for type 2 diabetes is usually **metformin (Glucophage)**. This drug can be used alone or in combination with other agents and works by inhibiting excess hepatic glucose production, a process that normally occurs at a slow rate overnight.

Metformin also increases insulin sensitivity in muscle and other body tissues. Metformin is typically taken two to three times a day with food or meals. When treatment begins, a low dose is prescribed to prevent upset stomach, abdominal cramps, and diarrhea. Slowly, the dose is increased. Metformin can take as long as three weeks to reach full effect. It usually does not cause hypoglycemia unless it is taken in combination with other agents for diabetes. In addition, metformin can promote mild weight loss (five to six pounds) and improve cholesterol profiles. The best time to test blood glucose when taking metformin is in the morning, just after waking. See Table 14.15 for metformin products. Metformin is paired with other antidiabetic agents into several combination products, which are not discussed in this text.

Common side effects of metformin include upset stomach, abdominal cramps, nausea, diarrhea, flatulence, and a metallic taste. These effects can be diminished or avoided by taking the medication with food and increasing the dose slowly. Over time, these side effects will decrease.

Serious but rare side effects include **lactic acidosis**, a potentially fatal condition that requires medical care and hospitalization. This side effect can usually be avoided if patients stop taking metformin when they are severely ill or hospitalized. The risk for lactic acidosis increases under the following circumstances:

- severe dehydration or altered fluid balance
- excessive alcohol consumption
- liver or kidney impairment (or taking other drugs that contribute to impairment)
- sepsis (a serious, acute infection in the bloodstream that requires intravenous [IV] antibiotics)
- unstable or acute heart failure

Contraindications Metformin is contraindicated for patients who have kidney dysfunction, liver problems, or heart failure because these conditions raise the risk for lactic acidosis. Metformin should also be avoided in the presence of shock, sepsis, or metabolic acidosis. This medication should also not be used in patients 80 years or older unless they have normal kidney function. The dose generally should not be increased to the maximum dose in older adults (over 80 years old).

Cautions and Considerations Metformin contains a boxed warning for increased risk of lactic acidosis. Patients who are taking metformin should temporarily discontinue the medication when undergoing procedures in which contrast dye or iodine substances are used. Such patients are usually instructed to stop taking metformin the day before the procedure and resume the medication 48 hours after the procedure. Drug interactions between these substances and metformin can precipitate kidney failure and lactic acidosis.

Drug Interactions The lactic acidosis side effect of metformin may be exacerbated by other drugs that can cause lactic acidosis (such as alcohol, carbonic anhydrase inhibitors, and topiramate).

TABLE 14.15 Metformin Products

Generic (Brand)	Pronunciation	Dosage Form	Dispensing Status
metformin (Glucophage)	met-FOR-min	Oral solution, tablet	Rx
Combination Products			
glipizide-metformin (Metaglip)	GLIP-i-zide met-FOR-min	Tablet	Rx
glyburide-metformin (Glucovance)	GLYE-byoo-ride met-FOR-min	Tablet	Rx
pioglitazone-metformin (Actoplus Met)	pye-oh-GLIT-a-zone met-FOR-min	Tablet	Rx
repaglinide-metformin (PrandiMet)	re-PAG-lin-ide met-FOR-min	Tablet	Rx
rosiglitazone-metformin (Avandamet)	roe-see-GLIT-a-zone met-FOR-min	Tablet	Rx
saxagliptin-metformin (Kombiglyze XR)	sax-a-GLIP-tin met-FOR-min	Tablet	Rx
sitagliptin-metformin (Janumet)	i-ta-GLIP-tin met-FOR-min	Tablet	Rx

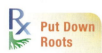

Put Down Roots

To recognize a meglitinide, look at the ending. They end in -glinide.

Safety Alert

Quinolone antibiotics and diabetes medications can interact and cause serious hypoglycemia. The pharmacy technician should always watch for these two drugs when dispensing.

Insulin Secretagogues

Agents that stimulate insulin production from the pancreas to directly lower blood glucose levels are known as **insulin secretagogues**. Two common classes of insulin secretagogues are **sulfonylureas** and **meglitinides**. Sulfonylureas include **glimepiride (Amaryl)**, **glipizide (Glucotrol)**, **glipizide ER (Glucotrol XL)**, and **glyburide (DiaBeta, Glynase, Micronase)**. Nateglinide (Starlix) and **repaglinide (Prandin)** are meglitinides.

Sulfonylureas and meglitinides differ in their onset and duration of action. Sulfonylureas can take 30 minutes or more to start working and can last for 8 hours or longer. Meglitinides act within 10 minutes and last around 2 hours. Sulfonylureas are used alone or in combination with other agents to treat type 2 diabetes. They are taken before breakfast each day and sometimes again before dinner. Meglitinides are used in combination with other agents to treat type 2 diabetes. They are taken just before eating and provide an extra boost of insulin for a specific meal. Table 14.16 provides information on common insulin secretagogues.

Low blood glucose reactions (hypoglycemia) are the most common side effect of these medications. Symptoms of hypoglycemia include shakiness, headache, blurred vision, dizziness, confusion, irritability, hunger, and tiredness. Hypoglycemia tends to occur when a patient takes the medication but then skips a meal or does more physical activity than usual. Patients can avoid this effect by not skipping meals or omitting a dose when they anticipate eating significantly less than usual on a particular day. Other side effects include nausea, diarrhea, and constipation.

Contraindications All sulfonylureas and meglitinides are contraindicated in the presence of diabetic ketoacidosis. Glipizide, glyburide, nateglinide, and repaglinide should not be used to treat type 1 diabetes mellitus. In addition, glyburide use is contraindicated with bosentan use, and repaglinide should not be used with gemfibrozil.

TABLE 14.16 Common Insulin Secretagogues

Generic (Brand)	Pronunciation	Dosage Form	Dispensing Status
Sulfonylureas			
glimepiride (Amaryl)	GLYE-me-pye-ride	Tablet	Rx
glipizide, glipizide ER (Glucotrol, Glucotrol XL)	GLIP-i-zide	Tablet	Rx
glyburide (DiaBeta, Glynase, Micronase)	GLYE-byoo-ride	Tablet	Rx
Meglitinides			
nateglinide (Starlix)	na-TEG-li-nide	Tablet	Rx
repaglinide (Prandin)	re-PAG-lin-ide	Tablet	Rx

Safety Alert

Do not confuse Glucotrol and Glucotrol XL.

Safety Alert

Do not confuse glyburide and glipizide.

Cautions and Considerations Because sulfonylureas and meglitinides increase the risk of hypoglycemia, patients should be informed of the symptoms of low blood glucose and know how to treat it. Patients should monitor their blood glucose level at home regularly and whenever they feel their level may be low. The best times to check blood glucose when taking sulfonylureas are first thing in the morning before eating (fasting) and then occasionally before other meals during the day. The best time to check blood glucose when taking meglitinides is one to two hours after meals. Patients with liver or kidney disease may not be able to take sulfonylureas depending on the agent chosen. Patients with these conditions should talk with their prescribers before taking one of these agents.

Drug Interactions Diabetes medications, androgens, and beta blockers increase the risk of hypoglycemia of other blood glucose lowering products. Loop diuretics may diminish the therapeutic effects of diabetes agents.

Sulfonylureas may enhance the adverse effects of alcohol (flushing is commonly seen). Cimetidine and fluconazole may increase the serum concentrations of sulfonylureas.

Calcium channel blockers, estrogens, isoniazid, nicotinic acid and phenothiazines may decrease the blood glucose lowering effects of meglitinides. Chloramphenicol, cyclosporine, probenecid, sulfonamide, and warfarin may increase the hypoglycemic effects of meglitinides.

Gemfibrozil increases serum concentrations of repaglinide, and coadministration is not recommended.

Thiazolidinediones

Agents known as **thiazolidinediones (TZDs)**—or **glitazones**—are used in combination with metformin or sulfonylureas to treat type 2 diabetes (see Table 14.17). The TZDs—**pioglitazone (Actos)** and **rosiglitazone (Avandia)**—work by directly increasing insulin sensitivity in cells of the body. TZDs connect with intracellular receptors to stimulate production of more insulin receptors. This process can take weeks to months to occur, and thus onset of effect is not immediate. The best time to check blood glucose levels when using TZDs is first thing in the morning before eating (fasting), and occasionally after meals during the day.

TABLE 14.17 Commonly Used TZDs

Generic (Brand)	Pronunciation	Dosage Form	Dispensing Status
pioglitazone (Actos)	pye-oh-GLIT-a-zone	Tablet	Rx
rosiglitazone (Avandia)	roe-zi-GLIT-a-zone	Tablet	Rx

Common side effects of TZDs include fluid accumulation (edema) and weight gain. If patients notice rapid weight gain or swelling, especially with shortness of breath, they should talk with their prescribers right away.

Rare but serious effects include liver toxicity and macular edema (swelling of the eye, resulting in distorted vision). If patients experience unexplained nausea, vomiting, abdominal pain, fatigue, or dark urine, they should report these symptoms to their healthcare prescribers. Regular blood tests are conducted to monitor liver function.

Patients with diabetes should see an eye doctor annually for an eye examination in which their pupils are dilated and their retinas are examined.

Contraindications Because TZDs can cause fluid retention and edema, pioglitazone and rosiglitazone therapies should not be initiated in patients with New York Heart Association (NYHA) class III or class IV heart failure.

Cautions and Considerations TZDs can worsen heart failure and have a boxed warning regarding this issue. Patients with heart failure should not take TZDs. Patients with edema or other heart problems may not be good candidates for TZD therapy. In some women with fertility problems, TZDs increase ovulation and pregnancy rates. Patients who are sexually active but do not want to become pregnant should use a contraceptive to prevent pregnancy.

Drug Interactions Diabetes medications, androgens, and beta blockers increase the risk of hypoglycemia of other blood glucose lowering products. Loop diuretics may diminish the therapeutic effects of diabetes agents.

Rosiglitazone should not be used with insulin because of the increased risk of fluid retention, heart failure, and hypoglycemia.

Sodium-Glucose Linked Transporter-2 Inhibitors

Sodium-glucose linked transporter-2 (SGLT-2) inhibitors, such as **canagliflozin (Invokana)**, **dapagliflozin (Farxiga)** and **empagliflozin (Jardiance)**, are a class of new medications used for type 2 diabetes (see Table 14.18). SGLT-2 inhibitors are taken once a day, often in combination with other oral agents such as metformin. They work by blocking the reabsorption of glucose that the kidney filters out of the bloodstream, thus increasing the excretion of glucose in the urine.

TABLE 14.18 Commonly Used SGLT-2 Inhibitors

Generic (Brand)	Pronunciation	Dosage Form	Dispensing Status
canagliflozin (Invokana)	kan-a-gli-FLOE-zin	Tablet	Rx
dapagliflozin (Farxiga)	dap-a-gli-FLOE-zin	Tablet	Rx
empagliflozin (Jardiance)	em-pag-gli-FLOE-zin	Tablet	Rx

Patients taking SGLT-2 inhibitors can experience urinary tract infections and genital fungal infections such as yeast infections. Patients who have a history of these types of infections prior to taking these medications should talk with their healthcare prescribers before taking SGLT-2 inhibitors. Some patients have experienced low blood pressure and high potassium blood levels from taking these drugs.

Contraindications The use of canagliflozin, dapagliflozin, and empagliflozin is contraindicated for patients with severe kidney impairment and end-stage renal disease, as well as for patients who are on dialysis.

Cautions and Considerations SGLT-2 inhibitors are not for use in patients with type 1 diabetes. They may cause hypotension. This effect may be pronounced in older adults and those who have kidney dysfunction or are using antihypertensive drugs. Kidney toxicity is a concern with use of SGLT-2 inhibitors. Hyperkalemia may occur with use. Patients using SGLT-2 inhibitors are at increased risk of certain fungal infections. Use with caution in patients with kidney or liver impairment.

Drug Interactions SGLT-2 inhibitors are associated with many drug interactions, only some of which are covered in this text.

Diabetes medications, androgens, and beta blockers increase the risk of hypoglycemia of other blood glucose lowering products. Loop diuretics may diminish the therapeutic effects of diabetes agents.

SGLT-2 inhibitors can increase the potassium-increasing effects of other drugs that increase potassium (such as ACE inhibitors, aliskiren, angiotensin receptor blockers, eplerenone, heparin, and potassium-sparing diuretics).

Carbamazepine, efavirenz, fosphenytoin, phenobarbital, phenytoin, primidone, and rifampin may decrease the serum concentration of canagliflozin.

Canagliflozin may increase the hypotensive effects of loop diuretics. Pimozide levels may be increased by canagliflozin.

Growth Disorders

From childhood to adulthood, **growth hormone (GH)** plays a fundamental role in metabolism. Measurements of height and weight over time serve as an index of physical and emotional health. Growth failure is a well-recognized disorder of childhood. In many children, a deficiency of endogenous growth hormone causes retardation of growth, which may be treated with exogenous hormone replacement.

Growth rates vary by sex and age throughout childhood. Growth delay may be caused by various factors including family growth patterns, genetic disorders, malnutrition, systemic or chronic illness, psychosocial stress, or a combination of these. In addition, growth delay may be due to an endocrine deficiency. Thyroxine, cortisol, insulin, and growth hormone all affect skeletal and somatic growth.

Nonendocrine-related disorders that can cause growth delay include intrauterine growth retardation, chromosomal defects, abnormal growth of cartilage or bone, poor nutrition, and a variety of systemic diseases. Some patients show a variation from normal growth (constitutional growth delay); these patients include those who are small for their age and those who have delay in skeletal growth, in the onset of puberty, and in adolescent development. Another type of growth delay is a family trait (i.e., it is inherited). These patients are shorter than their peers, but are comparable in height with other family members and grow at a parallel rate. Puberty occurs at the expected time and progresses as usual. However, adult height is short (less than 5 feet 4 inches for men, and less than 4 feet 11 inches for women).

Growth hormone is a mixture of peptides (short protein molecules) from the anterior pituitary gland released in response to **growth hormone-releasing factor (GHRF)**. The major component is the peptide somatotropin. The pituitary releases GH in response to stimulation by GHRF, which is secreted by the hypothalamus. GH release occurs irregularly throughout the day and during sleep stages III and IV (the deepest stages of non-REM sleep). GH stimulates the growth of skeletal muscle and connective tissue. It increases the rate of protein synthesis and fatty acid mobilization from adipose tissue and decreases the rate of glucose utilization. It is inhibited by glucocorticoids, obesity, depression, progesterone, hypokalemia, and altered thyroid function.

Growth Hormone Deficiency

Growth hormone deficiency, a disorder that occurs when the pituitary gland does not produce enough growth hormone, occurs in 1 in 5,000 children in a male-to-female ratio of 4:1. Among the known causes are intracranial infection (from tuberculosis and meningitis), skull fracture, radiation, and cancer. It can be treated by the administration of somatropin or other growth promotion agents.

Treatment of Growth Hormone Deficiency

Originally, **somatotropin** (as GH is called when produced naturally by the human body) was recovered from the pituitaries of human cadavers, a process that required 20 to 30 cadavers to obtain sufficient hormone to treat one patient. Today, the drug **somatropin (Genotropin, Humatrope, Omnitrope, Saizen, Serostim, Zomacton, Zorbtive)** is supplied through recombinant DNA technology. Genetic material from human cells is inserted into microorganisms, which then reproduce with the added genes and produce the hormone. The hormone is recovered, purified, and packaged. Table 14.19 presents the synthetic human growth hormones most commonly used as growth-promotion agents.

GH replacement therapy is most successful when begun at a young age. That is, the younger the patient at the time of GH treatment, the greater the height that may be achieved through replacement. Bone age and the extent of epiphyseal fusion at the time of treatment also influence the eventual response to GH. GH treatment is minimally effective if employed after ages 15 to 16 years old in boys or 14 to 15 years old in girls. Approximately 80%–90% of patients who receive GH experience "catch up" growth. Maximum increases in growth occur within the first 6 to 12 months of therapy, with a decline in response after that. GH therapy should be continued throughout childhood and adolescence to prevent slowing of growth velocity. When epiphyseal closure has occurred, little further response occurs. Treatment duration usually

TABLE 14.19 Most Commonly Used Synthetic Human Growth Hormones

Generic (Brand)	Pronunciation	Dosage Form	Dispensing Status
somatropin (Genotropin, Humatrope, Omnitrope, Saizen, Serostim, Zomacton, Zorbtive)	soe-ma-TROE-pin	Injection	Rx

ranges from 2 to 10 years. GH has not been effective for patients under the following conditions: other family members have short stature; growth retardation associated with psychosocial dwarfism; steroid-induced short stature; Down syndrome; bone and cartilage disorders; or renal, GI, or cardiac disease.

Contraindications Somatropin is contraindicated in pediatric patients with closed epiphyses, progression or recurrence of any underlying intracranial lesion or actively growing intracranial tumor, acute critical illness, acute respiratory failure, evidence of active malignancy, and active diabetes-related retinopathy. Patients with Prader-Willi syndrome who are obese, have a history of airway obstruction, or respiratory impairment should also not receive somatropin.

Cautions and Considerations Somatropin should be used with caution in patients with diabetes or with risk factors for impaired glucose tolerance. Insulin sensitivity may be decreased.

Intracranial hypertension has been reported with somatropin use. Fluid retention may also occur with use.

Scoliosis may progress in patients using somatropin who experience rapid growth.

Some somatropin formulations may contain benzyl alcohol. Large amounts of benzyl alcohol may be associated with neonatal gasping syndrome.

Hypothyroidism has been observed in less than 5% of treated patients. Thyroid supplementation is unnecessary, however, unless the patient has thyroid deficiency during treatment. The hypothyroidism appears to result from a change in the conversion of thyroxine or thyroid-controlling hormone rather than a true deficiency.

Drug Interactions Somatropin may decrease the hypoglycemic effect of diabetes medications. Cortisone and prednisone effectiveness may be diminished by somatropin use. Estrogen derivatives may decrease the effectiveness of somatropin.

Complementary and Alternative Therapies

Hormonal disorders are often treated with complementary and alternative medicine. A discussion of commonly used therapies is provided here.

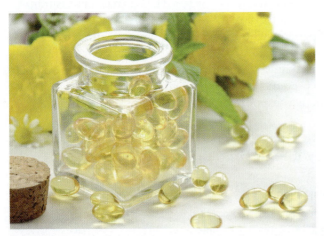

Evening primrose oil is available as a liquid and capsules, as pictured.

Therapies for Female Hormones

Soy, also known as isoflavone or **phytoestrogen**, is a plant source of protein used to treat several conditions. In the United States, it is used most frequently for hot flashes associated with menopause. Soy is a source of fiber and protein found most commonly in milk and dairy substitutes. It can be obtained from dietary sources alone or from a combination of food and oral supplements. It has estrogenic effects that can be beneficial for menopausal symptoms, diabetes, high cholesterol, osteoporosis, kidney disease, and, possibly, breast cancer prevention.

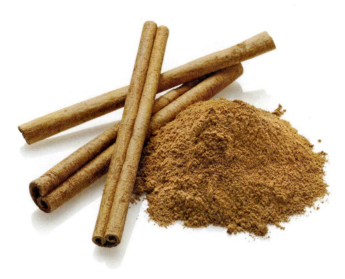

Although studies on its benefits have conflicting results, cinnamon may be used by patients with diabetes.

Soy is usually well tolerated but can cause upset stomach, diarrhea, constipation, bloating, nausea, and even insomnia in some cases. It can also worsen migraine headaches, especially for women whose headaches are related to hormonal fluctuations of the menstrual cycle.

Black cohosh is a plant product with estrogenic effects used for menopausal symptoms such as hot flashes. It is sometimes used in combination with St. John's wort for psychological symptoms that may be associated with menopause, such as depression and mood swings. Studies have not produced standard dosing, so success varies. Side effects of black cohosh include upset stomach, rash, headache, dizziness, weight gain, cramping, breast tenderness, and vaginal spotting (bleeding). Some concern exists about black cohosh and liver disease because some women have experienced hepatitis-type symptoms after taking black cohosh. Women with liver disease or those who are pregnant or breastfeeding should probably avoid black cohosh.

Evening primrose oil is sometimes used to reduce symptoms of menopause or premenstrual syndrome (PMS). However, studies have found mixed results and do not currently support its effectiveness for these conditions. Evidence for the use of evening primrose oil for osteoporosis is also mixed. It is considered safe to take, and few side effects have been reported.

Wild yam, also called Mexican yam, contains a phytoestrogen similar to soy, and it has mild estrogenic effects. It is applied topically or ingested orally as a tincture. Some women use it for menopausal symptoms such as hot flashes. Published research does not recommend a formulation or dose that is consistently effective. Ingestion of large amounts can cause vomiting. More research is needed to determine the clinical usefulness of wild yam.

Therapies for Diabetes

Chromium is an essential trace element that has been used for diabetes prevention and treatment. Its effectiveness is somewhat controversial, in that patients should not expect dramatic reductions in blood glucose levels from taking it. Patients with diabetes have been found to be deficient in chromium, but little definitive evidence is available to verify that correcting chromium deficiency is beneficial for improving blood glucose levels. Typical doses range from 200–1,000 mg a day. Side effects are rare but may include headache, insomnia, diarrhea, and hemorrhage. Patients with kidney or liver disease should not take chromium.

Cinnamon is often taken for type 2 diabetes. One initial study showed potential benefits, but all subsequent trials have shown that cinnamon has little effect on blood glucose levels. Although manufacturers of cinnamon products claim benefits, patients should know that taking cinnamon may not produce any noticeable effect on their blood glucose or hemoglobin A1c results. Patients with liver disease probably should not take cinnamon, because it has the potential to exacerbate hepatic conditions.

Therapies for Osteoporosis

When patients take prescription drugs for osteoporosis, they should also take calcium and vitamin D. Without calcium, osteoblasts cannot build more bone. Vitamin D improves calcium absorption from the GI tract. Therefore, calcium and vitamin D supplementation helps other osteoporosis agents work more effectively. Supplementation of calcium and vitamin D is also useful for patients with **osteopenia** (bone weakening), who are at high risk for developing osteoporosis. Often, vitamin D comes as a combination product with calcium. Vitamin D can be found in fish and is added to milk and breakfast cereals.

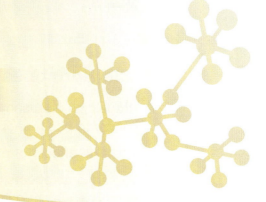

CHAPTER SUMMARY

The Endocrine System

- The endocrine system maintains the homeostasis by regulating physiologic functions involved in normal daily living and stress. The tissue affected by a hormone is called the target.

- Regulation of hormone synthesis is achieved via an intricate negative feedback mechanism involving the gland, the hypothalamic-pituitary axis, and autoregulation.

Thyroid Disorders

- The thyroid gland produces hormones that stimulate various body tissues to increase the level of activity.

- Thyroid replacement therapy should not be aimed at treating obesity.

- Hypothyroidism is treated with levothyroxine (Levoxyl, Synthroid, Tirosint, Unithroid), liothyronine (Cytomel, Triostat), or thyroid extract (Armour Thyroid).

- Hyperthyroidism is treated with propylthiouracil and methimazole (Tapazole).

Male Hormones and Sexual Dysfunction

- Testosterone undergoes extensive first-pass metabolism in the gastrointestinal tract and liver after oral administration. To overcome this problem, various testosterone derivatives and innovative dosage forms have been developed.

- Testosterone compounds are classified as Schedule III-controlled substances.

- Erectile dysfunction (ED) may have many causes, including testosterone deficiency, alcoholism, cigarette smoking, medications, and psychological factors.

- The following drugs may cause ED: alcohol, amphetamines, antidepressants, antihypertensives, corticosteroids, estrogens, H_2 blockers, haloperidol, lithium, and opiates.

- ED is treated primarily with phosphodiesterase-5 inhibitors sildenafil (Viagra), tadalafil (Cialis), and vardenafil (Levitra).

Female Hormones and Sexual Dysfunction

- Progestins are used primarily in oral contraceptive pills and to prevent uterine cancer in postmenopausal women taking hormone replacement therapy (HRT).

- The side effects of progestin are acne, depression, fatigue, and weight gain.

- The adverse effects of estrogen are nausea, fluid retention, breast tenderness, vomiting, weight gain, and breakthrough bleeding. Hypercoagulability is also attributed to estrogen use, especially if combined with nicotine.

- The decision to take HRT is personal and requires consultation between a woman and her physician. The advantages must be weighed against the disadvantages. The risks and benefits are different for each woman, depending on her family history and her own physical condition.

Contraceptives, Pregnancy, and Childbirth

- The advantages of oral contraceptives include ease of use, high efficacy rate, and relative safety. Most oral contraceptives are a combination of estrogen and progestin. They suppress ovulation by interfering with the production of hormones that regulate the menstrual cycle. They also alter the cervical mucus to prevent penetration of sperm, and they change the composition of the endometrium to inhibit implantation. The progestin-only pills rely on the effects of progestin on the cervical mucus and endometrium.

- Some studies indicate that oral contraceptives should not be prescribed to women who have hypertension, diabetes mellitus, or elevated cholesterol. Women should not smoke while taking oral contraceptives.

- Many forms of contraceptives are on the market. They are available in pill form, patches, rings, injections, implants, and intrauterine devices.

- Emergency contraceptives are available over the counter and by prescription.

- Oral contraceptives can interact with the following classes of drugs: antibiotics, anticonvulsants, antifungals, benzodiazepines, bronchodilators, corticosteroids, lipid-lowering agents, and tricyclic antidepressants (TCAs).

- Pregnancy tests detect the presence of the hormone human chorionic gonadotropin (hCG). The home pregnancy tests on the market are very simple to use.

Osteoporosis

- Lifestyle changes to decrease bone loss include increasing calcium intake, ceasing cigarette smoking and heavy caffeine use, and engaging in weight-bearing exercises.

- Bisphosphonates are the drug class most commonly used to treat osteoporosis.

- Alendronate (Fosamax) is a bisphosphonate approved by the FDA for the treatment of osteoporosis. It should be taken 30 minutes before the first meal of the day with a full glass of water; the patient must not lie down or eat for 30 minutes after taking it.

- Calcitonin (Miacalcin) suppresses the bone resorption activity of osteoclasts.

Adrenal Gland Disorders and Corticosteroid Therapy

- Corticosteroids are used as anti-inflammatories, immunosuppressants, and in treating diseases of hematologic, allergic, neoplastic, and autoimmune origin.

- Addison's disease is a deficiency of glucocorticoids and mineralocorticoids; Cushing's disease is caused by an overproduction or excessive administration of steroids over an extended period.

- Corticosteroids have adverse effects with metabolic, cardiovascular, gastrointestinal, immunologic, dermatologic, musculoskeletal, ophthalmic, and neuropsychiatric implications. They should be used with great caution in treating patients with diabetes, hypertension, heart failure, severe infections, and ulcers. If possible, patients should take the dose in the morning to minimize hypothalamic-pituitary axis suppression and side effects. This more closely mimics the circadian rhythm of the body's release of corticosteroids.

Diabetes

- The four types of diabetes are type 1, type 2, gestational, and secondary.

- Type 1 diabetes patients must have insulin. Type 2 diabetes patients may be able to control the disease through diet and exercise, but often they have to add drug therapy (including insulin). Gestational diabetes usually goes away after the baby's birth, but the mother is at high risk of developing type 2 diabetes. Secondary (drug-induced) diabetes can return to normal when the drug is discontinued.

- Short-term hypoglycemia is dangerous, but long-term hyperglycemia has devastating complications. Retinopathy, neuropathy, nephropathy, and vascular and dermatologic complications can affect the quality and length of life.

- In an emergency situation, insulin may not require a prescription. Most insulins require a prescription. Some states require a prescription for needles.

- Insulin lispro (Humalog) is a rapid-onset insulin, so patients can inject it immediately before or after meals.

- Insulin glargine (Lantus, Toujeo SoloStar) is a long-acting insulin that provides a constant concentration over 24 hours. It more closely approximates physiologic insulin release.

Growth Disorders

- Measurement of height and weight over time serves as an index of physical and emotional health. A deficiency of growth hormone causes growth failure.

- Human growth hormone is manufactured with recombinant DNA technology.

- Once epiphyseal closure has occurred, little further response to GH treatment can be expected.

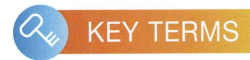

KEY TERMS

AB rated when a generic and a brand name drug are rated as bioequivalent by the FDA, as shown by an experimental study and listed in the Orange Book

ablation the removal or reduction of a malfunctioning gland

Addison's disease a life-threatening deficiency of glucocorticoids and mineralocorticoids that is treated with the daily administration of corticosteroids

alopecia hair loss

amylin a hormone coproduced with insulin that reduces glucagon production, slows gastric emptying, and produces satiety

androgen hormone promoting development and maintenance of male characteristics

basal insulin insulin released throughout the day to allow energy for basic cellular function

bisphosphonate drug used with estrogen to reduce osteoporosis

bolus insulin insulin released at mealtimes to react with glucose entering the body from food intake

bone mineral density (BMD) a machine that uses X-ray and ultrasound technology to determine bone density measurements

cervical cap a contraceptive device inserted inside the vagina that fits over the cervix to prevent sperm from entering the uterus

circadian regularly recurring on a cycle of 24 hours

climacteric the syndrome of endocrine, somatic, and psychological changes occurring at the end of the reproductive period in females

contraception medicines or devices used to prevent pregnancy

corticosteroid steroid hormone produced by the adrenal cortex

Cushing's syndrome a disease caused by overproduction of steroids or by excessive administration of corticosteroids over an extended period

diabetes a disease characterized by high blood glucose due to insufficient levels of insulin

diaphragm a contraceptive device inserted inside the vagina to prevent sperm from entering the uterus

dipeptidyl peptidase-4 (DPP-4) inhibitors a class of oral hypoglycemics that are used to treat type 2 diabetes

dispense as written (DAW) instruction in a prescription to prevent substitution of generic drugs for the branded drug

dyspareunia a condition of the female in which normal intercourse is painful

emergency contraceptives drugs taken within 120 hours of having sex that stop the release of an egg from the ovary to prevent fertilization by sperm; if the patient is already pregnant, the drug will have no effect

endocrine system glands and other structures that control internal secretions, called hormones, that are released directly into the circulatory system

endometrium the inner lining of the uterus, which grows in the early part of the menstrual cycle to be ready to receive a fertilized egg and breaks down at the end of the cycle, leading to menstruation

erectile dysfunction (ED) failure of the male to initiate or maintain an erection until ejaculation

estrogen one of the group of hormones that stimulate the growth of reproductive tissue in women

exophthalmos a condition in which fat collects behind the eyeball

feedback mechanism the return of some of the output of a system as input to exert some control on the process

female condom worn by a woman and forms a physical barrier between the penis and the vagina

female sexual dysfunction marked by persistent recurrent problems with sexual response, including decreased desire, reduced arousal, inability to achieve orgasm, and pain during sexual intercourse

female-to-male (FTM) gender reassignment that involves terminating menstruation and inducing the development of traditionally male appearance

gender reassignment the process of using drug therapy and/or surgery to change a person's body to match their gender identity

gestational diabetes diabetes that occurs during pregnancy when insufficient insulin is produced

glitazone thiazolidinediones that lower blood glucose

glucagon-like peptide-1 (GLP-1) a class of endogenous incretin hormones; used to treat diabetes

glucocorticoid corticosteroid involved in metabolism and immune system regulation

gluconeogenesis the process of forming new glucose, in which protein and fatty acids are converted into immediate energy sources

glucose-dependent insulinotropic polypeptide a class of endogenous incretin hormones; used to treat diabetes

glycosylated hemoglobin (HbA1C) an "average" of the sugar measured in blood glucose over a period of time (*Hb* stands for hemoglobin)

Graves' disease a condition in which the production of the thyroid hormone is increased

growth hormone (GH) a fundamental hormone that affects metabolism, skeletal growth, and somatic growth; deficiency causes growth retardation

growth hormone deficiency a condition when the body doesn't produce the regular amount of growth hormone, which leads to stunted height or muscle development

growth hormone-releasing factor (GHRF) a neuropeptide secreted by the hypothalamus that stimulates the secretion of growth hormone by the pituitary

gynecomastia excessive development of the male mammary glands, with or without tenderness

hip fractures breaks and cracks in the hip bone

hirsutism abnormal hairiness, especially in women

hormone therapy (HT) replacement of deficient hormones such as estrogen

hormones secretions released by glands into the circulatory system that have specific regulatory effects on organs and other tissues

human chorionic gonadotropin (hCG) glycoprotein produced by trophoblastic cells and their descendants in the placenta

hydrocortisone the pharmaceutical term for cortisol

hyperglycemia elevated blood sugar level

hyperthyroidism a condition caused by excessive thyroid hormone and marked by increased metabolic rate; also called *thyrotoxicosis*

hypoglycemia low blood glucose level (less than 70 mg/dL)

hypogonadism a deficiency of hormone production and secretion

hypothyroidism a deficiency of thyroid activity that results in a decreased metabolic rate, tiredness, and lethargy in adults, and causes cretinism in children

insulin a hormone that helps cells burn glucose for energy

insulin pumps devices that deliver insulin through a tiny tube inserted just under the skin

insulin secretagogues agents that stimulate insulin production from the pancreas to directly lower blood glucose levels

intermediate-acting insulin begins to be effective in 30–60 minutes and lasts 6 to 8 hours in most cases

intrauterine device (IUD) a small contraceptive device placed into the uterus by a healthcare practitioner every 5–10 years

lactic acidosis a potentially fatal condition that requires medical care and hospitalization

long-acting insulin works for approximately 24 hours and is injected once a day

male condom placed over the erect penis before sexual intercourse

male-to-female (MTF) gender reassignment that involves the reduction of the effects of androgen

meglitinides drugs that stimulate insulin release from the pancreatic cells

melasma dark skin patches on the face

mineralocorticoid corticosteroid involved in electrolyte and water balance

neuropathy a lack of blood flow to nerves that leaves them unable to function

nonvirilized description of people born with a Y chromosome lacking male secondary sex characteristics

oral contraceptive (OC) a combination of one or more hormonal compounds taken orally to prevent the occurrence of pregnancy

oral thyroid supplementation drug given to artificially provide adequate hormone levels

Orange Book a government-approved listing of drugs that are therapeutically equivalent to each other (e.g., brand and generic); officially known as the *Approved Drug Products with Therapeutic Equivalence Evaluations*

osteoblast a cell that forms bone

osteoclast a cell that resorbs bone

osteopenia bone weakening

osteoporosis the condition of reduced bone mineral density, disrupted microarchitecture of bone structure, and increased likelihood of fracture

oxytocic agent a drug that promotes contraction of uterine muscle at term of pregnancy

phase I insulin response the immediate burst of insulin that occurs with the first bite of food

phase II insulin response the continued but somewhat slower release of insulin in the hours after eating

phosphodiesterase-5 (PDE-5) inhibitors the class of drugs most frequently used to treat ED

phytoestrogen an estrogen occurring naturally in certain seedpod plants

prandial mealtime

progesterone the hormone that prepares the uterus for the reception and development of the fertilized ovum

progestin a synthetic hormone that emulates the effects of progesterone

rapid-acting insulin insulin that begins to work in 10 minutes and lasts as long as 2 hours

retinopathy when the blood vessels in the eyes become damaged and rupture, causing loss of sight

satiety a sensation of fullness and satisfaction

secondary diabetes diabetes caused by drugs

selective estrogen receptor modulators (SERMs) estrogen receptors that mimic the beneficial effects of estrogen on bone mineral density

self-injector pens a syringe that only needs to pierce the skin to pump medicine into the body

short-acting insulin insulin that begins to work in around 30 minutes and lasts up to 4 hours

sodium-glucose linked transporter-2 (SGLT-2) inhibitors a class of medications used for type 2 diabetes that are taken once a day

somatotropin the agent synthesized with recombinant DNA technology to produce synthetic human growth hormones

spermicide an agent that kills sperm cells on contact

sulfonylureas diabetes medications that increase secretion of insulin from the pancreas

syringes a tube with a hollow needle attached used for ejecting liquid in a thin stream

T-score the estimate of risk (not a diagnosis) for bone density issues

target a cell, tissue, or organ that is affected by a particular hormone

testosterone a hormone that is responsible for sperm production, sexual potency, and the maintenance of muscle mass and strength, among other functions

thiazolidinediones (TZDs) drugs that lower blood glucose by improving cellular response to insulin

thyroid gland a gland that produces hormones that stimulate various body tissues to increase their activity level

thyroid storm a life-threatening medical emergency with the symptoms of thyrotoxicosis, but more exaggerated

thyroxine (T_4) a hormone produced by the thyroid gland that can increase metabolic activity; tends to be less active than triiodothyronine (T_3)

tocolytic agent a drug that slows labor in pregnancy; used to treat premature labor

transdermal contraceptives the use of a stick-on patch to deliver a combination of estrogen and progesterone in a steady supply through the skin

transgender an umbrella term for people who express discomfort or dissatisfaction with the gender identity and roles assigned to them at birth

transsexual a subset of transgender; people who have gone through the process of gender reassignment

triiodothyronine (T_3) a hormone produced by the thyroid gland that can increase metabolic activity; tends to be more active than thyroxine (T_4)

type 1 diabetes insulin-dependent diabetes, in which the pancreas has no ability to produce insulin

type 2 diabetes a type of diabetes characterized by insulin insufficiency or by the resistance of the target tissues to the insulin produced

vaginal ring is a combination contraceptive that is inserted into that vagina, contains synthetic estrogen and progesterone

vasomotor affecting constriction and dilation of blood vessels

vials long tubes to hold medicine

virilization the development of male characteristics

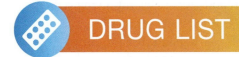

DRUG LIST

Thyroid Preparations

Drugs to Treat Hypothyroidism

levothyroxine, T_4 (Levoxyl, Synthroid, Tirosint, Unithroid)
liothyronine (Cytomel, Triostat)
thyroid extract (Armour Thyroid)

Drugs to Treat Hyperthyroidism

methimazole (Tapazole)
propylthiouracil (PTU)

Drugs to Treat Erectile Dysfunction

alprostadil (Caverject, Edex, Muse, Prostin)
avanafil (Stendra)
sildenafil (Viagra)
tadalafil (Cialis)
testosterone (Androderm, AndroGel, Striant, Testoderm)
vardenafil (Levitra)

Hormone Replacement Therapy Products

Progestin-Only

progesterone (Crinone, Endometrin, First-Progesterone, Prometrium)

Estrogen-Only Hormone Therapy Products

conjugated estrogen (Premarin)
estradiol (Alora, Climara, Divigel, Elestrin, Estrogel, Evamist, Femring, Menostar, Minivelle, Vivelle-Dot)
estropipate (Ogen, Ortho-Est)

Estrogen-Progestin Hormone Therapy Products

conjugated estrogen-medroxyprogesterone (Premphase, Prempro)
estradiol-levonorgestrel (Climara Pro)

estradiol-norethindrone (Activella, CombiPatch)
estradiol-norgestimate (Prefest)
ethinyl estradiol-norethindrone (femhrt)

Contraceptives

Combination Oral Contraceptives

ethinyl estradiol-desogestrel (Apri, Azurette, Caziant, Cyclessa, Desogen, Emoquette, Enskyce, Kariva, Mirecette, Orth-Cept, Reclipsen, Solia, Velivet, Viorele)
ethinyl estradiol-drospirenone (Beyaz, Gianvi, Loryna, Nikki, Ocella, Syeda, Vestura, Yasmin, Yaz, Zarah)
ethinyl estradiol-ethynodiol diacetate (Kelnor, Zovia)
ethinyl estradiol-levonorgestrel (Traditional: Altavera, Amethyst, Aviane, Enpresse, Falmina, Lessina, Levora, Lutera, Lybrel, Marlissa, Myzilra, Orsythia, Portia, Trivora; Extended combinations: Amethia, Camrese, Introvale, Jolessa, Quasense, Quartette, Seasonique)
Ethinyl estradiol-norethindrone (Alyacen, Aranelle, Brevicon, Cyclafem, Dasetta, Estrostep, femhrt, Leena, Junel, Loestrin, Lo Minastrin, Microgenstin, Necon, Norinyl, Nortrel, Ortho-Novum, Ovcon, Tilia, Tri-Legest, Tri-Norinyl)
ethinyl estradiol-norgestimate (MonoNessa, Ortho-Cyclen, Ortho-TriCyclen, Ortho-TriCyclen Lo, Previfem, Sprintec, TriNessa, Tri-Previfem, Tri-Sprintec)
ethinyl estradiol-norgestrel (Cryselle 28, Elinest, Low-Ogestrel, Norgestrel, Ogestrel, Ovral)

Progestin-Only Contraceptives

norethindrone (Camila, Errin, Heather, Jolivette, Lyza, Micronor, Nora-BE, Nor-QD)

Emergency Contraceptives

levonorgestrel (Plan B, Plan B One-Step, Next Choice, Next Choice One Dose, Take Action)
ulipristal (ella)

Other Hormonal Contraceptives

ethinyl estradiol etonogestrel (NuvaRing)
ethinyl estradiol-norelgestromin (Ortho Evra)
medroxyprogesterone (Depo-Provera, Provera)

Implant Device

etonogestrel (Implanon)

Intrauterine Devices

copper (ParaGard)
levonorgestrel (Liletta, Mirena, Skyla)

Drugs Used for Female Sexual Dysfunction

flibanserin (Addyi)

Drugs Used for Heavy Menstrual Bleeding

estradiol-dienogest (Natazia)
tranexamic acid (Lysteda)

Drugs Used at Birth

dinoprostone (Cervidil, Prepidil, Prostin E)
magnesium sulfate
misoprostol (Cytotec)
nifedipine (Procardia)
oxytocin (Pitocin)

Agents for Bone Diseases

Bisphosphonates

alendronate (Fosamax, Fosamax Plus D)
ibandronate (Boniva)
pamidronate (Aredia)
risedronate (Actonel)
zoledronic acid (Reclast)

Selective Estrogen Receptor Modulators (SERMs)

raloxifene (Evista)

Other Drugs for Osteoporosis

calcitonin (Miacalcin)
denosunab (Prolia)
teriparatide (Forteo)

Corticosteroids

budesonide (Entocort EC)
cortisone
dexamethasone (Baycadron, Dexamethasone, DexPak)
hydrocortisone (A-Hydrocort, Cortef, Solu-Cortef)
prednisone
triamcinolone

Agent for Diabetic Ulcers

becaplermin gel (Regranex)

Agents for Diabetes

Rapid-Acting

inhaled regular insulin (Afrezza)
insulin aspart (NovoLog)
insulin glulisine (Apidra)
insulin lispro (Humalog)

Short-Acting

Regular insulin (Humulin R, Novolin R)

Intermediate-Acting

neutral protamine Hagedorn (NPH) insulin (Humulin N, Novolin N)
regular insulin U-500 (Humulin R U-500)

Long-Acting

insulin degludec (Tresiba)
insulin detemir (Levemir)
insulin glargine (Lantus, Toujeo SoloStar)

Premixed

insulin NPH/regular 70/30 (Humulin 70/30, Novolin 70/30, ReliOn Novolin 70/30)
insulin lispro protamine/lispro 75/25 (Humalog 75/25)

insulin aspart protamine-aspart 70/30
(Novolog 70/30)
insulin lispro protamine-lispro 50/50
(Humalog 50/50)

Incretin Therapies

GLP-1 Agonists

abiglutide (Tazeum)
dulaglutide (Trulicity)
exenatide (Byetta)
exenatide ER (Bydureon)
liraglutide (Victoza)
pramlintide (Symlin)

DPP-4 Inhibitors

alogliptin (Nisena)
linagliptin (Tradjenta)
saxagliptin (Onglyza)
sitagliptin (Januvia)

Metformin

metformin (Glucophage)

Sulfonylureas

glimepiride (Amaryl)
glipizide, glipizide ER (Glucotrol,
Glucotrol XL)
glyburide (DiaBeta, Glynase, Micronase)

Meglitinides

nateglinide (Starlix)
repaglinide (Prandin)

Thiazolidinediones (TZDs)

pioglitazone (Actos)
rosiglitazone (Avandia)

SGLT-2 Inhibitors

canagliflozin (Invokana)
dapagliflozin (Farxiga)
empagliflozin (Jardiance)

Metformin Combinations

glipizide-metformin (Metaglip)
glyburide-metformin (Glucovance)
pioglitazone-metformin (Actoplus Met)
repaglinde-metformin (Prandimet)
rosiglitazone-metformin (Avandamet)
saxagliptin-metformin (Kombiglyze XR)
sitagliptin-metformin (Janumet)

Synthetic Human Growth Hormones

somatropin (Genotropin, Humatrope,
Omnitrope, Saizen, Serostim, Zomacton,
Zorbtive)

Black Box Warnings

alprostadil (Caverject, Edex, Muse)
becaplermin gel (Regranex)
conjugated estrogen (Cenestin, Enjuvia,
Premarin)
conjugated estrogen-medroxyprogesterone
(Premphase, Prempro)
dinoprostone (Cervidil, Prepidil, Prostin E)
estradiol (Alora, Climara, Divigel, Elestrin,
Estrogel, Estring, Evamist, Femring,
Menostar, Minivelle, Vivelle, Vivelle-Dot)
estradiol-drospirenone (Angeliq)
estradiol-levonorgestrol (Climara Pro)
estradiol-norethindrone (Activella,
CombiPatch)
estradiol-norgestimate (Prefest)
estropipate (Ogen, Ortho-Est)
ethinyl estradiol (Estinyl)
ethinyl estradiol-desogestrel (Apri, Azurette,
Caziant, Cyclessa, Desogen, Emoquette,
Enskyce, Kariva, Mirecette, Orth-Cept,
Reclipsen, Solia, Velivet, Viorele)
ethinyl estradiol-drospirenone (Gianvi,
Loryna, Nikki, Ocella, Safyral, Syeda,
Vestura, Yasmin, Yaz, Zarah)
ethinyl estradiol-ethynodiol diacetate
(Kelnor, Zovia)
ethinyl estradiol-etonogestrel (NuvaRing)
ethinyl estradiol-levonorgestrel (Traditional:
Altavera, Amethyst, Aviane, Enpresse,
Falmina, Lessina, Levora, Lutera, Lybrel,
Marlissa, Myzilra, Orsythia, Portia,
Trivora;
Extended combinations: Amethia,
Camrese, Introvale, Jolessa, Quasense,
Quartette, Seasonique)
ethinyl estradiol-norethindrone (Aranelle,
Brevicon, Cyclafem, Dasetta, Estrostep,
Femhrt, Leena, Junel, Loestrin, Lo
Minastrin, Microgenstin, Necon, Norinyl,
Nortrel, Ortho-Novum, Ovcon, Tilia,
Tri-Legest, Tri-Norinyl)

ethinyl estradiol–norgestimate (MonoNessa, Ortho-Cyclen, Ortho-TriCyclen, Ortho-TriCyclen Lo, Previfem, Sprintec, TriNessa, Tri-Previfem, Tri-Sprintec)

ethinyl estradiol–norgestrel (Cryselle 28, Elinest, Low-Ogestrel, Norgestrel, Ogestrel, Ovral)

flibanserin (Addyi)

glipizide-metformin (Metaglip)

glyburide-metformin (Glucovance)

inhaled regular insulin (Afrezza)

levonorgestrel (Next Choice, Norplant, Norplant II, One Step, Plan B)

levothyroxine (Levothroid, Levoxyl, Synthroid, Tirosint, Unithroid)

linagliptin-metformin (Jentadueto)

liraglutide (Victoza)

medroxyprogesterone (Depo-Provera, Provera)

methimazole (Tapazole)

metformin (Glucophage)

metformin-sitagliptin (Janumet)

metronidazole (Flagyl)

misoprostol (Cytotec)

oxytocin (Pitocin)

pioglitazone (Actos)

pioglitazone-metformin (Actoplus Met)

pramlintide (Symlin)

progesterone (Crinone, Endometrin, First-Progesterone Prometrium)

propylthiouracil (PTU)

repaglinide-metformin (Prandimet)

rosiglitazone-glimepride (Avandryl)

rosiglitazone-metformin (Avandamet)

saxagliptin-metformin (Kombiglyze XR)

teriparatide (Forteo)

testosterone (Androderm, AndroGel, Striant, Testoderm)

thyroid extract (Armour Thyroid)

Medication Guides

alendronate (Fosamax)

alendronate-cholecalciferol (Fosamax Plus D)

alogliptin (Nesina)

canagliflozin (Invokana)

dapagliflozin (Farxiga)

denosumab (Prolia)

exenatide (Byetta)

flibanserin (Addyi)

ibandronate (Boniva)

inhaled regular insulin (Afrezza)

liraglutide (Victoza)

metformin-sitagliptin (Janumet)

pioglitazone (Actos)

pioglitazone-metformin (Actoplus Met)

pramlintide (Symlin)

raloxifene (Evista)

risedronate (Actonel)

rosiglitazone-glimepride (Avandaryl)

rosiglitazone-metformin (Avandamet)

saxagliptin-metformin (Kombiglyze XR)

sitagliptin (Januvia)

teriparatide (Forteo)

testosterone (Androderm, AndroGel, Striant, Testoderm)

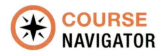

COURSE NAVIGATOR

Access interactive chapter review exercises, practice activities, flash cards, and study games.

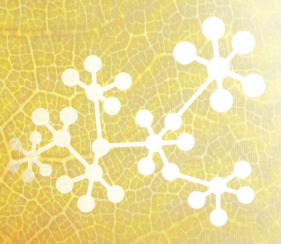

15

Topical, Ophthalmic, and Otic Medications

Learning Objectives

1 Describe the skin as an organ.

2 Describe the physiology of the skin.

3 Describe the classes of topical drugs and the skin conditions they treat.

4 Explain the action of topical corticosteroids and their application.

5 Recognize the classes of antiseptics and disinfectants.

6 Recognize ophthalmic and otic agents and their uses.

COURSE NAVIGATOR

Access additional chapter resources.

Topical, ophthalmic, and otic medications are used to treat a variety of conditions, such as skin disorders, allergic and inflammatory reactions, infections, infestations, glaucoma, conjunctivitis, and otalgia. These classes of drugs range from mild agents to stronger forms of antibiotics, antiseptics, disinfectants, and corticosteroids.

The Integumentary System

The integumentary system refers to the tissue that covers the body and includes skin, nails, and hair. This system protects the body from exposure to harmful pathogens and harsh substances and helps to regulate body temperature. Accounting for 16% of body weight, the skin is the largest organ. It is equipped to deal with microbial, chemical, and physical assaults on the body. It is also an important source of sensory input and is the main organ involved in temperature regulation. The correction of skin defects may be indicated, even when they do not pose a hazard to health, to aid the psychological well being of the affected person.

Figure 15.1 illustrates the anatomy of the skin. The **epidermis** is the top layer of the skin and is derived from embryonic ectoderm. It continually forms new cells in a basal layer; sheds old, dead cells; and also produces nails, hair, and glands. Pressure or friction on any part of the body stimulates skin growth, resulting in a thickening of cells called a *callus*. Melanocytes, cells that produce the pigment

FIGURE 15.1
**Anatomy of
the Skin**

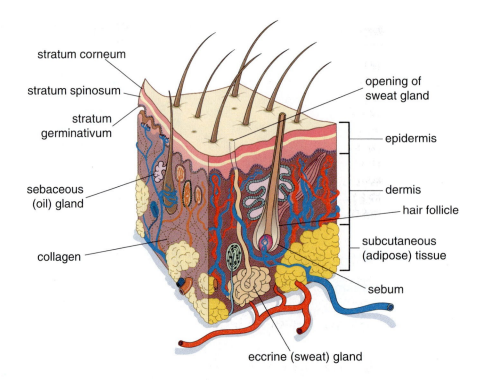

stratum corneum

stratum spinosum

stratum
germinativum

sebaceous
(oil) gland

collagen

opening of
sweat gland

epidermis

dermis

hair follicle

subcutaneous
(adipose) tissue

sebum

eccrine (sweat) gland

melanin, are interspersed throughout the epidermis, with most just slightly below the basal layer.

The **dermis**, which is below the epidermis, is composed of connective tissue with upward projections into the epidermis. It is supplied with capillaries and sensory nerve terminals that do not penetrate the epidermis. The dermis contains smooth muscle at hair follicles (arrector pili), in sheets in the areola of the nipple, and in the scrotum, where the muscle action causes wrinkled skin.

Two types of glands are widely distributed in the skin: sebaceous glands and sweat glands. **Sebaceous glands** secrete sebum, a substance that oils the skin and hair, preventing them from drying, and that is also toxic to certain types of bacteria. Most sebaceous glands develop from hair follicles and empty their secretions into the follicles. The other sebaceous glands empty their secretions directly onto the surface of the epidermis. The product of most of the body's **sweat glands** (called eccrine sweat glands) consists of water and salts. The larger, deeper sweat glands of the axillary, perineal, and genital regions (called apocrine sweat glands) produce sweat containing various organic materials that can produce an offensive odor when broken down by bacteria on the skin. The apocrine glands in the skin of the external ear canal produce cerumen (earwax), which has antibacterial and antifungal activity; it also contains squamous cells and dust.

The **subcutaneous tissue** is the innermost layer of the skin and connects the dermis to underlying organs and tissues. This layer is composed of elastic fibers, also called fascia, and a layer of fat cells, called **adipose tissue**. The thickness of the subcutaneous layer varies depending on the region of the body. Female breast tissue arises from the subcutaneous layer.

Sun Exposure and Skin Cancer

Energy from the sun reaches the earth as electromagnetic radiation. Familiar examples of electromagnetic radiation are radio waves, microwaves, visible light, ultraviolet light,

TABLE 15.1 Commonly Used Sunscreens

Sunscreen Active Ingredient	UV Coverage
Chemical	
Avobenzene	UVA-1, UVA-2
Homosalate	UVB
Octinoxate	UVB
Oxybenzone	UVA-2, UVB
para-Aminobenzoic acid (PABA)	UVB
Physical	
Titanium oxide	UVA-2, UVB
Zinc oxide	UVA-1, UVA-2, UVB

and X-rays. The energy from the sun not only enables us to see but also warms the planet, provides energy as food (beginning with photosynthesis), and plays a critical role in climate and weather patterns. The energy also interacts with our skin and produces suntans.

In contemporary Western culture, many people consider suntans attractive. Unfortunately, the rays of the sun that produce suntans are also very damaging to skin. Even with minimal sun exposure, skin will eventually show some signs of photoaging. With prolonged exposure, the skin undergoes hypermelanization and hyperkeratosis. The best way to prevent sun-damaged skin is to avoid excessive exposure to the sun and, while spending time outdoors, to protect the skin with sunscreen. To be effective, sunscreen should contain a rating of at least **SPF (sun protection factor)** 30.

The rays responsible for suntans and sunburns are ultraviolet (UV) radiation. Ultraviolet radiation is higher in energy than visible light. Humans cannot see UV radiation, but this energy does interact with the atoms in the cells of our epidermis. Ultraviolet A (UVA) radiation is informally referred to as the suntan region; there are two types of UVA (1 and 2). UVB is referred to as the sunburn region. To be effective, a sunscreen must protect against UVA and UVB rays. See Table 15.1 for a listing of available sunscreens and their UV coverage.

Even though sun exposure deleteriously affects everyone's skin, skin pigment does play a role. Fair-skinned persons are more likely to have atrophy and scaling of the epidermis than dark-skinned persons. Skin cancer is also more prevalent in lightly pigmented people than in those with dark skin. For all skin cancer victims, tumor growth is more common in areas exposed to the sun than in covered or shaded areas of the body.

The following are several categories of skin cancer:

- **Actinic keratosis:** a precancerous condition resulting from overexposure to sunlight
- **Basal cell carcinoma:** a slow-growing tumor that usually forms polyps and rarely metastasizes
- **Melanoma:** a highly malignant cancer that forms from melanocytes; sunburn greatly increases the risk of this skin disorder
- **Squamous cell carcinoma:** a type of cancer that grows more rapidly than basal cell carcinoma; cells tend to keratinize; metastasis is uncommon

Drug Therapies for Sun Exposure

Pharmacologic treatment can help improve the condition of skin overexposed to the sun (see Table 15.2). For severe sunburn, corticosteroids are usually used. Aspirin can reduce irritation, pain, and edema.

Benzocaine (Dermoplast, Hurricaine) and **lidocaine (Lidoderm, Lidopin, Topicaine, Xolido, Xylocaine)** are topical anesthetics that provide temporary relief of sunburn pain. These should be used only on intact skin for short periods.

Hydrocortisone (Cortaid, Cortizone) can also be used on intact skin to decrease inflammation and accelerate healing. It also helps with pain relief.

Silver sulfadiazine (Silvadene, SSD) is a topical antiseptic product that can be used to prevent infection in serious burns. Silver sulfadiazine works on the bacterial cell wall and cell membrane. Silver sulfadiazine frequently darkens in its container or after being applied to the skin, but this color change does not interfere with its antimicrobial properties. Hypersensitivity to this drug is rare, and it is painless upon application.

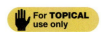
For TOPICAL use only

Contraindications Benzocaine is contraindicated in patients with hypersensitivity to similar (ester-type classification) local anesthetics and in patients with secondary bacterial infections in the area of use. It should not be used in the eyes.

Topical lidocaine is contraindicated for the treatment of dermatitis associated with diaper use.

Pregnant women and infants in the first two months of life should not use silver sulfadiazine products.

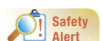
Safety Alert

Stickers warning patients to apply drugs appropriately should be placed on all topical drugs, especially the liquids. It is not uncommon for someone to ingest a topical. This can be very dangerous.

Cautions and Considerations Benzocaine is associated with **methemoglobinemia**, a disorder where an abnormal form of hemoglobin is produced. Methemoglobinemia can be a medical emergency. For this reason, benzocaine use is not recommended in patients below the age of two years.

Topical hydrocortisone may result in allergic contact dermatitis and local sensitization.

Patients who are allergic to sulfonamides can have an allergic reaction to silver sulfadiazine, so careful consideration must be given before its use. Because tissue necrosis (death) in the area of application has occurred, careful wound care and monitoring are necessary. Silver sulfadiazine does not protect against fungal organisms, so the wound should be monitored for development of a fungal infection.

Drug Interactions In general, drugs that are applied topically have few drug interactions.

TABLE 15.2 Most Commonly Used Drugs to Treat Sun-Damaged Skin

Generic (Brand)	Pronunciation	Dosage Form	Dispensing Status
benzocaine (Dermoplast, Hurricaine)	BEN-zoe-kayn	Aerosol, gel, liquid, lozenge, ointment, swab	OTC
hydrcortisone (Cortaid, Cortizone)	hye-droe-KOR-ti-sone	Cream, gel, lotion, ointment, solution	OTC, Rx
lidocaine (Lidoderm, Lidopin, Topicaine, Xolido, Xylocaine)	LYE-doe-kayn	Cream, gel, ointment, patch	OTC, Rx
silver sulfadiazine (Silvadene, SSD)	SIL-ver sul-fa-DYE-a-zeen	Cream	Rx

Photosensitivity

Photosensitivity is an abnormal sensitivity to light, especially of the eyes, but can also include increased sensitivity of the skin to sunlight. Photosensitivity can increase the patient's susceptibility to phototoxicity. Drugs in certain classes cause photosensitivity through biochemical interactions in the body, so it is important to alert a patient to this side effect when dispensing such a drug. The following classes have drugs that may cause photosensitivity: antihistamines, antibiotics, antifungals, antiretrovirals, antimalarials, antivirals, antineoplastics (chemotherapeutic agents), antiplatelets, diuretics, angiotensin-converting-enzyme (ACE) inhibitors, statins, anticonvulsants, antipsychotics, antidepressants, sedatives, hypnotics, analgesics, nonsteroidal anti-inflammatory drugs (NSAIDs), hormones, diabetes agents, topicals, and vitamins. Table 15.3 lists some of the drugs that cause photosensitivity.

The technician will need to watch for computer prompts on the pharmacy's computer system to know whether a particular drug will need a sticker to warn the patient to avoid exposure to sunlight while taking the medication. Because photosensitivity is common and occurs in various ways, individual patients may react differently to a particular drug.

TABLE 15.3 Some Drugs That Cause Photosensitivity

Drug Class	Drug Example	Drug Class	Drug Example
ACE inhibitors	All agents	Chemotherapeutic agents	Dacarbazine
Antibiotics	Griseofulvin		Fluorouracil, 5-FU
	Quinolones		Methotrexate
	Sulfas		Procarbazine
	Tetracyclines		Vinblastine
Antidepressants	Clomipramine	Diuretics	Acetazolamide
	Maprotiline		Furosemide
	Sertraline		Metolazone
	Tricyclic antidepressants (TCAs)		Thiazides
Antihistamines	Cyproheptadine	Hypoglycemics	Sulfonylureas
	Diphenhydramine	NSAIDs	All agents
Antipsychotics	Haloperidol		
	Phenothiazines		
Cardiovascular drugs	Amiodarone		
	Diltiazem		
	Quinidine		
	Simvastatin		
	Sotalol		

Acne, Wrinkles, and Rosacea

In the United States, acne is the most common skin condition for which treatment, either over-the-counter (OTC) or prescription, is sought. Acne is initiated by the overproduction of **sebum**, which is produced from glands around hair follicles. Such overproduction is most often stimulated by the hormonal changes encountered during puberty. **Pimples**, **blackheads**, and **whiteheads** appear as pores and follicles become clogged with oily material, dead skin cells, and dirt from the skin's surface. Mild forms of acne can be treated with OTC products. However, acne in its most severe forms, such as **nodular acne** or **acne vulgaris**, can cause deep cysts that permanently damage the dermal layer. Visible scars and pockmarks can form. Prescription drug therapy is needed to treat moderate to severe acne.

Wrinkles are another skin concern that affects many patients. A **wrinkle** is a line or crease in the skin. They usually happen on parts of the body that receive the most sun exposure, such as the face, hands, and neck. Other factors such as smoking, lighter skin, and genetics can promote wrinkling.

Rosacea is a chronic inflammatory disorder seen in adults and is characterized by redness, visible surface blood vessels, and raised bumps or pustules on the face and cheeks. Triggers of rosacea include stress, temperature, hot drinks, exercise, spicy food, alcohol, or any topical product that irritates the skin. Sunlight exposure is a major exacerbating factor of rosacea.

Drug Therapy for Acne, Wrinkles, and Rosacea

First-line treatment for mild to moderate acne is to cleanse the affected area twice a day. Although this cleansing will not eliminate acne, it can help prevent new blackheads and pimples from forming. Mild soap or cleanser is used twice a day to remove excess oil, dirt, and dead skin cells that clog pores.

Treatment of repeated acne lesions starts with OTC products, such as benzoyl peroxide. Moderate to severe acne requires the use of prescription products, starting with topical agents and progressing to oral agents when needed. Oral agents include antibiotics such as erythromycin, tetracycline, doxycycline, minocycline, and clindamycin (see Chapter 4). Some women may use oral contraceptives to decrease acne (see Chapter 14). The use of oral agents is associated with more side effects, so these medications are reserved for patients who do not gain adequate control with topical treatments.

Wrinkles are typically treated with retinoids.

When rosacea drug therapy is initiated, the specific triggers should be identified and then avoided. Because the disorder is not curable, only its symptoms are treated with antibiotics. Topical agents used for treatment are azelaic acid, brimonidine, and metronidazole. Systemic tetracycline antibiotics (covered in Chapter 4) are oral treatments of rosacea.

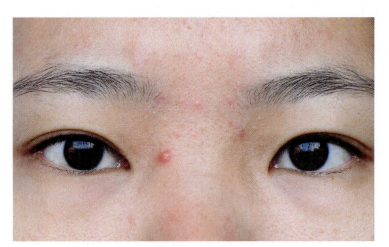

Acne is characterized by clogged pores and follicles.

Topical Antibiotics

Topical antibiotics (see Table 15.4) are used alone to treat mild acne and may be used in combination with oral agents to treat moderate to severe acne. Benzoyl peroxide is a mainstay of treatment for mild acne.

Common side effects of topical acne products include dryness, redness, burning, and flaking or peeling skin. Moisturizers can be applied to control these side effects. In general, less frequent use of these acne products is recommended if side effects are bothersome.

Azelaic acid (Azelex, Finacea) is a topical treatment for mild to moderate inflammatory acne vulgaris. After the skin is washed and patted dry, a thin film should be gently applied to the affected area twice daily. Hands should be washed after each application. Improvement usually occurs within four weeks.

Benzoyl peroxide (Benzac, Brevoxyl, Clearasil, Desquam-X, NeoBenz, Neutrogena, Oxy, PanOxyl, Triaz, ZoDerm) is another drug used to treat acne. It has antibacterial and mild drying effects, which help remove excess oils. Benzoyl peroxide produces oxygen, which is toxic to the bacteria that cause pimples. Benzoyl peroxide is available in both OTC and prescription strengths.

Clindamycin (Cleocin T, Clindagel, ClindaMax, Clindets, Evoclin) is a topical drug product used to treat acne. It is available as a foam, gel, lotion, and topical solution.

TABLE 15.4 Commonly Used Agents for Acne, Wrinkles, and Rosacea

Generic (Brand)	Pronunciation	Dosage Form	Dispensing Status
Topical Antibiotics			
azelaic acid (Azelex, Finacea)	ay-ze-LAY-ik AS-id	Cream, foam, gel	Rx
benzoyl peroxide (Benzac, Brevoxyl, Clearasil, Desquam-X, NeoBenz, Neutrogena, Oxy, PanOxyl, Triaz, ZoDerm)	BEN-zoe-il per-OX-ide	Bar, cleanser, cream, gel, liquid	OTC
clindamycin (Cleocin T, Clindagel, ClindaMax, Clindesse, Evoclin)	klin-da-MYE-sin	Foam, gel, lotion, topical solution	Rx
dapsone (Aczone)	DAP-sone	Gel	Rx
erythromycin (Ery, Erygel)	eh-rith-roe-MYE-sin	Gel, ointment, pads, solution	Rx
metronidazole (MetroCream, MetroGel, MetroLotion, Noritate, Rosadan)	me-troe-NI-da-zole	Cream, gel, lotion	Rx
Retinoids			
adapalene (Differin)	a-DAP-a-leen	Cream, gel, lotion	Rx
isotretinoin (Accutane, Claravis)	eye-soe-tret-i-NOE-in	Capsule	Rx
tazarotene (Avage, Tazorac)	ta-ZAR-oh-teen	Cream, gel	Rx
tretinoin (Atralin, Avita, Renova, Retin-A)	tret-i-NOE-in	Cream, gel	Rx
Miscellaneous			
brimonidine (Mirvaso)	bri-MOE-ni-deen	Gel	Rx
salicylic acid (Clearasil, Fostex, Neutrogena, Oxy, PROPA pH, Sal-Clens, Stridex)	sal-ah-SIL-ic AS-id	Cleanser, cream, lotion, pads, stick	Topical

Dapsone (Aczone) is a topical antibiotic gel used for acne. It can also be used orally to treat leprosy, spider bites, and other skin conditions. The oral form of the drug has serious side effects, but the topical form is free of many of these side effects because it is not absorbed systemically. Dapsone should not be used by anyone younger than 12 years old. A pea-sized amount of gel should be applied to clean skin of the affected area. Hands should be thoroughly washed after use.

Erythromyin (Emgel, Eryderm, Ery Pads) is a topical antibiotic used for acne. It is available as a gel, ointment, pads, and solution. It should be applied sparingly as a thin layer to affected areas once or twice daily.

Metronidazole (MetroCream, MetroGel, MetroLotion, Noritate, Rosadan) is a topical antibiotic used for rosacea. It is available as a gel and should be applied to clean, dry skin.

Contraindications Acne products should not be used on moles, warts, or areas of skin that are infected, red, or irritated. In addition, topical acne products should not be used to treat infants or patients with impaired circulation, because their skin is more fragile.

Topical metronidazole is contraindicated in patients with hypersensitivity to parabens. It should not be used in patients who have used disulfiram within the last two weeks or recently used alcohol or propylene glycol.

Cautions and Considerations All of these products are for external use only. Some of the topical antibiotic products are flammable. Products should be kept away from intense heat.

Drug Interactions Topical antibiotics are generally not associated with serious drug interactions.

Topical metronidazole may increase the adverse effects of alcohol, disulfiram, and lopinavir.

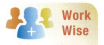
Work Wise

Pharmacy technicians should be aware that the use of retinoids to minimize the signs of aging is considered by many insurance companies to be a cosmetic rather than a therapeutic indication. Consequently, these companies deny insurance coverage for the cost of these medications. It can be helpful to warn patients that these products can be costly before they have their prescriptions filled.

Retinoids

Vitamin A derivatives including **retinoids** work by increasing cell turnover in follicles, which pushes clogged material out of the pores. In acne, retinoids alter cell development and inflammatory processes to reduce swelling and redness.

Retinoids are used to treat moderate to severe acne and to reduce the appearance of fine lines and wrinkles that accompany aging. Because of severe side effects and toxicities, oral retinoid agents are reserved for use in the most severe forms of acne or psoriasis. Refer back to Table 15.4 for more information on retinoids.

Common side effects of topical retinoid agents include burning, dry skin, itching, peeling, and redness. Sensitive skin may be especially prone to these effects. If these effects are severe or bothersome, the patient should stop using the product. In addition, retinoids also should not be used along with topical antibiotics such as tetracycline because the antibiotics can increase these side effects.

Oral agents, such as isotretinoin, have systemic side effects that can include depression, psychosis, pancreatitis, high triglyceride levels, and hepatotoxicity. Patients who already have these conditions should not take isotretinoin. Patients must be monitored closely for mental status changes, and regular laboratory blood tests must be performed to watch for pancreas or liver problems.

Adapalene (Differin) is a retinoid for acne treatment. It is less likely to cause skin irritation than tretinoin because it is water-based, whereas tretinoin contains alcohol. It is applied once daily, usually at night.

Isotretinoin (Accutane, Claravis), a retinoid, should be used as a treatment of last resort for severe acne. Isotretinoin is a known teratogen, which means it causes birth defects. For isotretinoin to be used by a patient, participation in a special program called iPLEDGE is mandated by the FDA. Both male and female patients must sign an agreement to use birth control, and females must undergo pregnancy testing while receiving isotretinoin. The prescriber must initiate enrolling the patient with the iPLEDGE program, and then the patient must go online and register. Finally, the dispensing pharmacy must re-register the patient online. Failure of any of the parties to follow protocol will halt the dispensing of the drug by the pharmacist. In the pharmacy, a pharmacy technician is responsible for setting up the iPLEDGE program. A patient must have his or her iPLEDGE card to receive a prescription. Furthermore, if a patient has any form of mental illness, he or she will most likely not be accepted into the program. A depressed mood is a major side effect of this drug. Isotretinoin must always be taken with a full glass of water to prevent the capsule from dissolving in the esophagus.

Tazarotene (Avage, Tazorac), a synthetic retinoid, has been approved for acne and psoriasis treatment. It modulates epithelial tissue and exerts some anti-inflammatory and immunological activity. Tazarotene is a prodrug that is converted to its active form, tazarotenic acid, by de-esterification. A thin layer should be applied to very dry skin in the evening, since this drug makes the skin highly sensitive to sunlight. Some systemic absorption occurs with tazarotene, and because of the prolonged retention of the drug within the body, the therapeutic effects can last up to three months after discontinuation.

Tretinoin (Atralin, Avita, Renova, Retin-A), a retinoid, is a topical medication approved for the treatment of acne. It is also used to treat photodamaged skin and some skin cancers. Epidermal cells in the sebaceous follicle become less adherent, and tretinoin works by removing these cells (keratinocytes) and loosening the keratic (thickening) cells at the mouth of the duct, causing easy sloughing and sebum discharge. Thus, the drug helps the skin to renew itself more quickly, improving its texture and appearance. Patients should avoid direct sunlight when using tretinoin.

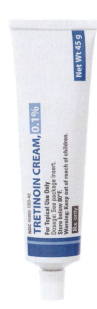

Tretinoin is a topical product used for acne.

Contraindications Retinoids should not be used by patients with liver or kidney impairment. Because of their side effects, they should be used with caution in patients with depression or hypertriglyceridemia. Isotretinoin cannot be used by women who are or might become pregnant. Severe birth defects are highly likely if a woman becomes pregnant while taking isotretinoin.

Cautions and Considerations As with all acne products, retinoids should not be used on areas of skin that are infected, red, or irritated. Care should also be taken to avoid applying these products close to the eyes or around the mouth.

Drug Interactions Topical products are generally not associated with serious drug interactions.

Alcohol, multivitamins, tetracyclines, and vitamin A may enhance the adverse effects of isotretinoin. Isotretinoin may decrease the effectiveness of oral contraceptives.

Miscellaneous Products

Brimonidine (Mirvaso) is a topical alpha agonist used for rosacea. It decreases redness by causing constriction of blood vessels. A pea-sized amount should be applied to the face.

Salicylic acid (Clearasil, Fostex, Neutrogena, Oxy, PROPA pH, Sal-Clens, Stridex) is a **keratolytic** agent that breaks down and peels off dead skin cells, thereby preventing them from clogging pores. Salicylic acid is a mainstay of treatment for mild acne. It is available in various dosage forms and is commonly used.

Contraindications Brimonidine does not have contraindications.

Salicylic acid should not be used on moles, warts, or areas of skin that are infected, red, or irritated. In addition, it should not be used to treat infants or patients with impaired circulation because their skin is more fragile.

Cautions and Considerations Worsening of erythema may occur with use of brimonidine. Serious adverse effects (such as cardiac and respiratory problems) may occur with ingestion of topical brimonidine.

Drug Interactions Topical brimonidine may increase the antihypertensive effects of other drugs that reduce blood pressure. The central nervous system (CNS) depressant side effects of other drugs may be enhanced by brimonidine

Dermatitis, Eczema, Psoriasis, and Dandruff

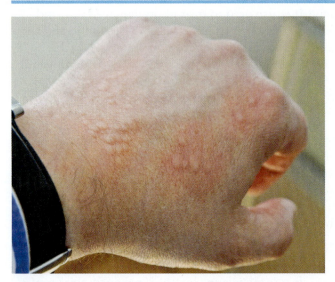

Irritant contact dermatitis is often caused by these common substances: soaps, cosmetics, rubbing alcohol, bleach, and solvents.

Dermatitis is **pruritic** (itchy), inflamed skin that can be caused by a variety of factors. The most severe cases can result in blisters and oozing erosions on the skin, but typical symptoms include areas of redness, dry flaky skin, raised or bumpy skin, and pruritus. Types of dermatitis include contact dermatitis, seborrheic dermatitis, diaper rash, and atopic dermatitis.

Contact dermatitis occurs in response to exposure to irritants or allergenic substances. Rash appears wherever skin has come into contact with the offending substance, such as soaps or detergents. Poison ivy, poison oak, and other plants can cause redness, itching, rash, and blisters when their oils come into contact with the skin.

Seborrheic dermatitis, also called **cradle cap**, is a greasy, scaly area on the skin that sometimes appears red, brown, or yellow. It usually occurs in infants and in areas where sebaceous follicles are concentrated, such as the scalp, ears, upper trunk, eyebrows, and around the nose. In adult men, it can occur in the beard area.

Another skin rash common in infants is **diaper rash**. This acute and easily treated condition occurs most frequently in children who are not yet toilet trained, but it can also occur in adults who must wear incontinence pads. When skin remains wet for long periods, tissue breakdown allows bacteria on the surface to enter deeper tissues. Diaper rash products are used for irritation and redness when skin frequently contacts urine, feces, or both. These products contain a variety of ingredients that combine to promote healing, protect skin from further insult, and prevent infection. Common ingredients include the following:

- balsam of Peru for wound healing and tissue repair
- camphor or menthol to provide local anesthetic action to relieve pain and itching
- eucalyptol (eucalyptus oil) for antimicrobial activity
- talc or kaolin for moisture absorption
- zinc oxide, a drying agent

These agents should be used as soon as redness appears in order to protect the skin from further damage and prevent infection from bacteria or fungi.

Atopic dermatitis, also called **eczema**, is a chronic condition that usually first occurs in childhood and can continue into adulthood. Atopic dermatitis is not well understood but has an immunologic component, in that patients tend to have elevated levels of immunoglobulin E (IgE) in their blood. Patients with atopic dermatitis have a greater tendency to develop asthma or hay fever sometime in life. Eczema appears as dry, flaky, red skin that is very itchy. Patients sometimes scratch enough to cause secondary skin infections. Unlike other types of dermatitis that are usually curable, atopic dermatitis is a chronic condition. Periods of severe symptoms (exacerbation) can cycle with periods of remission. Common triggers for exacerbations include stress, exposure to skin irritants, and food allergies.

Psoriasis is an immunologic condition affecting T-cell activity in the skin. It manifests on the skin as well-defined plaques (patches) that are raised, silvery or white, flaky, and pruritic. The plaques can appear anywhere on the body and may be very small or quite large and painful. Like eczema, psoriasis is characterized by periods of exacerbation that cycle with periods of remission. Stress and exposure to environmental factors that dry out skin can trigger exacerbation.

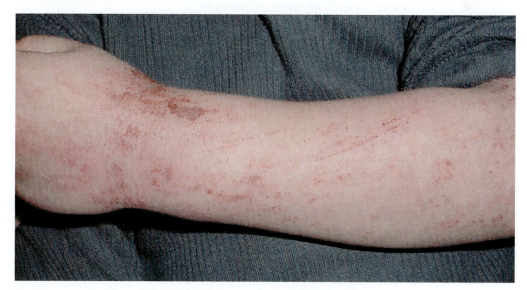

Atopic eczema can have allergic, hereditary, or psychogenic causes.

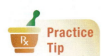
Drug Therapy for Dermatitis, Eczema, and Psoriasis

Corticosteroids are usually first-line therapy for dermatitis and eczema. Therapy starts with topical medications but may include oral corticosteroids if severe. Seborrheic dermatitis can be treated with attention to good hygiene and topical antihistamines, anti-inflammatory agents, and moisturizing creams. Eczema treatment involves constant maintenance of skin with moisturizers to prevent exacerbations, along with topical corticosteroids for flare-ups. If the affected skin becomes infected, topical antibiotics may be used.

Psoriasis can be difficult to treat and does not always respond well to drug therapy. Like dermatitis and eczema, corticosteroids are the first-line treatment for psoriasis. Immunosuppressants and immunomodulators are sometimes required.

Immunosuppressants used to treat psoriasis include azathioprine, cyclosporine, and methotrexate. Immunomodulators used include biologic therapies such as adalimumab (Humira) and etanercept (Enbrel). Biologic agents, such as these tumor necrosis factor alpha (TNF-alpha) inhibitors, are a costly but effective treatment for severe psoriasis. Immunosuppressants and immunomodulators are covered in Chapters 13 and 16.

Topical Corticosteroids

Anti-inflammatory agents that work by inhibiting redness, swelling, itching, and pain in the dermal layer of the skin, are **topical corticosteroids**, which are used to treat contact dermatitis, eczema, psoriasis, and allergic reactions (see Table 15.5). A thin layer of medication is applied to affected skin for a limited period. Because corticosteroids can penetrate the skin and be absorbed systemically, they should be used sparingly. Systemic absorption can cause **hypothalamic-pituitary-adrenal (HPA) axis suppression**, which is associated with appetite changes, weight gain, fat redistribution, fluid retention, and insomnia.

Treatment with topical corticosteroids starts with OTC-strength products, such as 0.5% or 1% hydrocortisone. Both strengths are usually effective for treatment of poison ivy and diaper rash (the lower strength should be used for infants and children). Combination products that contain an antifungal along with a corticosteroid can be useful for treating severe diaper rash.

Corticosteroid products vary in potency, depending on the formulation. Ointments are typically more potent than creams. Ointments are most appropriate for treating dry, scaly lesions, whereas creams are most effective for treating moist or oozing lesions. When using gels, patients should follow package and prescription instructions. Creams, gels, and ointments are not interchangeable and should not be substituted for each other.

Common side effects of topical corticosteroids include burning, itching, dryness, excessive hair growth, dermatitis, acne, hypopigmentation, and thinning of the skin. Use of the least amount over the smallest area for the shortest period possible is recommended to minimize these effects.

Contraindications Topical corticosteroids have no contraindications.

Cautions and Considerations Occlusive wound dressings should not be applied over topical corticosteroid products, especially the high potency ones. To reduce the potential for systemic absorption and HPA axis suppression, super potent corticosteroid products are restricted in the length of treatment or total amount used. These agents should not be used for longer than two consecutive weeks. The total amount used in one week should not exceed 45–50 g, and these products should not be applied close to the eyes or mucous membranes.

TABLE 15.5 Commonly Used Topical Corticosteroids

Generic (Brand)	Pronunciation	Dosage Form	Dispensing Status
Low Potency			
alclometasone (Aclovate)	al-kloe-MET-a-sone	Cream, ointment	Rx
hydrocortisone (Cortaid, Cortizone-10, Dermolate, HydroSKIN, Procort, Scalpicin)	hye-droe-KOR-ti-sone	Cream, gel, liquid, lotion, ointment, spray	OTC
hydrocortisone (Acticort, Ala-Cort, Cetacort, Cort-Dome, Eldecort, Hi-Cor, Hycort, Hydrocort, Hytone, LactiCare, Penecort, Synacort, Texacort)	hye-droe-KOR-ti-sone	Cream, liquid, lotion, ointment, solution	Rx
hydrocortisone acetate (Cortaid, Cortef, Corticaine, Gynecort, Lanacort, Tucks)	hye-droe-KOR-ti-sone	Cream, ointment	OTC, Rx
hydrocortisone butyrate (Locoid)	hye-droe-KOR-ti-sone	Cream, lotion, ointment, solution	Rx
hydrocortisone probutate (Pandel)	hye-droe-KOR-ti-sone	Cream	Rx
prednicarbate (Dermatop)	pred-ni-KAR-bate	Cream, ointment	Rx
High Potency			
betamethasone dipropionate (Diprosone, Maxivate)	bay-ta-METH-a-sone	Aerosol, cream, lotion, ointment	Rx
betamethasone valerate (Beta-Val, Luxiq, Psorion)	bay-ta-METH-a-sone dye-PRO-pee-on-ate	Cream, foam, lotion, ointment	Rx
clocortolone (Cloderm)	kloe-KOR-toe-lone	Cream	Rx
desoximetasone (Topicort)	des-ox-i-MET-a-sone	Cream, gel, ointment	Rx
fluocinolone acetonide (Capex, Synalar)	floo-oh-SIN-oh-lone	Cream, oil, ointment, shampoo, solution	Rx
fluocinonide (Lidex, Vanos)	floo-oh-SIN-oh-nide	Cream, gel, ointment, solution	Rx
fluticasone (Cutivate)	floo-TIK-a-sone	Cream, lotion, ointment	Rx
halcinonide (Halog)	hal-SIN-oh-nide	Cream, ointment, solution	Rx
hydrocortisone valerate (Westcort)	hye-droe-KOR-ti-sone va-LAIR-ate	Cream, ointment	Rx
mometasone furoate (Elocon)	moe-MET-a-sone	Cream, lotion, ointment, solution	Rx
triamcinolone (Flutex, Kenalog, Kenonel)	trye-am-SIN-oe-lone	Aerosol, cream, lotion, ointment	Rx
Very High or Super Potency			
amcinonide (Cyclocort)	am-SIN-oh-nide	Cream, lotion, ointment	Rx
betamethasone dipropionate, augmented (Diprolene)	bay-ta-METH-a-sone dye-PRO-pee-on-ate	Cream, gel, lotion, ointment	Rx
clobetasol propionate (Clobex, Cormax, Olux, Temovate)	kloe-BAY-ta-sawl	Cream, foam, gel, lotion, ointment, shampoo, solution, spray	Rx
desonide (DesOwen, LoKara, Verdeso)	DESS-oh-nide	Cream, foam, gel, lotion, ointment	Rx
halobetasol propionate (Ultravate)	hal-oh-BAY-ta-sawl	Cream, ointment	Rx

Drug Interactions In general, topical corticosteroids do not have drug interactions.

Calcineurin Inhibitors

These medications are immunomodulators that work by inhibiting T-cell activation, which prevents release of chemical mediators that promote inflammation (see Table 15.6). **Calcineurin inhibitors** are used to treat severe eczema, especially when topical corticosteroids have not been effective. These agents are available in the following forms: capsule, cream, ointment, and solution.

Pimecrolimus (Elidel), a drug similar to antirejection drugs, is approved for the treatment of eczema. An immunosuppressant, it reduces itching and inflammation by suppressing the release of cytokines from the T cells. The patient should apply a thin layer to all areas of the skin diagnosed as having eczema. The drug should not be applied to areas that do not have eczema. Other skin products should not be applied to the areas with eczema.

Tacrolimus (Protopic) is also similar to antirejection drugs or topical immunomodulators (TIM). The advantage of this drug over a steroid is that tacrolimus will not cause thinning of the skin or other side effects of long-term steroid use. Tacrolimus may be used anywhere on the body, even the face. Products with a concentration of 0.03% tacrolimus are approved for use in children aged 2–15 years old, and products containing 0.1% tacrolimus can be used by adults.

Common side effects of calcineurin inhibitors include burning, itching, tingling, acne, and redness at the site of application. Other effects include headache, muscle aches and pains, sinusitis, and flu-like symptoms. To minimize these effects, these agents should be used sparingly for a short treatment period.

Contraindications No contraindications exist for topical calcineurin inhibitors.

Cautions and Considerations Calcineurin inhibitors have been associated with increased occurrences of cancer (skin cancer and lymphoma). Topical application is less likely to cause malignancy, but patients must be informed of this risk. Use of calcineurin inhibitors, even topical application, can cause alcohol intolerance. Facial flushing can occur when drinking alcohol and using these medications.

Drug Interactions Topical tacrolimus may increase the adverse effects of alcohol. Antidepressants, antifungals, calcium channel blockers, cyclosporine, and danazol may increase tacrolimus levels.

Immunosuppressant side effects may be enhanced by tacrolimus use. Topical tacrolimus may enhance the kidney-damaging effects of cyclosporine and sirolimus.

Pimecrolimus may enhance the adverse effects of immunosuppressants.

TABLE 15.6 Commonly Used Agents for Dermatitis, Eczema, and Psoriasis

Generic (Brand)	Pronunciation	Dosage Form	Dispensing Status
calamine	KAL-ah-mine	Lotion	OTC
calcipotriene (Calcitrene, Dovonex, Sorilux, Taclonex)	kal-si-poe-TRY-een	Cream, ointment, topical solution	Rx
pimecrolimus (Elidel)	pim-e-KROE-li-mus	Cream	Rx
tacrolimus (Protopic)	ta-KROE-li-mus	Ointment	Rx

A synthetic form of vitamin D, **calcipotriene (Calcitrene, Dovonex, Sorilux, Taclonex)** regulates cell growth and development of skin cells. In psoriasis, skin cells reproduce abnormally and rapidly to form plaques. Vitamin D naturally regulates this cell process.

Vitamin D analogs are available in several forms, including creams, foam, ointments, and solutions. Some dosage forms can be used to effectively treat psoriatic lesions on the scalp when other creams and ointments are too greasy and thick to use where hair is dense.

Common side effects of calcipotriene include burning, itching, and redness at the site of application. Less common effects include inflamed hair follicles (folliculitis), skin irritation, change in skin color at the site of application, and thinning of the skin. Patients who experience these problems should stop using calcipotriene and contact their healthcare practitioners.

Contraindications Patients who have hypercalcemia, vitamin D toxicity, or acute psoriasis should not use calcipotriene.

Cautions and Considerations Vitamin D analogs can cause alterations in calcium metabolism, so patients who have had problems with too much calcium in the blood (such as a history of kidney stones) should not use them without medical supervision. Periodic blood tests may be performed to monitor calcium levels.

Drug Interactions Calcipotriene may increase concentrations of aluminum hydroxide. It may decrease concentrations of sucralfate.

The toxic effects of calcipotriene may be enhanced by multivitamins and other vitamin D analogs.

Calamine

Mild itching from insect bites, rashes, hives, poison ivy or poison oak, and other allergic reactions can be relieved with **calamine** (see Table 15.6). It works through a counterirritant action that involves evaporation and cooling, which soothes the itchy sensation. Many calamine products also contain zinc oxide, an ingredient with antiseptic properties that protects against infection from repeated scratching.

Calamine can be used frequently and has few side effects.

Contraindications Calamine should not be used on broken or blistered skin. It is also not recommended for children younger than two years.

Cautions and Considerations If itching and rash are not relieved within a few days of using calamine, patients should see their healthcare practitioners. Stronger prescription products may be needed, or there may be an underlying problem that requires medical treatment.

Drug Interactions There are no known drug interactions to calamine.

Dandruff

Dandruff is a malfunction of the oil-producing glands around hair follicles on the scalp. Cell proliferation in the scalp is also accelerated. Overproduction of sebum and cells results in layers of epidermis sticking together and flaking off as they dry. Specks of skin become visible in the hair and on the scalp. Although unsightly, dandruff is not harmful.

Drug Therapy for Dandruff

The active ingredients used most in OTC dandruff products are **selenium sulfide (Head & Shoulders Intensive Treatment, Selsun Blue)** and **pyrithione zinc**. These products are used once a day or on a regular basis to control dandruff. Coal tar shampoos including Neutrogena T/Gel are also available over the counter but tend to be used in severe cases. Coal tar is safe, but its use can be messy and odorous, and most patients find long-term use unpleasant.

Nizoral shampoo is available in OTC and prescription strengths. It contains keto-conazole, which is typically considered an antifungal agent.

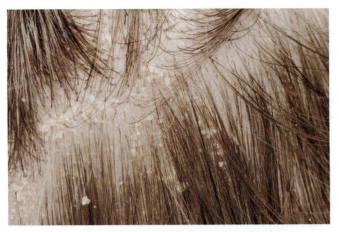

Dandruff is a cosmetic concern that appears as specks of skin in the hair and on the scalp.

All of these active ingredients work by slowing cell and oil production, which results in reduced skin flaking. In addition, these products have antipruritic properties that reduce the itching associated with dry, flaking skin.

Side effects of dandruff products are rare and mild. However, possible effects include contact dermatitis, photosensitivity, and aggravation of preexisting skin conditions such as acne or psoriasis. If such effects occur, the patient should stop using the product and these effects will subside.

Contraindications No contraindications exist for these products.

Cautions and Considerations If dandruff and scalp itching continue with repeated use of these products, patients should seek medical advice to see if there is an alternative cause.

Drug Interactions Topical products are generally not associated with serious drug interactions.

Skin Infections

Skin infections are common. Although most can be managed with nonprescription topical antimicrobial products, some do not respond to ordinary products, necessitating treatment with a prescription drug. The severity of a skin infection depends on the extent to which the skin and its structures are involved. There can be drainage, swelling, fever, and malaise.

Bacterial Infections

Bacterial skin infections most frequently involve *Staphylococcus aureus*, which is considered normal flora and is not generally harmful, unless overgrowth occurs or it is introduced internally through a cut or sore. Methicillin-resistant *Staphylococcus aureus* (MRSA), an organism that is particularly difficult to treat when introduced internally, is often found on the skin. Therefore, systemic antibiotics are given prior to surgery to prevent infection from an incision through the skin.

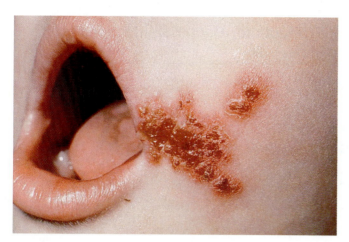
Imeptigo is a contagious skin infection that primarily affects young children.

Impetigo is another example of a skin infection caused by *S. aureus* or *Streptococcus*. It is a superficial but highly contagious skin infection that is common in early childhood, particularly in warm, humid climates and where hygiene is poor. It is uncommon in adults, but it may be seen, particularly in older adults and immunocompromised patients.

Erysipelas, a form of cellulitis, is characterized by redness and warmth, local pain, edematous plaques with sharply established borders, chills, malaise, and fever. The infection spreads progressively and rapidly through the superficial layers of the skin. On the face, erysipelas may assume a butterfly distribution. Erysipelas usually responds well to oral antibiotics. However, if systemic toxicity (high fever with elevated white blood cell count) results, parenteral antibiotics should be administered.

Folliculitis is an inflammation of a hair follicle that is characterized by a minute, red, pustulated nodule without involvement of the surrounding tissues. There is little pain. It commonly occurs in men on the bearded part of the face.

A **furuncle** (boil) is a staphylococcal infection beginning in a sebaceous gland and the associated hair follicle. The follicular infection is more extensive and deeper than in folliculitis. It begins with itching, local tenderness, and erythema, followed by swelling, marked local pain, and pus formation within the lesion. A **carbuncle** is a coalescent mass of infected follicles with deeper penetration than a furuncle. Pain, erythema, swelling, purulent drainage, fever, and systemic toxicity are common.

Drug Therapies for Bacterial Skin Infections

Bacterial skin infections can be treated with topical products and systemic therapies. Systemic antibiotics are covered in Chapter 4. Table 15.7 presents commonly used antibiotic drugs for treating bacterial skin infections.

Generic names for topical antibiotic agents differ from names of oral antibiotics, so familiarity with oral antibiotics does not automatically confer knowledge of topical products. Topical antibiotics are used to treat local skin infections such as cuts or scrapes, impetigo, and diaper rash.

Certain antibiotic combinations are available OTC. Bacitracin and **bacitracin-neomycin-polymyxin B (triple antibiotic ointment, Neosporin, Mycitracin)** are used to prevent or treat minor skin infections.

Mupirocin (Bactroban) is a common topical treatment for impetigo caused by *Staphylococcus aureus* or *Streptococcus pyogenes*. It should not be applied to the eye; use should be discontinued if rash, itching, or irritation occurs or if there is no improvement within five days. Mupirocin is applied three times a day for 12 days.

Retapamulin (Altabax) is an ointment approved for the topical treatment of impetigo for both adults and children. Retapamulin is one of several drugs from a new class of antibiotics. This class of antibiotics, the pleuromutilins, inhibits bacterial protein synthesis in the same way as mupirocin, but it binds at different sites. The active ingredient is derived from an edible mushroom. Retapamulin should be used twice a day for five days. Retapamulin is slower acting than mupirocin, the other topical agents used for impetigo.

TABLE 15.7 Commonly Used Topical Products for Bacterial Infections of the Integumentary System

Generic (Brand)	Pronunciation	Dosage Form	Dispensing Status
bacitracin	bas-i-TRAY-sin	Ointment	OTC
bacitracin-neomycin-polymyxin B (triple antibiotic ointment, Neosporin, Mycitracin)	bas-i-TRAY-sin nee-oh-MYE-sin pol-ee-MIX-in B	Ointment	OTC
mupirocin (Bactroban)	myoo-PEER-oe-sin	Cream, ointment	Rx
retapamulin (Altabax)	ret-a-PAM-yoo-lin	Ointment	Rx

Erythromycin and metronidazole, previously discussed in this chapter, may be used for bacterial skin infections.

Contraindications Patients with allergies to any of these antibiotics should not use any of these topical anti-infective products. Remember, when a patient is allergic to one antibiotic, they are allergic to all antibiotics in the same drug class. Patients can check with their pharmacists if they are not sure whether an allergy should prevent them from using one of these medications.

Cautions and Considerations These products are for external use only and should be kept away from the eyes and other mucous membranes during application. They should not be applied over large areas of skin, because systemic absorption can occur.

Drug Interactions Topical antibiotics are generally not associated with serious drug interactions.

Fungal Infections

Skin and nails are susceptible to various fungal infections. Recall from Chapter 4 that candidiasis is an infection by *Candida albicans*, a fungus that usually causes lesions in the vagina or the mouth (where it is called thrush). It may be treated with agents such as clotrimazole and miconazole. Swish-and-swallow nystatin is frequently used if the mouth is involved. Table 15.8 lists common products used for skin and nail fungal infections.

Drug Therapies for Fungal Skin Infections

Ringworm (also called *tinea*) is caused by a microscopic fungus that infects the horny (scaly) layer of the skin or the nails. The infection spreads outward as the center heals, leaving a ring. Ringworm responds to topical antifungal agents such as butenafine (Lotrimin Ultra, Mentax) and terbinafine (Lamisil AT), two drugs that are also used for athlete's foot and jock itch. Because they kill the fungus, butenafine and terbinafine are more effective than other antifungal agents that only terminate fungal growth.

Butenafine (Lotrimin Ultra, Mentax) is used to treat athlete's foot, ringworm, and jock itch. It is applied once daily for four weeks. After the last application, the drug may maintain its effect for an additional four weeks. This is why butenafine is the popular treatment for athlete's foot and ringworm. Lotrimin Ultra OTC is identical to Mentax, the prescription form of butenafine. It also remains active after the patient stops using it. It is important to know the generic and brand names of these drugs.

TABLE 15.8 Commonly Used Topical Products for Fungal Infections of the Integumentary System

Generic (Brand)	Pronunciation	Dosage Form	Dispensing Status
butenafine (Lotrimin Ultra, Mentax)	byoo-ten-a-feen	Cream	OTC, Rx
ciclopirox (Ciclodan, Penlac, Loprox)	sye-kloe-PEER-ox	Cream, gel, shampoo, solution, and suspension	Rx
clotrimazole (Alevazol, Desenex, FungiCure, Gyne-Lotrimin, Lotrimin AF, Mycelex)	kloe-TRIM-a-zole	Cream, ointment	OTC, Rx
ketoconazole (Extina, Ketodan, Nizoral, Xolegel)	kee-toe-KOE-na-zole	Cream, foam, gel, shampoo	OTC, Rx
miconazole (Desenex, Lotrimin AF, Micaderm, Neosporin AF)	mi-KON-a-zole	Aerosol powder, cream, lotion, ointment, powder, solution	OTC, Rx
sertaconazole (Ertaczo)	ser-ta-KON-a-zole	Cream	Rx
terbinafine (Lamisil, Lamisil AT)	ter-BI-na-feen	Cream, gel, solution	OTC, Rx
tolnaftate (Lamisil AF Defense, Tinactin)	tol-NAFF-tate	Aerosol, cream, powder, solution	OTC

Only Lotrimin Ultra is butenafine; Lotrimin AF cream is clotrimazole, and Lotrimin AF sprays and powder are miconazole.

Ciclopirox (Ciclodan, Penlac, Loprox) is probably the most effective topical medication for nail fungus (onychomycosis), which is extremely difficult to treat. The aging population in the United States is very prone to this infection, which causes the nail to thicken and can potentially lead to foot problems. Nail fungus infections are difficult to treat topically because it is so difficult to penetrate the nail or get the medicine under the nail to attack the fungus directly. Because of this, these infections are commonly treated with oral medications.

Clotrimazole (Alevazol, Desenex, FungiCure, Gyne-Lotrimin, Lotrimin AF, Mycelex) is available in topical forms OTC and by prescription. OTC dosage forms include creams, ointments, and topical solutions. Prescription forms include lozenges and cream.

Ketoconazole (Extina, Xolegel) is a 2% gel indicated for seborrheic dermatitis for persons 12 years and older. The **ketoconazole (Ketodan)** formula is a 2% foam. **Ketoconazole (Nizoral)** is available as a shampoo for patients with fungal infections of the scalp. It is used daily for two weeks. Patients should wait 20 minutes after application before using sunscreen or makeup on the affected areas.

Miconazole (Desenex, Lotrimin AF, Micaderm, Neosporin AF) is available as a powder or liquid spray. Note that Lotrimin AF spray or powder is miconazole, whereas Lotrimin AF cream is clotrimazole.

Sertaconazole (Ertaczo) is an imidazole antifungal agent. It is believed to inhibit the synthesis of ergosterol, which is a key component of the cell membrane of fungi. Sertaconazole is approved to treat ringworm that affects the scalp, feet, hands, groin, or toenails and also for athlete's foot. These infections are generally transmitted through close human contact or by indirect contact. Because the infections are superficial,

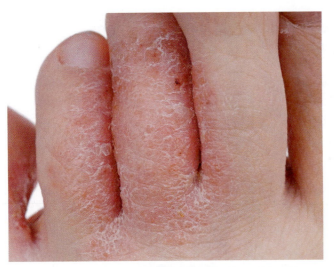

Athlete's foot causes scaling, flaking, and itching of the skin.

topical therapy is generally sufficient. Sertaconazole is applied to the affected area twice daily for four weeks. The most common side effect is contact dermatitis.

Terbinafine (Lamisil Advanced, Lamisil AT) is a topical cream that may be used to treat fungi. It inhibits the biosynthesis of fungal membrane sterols. For athlete's foot, it should be applied twice daily, and four times daily for ringworm and jock itch. The treatment course takes only one week, as opposed to four weeks for other antifungal agents. Systemic absorption of the topical medication is also low. Terbinafine remains active for one week or longer after the patient stops using it.

Tolnaftate (Lamisil AF Defense, Tinactin) is an OTC drug recommended for treatment of jock itch. It is not recommended for nail infections and should not be used around the eyes. Side effects are pruritus, contact dermatitis, irritation, and stinging. If skin irritation develops, infection worsens, or there is no improvement within 10 days, the patient should consult a physician.

Contraindications The topical antifungals presented do not have contraindications.

Cautions and Considerations Discontinue use of these products if sensitivity or skin irritation occurs. Ciclopirox may cause a burning sensation upon application.

Ketoconazole is for external use only and should not be used on mucous membranes. Ketoconazole cream contains sulfites and should be avoided in patients with sulfite-sensitivity.

Drug Interactions There are no known significant interactions with topical antifungals.

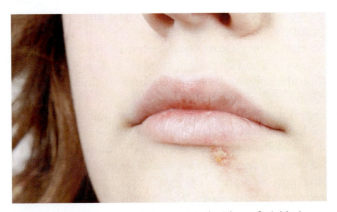

Herpes simplex virus type 1 is associated with orofacial lesions, as shown.

Viral Infections

Viral infections can cause several skin disorders, including herpes labialis (cold sores) and warts. Herpes simplex virus (HSV) is associated with painful dermatitis and vesicles. HSV type 1 is usually associated with orofacial disease (herpes labialis), and HSV type 2 is usually associated with genital infection.

A **wart** is a virally caused epidermal tumor. Remission is due to developing immunity, but the virus may lie dormant and later cause reinfection. Genital warts are transmitted by sexual contact.

Drug Therapies for Viral Infections

Topical treatment of HSV is palliative; it affords relief but does not cure, although antivirals such as acyclovir (see Chapter 5), if initiated early enough, may prevent recurrent outbreaks. Warts can be removed by surgery or destroyed by local freezing. Some OTC products may be effective if the wart is small. Most agents contain salicylic acid (discussed previously) as an active ingredient.

Table 15.9 lists commonly used topical products for viral infections.

TABLE 15.9	Commonly Used Topical Products for Viral Infections of the Integumentary System		
Generic (Brand)	**Pronunciation**	**Dosage Form**	**Dispensing Status**
acyclovir (Zovirax)	ay-SYE-kloe-veer	Cream, ointment	Rx
docosanol (Abreva)	doe-KOE-sa-nole	Cream	OTC

Acyclovir (Zovirax) is a prescription topical antiviral medication. It is used for genital herpes simplex virus, herpes labialis, and mucocutaneous HSV. **Docosanol (Abreva)** is another OTC topical medication that is indicated for the treatment of cold sores. It blocks the virus from invading the cells and is most effective when administered at the first sign of an outbreak. It must be applied five times a day to be effective.

Contraindications Topical acyclovir is contraindicated in patients with hypersensitivity to valacyclovir. There are no contraindications to docosanol.

Cautions and Considerations Docosanol may contain benzyl alcohol, which is associated with potentially fatal neonatal gasping syndrome.

Drug Interactions There are no known significant interactions with acyclovir or docosanol.

External Parasites

Two common types of external parasites use the human body as a host: lice and scabies mites. Lice spend their entire life cycle on the skin surface, hair, and clothing fibers of their host. An infestation of lice is called **pediculosis**. The mites that cause scabies may spend part of their life cycle on the skin surface and the remainder burrowed in the host's skin.

Lice

Lice are wingless insects that live parasitically on various animals, including most mammals. Human lice exist in all climate zones, from arctic conditions to the tropics, and may infest persons of any walk of life. They live up to 45 days, but may die prematurely because of scratching, combing, or disease. Injured or weak lice fall off the host. Human blood is their only source of nourishment. Lice are spread by direct contact with the infested person's head, body, or personal items such as hats, hairbrushes, combs, or bedding. The symptom of an infestation of lice is itching.

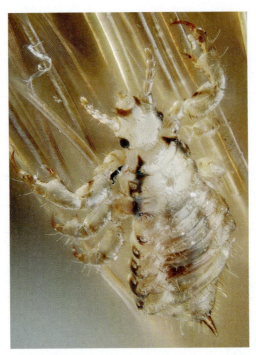

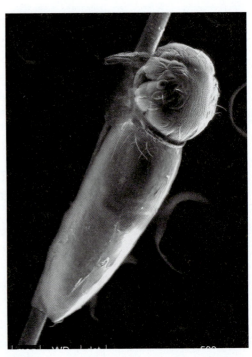

An adult head louse (left) can live for up to 45 days on the scalp. The heat from the scalp helps nits (right) to hatch in just eight days.

Humans can be infested by three types of lice: body lice, head lice, and pubic lice. DNA studies suggest that body lice evolved from head lice, possibly when *Homo sapiens* first began to wear clothing (possibly 70,000 years ago). In contrast, pubic lice are more closely related to lice that live on nonhuman primates, such as gorillas, than to human head or body lice.

Body lice are 2 to 4 mm long and live in clothing and moist areas of the body, such as the waistline and armpits. Body lice do not always require treatment with drugs. Instead, they can often be treated by removing clothing, bathing the patient, and putting on clean bedding and clothes. Body lice are sensitive to heat, so washing clothes in hot water or using a clothes dryer can eliminate both adult lice and eggs.

The head louse, *Pediculus humanus capitis*, is 1 to 2 mm long and lives on the scalp and hair, but not on eyebrows or eyelashes. Head lice are not generally believed to transmit any viral or bacterial diseases. They feed on blood from the scalp, which produces the intense pruritus. A female head louse has a life span of 40 days, during which she lays approximately 10 eggs (nits) per day. These nits are cemented to hair shafts close to the scalp and take advantage of body heat, which helps them to hatch in approximately eight days. This is why the treatment must be repeated. The nits are best seen by shining a bright light on the scalp. They appear white and look like dandruff. They cannot be shaken off.

Pubic, or crab, lice are 0.8 to 1.2 mm long and live in the pubic area. The infestation may resemble dermatitis and be very itchy; corticosteroids worsen this condition. Pubic lice are transmitted by sexual contact and should be treated to eliminate the parasite. In rare cases, pubic lice may inhabit the scalp.

Drug Therapy for Lice

Table 15.10 presents the most commonly used agents for lice. Instructions to the patient vary with the type of lice infestation:

- Body lice: Shower or bathe, and apply 20–30 g of cream or lotion to the whole body from the neck down; then wash off in 24 hours. Repeat in one week.

- Head lice: Massage two ounces or less of cream or lotion into premoistened hair for four minutes, and rinse out. Repeat after one week. The repetition is important to eliminate eggs.

- Pubic lice: Apply a thin layer of cream or lotion that extends to the thighs, trunk, and axillary regions; wash off within 24 hours. Repeat in one week.

For both head and pubic lice, it is important to comb the hair with a clean, fine-tooth comb to remove the nits.

Ivermectin (Sklice, Soolantra) is a topical product used for head lice. It may also be used for inflammatory lesions of rosacea in adults. This drug requires a prescription.

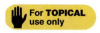

Lindane in shampoo form is used for treating head, body, and pubic lice. It is directly absorbed by the parasites and ova through the exoskeleton; it stimulates their nervous systems, causing seizures and death. This drug requires a prescription and is for topical use only. Very specific instructions come with the product. Clothing and bedding should be washed in hot water or dry-cleaned. Combs and brushes may be washed with lindane shampoo and then thoroughly rinsed with water. This drug should be used as a second-line effort after first trying an OTC medication.

Permethrin (Acticin, Elimite, Nix) is at least as effective as lindane, with the advantage that, unlike lindane, it produces virtually no effects on the CNS. A 1% concentration is the drug of choice for treating head lice. It has residual action lasting up to 14 days that continues to kill any lice hatched after the initial application. It is available as an OTC drug.

Pyrethrin (Rid), which is extracted from chrysanthemum seeds, is an OTC drug usually used for head lice. The mechanism of action involves disruption of lice neuronal transmission and is similar to the action of the now-banned insecticide DDT. Pyrethrin and lindane are similarly efficacious, but pyrethrin is less neurotoxic. Pyrethrin must be applied to premoistened hair and scalp for 10 minutes and then rinsed off; treatment is repeated in one week.

TABLE 15.10 Commonly Used Topical Agents for Lice

Generic (Brand)	Pronunciation	Dosage Form	Dispensing Status
ivermectin (Sklice, Soolantra)	eye-ver-MEK-tin	Cream, lotion	Rx
lindane	LIN-dane	Lotion, shampoo	Rx
permethrin (Acticin, Elimite, Nix)	per-METH-rin	Cream, lotion	OTC, Rx
pyrethrin (Rid)	pye-REE-thrin	Shampoo, spray	OTC

Contraindications Lindane is contraindicated in premature infants and individuals with known uncontrolled seizure disorders. Permethrin use is contraindicated in patients with hypersensitivity to pyrethroids or pyrethrin. OTC pyrethrin should not be used near eyes; inside the nose, mouth, or vagina; or on infestations in eyebrows or eyelashes.

Cautions and Considerations Topical ivermectin should only be used on the scalp and hair.

Lindane has box warnings because it can cause neurotoxicity. Preparations can be irritating to the eyes, mucous membranes, and skin. Overuse may cause dermatitis. Lindane is banned in the state of California due to concerns surrounding adverse effects.

Permethrin may cause difficulty breathing in patients with asthma.

Patients sensitive to ragweed may be sensitive to impurities in pyrethrins.

Drug Interactions Use lindane with caution in combination with drugs that lower seizure threshold (such as antipsychotics, antidepressants, and meperidine).

Scabies

Scabies is produced by small (0.2–0.4 mm long), eyeless, white, flattened, oval mites. Along with spiders and ticks, mites belong to the class of animals called arachnids (similar to insects, but having eight legs rather than six).

The female mite burrows into the epidermis and secretes substances that disintegrate the skin; she then digests the skin and sucks the intracellular fluid. No blood is consumed, because the capillaries are below the epidermis. The mite deposits fecal pellets that probably cause the intense itch.

When infected, the patient experiences an intense itching that worsens at night after the bed is warmed by body heat. This intense itching may be due to the mites' increased activity, feeding, and excretion of feces. Lesions appear as very small, wavy, threadlike, slightly elevated, grayish-white burrows, most often in the webs between the finger. Burrows usually range from 1–10 mm long. Figure 15.2 shows the common sites of scabies infestation. Drug treatment for scabies usually involves permethrin. Permethrin (discussed with lice) should be massaged thoroughly into the skin from the neck to the soles of the feet in adults. The hairline, neck, temples, and forehead may be infested in infants or older adults; in these patients permethrin should also be applied to the scalp and face with avoidance of the eyes. Permethrin should be washed off 8 to 12 hours later.

Further repeated treatment is rarely needed. Persistent inflammation and itching may be due to scratching, contact dermatitis, or a secondary infection rather than the mite infestation. Additional applications could cause dermatitis.

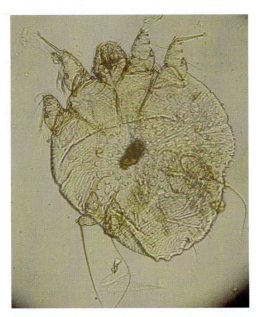

Mites cause intense itching while they are living on the skin.

FIGURE 15.2
Sites of
Scabies
Infestation

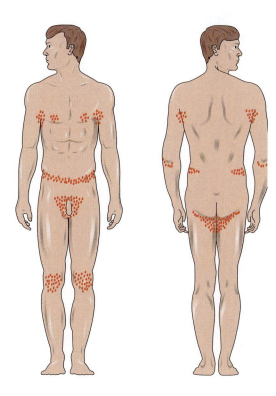

Antiseptics and Disinfectants

Chemicals have long been used to control **suppuration** (formation or discharge of pus), prevent the spread of disease, and preserve food. In the mid-19th century, scientists such as Robert Koch and Louis Pasteur showed that infection and putrefaction were due to microorganisms. Nevertheless, it was only after Joseph Lister developed techniques for antiseptic surgery and the control of postoperative sepsis in the 1860s and 1870s that physicians began to appreciate the importance of disinfecting the skin of the patient undergoing surgery, the hands of the surgeon, the instruments, and the operating theater.

Uses of Disinfectants

Antiseptics and disinfectants have two uses. They are used to disinfect instruments and to treat accessible infections in the oral cavity and on body surfaces. The ideal antiseptic must possess the ability to inhibit all forms of infectious organisms without being toxic to the patient or inducing sensitization of human tissues. It should be capable of penetrating tissues and of acting in the presence of body fluids (i.e., serum, pus, and mucus). It should be soluble in water, stable, noncorrosive, and inexpensive. No agent meets all these requirements. If an antiseptic is to be used to clean instruments or to maintain sterility in a cleanroom, it is always best to use two separate agents with different mechanisms of action. Table 15.11 lists the most commonly used antiseptics and disinfectants. The oral cavity is very difficult to disinfect. Very few drugs will adhere to the mucosal lining long enough to overcome bacteria or ease pain.

TABLE 15.11   Most Commonly Used Antiseptics and Disinfectants

Generic (Brand)	Pronunciation	Dosage Form	Dispensing Status
Topical Products			
benzalkonium chloride (Viroxyn)	benz-al-KOE-nee-um KLOR-ide	Solution	OTC
hexachlorophene (pHisoHex)	hex-a-KLOR-oh-feen	Liquid antiseptic	OTC
hydrogen peroxide (various brands)	HYE-droe-jen per-OX-ide	Solution	OTC
isopropyl alcohol (various brands)	eye-so-PROE-pil AL-koe-hawl	Liquid disinfectant	OTC
povidone-iodine (Betadine)	POE-vi-done EYE-oh-dyne	Aerosol, gel, ointment, solution	OTC
sodium hypochlorite (Clorox)	SOE-dee-um hye-poe-KLOR-ite	Liquid disinfectant	OTC
zinc oxide (Desitin Maximum Strength Original, Desitin Rapid Relief)	ZINK OX-ide	Ointment	OTC
Other Products			
benzocaine (Hurricaine)	BEN-zoe-kayn	Gel, liquid, spray	OTC, Rx
carbamide peroxide (Gly-Oxide Oral)	KAR-ba-mide per-OX-ide	Solution	OTC
chlorhexidine gluconate (Hibiclens)	klor-HEX-i-deen GLOO-koe-nate	Oral liquid antiseptic, external liquid	OTC

Types of Disinfectants

A variety of agents, listed in Table 15.12, are used as antiseptics and disinfectants. These chemicals have specific actions. The most desirable property of a germicide is its ability to destroy microorganisms rapidly and completely. No single germicide is equally effective against all types of organisms. Furthermore, many agents that rapidly destroy organisms may be too toxic to be applied to human or animal tissue cells.

Esthetic factors, such as odor, taste, and staining quality, may also influence germicide selection. If a germicide is used in or around the mouth, bad odor or taste may reduce patient adherence. Patients may also object to materials that stain the oral mucosa, skin, or clothing.

Heavy metal compounds, in concentrations as low as one part per million, inhibit microorganisms. These ions have a strong affinity for proteins. Heavy metals are irritating and astringent (causing a drying out feeling). They do not consistently kill bacteria. Since the advent of new chemicals with better properties, heavy metal compounds are infrequently used as antiseptics and disinfectants.

Benzalkonium chloride (Viroxyn) is used as a preoperative skin disinfectant and for storing instruments and hospital utensils.

Hexachlorophene (pHisoHex) is a surgical scrub and bacteriostatic skin cleanser that is especially effective if gram-positive bacteria are present. It should not be left on skin for long periods of time.

Hydrogen peroxide is a strongly disinfecting, cleansing, and bleaching agent. It is used to prepare dental surfaces before filling and to clean wounds. The release of oxygen provides the antiseptic action.

TABLE 15.12 Actions of Antiseptics and Disinfectants

Agent	Action
Antiseptic	A substance that inhibits growth and development of microorganisms, but does not necessarily kill them
Disinfectant	A chemical applied to objects to free them from pathogenic organisms or render such organisms inert
Fungicide	A substance that destroys fungi
Germicide	A substance that destroys bacteria, but not necessarily spores
Preservative	An agent that prevents decomposition by either chemical or physical means
Sanitizer	An agent that reduces the number of bacterial contaminants to a safe level
Sporicide	A substance that destroys spores

Isopropyl alcohol is supplied in 70%–90% concentrations. This alcohol is inexpensive, spreads well, dries slowly, and does not extract cutaneous fats. It primarily removes bacteria, but can also kill some bacteria. Isopropyl alcohol denatures proteins and produces a marked stinging reaction when applied to cuts or abrasions. To be effective, alcohol must dry and be left on the wound for at least two minutes.

Povidone-iodine (Betadine) is an aqueous solution that does not stain and causes little discomfort when applied to an open wound. It is among the most effective disinfectants available. It has a broad microbicidal spectrum against bacteria, fungi, viruses, protozoa, and yeasts.

Sodium hypochlorite (Clorox) disinfects and deodorizes by killing most germs and their odors. It is a common laundry and household product (chlorine bleach) that is used in cleaning and stain removal.

Zinc oxide (Desitin Maximum Strength Original, Desitin Rapid Relief) is a mild antiseptic and astringent used for some conjunctival and skin diseases. It is the main ingredient in calamine lotion. The oxide salt, a zinc salt, is combined with a petroleum jelly and a waxy lanolin base for use in treating diaper rash and other minor skin irritations.

Benzocaine (Hurricaine) is a local anesthetic, but it also forms a protective barrier over the mucosa. The patient should not eat for an hour after applying to oral mucosa. Benzocaine should not be applied to broken skin.

Carbamide peroxide (Gly-Oxide Oral) releases oxygen on contact with oral tissues and reduces inflammation, inhibits odor-forming bacteria, and relieves pain in periodontal pockets, oral ulcers, and dental sores. It is also used to **emulsify** (enable mixing with water) and disperse earwax.

Chlorhexidine gluconate (Hibiclens) is a skin cleanser for surgical scrub, skin wounds, germicidal hand rinse, and antibacterial dental rinse. It is active against gram-positive and gram-negative organisms and yeast. Studies show that patients on ventilators who have scheduled mouth cleansings throughout the day with chlorhexidine gluconate have significantly decreased incidences of pneumonia.

The Eyes

The eyes are sensory organs specially designed to sense light and produce vision. Light enters the eye through the pupil and is focused by the lens (see Figure 15.3). The lens is located just behind the **pupil**, the black center of the eye. The **lens** of the eye acts like a lens in a camera, focusing light onto the back of the eye. The **iris**, which surrounds the pupil, determines eye color. The **sclera** is the outer coating of the eyeball, commonly referred to as the white of the eye.

Sight begins with light that travels through the lens to the retina in the back of the eye. In the **retina**, photoreceptor cells detect light and color. These rod- and cone-shaped sensory cells send signals via the optic nerve to the brain, where sight is ultimately perceived and interpreted. **Rod cells** are sensitive to light in dimly lit conditions. They are responsible for night vision. Vitamin A deficiency can cause malfunctions in retinal rod cells, which then affects night vision. Rod cells are also considered responsible for black and white vision. **Cone cells** sense color and are responsible for day vision. **Color blindness** (usually a genetic trait that affects mostly male offspring) is a condition in which cone cells do not differentiate colors. The most common form of color blindness is being unable to differentiate red from green. Inside the **macula**, a yellowish spot near the center of the retina, is the focal point (fovea centralis) where light is concentrated for vision (see Figure 15.3). This part of the retina is rich in cone cells.

Other parts of the eye relevant to drug therapy include the cornea, anterior chamber, aqueous humor, ciliary muscle, and conjunctiva. The **cornea** covers the **anterior chamber**. The anterior chamber holds **aqueous humor**, a fluid that lubricates and protects the lens. **Vitreous humor** is the fluid inside the eye, behind the lens. The **ciliary muscle** holds the lens in place. The **conjunctiva** forms the mucous membranes of the socket that hold the eye in place.

Some eye disorders require chronic treatment, whereas others need only acute treatment. For example, glaucoma and chronic dry eye are managed primarily with long-term or chronic use of medications. Conversely, conjunctivitis requires acute treatment to resolve the eye infection.

Pharmacy technicians should also be aware of several medications that are used during eye examinations and procedures. These products are not usually used to treat ophthalmic disorders and are rarely dispensed in pharmacies. Still, it can be useful to be familiar with them (see Table 15.13).

TABLE 15.13 Ophthalmic Products for Eye Examinations and Procedures

Drug Class	Generic (Brand)	Common Use
Mydriatics	atropine ophthalmic (Atropine Care, Isopto Atropine), cyclopentolate ophthalmic (Cyclogyl), Homatropine ophthalmic (Homatropaire, Isopto Homatropine), scopolamine ophthalmic (Isopto Hyoscine), tropicamide ophthalmic (Mydral, Mydriacyl)	Pupil dilation during eye examinations
Ophthalmic local anesthetics	lidocaine ophthalmic (Akten), proparacaine ophthalmic (Alcaine, Parcaine), tetracaine ophthalmic (Altacaine, Tetcaine, TetraVisc)	Ocular surface analgesia during procedures

FIGURE 15.3 The Structures of the Eye

(a) The external eye   (b) Cross section of the internal eye

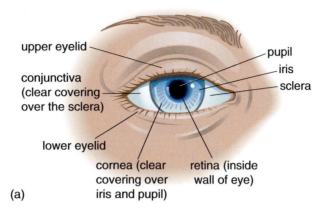

(a)

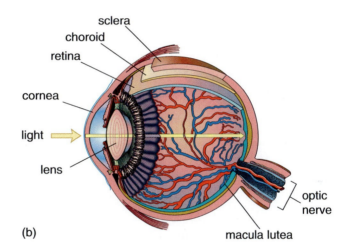

(b)

Glaucoma

Glaucoma is a condition in which abnormally high **intraocular pressure** pushes on the **optic nerve** and damages it. Glaucoma can lead to blindness if it is not treated. The increased pressure comes from either overproduction of aqueous humor or blockage of its outflow from the anterior chamber. (See the parts of the eye in Figure 15.3.) As fluid builds up in the anterior chamber, intraocular pressure increases, and pressure is applied to the optic nerve. **Open-angle glaucoma** is a slowly progressing, chronic condition managed with medication alone. **Narrow-angle glaucoma** is an acute condition that comes on quickly and is resolved with surgery followed by drugs.

Drug Therapies for Treat Glaucoma

Ophthalmic glaucoma agents work by reducing aqueous humor production and, in some cases, enhancing its drainage from the anterior chamber. Miotic agents constrict the pupil slightly by contracting the ciliary muscle. This contraction enhances aqueous humor outflow. Beta blockers are first-line therapy for glaucoma and tend to be used

TABLE 15.14　Ophthalmic Agents for Glaucoma

Generic (Brand)	Pronunciation	Dosage Form	Dispensing Status
Prostaglandin Agonists			
bimatoprost (Lumigan)	bye-MAT-oe-prost	Ophthalmic solution	Rx
latanoprost (Xalatan)	la-TAN-oe-prost	Ophthalmic solution	Rx
tafluprost (Zioptan)	TA-flu-prost	Ophthalmic solution	Rx
travoprost (Travatan-Z)	TRAV-oe-prost	Ophthalmic solution	Rx
unoprostone (Rescula)	yoo-noe-PROS-tone	Ophthalmic solution	Rx
Beta Blockers			
betaxolol (Betoptic-S)	be-TAX-oe-lawl	Ophthalmic solution and suspension	Rx
levobunolol (Betagan)	LEE-voe-BYOO-no-lahl	Ophthalmic solution	Rx
metipranolol (OptiPranolol)	MET-i-PRAN-oh-lol	Ophthalmic solution	Rx
timolol (Timoptic)	TYE-moe-lawl	Ophthalmic solution	Rx
Alpha Receptor Agonists			
brimonidine (Alphagan P)	bri-MOE-ni-deen	Ophthalmic solution	Rx
Miotics			
carbachol (Miostat)	KAR-ba-kawl	Ophthalmic solution	Rx
echothiophate (Phospholine Iodide)	ek-oh-THYE-oh-fate	Ophthalmic powder for reconstitution	Rx
pilocarpine (Isopto Carpine)	pye-loe-KAR-peen	Ophthalmic gel and solution	Rx

Safety Alert

Betoptic and Betagan are easily confused. Also, Betoptic and Betoptic S could be confused.

most frequently (see Table 15.14). Other agents for glaucoma include prostaglandin agonists and ophthalmic alpha receptor agonists. (Oral dosage forms of beta blockers and alpha receptor agonists are covered in Chapter 12.)

Glaucoma agents are usually well tolerated. Side effects include mild stinging, tearing, itchiness, and dryness of the eyes. These effects generally improve with time. Many glaucoma agents have the potential to cause systemic effects if enough medication is absorbed into the bloodstream. These effects are primarily associated with beta blockers and include slowed heart rate, heart problems, insomnia, dizziness, vertigo, headaches, tiredness, and difficulty breathing. If any of these effects occur, patients should contact their prescribers right away. A change in drug therapy will be needed.

Contraindications The prostaglandin agonists do not have contraindications.

The beta blocker ophthalmic products are contraindicated in patients with heart problems including sinus bradycardia, heart block greater than first degree, cardiogenic shock, and uncompensated heart failure. Carteolol and levobunolol should not be used in patients with respiratory problems such as chronic obstructive pulmonary disease (COPD), bronchial asthma, and pulmonary edema.

The alpha receptor agonist brimonidine should not be used in children younger than two years.

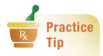

Practice Tip

Use color-coded flash cards to help you learn the generic and brand names of eye and ear products. Choose one color card for eye products and another for ear products. You may also want to use different colored pens to represent the various drug classes.

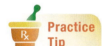

Practice Tip

Eye drops are sterile medications. Tell patients to keep the dropper bottle in a clean place and avoid touching the drop applicator to surfaces, fingers, or the eye itself. If the drop applicator accidentally touches a surface, instruct patients to use an alcohol swab to clean the applicator.

Work Wise

Eye drops are typically solutions, but a few are suspensions that should be shaken well before use. Prior to instilling eye drops, patients must remove their contact lenses and leave them out for at least 15 minutes.

In terms of the miotic ophthalmic products, carbachol use is contraindicated in acute iritis and acute inflammatory disease of the anterior eye chamber.

Echothiophate should not be used in narrow-angle glaucoma and acute uveal inflammation. Acute inflammatory disease of the anterior chamber of the eye contraindicates pilocarpine use.

Cautions and Considerations Patients with heart or thyroid problems should discuss their choices for glaucoma treatment with their prescribers before selecting and using these products. Specifically, the systemic effects of beta blockers can interfere with these conditions and other drug therapies used to treat them.

Prostaglandin agonists have a unique effect in that they cause the iris of the eye to turn brown. Patients should be informed of this effect because their eye color will likely change.

Drug Interactions The effectiveness of prostagladin may be reduced by NSAIDs.

Beta agonists may decrease the effectiveness of beta blockers.

Alpha agonists may decrease the effectiveness of alpha blockers.

Conjunctivitis

Conjunctivitis (commonly called pinkeye) is an inflammation caused by bacteria or viruses in the mucous membranes surrounding the eye. Symptoms include redness of the sclera and the insides of the eyelids, itching, pain, tearing, and the release of exudate. This exudate can be white, yellow, or green. Treatment with antibiotics is relatively easy.

Newborns of mothers with untreated gonorrhea are at high risk for gonococcal conjunctivitis. Treatment for newborns suspected to be infected includes topical ophthalmic anti-infectives for prevention and systemic antibiotics. Pregnant women should be tested for gonorrhea and treated before giving birth, if possible.

Drug Therapy for Conjunctivitis

The number of ophthalmic anti-infective agents is large and can be intimidating to learn. However, this extensive number of products ensures that proper treatment of eye infections can be achieved easily. Many of these medications are given as **ophthalmic ointments** (eye ointments) and, therefore, require patients to learn a specific administration technique.

Common side effects of topically administered anti-infectives are few, and, if present, they are usually mild and tolerable. Although systemic absorption is typically low with these dosage forms, systemic side effects are possible. To learn more about the systemic side effects of anti-infectives, see Chapters 4 and 5.

Contraindications Certain aminoglycosides have contraindications. Tobramycin should not be used in patients with hypersensitivities to other aminoglycosides. Gentamicin does not have contraindications.

Ophthalmic erythromycin, a macrolide, does not have contraindications.

Sulfacetamide, a sulfonamide, is contraindicated in patients with a hypersensitivity to sulfonamides. Trimethoprim–polymyxin B does not have contraindications.

All of the miscellaneous combination products (see Table 15.15) that contain an aminoglycoside or steroid are contraindicated in patients with a hypersensitivity to aminoglycosides or corticosteroids. In addition, all of the miscellaneous combination products are contraindicated in viral disease of the cornea and conjunctiva and in a mycobacterial or fungal infection of the eye.

Cautions and Considerations Anti-infectives are drugs to which many patients have allergies. Therefore, you should ask each patient about allergies and document them in the patient's record. Even topical anti-infective agents can cause serious allergic reactions, so updated allergy information is important for patient safety.

Drug Interactions In general, ophthalmic anti-infectives do not have significant interactions.

TABLE 15.15 Commonly Used Ophthalmic Anti-Infectives

Generic (Brand)	Pronunciation	Dosage Form	Dispensing Status
Aminoglycosides			
gentamicin (Gentak, Genoptic)	jen-ta-MYE-sin	Ophthalmic ointment, ophthalmic solution	Rx
tobramycin (Tobrex)	toe-bra-MYE-sin	Ophthalmic ointment, ophthalmic solution	Rx
Macrolides			
erythromycin (Ilotycin)	eh-rith-roe-mye-sin	Ophthalmic ointment	Rx
Sulfonamides			
sulfacetamide (Bleph-10)	SUL-fa-SET-a-mide	Ophthalmic ointment, ophthalmic solution	Rx
Quinolones			
ciprofloxacin (Ciloxan)	sip-roe-FLOX-a-sin	Ophthalmic ointment, ophthalmic solution, solution	Rx
levofloxacin (Iquix, Quixin)	le-voe-FLOX-a-sin	Ophthalmic solution	Rx
ofloxacin (Ocuflox)	oh-FLOX-a-sin	Ophthalmic solution	Rx
Miscellaneous Combinations			
gentamicin-prednisolone (Pred-G)	jen-ta-MYE-sin pred-NIS-oe-lone	Ophthalmic ointment, ophthalmic suspension	Rx
neomycin–polymyxin B–dexamethasone (Maxitrol)	nee-oh-MYE-sin pol-i-MIX-in dex-a-METH-a-sone	Ophthalmic ointment, ophthalmic suspension	Rx
sulfacetamide-fluorometholone (FML-S)	sul-fa-SEE-ta-mide flor-oh-METH-oe-lone	Ophthalmic solution, suspension	Rx
sulfacetamide-prednisolone (Blephamide)	sul-fa-SEE-ta-mide pred-NIS-oe-lone	Ophthalmic ointment, ophthalmic solution, ophthalmic suspension	Rx
tobramycin-dexamethasone (TobraDex)	toe-bra-MYE-sin dex-a-METH-a-sone	Ophthalmic ointment, ophthalmic suspension	Rx

The Ears

The ears are sensory organs designed to sense sound waves and produce hearing. As seen in Figure 15.4, the ear is divided into three parts: external, middle, and inner. The **external ear** captures **sound waves** and directs them through the **auditory canal** to the **tympanic membrane** (eardrum). **Cerumen** (earwax) is produced by follicles lining the auditory canal.

)) For the EAR

The eardrum separates the **middle ear** from the external ear. It vibrates in response to sound waves, causing the three bones (**malleus**, **incus**, and **stapes**) of the middle ear to move. The stapes taps on the **oval window**, the entrance to the inner ear. The **eustachian tube** connects the middle ear to the throat to allow fluid to drain and to allow equalization of the pressure in the middle ear when atmospheric air pressure changes. The **inner ear** includes the semicircular canals and the cochlea. Fluid in the **cochlea** responds to the tapping on the oval window, producing pressure waves that flow through the spiral-shaped organ (see Figure 15.4). Sensory hairs line the surface of the cochlea in what is called the **organ of Corti**. Sound is perceived and interpreted when corresponding vibrations in these tiny hairs send signals via nerves to the brain. Damage to sensory hairs in the inner ear occurs naturally with age and exposure to loud noise. This kind of hearing loss is called **presbycusis**. The first sounds lost to perception are those produced by high-pitched sound waves.

Fluid in the **semicircular canals** maintains balance and orientation. Gravity pulls the fluid in these channels downward, signaling to the **vestibular nerves** when the body is vertical, horizontal, or upside down. **Vertigo** is a malfunction of these semicircular canals, resulting in balance problems and dizziness.

FIGURE 15.4
The Structural Components of the Ear

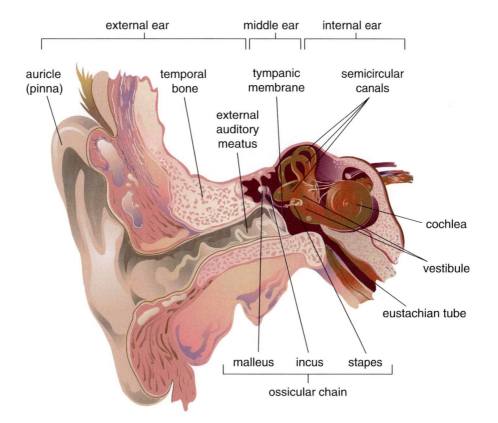

external ear   middle ear   internal ear

auricle (pinna)   temporal bone   tympanic membrane   semicircular canals

external auditory meatus

cochlea

vestibule

eustachian tube

malleus   incus   stapes

ossicular chain

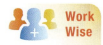

Infections make up the majority of ear disorders that require drug therapy. Oral drug therapy is usually necessary for middle ear infections (see Chapter 4). Antibiotic eardrops will not effectively treat an infection of the middle ear because medication applied to the external ear will not reach the intended site of action unless the tympanic membrane is ruptured.

Otitis Media

Middle ear infection (otitis media) is most common in children. Because the eustachian tube is more horizontal than vertical in children as compared with adults, fluid from the middle ear does not drain well, allowing bacteria and viruses to flourish. Most middle ear infections are viral and clear on their own. Often, otitis media develops after a viral respiratory tract infection in which mucus and fluid build up and provide a growing medium for bacteria. Symptoms of an ear infection include ear pain, jaw pain, sinus pain, itching, and fever. Pain is often intense enough to cause patients (or their parents) to seek medical attention. Sometimes, congestion in the ear can cause fluid pressure on the semicircular canals and cause dizziness (vertigo).

Drug Therapy for Otitis Media

To treat otitis media, healthcare practitioners prescribe oral antibiotics to eradicate the infection and topical analgesics to relieve the pain. To reduce antibiotic resistance, these practitioners attempt to be judicious when prescribing antibiotics for ear infections. Patients experiencing dizziness can use decongestants to reduce pressure in the middle ear.

There are not as many otic antibiotics as there are oral antibiotics. These preparations are usually used as adjunct therapy to oral antibiotics for severe ear infections in which the eardrum is ruptured or tubes have been placed (see Table 15.16). Topical, otic analgesics are used for patients with severe ear pain associated with infection. These products work by temporarily numbing the ear canal (see Table 15.17).

TABLE 15.16 **Commonly Used Antibiotics for Otitis Media**

Generic (Brand)	Pronunciation	Dosage Form	Dispensing Status
Quinolones			
ciprofloxacin (Cetraxal)	sip-roe-FLOX-a-sin	Otic solution, otic suspension	Rx
ofloxacin (Floxin Otic)	oh-FLOX-a-sin	Otic solution	Rx
Combinations			
ciprofloxacin-dexamethasone (Ciprodex)	sip-roe-FLOX-a-sin dex-a-METH-a-sone	Otic suspension	Rx
ciprofloxacin-hydrocortisone (Cipro HC)	sip-roe-FLOX-a-sin hye-droe-KOR-ti-sone	Otic suspension	Rx
neomycin-polymyxin B-hydrocortisone (Cortisporin, Otosporin)	nee-oh-MYE-sin pol-i-MIX-in hye-droe-KOR-ti-sone	Otic solution, otic suspension	Rx

TABLE 15.17   Miscellaneous Otic Products

Generic (Brand)	Pronunciation	Dosage Form	Dispensing Status
Drying Agents			
isopropyl alcohol-glycerin (Auro-Dri, Ear Dry)	Eye-SOH-pro-pill al-COH-hall gleh-SER-in	Otic solution	OTC
Earwax Removers			
carbamide peroxide (Debrox)	KAR-ba-mide per-OX-ide	Otic solution	OTC
Analgesics			
antipyrine-benzocaine (Auralgan)	an-tee-PYE-reen BEN-zoe-kayn	Otic solution	Rx

The few side effects of otic agents are rarely experienced. Although systemic absorption is seldom seen with otic agents, allergic reactions are still possible. Be sure to update the patient's allergy profile each time new orders are written.

Contraindications The quinolone otic products are contraindicated in patients with a sensitivity to other quinolones. Ciprofloxacin-dexamethasone (Ciprodex) should not be used in patients with a quinolone or steroid hypersensitivity and viral infection of the external ear canal. Neomycin-polymyxin B-hydrocortisone (BenzaClin) should not be used in patients with viral infections, fungal diseases, or mycobacterial infections.

Cautions and Considerations Few problems are encountered with otic antibiotics. In severe cases, children can have conjunctivitis along with an ear infection. If both eye drops and eardrops are prescribed, be sure to inform the patient about the difference between these medications.

Drug Interactions In general, otic antibiotics do not have significant interactions.

Otitis Externa

External ear infection (otitis externa) is an infection of the ear canal and involves bacteria or fungi that thrive in moist environments such as that found in cerumen (earwax). When cerumen builds up, hearing can become impaired, and infection can follow. Regular swimmers have the highest propensity to develop external ear infections because pool water and moisture may not properly drain. For that reason, otitis externa is commonly known as *swimmer's ear*.

Drug Therapy for Otitis Externa

Treating external ear infections calls for removing moisture, wax, and any bacteria present from the ear canal. Topical otic preparations are necessary, as oral administration would not reach the desired site of action. These preparations, commonly known as **eardrops**, are effective only for otitis externa. If an infection is in the middle ear or inner ear, medication applied to the external ear will not reach the intended site of action. Systemic absorption of otic preparations usually is not possible.

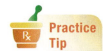

FIGURE 15.5
**Administering
Otic Drops**

(a) Children ages
three and older
and adults should
have the earlobe
pulled up and
back when otic
medications are
administered.

(b) Children under
age three should
have the earlobe
pulled down and
back.

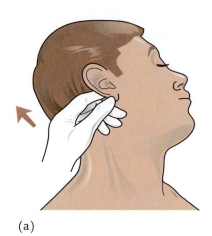

(a)

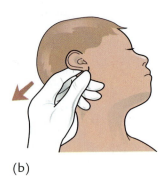

(b)

**Practice
Tip**

Special instruc-
tions should be
given to patients
who have tubes
in their ears. This
patient popula-
tion should only
instill suspensions
and should be
extra careful to
keep otic prepa-
rations sterile to
prevent introduc-
ing infection in
the ears.

Drying agents are used for treatment or prevention of otitis externa. Treatment may be given on a short-term basis for active infection or taken on a regular (even daily) basis to prevent potential infection. **Earwax removers** are used for patients with cerumen impaction. Earwax removers first loosen and dissolve cerumen, after which irrigation with warm water flushes it out. To become familiar with these two drug classes, refer to Table 15.17. Side effects from the instillation of otic drying agents and earwax removers are rare.

Contraindications Drying agents are contraindicated in patients with a perforated tympanic membrane. Carbamide peroxide is also contraindicated in patients with a perforated tympanic membrane as well as ear drainage, ear pain, or rash in the ear. Antipyrine-benzocaine should not be used in patients with a perforated tympanic membrane or with ear discharge.

Cautions and Considerations Other than the contraindications described previously, there are no other notable cautions and considerations associated with the use of otic drying agents and earwax removers.

Drug Interactions In general, otic drying agents and earwax removers do not have significant interactions.

Complementary and Alternative Therapies

Aloe gel has soothing and wound-healing properties. It inhibits bradykinin, a pain-inducing agent, and the synthesis of thromboxane, which may speed the healing of burns. Aloe gel also has antibacterial and antifungal properties. When combined with lidocaine, aloe gel is especially soothing.

Clove oil is an antiseptic used on exposed dentin. Mixed with zinc oxide or zinc acetate, it is used as a dental application in temporary fillings and cements, and in periodontal and intra-alveolar packs.

Vitamin A or **beta-carotene** is essential for photoreceptor cell growth and regeneration. Deficiency in vitamin A can cause night blindness. Vitamin A, vitamin C, vitamin E, and zinc may slow disease progression of age-related macular degeneration.

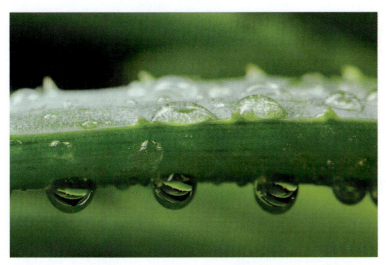

Aloe gel comes from the aloe plant and may be used for its soothing properties.

Ocuvite is the brand name product containing a combination of vitamins and minerals made especially for this use. Ocuvite is taken in doses of two tablets each morning and evening with food. This combination of vitamins does not cure or prevent macular degeneration. Patients who smoke or have a high risk of certain types of cancer may not be good candidates for therapy with this product. Patients should talk with their healthcare practitioners before starting to take any vitamin products to treat eye conditions.

Olive oil is an ingredient in some natural otic products used to soften earwax to remove it from the ears. Docusate sodium, a common stool softener, is combined with olive oil as a base and applied in the ear to soften earwax.

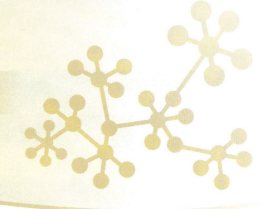

CHAPTER SUMMARY

Skin Ailments and Their Treatment

- The skin is a major organ in the human body and accounts for 16% of body weight. It is the main organ involved in temperature regulation.

- The dermis is composed of connective tissue with upward projections into the epidermis.

- Two types of glands receive widespread distribution in the skin: sebaceous glands and sweat glands.

- When filling a prescription, creams, gels, and ointments are not interchangeable.

Burns and Photosensitivity

- A suntan may look good but can permanently damage the skin.

- A sunscreen should protect against both UVA and UVB rays.

- Sun-damaged skin can be a precursor to skin cancer.

Skin Disorders and Their Pharmaceutical Treatment

- Acne is treated with cleansers, antibiotics, retinoids, brimonidine, and salicylic acid.

- Isotretinoin cannot be used by women who are or may become pregnant.

- Dermatitis is itchy, inflamed skin.

- Topical corticosteroids are commonly used for dermatitis.

- Topical corticosteroids should be applied sparingly as a very thin film. Significant quantities may reach systemic circulation because they can penetrate the skin.

- Eczema may be treated with the calcineurin inhibitors pimecrolimus (Elidel) and tacrolimus (Protopic).

- Dandruff is caused by a malfunction of oil producing glands on the scalp and over-proliferation of cells.

- Dandruff is treated with selenium sulfide.

Skin Infections

- Skin infections are common, and many can be managed with topical antimicrobial products.

- Impetigo is a highly contagious skin infection common in early childhood.

- Fungal infections of the skin and nails may occur.

- Ringworm is caused by a fungus. It may be treated with butenafine, ciclopirox, clotrimazole, ketoconazole, miconazole, sertaconazole, terbinafine, and tolnaftate.

- Viral infections may cause skin disorders such as herpes simplex virus types 1 and 2.

- Patients with herpes simplex type 1 may use topical acyclovir (Zovirax) or OTC docosanol (Abreva) to treat but not cure an outbreak.

External Parasites

- Head lice infestations are among the most common contagious diseases in the United States.

- Lice are insects that live on mammals. They can live on the scalp, skin, and pubic area.

- A lice infestation is treated with OTC products and prescription products.

- Scabies is caused by mites that burrow into the epidermis.

Antiseptics and Disinfectants

- When an antiseptic is used to disinfect instruments or to maintain sterility in a cleanroom, it is always best to use two separate cleansers with different mechanisms of action.

The Eyes

- Conjunctivitis is a common eye disorder, and treatments include topical antibiotics and steroids.

- Eye drops can be used to treat glaucoma.

- Glaucoma can lead to blindness if left untreated.

- Topical prostaglandins, beta blockers, alpha receptor agonists, and miotics are used to treat glaucoma.

The Ears

- Ophthalmics (eye drops) are often prescribed for use in the ear, but otics (eardrops) should never be used in the eye. Antibiotic eye drops are frequently dispensed for ear infections.

- Antipyrine-benzocaine (Auralgan) is a topical anesthetic dispensed as an eardrop; it can be very effective for ear pain.

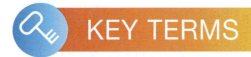 KEY TERMS

acne vulgaris an inflammation of the skin, usually on the face and neck, that is caused by increased activity of the sebaceous glands at puberty

actinic keratosis a scaly skin lesion that is caused by too much sun and can lead to skin cancer

adipose tissue the layer of skin consisting of fat cells

anterior chamber container behind eye that holds aqueous humor of the eye

aqueous humor the liquid in the front portion of the eye

atopic dermatitis a chronic itchy eruption of unknown origin, although allergic, hereditary, and psychogenic factors may be involved; also called *eczema*

auditory canal the part of the ear that sound travels through to reach the inner ear

basal cell carcinoma a slow-growing skin cancer that usually forms polyps and rarely metastasizes

calamine a treatment for mild itching from insect bites, rashes, hives, and poison ivy or poison oak

calcineurin inhibitors used to treat severe eczema

carbuncle a coalescent mass of infected hair follicles that is deeper than a furuncle

cerumen earwax

ciliary muscle part of the eye that holds the lens in place

cochlea part of the ear that produces pressure waves that flow through the spiral-shaped organ

color blindness a condition in which cone cells do not differentiate colors

cone cells the part of the eye responsible for day vision

conjunctiva the mucous membranes of the socket that hold the eye in place

conjunctivitis pinkeye; inflammation of the membrane covering the inside of the eyelid and the outside of the eyeball

contact dermatitis an inflammatory reaction produced by contact with an irritating agent

cornea the protective cover for the anterior chamber of the eye

cradle cap colloquial term for seborrheic dermatitis

dandruff a malfunction of the oil-producing glands around hair follicles on the scalp

dermatitis a condition of inflamed skin

dermis layer of skin below the epidermis

diaper rash common with infants, when skin remains wet for long periods and bacteria growing on the skin turns into a rash

drying agents used for treatment or prevention of otitis externa

eardrops topical otic preparations

earwax removers used to loosen and dissolve cerumen in patients with cerumen impaction

eczema a hot, itchy, red, oozing skin inflammation; also called *atopic dermatitis*

emulsify to break a liquid that does not dissolve in water into small globules that can be suspended in water

epidermis the top layer of the skin

erysipelas a skin infection characterized by redness and warmth, local pain, edematous plaque with sharply established borders, chills, malaise, and fever; a form of cellulitis

eustachian tube part of the ear that connects to the throat to allow fluid to drain

external ear the part of the ear that captures sound waves

external ear infection (otitis externa) an infection of the ear canal that involves bacteria or fungi that thrive in moist environments

folliculitis an inflammation of a hair follicle by a minute, red, pustulated nodule without involvement of the surrounding tissue

furuncle a boil; caused by a staphylococcal infection of a sebaceous gland and the associated hair follicle

glaucoma a chronic eye disorder characterized by abnormally high internal eye pressure that destroys the optic nerve and causes partial or complete loss of vision

hypothalamic-pituitary-adrenal (HPA) axis suppression a condition that causes appetite changes, weight gain, fat redistribution, fluid retention, and insomnia

impetigo a superficial, highly contagious skin infection; characterized by small red spots that evolve into vesicles, break, become encrusted, and are surrounded by a zone of erythema

inner ear part of the ear that includes the semicircular canals and the cochlea

intraocular pressure the buildup of force inside the eye

iris the coloring around the pupil of the eye

keratolytic an agent that breaks down and peels off dead skin cells to keep them from clogging pores

lens the part of the eye that focuses light onto the back of the eye, much like the lens of a camera

lice wingless insects that live parasitically on various animals, including most mammals

macula the focal point of the eye where light is concentrated for vision

malleus, incus, and stapes bones of the middle ear that vibrate in response to sound waves

melanoma a highly malignant skin cancer formed from pigmented skin cells

methemoglobinemia a disorder where an abnormal form of hemoglobin is produced

middle ear the part of the ear beyond the eardrum

middle ear infection (otitis media) when fluid from the middle ear does not drain well, allowing bacteria and viruses to flourish

narrow-angle glaucoma an acute condition that comes on quickly and is resolved with surgery followed by drugs

nodular acne a severe form of acne that can permanently damage skin

open-angle glaucoma a slowly progressing, chronic condition managed with medication alone

ophthalmic glaucoma agents reduce aqueous humor production and may enhance its drainage from the anterior chamber

ophthalmic ointments eye ointments

optic nerve the nerve connecting the eye to the brain

organ of Corti the sensory hairs lining the surface of the cochlea

oval window the entrance to the inner ear

pediculosis an infestation of lice

photosensitivity an abnormal response of the skin or eye to sunlight

pimples, blackheads, and whiteheads pores and follicles clogged with oily material, dead skin cells, and dirt from the skin's surface

presbycucis hearing loss due to damage to the organ of Corti

pruritic to be itchy

psoriasis a skin disorder characterized by patches of red, scaly skin that are slightly raised with defined margins; usually occurs on the elbows and knees but can affect any part of the body

pupil the black center of the eye

retina the photoreceptor cells that detect light and color in the eye

retinoid compound related to vitamin A that helps to regulate skin cell growth

ringworm a fungus that infects the horny (scaly) layer of skin or the nails; also called *tinea*

rod cells part of the eye responsible for night vision

rosacea chronic dermatologic disorder involving inflammation of the skin of the face; also called *acne rosacea*

sclera the outer coating of the eyeball, the whites of the eye

sebaceous glands secrete sebum, a substance that oils the skin and hair

seborrheic dermatitis greasy, scaly area on the skin that appears red, brown, or yellow

sebum an oil produced from glands around hair follicles that when overproduced creates acne

semicircular canals full of fluid, they maintain balance and orientation

sound waves vibrations in air that are interpreted by ears as noise

squamous cell carcinoma a skin cancer that grows more rapidly than basal cell carcinoma but in which metastasis is uncommon

Staphylococcus aureus a bacteria that causes infections on the skin and require antibiotics to treat

subcutaneous tissue the innermost layer of skin connecting the dermis to underlying organs and tissues

sun protection factor (SPF) a measurement of the effectiveness of a sunscreen

suppuration formation or discharge of pus

sweat glands water-salt producing glands found in the skin

topical corticosteroids used to treat contact dermatitis, eczema, psoriasis, and allergic reactions

tympanic membrane eardrum

vertigo a malfunction of the semicircular canals resulting in balance problems and dizziness

vestibular nerves part of the ear that signals when the body is vertical, horizontal, or upside down

vitamin A a vitamin essential to photoreceptor cell growth and regeneration

vitamin D analog a treatment for psoriasis

vitreous humor the fluid inside the eye behind the lens

wart a virally caused epidermal tumor

wrinkle a line or crease in the skin

DRUG LIST

Sun-Damaged Skin

aloe gel
benzocaine (Dermoplast, Hurricaine)
hydrocortisone (Anusol-HC, Cortaid)
lidocaine (Lidoderm, Lidopin, Topicaine,
    Xolido, Xylocaine)
silver sulfadiazene (Silvadene, SSD)

Skin Diseases and Disorders

Acne Vulgaris—Topical Antibiotics

azelaic acid (Azelex, Finacea)
benzoyl peroxide (Benzac, Brevoxyl,
    Clearasil, Desquam-X, NeoBenz,
    Neutrogena, Oxy, PanOxyl, Triaz,
    ZoDerm)
clindamycin-benzoyl peroxide (BenzaClin)
dapsone (Aczone)
erythromycin (Ery, Erygel)

Acne Vulgaris—Retinoids

adapalene (Differin)
isotretinoin (Accutane, Claravis)
tazarotene (Avage, Tazorac)
tretinoin (Atralin, Avita, Renova, Retin-A)

Acne Vulgaris—Miscellaneous

salicylic acid (Clearasil, Neutrogena, Oxy,
    Stridex)

Actinic Keratosis

fluorouracil (Efudex)

Bacterial Skin Infections

bacitracin
bacitracin-neomycin-polymyxin B
    (triple antibiotic ointment, Neosporin,
    Mycitracin)
mupirocin (Bactroban)
retapamulin (Altabax)

Dandruff

nizoral
pyrithione zinc

selenium sulfide (Head & Shoulders
    Intensive Treatment, Selsun Blue)

Dermatitis, Eczema, and Psoriasis

calamine
calcipotriene (Calcitrene, Dovonex, Sorilux)
pimecrolimus (Elidel)
tacrolimus (Protopic)

Fungal Skin Infections

butenafine (Lotrimin Ultra, Mentax)
ciclopirox (Ciclodan, Penlac, Loprox)
clotrimazole (Alevazol, Desenex, FungiCure,
    Lotrimin AF)
ketoconazole (Extina, Ketodan, Nizoral,
    Xolegel)
miconazole (Desenex, Lotrimin AF,
    Micaderm)
sertaconazole (Ertaczo)
terbinafine (Lamisil, Lamisil AT)
tolnaftate (Tinactin Antifungal)

Rosacea

brimonidine (Mirvaso)
metronidazole (MetroCream, MetroGel,
    MetroLotion, Noritate, Rosadan)

Viral Skin Infections

acyclovir (Zovirax)
docosanol (Abreva)

Wrinkles

tretinoin (Renova, Retin-A, Vesanoid)

Topical Corticosteroids

Low Potency

alclometasone (Aclovate)
hydrocortisone (Cortaid, Cortizone-10,
    Dermolate, HydroSKIN, Procort,
    Scalpicin)
hydrocortisone (Acticort, Ala-Cort, Cetacort,
    Cort- Dome, Eldecort, Hi-Cor, Hycort,
    Hydrocort, Hytone, LactiCare, Penecort,
    Synacort, Texacort)

hydrocortisone acetate (Cortaid, Cortef,
Corticaine, Gynecort, Lanacort, Tucks)
hydrocortisone butyrate (Locoid)
hydrocortisone probutate (Pandel)
prednicarbate (Dermatop)

High Potency

betamethasone dipropionate (Diprosone,
Maxivate)
betamethasone valerate (Beta-Val, Luxiq,
Psorion)
clocortolone (Cloderm)
desoximetasone (Topicort)
fluocinolone acetonide (Capex, Synalar)
fluocinonide (Lidex, Vanos)
fluticasone (Cutivate)
halcinonide (Halog)
hydrocortisone valerate (Westcort)
mometasone furoate (Elocon)
triamcinolone (Flutex, Kenalog, Kenonel)

Very High or Super Potency

amcinonide (Cyclocort)
betamethasone dipropionate, augmented
(Diprolene)
clobetasol propionate (Clobex, Cormax,
Olux, Temovate)
desonide (DesOwen, LoKara,Verdeso)

Topical Antivirals

acyclovir (Zovirax)
docosanol (Abreva

Treatments for Lice

ivermectin (Sklice, Soolantra)
lindane
permethrin (Elimite, Nix)
pyrethrin (Rid)

Topical Products

benzalkonium chloride (Viroxyn)
hexachlorophene (pHisoHex)
hydrogen peroxide
isopropyl alcohol
povidone-iodine (Betadine)
sodium hypochlorite (Clorox)
zinc oxide (Desitin Maximum Strength
Original, Desitin Rapid Relief)

Other

benzocaine (Dermoplast, Hurricaine)
carbamide peroxide (Gly-Oxide Oral)
chlorhexidine gluconate (Hibiclens)

Ophthalmics

Corticosteroids and Combinations

neomycin-polymyxin B-dexamethasone
(Maxitrol)
sulfacetamide-prednisolone (Blephamide)
tobramycin-dexamethasone (TobraDex)

Glaucoma Treatments

Ophthalmic Agents—Alpha Receptor Agonists

brimonidine (Mirvaso)

Ophthalmic Agents—Beta Blockers

betaxolol (Betoptic-S)
levobunolol (Betagan)
metipranolol (OptiPranolol)
timolol (Timoptic)

Ophthalmic Agents—Miotics

carbachol(Miostat)
echothiophate (Phospholine Iodide)
pilocarpine (Isopto Carpine)

Ophthalmic Agents—Prostaglandin Agonists

bimatoprost (Lumigan)
latanoprost (Xalatan)
tafluprost (Zioptan)
travoprost (Travatan-Z)
unoprostone (Rescula)

Ophthalmic Anti-Infectives

Aminoglycosides

gentamicin (Gentak, Genoptic)
gentamicin-prednisolone (Pred-G)

Quinolones

levofloxacin (Iquix, Quixin)
ofloxacin (Ocuflox)
tobramycin (Tobrex)

Sulfonamides

sulfacetamine
spfacetamine
sulfacetamide-fluorometholone (FML-S)

Otics

Analgesic

antipyrine-benzocaine (Auralgan)

Antibiotics

ciprofloxacin (Cetraxal)
ciprofloxacin-dexamethasone (Ciprodex)
ciprofloxacin-hydrocortisone
    (Cipro HC)
neomycin-polymyxin B-hydrocortisone
    (Cortisporin Otic)
ofloxacin (Floxin Otic)

Earwax Dissolvers

carbamide peroxide (Debrox)

Drying Agents

isopropyl alcohol-glycerin (Auro-Dri,
    Ear Dry)

Black Box Warnings

isotretinoin (Accutane, Claravis)
pimecrolimus (Elidel)
tacrolimus (Protopic)
tretinoin (Renova, Retin-A, Vesanoid)

Medication Guides

isotretinoin (Accutane, Claravis)
lindane
tacrolimus (Protopic)

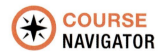

COURSE NAVIGATOR

Access interactive chapter review exercises, practice activities, flash cards, and study games.

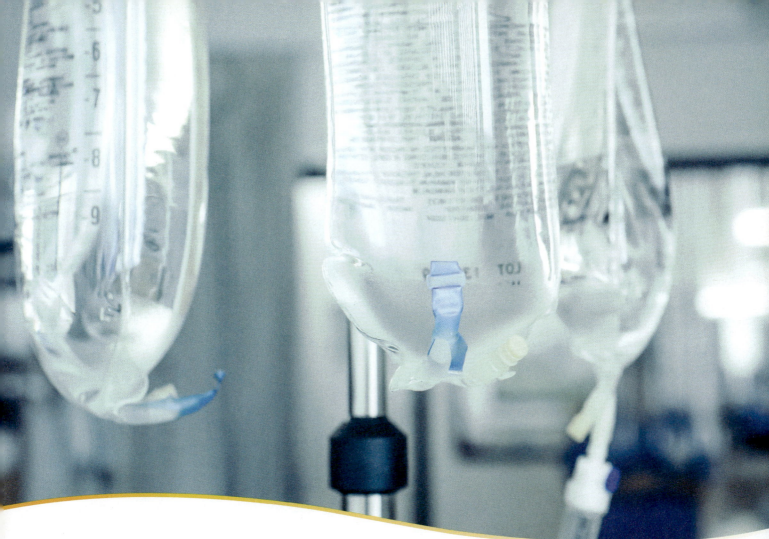

Chemotherapy and Miscellaneous Pharmaceutical Products

665

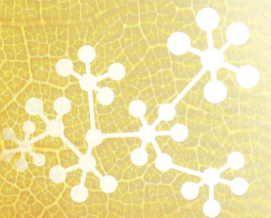

16

Cancer Drugs and Chemotherapy

Andrea Iannucci and Tanja Monroe

Learning Objectives

1 Explain the basic physiology of malignancy and tumor cell growth.

2 Identify and provide examples of traditional chemotherapy and cytotoxic drugs, hormonal drug therapies, and targeted drug therapies.

3 Identify the generic names, brand names, indications, dosage ranges, side effects, and cautions and considerations associated with the drugs commonly used to treat cancer.

4 Explain strategies that help prevent chemotherapy-related errors.

5 Identify current investigational therapies and alternative therapies used to treat cancer.

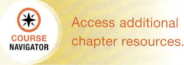

Access additional chapter resources.

E ach year, approximately 1.6 million individuals in the United States are diagnosed with cancer, and more than 500,000 patients will die from this disease. In fact, cancer is now the second-leading cause of death (behind heart disease) in the United States. These grim statistics are a reminder of the overwhelming impact cancer has on individuals, their families and caregivers, and the healthcare system. As part of this system, pharmacy technicians will most certainly be involved in caring for patients with cancer.

This chapter provides an overview of cancer and the arsenal of chemotherapy drugs used in the treatment of this disease. Chemotherapy drugs represent a complicated group of medications with a narrow window between safe therapeutic use and the potential for great toxicity. These medications are traditionally administered in a hospital or an outpatient chemotherapy infusion center by the intravenous (IV) route. Most IV chemotherapy drugs are prepared by pharmacists or pharmacy technicians in these settings. Over the past 10 years, however, the number of orally administered chemotherapy agents has increased; consequently, the care of patients with cancer is expanding into the community practice setting.

In addition to having a good understanding of chemotherapy medications, pharmacy technicians must be cognizant of the safety measures that must be implemented during the preparation, and handling of these medications.

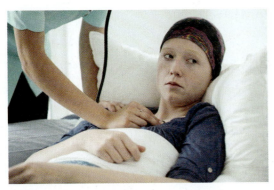

In the United States, breast cancer is the most common cancer among women.

Cancer and Its Development

Cancer is a term that describes a group of diseases characterized by the uncontrolled growth of dysfunctional cells. Normally, cells multiply only until there are enough of them to meet the needs of the body (for example, epidermal cells multiply to replace skin cells lost because of damage or aging). Cancer is thought to originate from a single cell (defined as **monoclonal**) that has lost its ability to control growth and proliferation.

This abnormal cell growth is caused by genetic changes that result from both external factors and internal factors. External factors include some lifestyle choices such as tobacco or heavy alcohol use, sun exposure, diet, physical inactivity, infectious disease processes; or exposure to environmental carcinogens, such as pesticides or asbestos. Internal factors include immune disorders, hormones, and genetic mutations. Although some cancers are hereditary, many more cancers result from some combination of lifestyle, environment, and genetic factors.

Pathophysiology of Cancer and Malignancy

In the past 20 years, scientists have discovered the role of genes in cancer development. Their research has established correlations between certain genetic mutations and the development of particular cancers. Identifying these correlations has been a catalyst for developing early cancer screening methods as well as targeting drug therapy for specific cancers. Both strategies continue to improve the early diagnosis and treatment of patients with cancer.

"Drivers" of Cancer

The two major classes of genes that play a role in cancer development are oncogenes and tumor suppressor genes. Changes to these genes have been identified by scientists as the **"drivers" of cancer**, or genetic alterations that promote cancer progression.

Oncogenes

Oncogenes are genes that promote cancer formation. Oncogenes develop from **proto-oncogenes**, or genes that code for growth factors or their receptors (see Figure 16.1). All cells possess proto-oncogenes for normal function. Alterations of proto-oncogenes via exposure to chemicals, viruses, radiation, or hereditary factors can activate the oncogene that promotes abnormal cell growth. One example of an oncogene is the ERBB2 gene (also called the HER2/neu gene), which codes for a growth-factor receptor found in some forms of breast cancer.

Tumor Suppressor Genes

Tumor suppressor genes turn off or down-regulate the proliferation of cancer cells. These genes are the brakes that inhibit inappropriate cell growth. Mutations or deletions of tumor-suppressor genes can also result in uncontrolled cell growth. One of the most common tumor suppressor genes is *p53*. The normal gene product of *p53* halts cell division and induces **apoptosis**, or programmed cell death, in abnormal or aging cells. Mutations of *p53* are linked to resistance to many chemotherapy drugs.

FIGURE 16.1 **Oncogenes and Cancer Formation**

The activation of an oncogene converts a normal cell to a cancer cell.

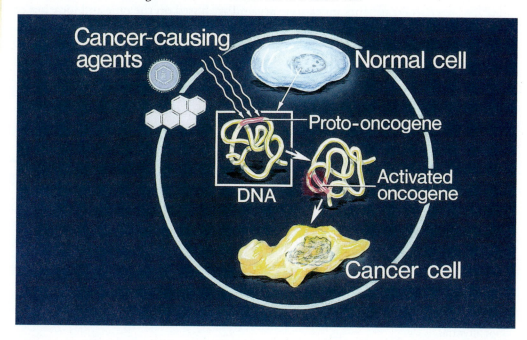

Tumor Cell Proliferation

In general, tumor cells grow and divide with a high rate of proliferation. Growth of tumor cells is not, however, linear. Tumor cells exhibit an exponential rate of growth early on in tumor development, but the growth rate gradually slows over time. A model for **tumor cell proliferation** was developed by German mathematician Benjamin Gompertz. This model is now widely accepted as an approximation of tumor cell proliferation (see Figure 16.2). One cell divides into two cells; two cells divide into four cells; and so on. It typically takes about 30 divisions to make 1 g (about 1 cm^3) of tumor mass, which is the smallest clinically detectable tumor (1 g = 1 cm^3 = 10^9 = 1 billion cells).

During the exponential phase, a tumor is most sensitive to chemotherapy agents that attack and destroy rapidly dividing cells. After a tumor has reached a certain size, growth slows, possibly due to restrictions in space, decreased blood supply, and decreased nutritional supply. However, note that only 10 more divisions will make a 1-kg mass (about 10^{12} cells), which is considered a lethal tumor burden.

Tumor Burden

Tumor burden is the number of cancer cells or the size of the tumor tissue. This measurement is a determining factor in the effectiveness of chemotherapy: The smaller the tumor burden, the more effective chemotherapy will be. A predominant hypothesis applied in cancer treatment is the **cell kill hypothesis**. This hypothesis presumes that each cycle of chemotherapy kills a certain percentage of cancer cells. If a tumor has 10 billion cells and a chemotherapy cycle kills 95% of them, then 0.5 billion cells remain. The second cycle kills 95% more, leaving 25 million cells, and the third cycle would leave 1.25 million cells. Using this theory, tumor cell count will never reach zero from treatment alone, but once the number of cancer cells is low enough, normal host defense mechanisms take over to eradicate the remaining cells.

Treatments for Cancer

Treatments for cancer vary and are based on the type and location of the tumor as well as the extent of the disease. Tumors that are localized are generally easier to treat than tumors that have spread from the primary site to other parts of the body, which is a process known as **metastasis**.

There are four major modalities (methods) used to treat cancer. These methods include surgery, radiation therapy, immunotherapy, and chemotherapy. These treatments may be used alone or in combination to treat cancer.

FIGURE 16.2
Tumor Cell Growth

A tumor must reach a certain size before it can be detected. Unfortunately, chemotherapy drugs can kill only a percentage of cancer cells in the tumor after this point, instead of completely eradicating it.

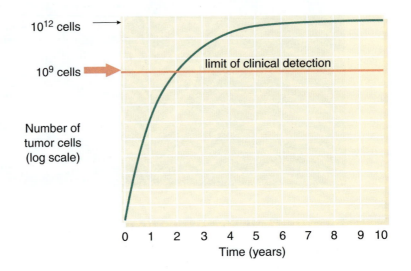

10^{12} cells

10^9 cells

limit of clinical detection

Number of tumor cells (log scale)

0 1 2 3 4 5 6 7 8 9 10
Time (years)

Surgery

The most curable types of cancer are localized tumors that can be surgically removed or **resected**. Ideally, the tumor can be removed without leaving any cancer cells at the site of the resection. The surgeon typically removes a little bit of normal tissue around the site of the tumor, an area known as the **margin**. Once the tumor is completely resected, the surgeon assesses the site of removal for residual tumor cells. The absence of these tumor cells, a condition known as a **negative margin**, lowers the risk of tumor regrowth.

Radiation Therapy

Some tumors occur in locations that are difficult to reach with surgery (e.g., brain tumors). Other tumors may be too extensive to remove without damaging normal tissue or structures. In these situations, radiation therapy may be a better option. **Radiation therapy** involves the use of external beam radiation delivered from a machine outside the body to the site of a tumor. Radiation therapy may be used to rapidly shrink the mass of a tumor that is causing pain or impinging on vital organs or structures, such as the spinal cord. Sometimes, radiation therapy is used with surgery to "clean up" areas of residual tumor that might have been left behind after surgery. This type of radiation therapy is called **adjuvant radiation therapy**.

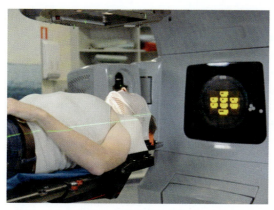

Almost half of all patients who have cancer undergo radiation therapy.

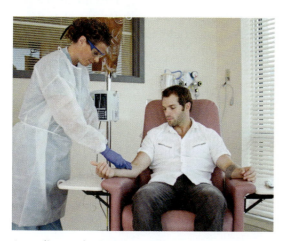

According to the American Cancer Society, prostate cancer is the most common cancer among men. Chemotherapy is sometimes used if the cancer has metastasized to other organs.

Immunotherapy

Immunotherapy is a type of cancer treatment that stimulates the immune system to stop or slow the growth of cancer cells. Two commonly used immunotherapy drugs are interferons and interleukins, which are used to treat **melanoma** (a frequently fatal type of skin cancer) and renal cell carcinoma (an aggressive type of kidney cancer).

Immunotherapy in cancer treatment is being heavily researched. Newer immune-based therapies are being developed to prevent immune cells from being turned off by cancer cells. These novel therapies are called **immune checkpoint inhibitors** and represent a broad category of antineoplastic agents that are being studied on a number of tumor types.

Chemotherapy

Chemotherapy is the modality of administering drugs to treat cancer. This treatment method provides systemic exposure to anticancer therapy as a means of affecting the primary tumor as well as migrating tumor cells. Chemotherapy may be described as primary, adjuvant, or palliative, depending on the goals of therapy.

Primary Chemotherapy

Primary chemotherapy refers to the initial treatment of cancer with chemotherapy with **curative** intent. Examples of some of the cancers that can be cured with primary chemotherapy are Hodgkin's disease, lymphoma, leukemias, and testicular cancer.

Adjuvant Chemotherapy

Adjuvant chemotherapy refers to the treatment of residual cancer cells after removal or reduction of the tumor by surgery. Sometimes, if the tumor is too large to remove, a patient may be given **neoadjuvant chemotherapy** in an attempt to shrink the tumor so that it can be safely and completely removed with surgery. Both adjuvant and neoadjuvant chemotherapy can be curative if the tumor is effectively removed. One example of adjuvant therapy is administering chemotherapy and/or hormone therapy following a lumpectomy or mastectomy (types of surgical removal) in breast cancer. The patient is given adjuvant chemotherapy and radiation after surgery to ensure that any remaining cancer cells are eradicated.

Palliative Chemotherapy

Palliative chemotherapy is given for cancer that is not curable. The usual purpose of palliative chemotherapy is to prolong a patient's life and to improve his or her quality of life by decreasing the tumor size and reducing the symptoms caused by the tumor.

Chemotherapy Drugs

Multiple factors affect tumor response to chemotherapy drugs. Examples include the size of the tumor (tumor burden), cell resistance to the chemotherapy agent, the amount of chemotherapy administered, and the condition of the patient prior to chemotherapy. To reduce the potential for the cancer to become resistant to treatment, **combination chemotherapy** is usually administered. This type of regimen is designed to include drugs with the following characteristics:

- proven efficacy against the tumor being treated
- nonoverlapping toxicities
- different mechanisms of action

Sometimes, combinations of drugs may have an enhanced response because the agents work together to amplify the individual effects of each drug. This is called a **synergistic effect**. The most important thing to know about combinations of anticancer drugs is that you cannot always predict the potential benefits or effects of the combination. Combination chemotherapy regimens must be selected based on proven safety and efficacy of the combination.

Pharm Facts

In the late 19th century, German bacteriologist Paul Ehrlich used methylene blue stain to demonstrate cell pathology. His research in the use of chemical compounds to identify and treat diseases paved the way for genetic studies in cancer research and the development of drugs that interfere with the cell cycle. These drugs became known as chemotherapy, a term Ehrlich coined from the words chemical and therapy. For his pioneering work, Ehrlich won a Nobel Prize in 1908. Today, he is considered to be the father of chemotherapy.

Cell Cycle and Mechanism of Action

Grasping how chemotherapy drugs work requires an understanding of the cell cycle. The **cell cycle** is the process by which both normal cells and cancer cells divide. Because most cancer cells have lost their checks and balances on the rate of cellular replication, chemotherapy drugs are designed to interfere with the cell cycle at specific points.

Cell Cycle–Specific Drugs

Cell cycle–specific drugs exert their effects on rapidly dividing cancer cells, which are the most sensitive to the effects of chemotherapy. These drugs target cancer cells as they move into the susceptible phase of the cell cycle, while minimizing exposure to normal cells that may be in the resting phase of the cell cycle (see Figure 16.3). For this reason, these drugs are considered schedule dependent and are administered as continuous infusions (e.g., fluorouracil or cytarabine) or in repeated bolus doses (e.g., weekly bleomycin).

Cytotoxic Drugs

Chemotherapy drugs may be cytotoxic drugs (toxic to cells), hormonal therapies, immunotherapy, or one of the newer targeted anticancer therapies. However, many individuals consider cytotoxic drugs to be synonymous with the term *chemotherapy*.

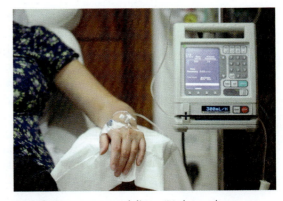

An infusion pump set delivers IV chemotherapy to a patient. The pump delivers medication at a controlled IV flow rate specified by the prescriber or pharmacist.

FIGURE 16.3
Cell Cycle

Often, multiple agents (shown in colored type) acting on different phases of cell growth and proliferation are used together to increase effectiveness and kill more cancer cells.

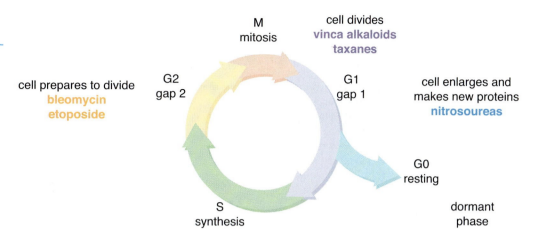

M
mitosis

cell divides
vinca alkaloids
taxanes

cell prepares to divide
bleomycin
etoposide

G2
gap 2

G1
gap 1

cell enlarges and
makes new proteins
nitrosoureas

G0
resting

dormant
phase

S
synthesis

DNA replication/synthesis
occurs
antimetabolites

Cytotoxic drugs work by interfering with some normal process of cell function or proliferation. Table 16.1 outlines the various categories of cytotoxic drugs and lists examples and major side effects of drugs within each category. Although cytotoxic drugs exert the majority of their effects on cancer cells, these agents do not target tumor cells specifically. As a result, chemotherapy drugs cause numerous side effects related to normal cell function. Side effects from traditional chemotherapy drugs include **bone marrow suppression** (decreased production of blood cells, increased risks of infections and bleeding), **alopecia** (hair loss), nausea and vomiting, and **mucositis** (inflammation and ulceration of the mucous membranes lining

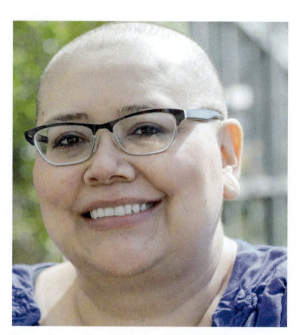

For patients with cancer, alopecia typically begins within the first two weeks of chemotherapy treatment and progressively worsens over the next two months.

the mouth and gastrointestinal [GI] tract). Table 16.2 describes some of the unique side effects of specific chemotherapy drugs as well as the measures taken to prevent these toxicities. Although there are many risks associated with traditional chemotherapy agents, the use of these powerful drugs continues to either cure many patients of cancer or slow the progression of their disease, which prolongs their lives. Cytotoxic drugs remain a critical component of cancer treatment.

TABLE 16.1 Traditional Chemotherapy and Cytotoxic Drug Categories

Category	Drugs	Major Side Effects	Dispensing Status
Alkylating agents	Bendamustine Busulfan Carboplatin Carmustine (BCNU) Chlorambucil Cisplatin Cyclophosphamide Dacarbazine Ifosfamide Lomustine Mechlorethamine Melphalan Oxaliplatin Procarbazine Temozolomid	Bone marrow suppression, alopecia, nausea and vomiting, infertility, secondary cancers	Rx
Antimetabolites	Capecitabine Cladribine Clofarabine Cytarabine Fludarabine Fluorouracil Gemcitabine Hydroxyurea Mercaptopurine Methotrexate Pemetrexed	Bone marrow suppression, immune system suppression, mucositis	Rx
Topoisomerase inhibitors	Daunorubicin Doxorubicin Epirubicin Etoposide Idarubicin Irinotecan Mitoxantrone Teniposide Topotecan	Bone marrow suppression, nausea and vomiting, mucositis, alopecia, diarrhea	Rx
Antimicrotubule agents	Docetaxel Eribulin Paclitaxel Vinblastine Vincristine Vinorelbine	Bone marrow suppression, mucositis, alopecia, nerve toxicity	Rx

TABLE 16.2　Unique Toxicities of Chemotherapy Agents

Category	Toxicity	Preventive Measures
Alkylating Agents		
Cisplatin	Kidney damage	• Administer aggressive IV fluids before and after each dose.
	Potassium and magnesium loss	• Provide potassium and magnesium supplements.
	Nerve pain and/or nerve damage	• Assess level of nerve damage with each treatment. Stop treatment at onset of symptoms. • Limit doses to ≤100 mg/m^2 for a cycle of treatment.
Ifosfamide	Hemorrhagic cystitis	• Administer IV fluids during and after treatment. • Give mesna (a bladder protectant) during and after treatment.
Oxaliplatin	Nerve pain and/or nerve damage (hands, feet, throat)	• Caution patients to avoid cold temperatures. • Advise patients to avoid cold beverages. • Limit doses or stop treatment if symptoms do not reverse.
Antimetabolites		
Capecitabine	Hand-foot syndrome Diarrhea	• Advise patients to use emollients on hands and feet. • Limit doses or stop therapy if symptoms develop.
Cytarabine	Conjunctivitis	• Administer steroid eyedrops during treatment whenever patients receive doses >1,000 mg/m^2.
Methotrexate	Kidney damage	• Administer aggressive IV fluids. • Provide urinary alkalinization using sodium bicarbonate.
	Severe bone marrow and mucosal toxicity	• Provide leucovorin rescue during the administration of methotrexate.
Pemetrexed	Severe bone marrow suppression	• Administer folic acid and vitamin B$_{12}$ supplements, starting 5–7 days before treatment.
	Skin rash	• Give dexamethasone, starting 1 day before treatment
Topoisomerase Inhibitors		
Anthracyclines: daunorubicin, doxorubicin, epirubicin, idarubicin	Cardiac toxicity: cardiomyopathy, congestive heart failure	• Track and limit cumulative doses. • Monitor heart function. • Stop treatment if symptoms develop.
Irinotecan	Severe diarrhea	• Administer atropine for diarrhea that occurs during drug administration. • Educate patients about how and when to take antidiarrheal agents (e.g., loperamide [Imodium], atropine-diphenoxylate [Lomotil]) after treatment.
Antimicrotubule Agents		
Paclitaxel	Allergic reaction	• Premedicate patients with diphenhydramine, famotidine, or another H$_2$ blocker or with dexamethasone.
	Nerve pain and/or nerve damage	• Decrease dose or stop treatment if symptoms occur.
Vincristine	Nerve damage	• Cap individual doses at 2 mg. • Stop treatment if symptoms develop.
Miscellaneous Agent		
Bleomycin	Lung damage	• Track and limit cumulative doses to <400 units. • Limit individual doses to ≤30 units. • Avoid giving to patients with kidney dysfunction.

Alkylating Agents

The oldest category of traditional cytotoxic drugs contains the **alkylating agents**. The first drug identified in this category as having anticancer activity was **mechlorethamine (Mustargen)**, or nitrogen mustard, a derivative of mustard gas. The accidental release of mustard gas during World War II was only later discovered to play a role in decreasing the activity of lymphocytes in soldiers who were exposed to the gas. The discovery of this reaction led to the development of this agent as a treatment for lymphoma, a cancer of the lymphatic system.

Alkylating agents work by binding to and damaging deoxyribonucleic acid (DNA) during the cell division process, ultimately preventing cell replication. Examples of alkylating agents are listed in Table 16.1. Alkylating agents have a broad spectrum of anticancer activity and are used to treat a variety of cancer types. **Cisplatin (Platinol)** is an alkylating agent that is used to treat many diseases, including lung, ovarian, and bone cancers. In addition, cisplatin is a critical component of the chemotherapy regimens for testicular cancer. **Cyclophosphamide (Cytoxan)** is an alkylating agent that plays an important role in treating lymphomas, leukemias, and breast cancer. **Carmustine (BCNU)**, and **lomustine (Gleostine)** are in the category of alkylating agents known as **nitrosoureas**. These agents have the ability to penetrate the central nervous system (CNS) and are frequently used in the treatment of brain tumors. See Tables 16.3 and 16.4 for examples of other types of cancer that are treated with oral and injectable alkylating agents.

The most common side effect of alkylating agents is bone marrow suppression. Alkylating agents also cause nausea, vomiting, and alopecia.

TABLE 16.3 Commonly Used Oral Chemotherapy Drugs

Generic (Brand)	Pronunciation	Common Indication	Dispensing Status
Alkylating Agents			
busulfan (Myleran)	byoo-sul-fan	Leukemia	Rx
chlorambucil (Leukeran)	klor-am-byoo-sill	Chronic lymphocytic leukemia	Rx
cyclophosphamide (Cytoxan)	sye-kloe-fos-fa-mide	Breast cancer, immune system diseases (e.g., arthritis, lupus)	Rx
lomustine (Gleostine)	loe-mus-teen	Brain tumor	Rx
melphalan (Alkeran)	mel-fa-lan	Multiple myeloma	Rx
procarbazine (Matulane)	proe-kar-ba-zeen	Brain tumor, Hodgkin's disease	Rx
temozolomide (Temodar)	te-mo-zole-oh-mide	Brain tumor, melanoma	Rx
Antimetabolites			
capecitabine (Xeloda)	kap-pe-site-a-been	Breast cancer, colon cancer	Rx
hydroxyurea (Droxia, Hydrea)	hye-drox-ee-yoor-ee-a	Leukemia, sickle-cell anemia	Rx
mercaptopurine (Purinethol)	mer-kap-toe-pyoor-een	Leukemia	Rx
methotrexate (various brands)	meth-o-trex-ate	Psoriasis, rheumatoid arthritis, systemic lupus erythematosus	Rx

Many alkylating agents cause unique toxicities. Cisplatin is notorious for causing kidney damage and depleting potassium and magnesium levels. These side effects are minimized by providing patients with potassium and magnesium supplements as well as 1–2 L of IV fluid before and after administration of cisplatin. Cisplatin may also cause **peripheral neuropathy** (extremely painful damage to the nerves that affect the hands and feet) and **ototoxicity**, which is damage to the nerves that affect hearing. Patients must be carefully assessed for these side effects between cycles of treatment, and doses should be decreased or stopped when symptoms develop. Maximum limits are placed on dosing cisplatin to avoid overdose and severe toxicities. **Ifosfamide (Ifex)** is known to cause **hemorrhagic cystitis**, which is damage to and bleeding of the urinary bladder. The physician may prescribe the bladder-protective medication, **mesna**, for coadministration to counteract hermorrhagic cysititis. Other unique toxicities of alkylating agents are outlined in Table 16.2.

Because alkylating agents damage DNA, they are also **mutagenic**, meaning that they have the ability to cause changes in genetic material. As mutagens, these drugs have the potential to cause certain types of **secondary cancers** in patients who have received the drugs. The potential to cause secondary cancers is a rare but very serious side effect.

Alkylating agents are also known to damage reproductive tissue, and patients who receive these medications may become infertile.

Contraindications Although alkylating agents are associated with several potential toxicities, there are very few absolute contraindications to the use of these agents in cancer treatment. Treatment decisions are always based on a risk/benefit assessment.

A history of allergic reaction would be one contraindication to the use of specific alkylating agents. Some alkylating agents such as cisplatin, **carboplatin (Paraplatin)**, and **oxaliplatin (Eloxatin)** are associated with a higher risk of allergic or hypersensitivity reaction. Patients who have exhibited an allergy to one of these agents may not be able to be treated with another agent in the *-platin* category. Skin tests to assess the risk of an allergic reaction and/or a protocol for administering sequentially escalating doses in a "desensitization" regimen may be ordered as a means of managing patients who do not have other treatment options.

Other relative considerations to alkylating agents relate to avoiding some of the unique toxicities of these drugs. For example, patients with kidney dysfunction may not be good candidates for cisplatin therapy, which could worsen their kidney function, or ifosfamide therapy, which can cause serious CNS toxicity when given to patients with kidney dysfunction.

Cautions and Considerations Alkylating agents are hazardous drugs and require special handling precautions for personnel who prepare them. Some alkylating agents are absorbed through the skin, so extreme caution must be used when handling them.

Drug Interactions Alkylating agents may increase the adverse effects of immunosuppressants (such as steroids and other cancer therapies). Caution should be exercised with concurrent use of alkylating agents and other immunosuppressants.

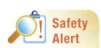

Safety Alert

Ifosfamide can cause severe hemorrhagic cystitis and is always prescribed with the bladder-protective agent, mesna. Orders for administration of ifosfamide without mesna should always be questioned.

TABLE 16.4   Commonly Used Injectable Chemotherapy Drugs

Generic (Brand)	Pronunciation	Common Indication	Dispensing Status
Alkylating Agents			
bendamustine (Treanda)	ben-da-MUSS-teen	Chronic lymphocytic leukemia, lymphoma	Rx
carboplatin (Paraplatin)	kar-boe-PLA-tin	Breast cancer, lung cancer, ovarian cancer	Rx
carmustine (BCNU)	kar-MUS-teen	Brain tumor, lymphoma	Rx
cisplatin (Platinol)	sis-PLA-tin	Bladder cancer, cervical cancer, ovarian cancer, sarcoma, testicular cancer	Rx
cyclophosphamide (Cytoxan)	sye-kloe-FOS-fa-mide	Breast cancer, immune system diseases, leukemia, lymphoma	Rx
ifosfamide (Ifex)	EYE-foss-fam-ide	Lymphoma, sarcoma, testicular cancer	Rx
mechlorethamine (Mustargen)	me-klor-ETH-a-meen	Hodgkin's disease, lymphoma	Rx
melphalan (Alkeran)	MEL-fa-lan	Multiple myeloma	Rx
oxaliplatin (Eloxatin)	ox-A-li-pla-tin	Colon cancer	Rx
Antimetabolites			
cytarabine (Cytosar-U)	sye-TARE-a-been	Leukemia, lymphoma	Rx
fludarabine (Fludara)	floo-DAR-a-been	Leukemia, lymphoma	Rx
fluorouracil (Adrucil)	flure-oh-YOOR-a-sill	Breast cancer, colon cancer, premalignant skin conditions (some), skin cancers (some)	Rx
gemcitabine (Gemzar)	jem-SITE-a-been	Bladder cancer, breast cancer, lung cancer, ovarian cancer, pancreatic cancer	Rx
methotrexate (various brands)	meth-o-TREX-ate	Bone cancer, immune system diseases, leukemia, lymphoma	Rx
pemetrexed (Alimta)	pe-me-TREX-ed	Lung cancer	Rx
Topoisomerase Inhibitors			
daunorubicin (Cerubidine, Daunomycin)	daw-noe-ROO-bi-sin	Leukemia	Rx
doxorubicin (Adriamycin)	dox-oh-ROO-bi-sin	Bone cancer, breast cancer, leukemia, lymphoma, multiple myeloma, sarcomas	Rx
epirubicin (Ellence)	ep-i-ROO-bi-sin	Breast cancer, esophageal/stomach cancers	Rx
etoposide (VePesid)	e-toe-POE-side	Leukemia, lung cancer, lymphoma, testicular cancer	Rx
idarubicin (Idamycin)	eye-da-ROO-bi-sin	Acute leukemia	Rx
irinotecan (Camptosar)	eye-ri-noe-TEE-kan	Brain tumor, colon cancer, lung cancer	Rx

mitoxantrone (Novantrone)	mye-toe-ZAN-trone	Breast cancer, leukemia, lymphoma	Rx
topotecan (Hycamtin)	toe-poe-TEE-kan	Lung cancer, ovarian cancer	Rx
Antimicrotubule Agents			
docetaxel (Taxotere)	doe-se-TAX-el	Breast cancer, lung cancer, prostate cancer	Rx
paclitaxel (Taxol)	PAK-li-tax-el	Breast cancer, lung cancer, ovarian cancer	Rx
vinblastine (Velban)	vin-BLASS-teen	Lymphoma, testicular cancer	Rx
vincristine (Oncovin)	vin-KRISS-teen	Leukemia, lymphoma	Rx
vinorelbine (Navelbine)	vine-oh-REL-been	Breast cancer, lung cancer	Rx

The risk of skin reactions with **bendamustine (Treanda)** may be enhanced by concurrent allopurinol use.

Metronidazole may increase the concentrations of busulfan.

Carboplatin's adverse effect of ototoxicity may be enhanced by use of aminoglycosides. Levels of fosphenytoin and phenytoin may be decreased by the use of carboplatin. Adverse effects of taxane derivatives may be enhanced by carboplatin.

Cisplatin's effects may be diminished by alpha-lipoic acid. Loop diuretics, such as furosemide, may increase the adverse kidney effects of cisplatin.

Cyclophosphamide has an active metabolite. The concentrations of the active metabolite may be increased by certain metabolic (cytochrome P450 2B6 [CYP2B6]) inducers. Conversely, concentrations may be decreased by inhibitors of the same metabolic enzyme. Etanercept may increase the risk of solid cancer development when used with cyclophosphamide.

Aprepitant, often used to help with nausea associated with chemotherapy, may increase the concentration of ifosfamide. Ifosfamide may enhance the anticoagulant effects of vitamin K antagonists (such as warfarin).

The adverse effects of melphalan may be enhanced by nalidixic acid; necrotic enterocolitis has been reported when the two agents are used together.

Oxaliplatin may decrease concentrations of fosphenytoin and phenytoin. Oxaliplatin may enhance the effects of other agents that prolong the QT interval.

Procarbazine may enhance the hypotensive effects of alpha and beta agonists. The combination should be avoided. The hypertensive effects of amphetamines may be enhanced by procarbazine use. Drugs that impact serotonergic activity (such as selective serotonin reuptake inhibitors [SSRIs] and serotonin antagonists) should be avoided in patients using procarbazine because of the risk of serotonin syndrome. Procarbazine may enhance the adverse effects of antipsychotic agents and enhance the effects of drugs that lower blood glucose level. The adverse effects of opioids may be enhanced when patients are using procarbazine.

Antimetabolites

Another class of cytotoxic drugs, known as **antimetabolites**, works in the synthesis phase of the cell cycle. These medications have differing mechanisms of action. Some antimetabolites inhibit enzyme production or activity that is needed for DNA or ribonucleic acid (RNA) synthesis. Methotrexate, cytarabine, and fluorouracil are antimetabolite drugs that interfere with the enzymes that are essential for tumor cell proliferation. Antimetabolites may also act as false **nucleotides** (the structural components of DNA and RNA) and, therefore, become incorporated into DNA during synthesis because they resemble DNA nucleotides. Their incorporation inhibits synthesis of normal DNA. **Mercaptopurine (Purinethol)** is an antimetabolite drug that interferes with cell synthesis by replacing normal nucleotides in DNA/RNA production.

Antimetabolite drugs are used to treat a variety of cancers (see Tables 16.3 and 16.4). **Fluorouracil (Adrucil)** and its oral counterpart, **capecitabine (Xeloda)**, are commonly used to treat colon cancer. A topical form of fluorouracil is used to treat some low-grade skin cancers and precancerous skin lesions. **Gemcitabine (Gemzar)** is an antimetabolite drug that is used to treat lung and pancreatic cancers, and **pemetrexed** is an antimetabolite drug that is critical to the treatment of certain types of lung cancer. **Cytarabine** and **fludarabine (Fludara)** are drugs that are primarily used to treat different types of leukemia and lymphoma. One unique feature of cytarabine is that this agent is able to be safely administered directly into the CNS via a lumbar puncture (or spinal tap) to patients who have leukemia cells in their cerebrospinal fluid. **Hydroxyurea (Droxia, Hydrea)** is an oral antimetabolite drug that is commonly used to rapidly lower white blood cell counts in patients who have leukemia. Hydroxyurea is also used to help decrease painful crisis episodes for individuals with sickle cell anemia.

Methotrexate is commonly used to treat leukemia, bone cancer, breast cancer, and lymphomas, as well as a variety of nonmalignant immunologic conditions, such as psoriasis, rheumatoid arthritis, and systemic lupus erythematosus. Methotrexate suppresses immune system function and is one of the most complicated antimetabolites to administer. Methotrexate may be prepared for administration by different routes, including oral, IV, intrathecal (IT), intramuscular, and subcutaneous. It is given in a wide range of doses, from 5 mg once a week for rheumatoid arthritis to 20 g once or twice a month when used for bone cancer. If administered incorrectly, methotrexate can result in serious and sometimes fatal toxicities.

The major overlapping side effects of antimetabolite drugs include bone marrow suppression, immune system suppression, and mucositis.

Antimetabolite drugs also exhibit some unique toxicities (see Table 16.2). For example, one of the most serious side effects of methotrexate is kidney damage. When methotrexate is administered in doses above 1,000 mg, it can accumulate in the kidneys and form damaging renal crystals. To prevent such accumulation, patients are given IV fluids containing sodium bicarbonate or sodium acetate to alkalinize (increase the pH) the urine. Increasing the urine pH makes methotrexate more soluble and prevents renal crystals from forming.

In high doses, methotrexate can also cause severe bone marrow suppression and mucosal injury in the GI tract. These side effects occur because methotrexate interferes with an enzyme that is important in normal bone marrow and mucosal cell development: dihydrofolate reductase. **Folinic acid** (also known as **leucovorin**) is a by-product of this enzyme. Therefore, the administration of folinic acid to patients who have received high-dose methotrexate rescues normal cells and allows the cells to resume their normal proliferation.

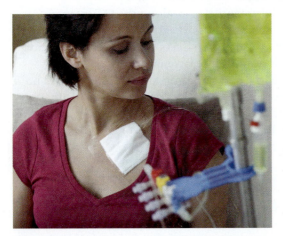

Methotrexate is often administered through a central venous catheter into the subclavian vein.

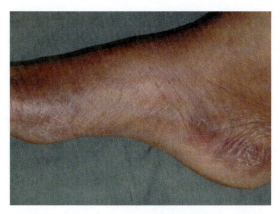

Hand-foot syndrome, a painful sloughing of the skin on the palms of the hands and soles of the feet, is a possible side effect of capecitabine.

This process, known as **leucovorin rescue**, is usually initiated 24–36 hours after the start of the methotrexate infusion, thus allowing methotrexate to exert its action on cancer cells. Timing is essential for leucovorin rescue because leucovorin cannot rescue cells that are exposed to high levels of methotrexate for more than 48 hours.

The oral antimetabolite capecitabine can cause a debilitating reaction called **palmar-plantar erythema**, better known as **hand-foot syndrome**. In hand-foot syndrome, patients experience painful sloughing and peeling of the skin on the palms of the hands and soles of the feet. The appearance of this condition in patients taking oral capecitabine necessitates a pause in treatment as well as a reduction in subsequent doses.

Cytarabine is an antimetabolite used in a wide range of doses. Overdosing of cytarabine results in **conjunctivitis**. To prevent this side effect, patients receiving high-dose cytarabine must also receive steroid eyedrops (e.g., dexamethasone, prednisolone) during therapy and for 24–48 hours after completion of therapy.

Contraindications Similar to alkylating agents, antimetabolite drugs have very few absolute contraindications to their use.

For individuals who have a deficiency or a lack of an enzyme called *dihydropyrimidine dehydrogenase* (an enzyme that helps to break down and eliminate fluorouracil and capecitabine), a significant reduction in doses or a selection of alternative agents may be necessary. These individuals are extremely susceptible to the side effects of fluorouracil and capecitabine.

Methotrexate should not be administered as part of an anticancer treatment regimen to women who are pregnant. Because of its unique toxicity profile, methotrexate also should not be administered to patients with severe kidney dysfunction. Lastly, because methotrexate accumulates in interstitial spaces (a condition known as *third-space fluid shift*), this medication should be avoided or administered with extreme caution in patients who have ascites or pleural effusions.

Cautions and Considerations Antimetabolites are hazardous drugs and require special handling precautions for all personnel who prepare them. As cell cycle–specific drugs, the cytotoxic effects of antimetabolite agents as well as their side effects may change, depending on how the agent is administered. Adjustments in the administration of these agents should only be made after considering the potential consequences.

Sometimes, the administration of these agents is manipulated to provide the best therapeutic effect. For example, in chemotherapy for patients with newly diagnosed acute leukemia, cytarabine is typically administered as a 24-hour continuous infusion for 7 days. By administering this cell cycle–specific agent continuously, the drug will be present in the synthesis phase of the cell cycle, where the cells are most susceptible to the toxic effects of this agent. In contrast, gemcitabine is a cell cycle–specific drug that is typically administered as a 30-minute infusion. Extending the duration of a gemcitabine infusion to 60 minutes might seriously increase the toxicity of this drug. Therefore, dosage schedules for antimetabolite drugs must be carefully followed to prevent excessive toxicity from these agents.

Drug Interactions Antimetabolites may increase the adverse effects of other immuno-suppressants. Caution should be exercised with concurrent use of antimetabolites and other immunosuppressants. Antimetabolites may increase the adverse effects and decrease the efficacy of live vaccines. Live vaccines should not be administered until at least three months after immunosuppressants have been discontinued.

Capecitabine and fluorouracil are CYP 2C9 inhibitors and may increase concentrations of drugs that are metabolized by CYP 2C9. Examples include diclofenac, lacosamide, ramelteon, and warfarin.

Clofarabine can decrease blood pressure and may enhance the hypotensive effects of other drugs.

Cimetidine may increase the serum concentration of fluorouracil. Gimeracil and metronidazole may increase the serum concentration of fluorouracil.

Gemcitabine may enhance the adverse effects of bleomycin, including the risk of pulmonary toxicity. Gemcitabine may enhance the effects of warfarin.

Hydroxyurea and didanosine may enhance the adverse effects of each other, including pancreatitis, liver toxicity, and neuropathy. Stavudine and hydroxyurea may enhance the adverse effects of each other.

Mercaptopurine concentrations may be increased by febuxostat. Sulfamethox-azole and trimethoprim may enhance the myelosuppressive effects of mercaptopurine.

Acitretin may enhance the liver toxicities associated with methotrexate use; foscarnet may enhance the kidney toxicities associated with methotrexate. Bile acid sequestrants may decrease the absorption of methotrexate. Ciprofloxacin, cyclosporine, nonsteroidal anti-inflammatory agents, penicillins, probenecid, and salicylates may increase the serum concentration of methotrexate. The effects of loop diuretics may be diminished by methotrexate.

Topoisomerase Inhibitors

Some enzymes important in the process of DNA synthesis and cell replication are topoisomerases. DNA structure is tightly coiled and must be unwound during the replication process. Topoisomerases produce temporary breaks and repairs in DNA strands, which help unwind the DNA and allow the transcription process to occur. There are two types of topoisomerase enzymes: **topoisomerase I enzymes** produce single-strand DNA breaks, and **topoisomerase II enzymes** produce double-strand DNA breaks. Topoisomerase inhibitors interfere with the DNA repair function of topoisomerases and disrupt the cell replication process. These agents are very important components of cancer treatment and are used to treat many different types of cancer (see Table 16.4).

Topoisomerase I inhibitors include topotecan and irinotecan, both of which are derived from a tree, *Camptotheca acuminata*, that is native to China. **Topotecan (Hycamtin)** is commonly used to treat ovarian cancer and lung cancer. **Irinotecan (Camptosar)** is most frequently used to treat lung cancer and colon cancer. Both of these agents are also used to treat brain tumors or brain metastases because of their ability to penetrate the CNS.

Anthracyclines represent a large category of **topoisomerase II inhibitors** that are commonly used. Anthracyclines inhibit topoisomerase activity by inserting themselves (or intercalating) into strands of DNA. Anthracyclines are also referred to as DNA **intercalating agents**. These agents include daunorubicin, doxorubicin, epirubicin, and idarubicin. They are derived from *Streptomyces* bacteria, which are found in soil and produce a red pigment.

Doxorubicin (Adriamycin) is part of curative chemotherapy regimens for breast cancer and lymphoma. It is also used in treating bone cancer, leukemia, multiple myeloma, and sarcomas. **Daunorubicin** and **idarubicin (Idamycin)** are primarily used to treat leukemia. **Epirubicin (Ellence)** is most frequently used to treat breast and esophageal/stomach cancers. Pharmacy technicians who work with chemotherapy patients may hear the acronym **CHOP** being used in the workplace. This acronym refers to a combination chemotherapy regimen:

- **Cyclophosphamide (Cytoxan)**
- **Hydroxy-daunorubicin** (better known as doxorubicin)
- **Oncovin** (brand name for vincristine)
- **Prednisone**

Etoposide and mitoxantrone are two other topoisomerase II inhibitors. **Etoposide (VePesid)** is derived from the American mayapple plant and is commonly used to treat leukemia, lung cancer, lymphoma, and testicular cancer. **Mitoxantrone (Novantrone)** is similar in activity to the anthracyclines but has an inky blue color. This medication is frequently used to treat breast cancer, leukemia, and lymphoma.

Topoisomerase inhibitors cause many of the same side effects common to other chemotherapy agents: bone marrow suppression, nausea and vomiting, mucositis, alopecia, and diarrhea.

Because these agents interfere with DNA synthesis, topoisomerase inhibitors also have the ability to cause secondary cancers such as acute leukemia. Although rare, the potential to cause secondary cancers is a serious side effect of topoisomerase inhibitors.

Another serious toxicity that can occur in patients who receive anthracyclines is **cardiac toxicity**, although it typically occurs many years after patients have received the drug. The risk of cardiac toxicity with anthracyclines is cumulative, increasing with each dose the patient receives. The best way to limit the risk of cardiac toxicity with these drugs is to track the patient's cumulative exposure and stop treatment after he or she has reached a **threshold dose**. The threshold dose is different for each anthracycline drug. For example, the lifetime cumulative dose limit for doxorubicin is approximately 450 mg/m², whereas the cumulative dose limit for idarubicin is approximately 225 mg/m².

Irinotecan causes the unique side effect of severe diarrhea (see Table 16.2). If not managed quickly, diarrhea from irinotecan can lead to serious complications. Patients who experience this type of diarrhea are treated with atropine, which is an injectable anticholinergic drug. The most serious form of diarrhea occurs in the days following administration of irinotecan. Patients must be adequately warned about the potential for this side effect and educated on how to appropriately administer antidiarrheal agents, such as loperamide, at the onset of symptoms.

Contraindications There are few absolute contraindications to the use of specific topoisomerase inhibitors. Patients who have a history of cardiac disease and/or evidence of congestive heart failure or cardiac dysfunction may not be good candidates for any of the anthracycline agents.

Many of the topoisomerase drugs are eliminated from the body through the liver and biliary systems. Therefore, patients who have significant liver dysfunction may not be able to tolerate drugs such as anthracyclines or irinotecan.

Topotecan is eliminated by the kidneys, so patients with significant kidney dysfunction are not good candidates for this agent.

Finally, patients who have a previous history of an allergic reaction to one of the topoisomerase inhibitors should not receive these medications.

Cautions and Considerations Patients who have a mutation in the liver enzyme UGT1a, which is responsible for breaking down irinotecan, are susceptible to increased toxicity from irinotecan when this agent is administered in high doses. A commercial test is available to identify patients who have this genetic mutation. However, the clinical utility of this test is not widely established; therefore, it is not recommended for routine use.

Anthracyclines, such as daunorubicin, doxorubicin, epirubicin, and idarubicin, cause severe tissue damage if the infusion leaks under the skin during administration. This leaking and the related damage is called **extravasation**. Drugs that cause extravasation injury are referred to as **vesicants** (see Table 16.5).

Some anthracycline drugs have been prepared in lipid formulations, known as **liposomal products**, to help decrease toxicity. Both daunorubicin and doxorubicin have liposomal formulations. Liposomal daunorubicin is known as DaunoXome, and liposomal doxorubicin is known as Doxil.

Drug Interactions Topoisomerase inhibitors may increase the adverse effects of other immunosuppressants. Caution should be exercised with concurrent use of topoisomerase inhibitors and other immunosuppressants. Topoisomerase inhibitors may increase the adverse effects and decrease the efficacy of live vaccines. Live vaccines should not be administered until at least three months after immunosuppressants have been discontinued.

Doxorubicin is a substrate, inhibitor, and inducer of different drugs. It is a substrate of CYP 2D6 and CYP 3A4, inhibitor of CYP 2B6, and inducer of P-glyco-protein. Doxorubicin concentrations may be increased by CYP 2D6 inhibitors (such as abiraterone acetate). Drugs that inhibit CYP 3A4 may increase concentrations of doxorubicin (such as conivaptan, fosaprepitant, and idelalisib). Doxorubicin may increase the serum concentration of drugs such as aripiprazole. Taxane derivatives may decrease the metabolism of doxorubicin. Doxorubicin may enhance the adverse effects of zidovudine.

Etoposide concentrations may be increased by atovaquone, conivaptan, cyclosporine, idelalisib, and mifepristone. Etoposide may enhance the anticoagulant effects of warfarin.

Irinotecan concentrations may be increased by aprepitant, conivaptan, fosaprepitant, idelalisib, and mifepristone.

Teniposide concentrations may be decreased by barbiturates, bosentan, enzalutamide, and phenytoin. Teniposide concentration may be increased by conivaptan, idelalisib, and mifepristone. Teniposide may increase the neurotoxic side effects of vincristine.

Topotecan concentrations may be increased by P-glycoprotein inhibitors.

TABLE 16.5 Chemotherapy Vesicant Drugs

• Daunorubicin	• Idarubicin	• Vinblastine
• Doxorubicin	• Mechlorethamine	• Vincristine
• Epirubicin	• Mitomycin	• Vinorelbine

Antimicrotubule Agents

Microtubules are important to cell function. They play a role in maintaining cell shape and structure and are critical elements in the process of cell division or mitosis. **Antimicrotubule agents** interfere with the formation and function of microtubules, ultimately preventing cell growth and division.

Most antimicrotubule drugs are derived from plant sources. **Paclitaxel (Taxol)** and **docetaxel (Taxotere)**—the **taxanes**—are derived from the bark and needles of yew trees. **Vincristine (Oncovin)**, **vinblastine (Velban)**, and **vinorelbine (Navelbine)**—the **vinca alkaloids**—are derived from periwinkle plants. Antimicrotubule agents are important components in the treatment of lung, breast, ovarian, prostate, and testicular cancers, as well as for some types of leukemia and lymphoma.

Similar to other traditional cytotoxic drugs, antimicrotubule agents cause bone marrow suppression, mucositis, and alopecia. The degree of alopecia varies with these chemotherapy agents. For example, patients receiving paclitaxel may experience total body alopecia, including loss of eyelashes, eyebrows, and pubic hair. Nausea and vomiting with antimicrotubule agents may occur but is generally mild.

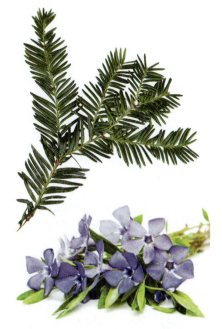

Yew needles (top) and periwinkle (bottom) are the plant sources for several antimicrotubule agents used in chemotherapy. The study of natural cancer-fighting sources is ongoing, as scientists have recently discovered that a berry from the blushwood tree (a species found only in North Queensland, Australia) holds promise for treating head and neck tumors and melanomas.

Because microtubules also play an important role in nerve function, many antimicrotubule agents cause peripheral neuropathy. Vincristine, in particular, can cause neurotoxicity to the GI tract. While on therapy with vincristine, patients must be closely monitored to make sure they do not develop **ileus**, a condition in which GI motility is severely reduced.

Other unique side effects of taxanes include bone and muscle aches, which can occur for several days after an infusion. These side effects are typically managed with an over-the-counter (OTC) pain reliever such as acetaminophen or ibuprofen.

Strontium-89 chloride (Metastron) may help reduce bone pain associated with breast and prostate cancer. Hot flashes and flushing are common side effects.

Contraindications The antimicrotubule agents paclitaxel and docetaxel are contraindicated in patients who have a history of a hypersensitivity reaction.

Vincristine should not be administered to patients who have a history of peripheral neuropathy. This medication may worsen the neuropathy.

Paclitaxel, docetaxel, vincristine, and vinblastine are contraindicated for patients with significant liver dysfunction because these agents are eliminated by the hepatic and biliary system.

Safety Alert

Vincristine and vinblastine must never be administered by the intrathecal (IT) route. This warning is critical. Fatalities have been reported around the world when vincristine was inadvertently administered as an IT agent.

Cautions and Considerations Because they are plant derivatives, paclitaxel and docetaxel are commonly associated with allergic reactions during drug administration. Patients typically require premedication with antihistamines and corticosteroids to prevent severe allergic reactions to these drugs. Patients who have had allergic reactions to one or both of these agents may require additional premedication with corticosteroids or may not be able to tolerate reexposure to the agent, depending on the severity of the reaction.

Drug Interactions Antimicrotubule agents may increase the adverse effects of other immunosuppressants. Caution should be exercised with concurrent use of antimicrotubule agents and other immunosuppressants. Antimicrotubule agents may increase the adverse effects and decrease the efficacy of live vaccines. Live vaccines should not be administered until at least three months after immunosuppressants have been discontinued.

Docetaxel concentrations may be increased by antifungal agents, dronedarone, idelalisib, ivacaftor, and mifepristone. Docetaxel concentrations may be decreased by dabrafenib, and enzalutamide.

Eribulin may enhance the effects of other agents that increase the QT interval.

Paclitaxel can decrease blood pressure and may enhance the antihypotensive effects of blood pressure lowering drugs. Paclitaxel concentrations may be increased by atazanavir, idelalisib, and mifepristone. Paclitaxel may decrease the metabolism of doxorubicin. Paclitaxel's adverse effects may be intensified by sorafenib. The adverse effects of vinorelbine may be enhanced by paclitaxel.

Vinblastine concentrations may be increased by conivaptan, idelalisib, macrolides, and mifepristone. Vinblastine concentrations may be decreased by vincristine. Vinblastine may decrease the concentrations of dabigatran, doxorubicin, and ledipasvir. Posaconazole and voriconazole may intensify the adverse effects of vinblastine.

Vincristine levels may be decreased by CYP 3A4 inducers and increased by CYP 3A4 inhibitors. Triazole antifungals may enhance the adverse effects of vincristine. Macrolides may increase the concentration of vincristine.

Vinorelbine's adverse effects may by increased by triazole antifungals.

Miscellaneous Cytotoxic Drugs

Two commonly used chemotherapy drugs that do not fit into the other cytotoxic drug categories are bleomycin and asparaginase.

Bleomycin (Blenoxane) works by cutting or breaking DNA strands, preventing the process of cell proliferation. It is part of the curative chemotherapy regimens used to treat testicular cancer and Hodgkin's disease (a type of lymphoma).

Asparaginase is a drug with a very narrow spectrum of activity. Asparaginase is used to treat acute lymphocytic leukemia, a common and often curable type of leukemia in children. Leukemia cells require a large amount of the amino acid **asparagine** to proliferate. Unlike normal cells, leukemia cells are not able to make asparagine. Asparaginase is an enzyme that breaks down asparagine, depriving leukemia cells of this essential amino acid.

Unlike many other cytotoxic drugs, one advantage to bleomycin is that it does not cause bone marrow suppression. However, this medication can cause a deadly type of lung toxicity known as **pulmonary fibrosis**. This condition occurs when the delicate tissue of the lung is damaged or scarred. It is important to track and limit cumulative doses of bleomycin to decrease the risk of pulmonary fibrosis.

Allergic reaction is one of the most common side effects of asparaginase therapy. Because asparaginase products are made from two different bacterial sources, patients who develop an allergic reaction to one product can often safely switch to the other product. Asparaginase can also interfere with normal protein synthesis in patients who are receiving it. Consequently, patients receiving asparaginase therapy have to be closely monitored for effects on clotting factors and might be at a higher risk for bleeding or clotting.

Contraindications Because of the risk for lung toxicity, patients older than age 60 years may not be good candidates for treatment with bleomycin. Young patients who are athletes may also choose to limit their exposure to bleomycin in an effort to preserve their lung function.

Cautions and Considerations Patients who have received bleomycin may be at a higher risk for respiratory problems during surgery with general anesthesia.

Drug Interactions Cytotoxic drugs may increase the adverse effects of other immunosuppressants. Caution should be exercised with concurrent use of cytotoxic drugs and other immunosuppressants. Cytotoxic drugs may increase the adverse effects and decrease the efficacy of live vaccines. Live vaccines should not be administered until at least three months after immunosuppressants have been discontinued.

Bleomycin's adverse effects may be enhanced by filgrastim and gemcitabine.

Asparaginase may increase concentrations of dexamethasone.

Hormonal Drug Therapies

Some types of cancer depend on naturally occurring hormones for growth. In tumors that are known to be dependent on specific hormones for proliferation, one treatment strategy is to block the activity of those hormones. Hormonal or endocrine drug therapies target the hormonal agent that is contributing to the growth of the specific type of tumor. For example, estrogen and progesterone are hormones that frequently stimulate breast tumors. Prostate cancer is often dependent on androgens, such as testosterone, for growth.

Antiestrogens

Antiestrogens, such as anastrazole, exemestane, letrozole and tamoxifen, are commonly used to treat breast cancer. **Tamoxifen** works by blocking the estrogen receptor and can be used in the treatment of breast cancer for women of any age.

Anastrazole, **letrozole**, and **exemestane** are **aromatase inhibitors**. These agents block the effects of estrogen by preventing synthesis of estrogen in the body. However, aromatase inhibitors only work in women who have experienced menopause. Younger women who have not undergone menopause will have too much ovarian production of estrogen that will counteract the effects of these agents.

Side effects of antiestrogen therapy are very similar to menopausal symptoms, such as hot flashes, mood swings, and depression. In addition, the use of these agents can increase a woman's risk for blood clots and endometrial cancer.

Contraindications A history of blood clots may be a relative contraindication for therapy with an antiestrogen agent. However, physicians and patients may decide that the potential benefits of therapy outweigh the risks and choose to initiate therapy with enhanced monitoring for signs and symptoms of blood clots. Antiestrogen agents should also be avoided in patients who are pregnant or trying to become pregnant.

Cautions and Considerations Although associated with an increased risk of endometrial cancer, tamoxifen is approved for the prevention of breast cancer in women who have very high risk factors for developing the disease. Women using tamoxifen for breast cancer prevention must be closely monitored for endometrial changes that are early indicators of cancer.

Drug Interactions Tamoxifen has an additive effect when combined with other drugs that prolong the QT interval (such as amiodarone, cisapride, disopyramide, dolasetron, moxifloxacin, quinidine, and ziprasidone). Drugs that decrease tamoxifen concentrations include CYP 2D6 inhibitors (such as bupropion), and rifamycins. Tamoxifen concentrations may be increased by bromocriptine. Tamoxifen can decrease concentrations of anastrozole and letrozole. Tamoxifen may increase the adverse effects (particularly bleeding) of anticoagulants. Coadministration of tamoxifen with sodium polystyrene sulfonate or other cation exchange resins may lead to serious gastrointestinal complications, and the combination should be avoided. Tamoxifen and mitomycin C enhance each other's adverse effects.

Estrogens may decrease the effects of anastrozole. Tamoxifen may decrease concentrations of anastrozole.

Letrozole levels may be decreased by tamoxifen.

Exemestane levels may be decreased by bosentan, dabrafenib, deferasirox, mitotane, siltuximab, and tocilizumab. Estrogens may decrease the efficacy of exemestane.

Antiandrogens

Antiandrogens work by blocking the activity of testosterone at the receptor level or interfering with the production of testosterone. These medications include **abiraterone**, **bicalutamide**, **enzalutamide**, and **flutamide**, and they are used to treat prostate cancer.

Side effects of antiandrogen agents include hot flashes, breast tenderness, **gynecomastia** (enlargement of the breasts), and decreased libido. Many antiandrogen agents also cause toxicity to the liver.

Contraindications There are no absolute contraindications to the use of antiandrogen agents.

Cautions and Considerations Patients taking antiandrogen agents must be educated by the pharmacist about the potential for these agents to interact with other drugs. For example, both bicalutamide and flutamide can increase the anticoagulant effects of warfarin. For this reason, patients must be instructed not to add new drugs to their regimen without consulting a healthcare professional who is aware of all of their medications.

Drug Interactions Abiraterone is a substrate of CYP 3A4, and levels are increased by CYP 3A4 inhibitors (such as bosutinib, eplerenone, ivabradine, and rivaroxaban) and decreased by CYP 3A4 inducers (such as budesonide and cannabis). Abiraterone may increase concentrations of enzalutamide.

Bicalutamide may increase the serum concentration of vitamin K antagonists such as warfarin. Midazolam levels may be increased when used with bicalutamide.

Enzalutamide is a substrate of CYP 2C8 and CYP 3A4; levels may be increased by inhibitors of these enzymes and decreased by inducers of these enzymes. In addition, enzalutamide is a strong inducer of CYP 3A4, and it decreases levels of drugs that are CYP 3A4 substrates (such as abiraterone acetate, apixaban, apremilast, aripiprazole, boceprevir, bosutinib, cannabinoids, corticosteroids, doxorubicin, irinotecan, itraconazole, ivabradine, nifedipine, quetiapine, rivaroxaban, saxagliptin, vincristine, warfarin, and zaleplon).

Flutamide is a substrate of CYP 1A2 and CYP 3A4; levels may be increased by inhibitors of the enzymes and decreased by inducers of these enzymes. When flutamide is used with nitric acid, the likelihood of methemoglobinemia increases.

Luteinizing Hormone–Releasing Hormone Agonists

Luteinizing hormone–releasing hormone (LHRH), also known as *gonadotropin-releasing hormone*, stimulates the production of both male and female reproductive hormones. LHRH initially stimulates the production of sex hormones; but over time, continuous exposure to LHRH ultimately shuts down the production of sex hormones through a negative feedback loop. **Leuprolide (Lupron)** and **goserelin (Zoladex)** are analogs of naturally occurring LHRH. These drugs are called **LHRH agonists** and are frequently given to patients with hormone-sensitive tumors, such as breast and prostate cancers, to eliminate the source of endogenous estrogen, progesterone, and testosterone production.

LHRH agonists cause many of the same side effects that are seen with antiandrogens. These side effects include hot flashes, gynecomastia, breast tenderness, decreased libido, and liver abnormalities. In addition, these agents can also cause local reactions or pain at the injection site.

Contraindications There are no absolute contraindications to the use of LHRH agonists in male patients. Women who are breastfeeding or pregnant should not be exposed to these drugs.

Cautions and Considerations Because LHRH analogs initially *stimulate* the production of testosterone, patients with prostate cancer may experience a flare of symptoms at the onset of therapy. This reaction can be significant if the tumor is close to vital structures (e.g., the spinal cord) or is associated with pain. To prevent this type of flare reaction, patients are commonly prescribed an antiandrogen such as bicalutamide to overlap with the first few weeks of LHRH agonist therapy.

LHRH agonists are available in a variety of dosage formulations that have different durations. For example, these medications are prepared as injections that are effective for days, weeks, or months. Pharmacy technicians who handle LHRH agonists must be cognizant of the different formulations of these agents.

Drug Interactions Goserelin and leuprolide have an additive effect when combined with other drugs that prolong the QT interval (such as amiodarone, cisapride, disopyramide, dolasetron, moxifloxacin, quinidine, and ziprasidone). Goserelin and leuprolide may decrease the effectiveness of drugs that are used to treat diabetes.

Targeted Anticancer Therapies

As scientists have learned more about the biology of cancer, they have identified features of certain types of cancer that are critical for tumor cell growth. These critical components have become targets for more sophisticated cancer treatments. **Targeted anticancer therapies**, for example, are directed at specific molecules that are required for tumor cell development, proliferation, and growth. By targeting specific features of tumor cells, these therapies exert fewer effects on normal cells and are usually better tolerated than traditional cytotoxic drugs.

Because targeted anticancer therapies are relatively new agents in the arsenal of cancer-fighting drugs, oncologists are still learning about them. Although these therapies have some serious and unusual side effects, they typically offer patients a much more direct treatment for their cancer, with fewer side effects than those that accompany

TABLE 16.6   Targeted Anticancer Therapies

Generic (Brand)	Pronunciation	Anticancer Effect	Dispensing Status
Angiogenesis Inhibitors			
bevacizumab (Avastin)	be-va-KIZ-oo-mab	Prevent formation of blood vessels that allow for tumor growth and invasion of surrounding tissue	Rx
lenalidomide (Revlimid)	LE-na-LID-o-mide		Rx
thalidomide (Thalomid)	tha-LID-oh-mide		Rx
Monoclonal Antibodies			
cetuximab (Erbitux)	se-TUX-i-mab	Target a specific marker or receptor on the surface of tumor cells, leading to destruction of those cells	Rx
panitumumab (Vectibix)	pan-i-TU-mu-mab		Rx
rituximab (Rituxan)	ri-TUX-i-mab		Rx
trastuzumab (Herceptin)	traz-TOO-zoo-mab		Rx
Signal Transduction Inhibitors			
axitinib (Inlyta)	ax-i-TI-nib	Prevent transmission of intracellular signals that stimulate cell proliferation	Rx
bosutinib (Bosulif)	boe-SUE-ti nib		Rx
dasatinib (Sprycel)	da-SAT-in-ib		Rx
erlotinib (Tarceva)	er-LO-ti-nib		Rx
imatinib (Gleevec)	i-MAT-i-nib		Rx
nilotinib (Tasigna)	ni-LO-ti-nib		Rx
sorafenib (Nexavar)	so-ra-FEN-ib		Rx
sunitinib (Sutent)	soo-NIT-in-ib		Rx

traditional cytotoxic drugs. Targeted anticancer therapies are the future of anticancer treatment. For an overview of these therapies, see Table 16.6.

Angiogenesis Inhibitors

Although some targeted anticancer therapies have narrow therapeutic applications, many agents have been developed to target a wider variety of cancers. **Angiogenesis inhibitors** work by preventing tumor cells from building blood vessels that will supply the tumor with vital nutrients. By inhibiting new blood vessel formation at the site of the tumor, the tumor cells will eventually die.

Bevacizumab (Avastin), for example, has significant anticancer activity in breast, lung, colon, and brain cancers. This medication also seems to enhance the effects of cytotoxic drugs when dispensed together.

Lenalidomide (Revlimid), another angiogenesis inhibitor, treats cancers of the blood. This medication targets mantle cell lymphoma and is used with dexamethasone to treat multiple myeloma. Like lenalidomide, **thalidomide (Thalomid)** is part of a combination drug therapy with dexamethasone for the treatment of multiple myeloma.

Although most side effects associated with targeted anticancer therapies are less severe and more manageable than those seen with cytotoxic drugs, some of these drugs can cause very serious reactions.

Bevacizumab has the potential to interfere with wound healing and normal blood vessel formation. Bevacizumab may also cause bleeding, such as such as in the GI tract, nose, and CNS. Bevacizumab can also cause **hypertension** (high blood pressure) and kidney damage, so blood pressure measurements and urine samples must be evaluated prior to treatment.

Contraindications Bevacizumab is contraindicated in patients who have active bleeding (e.g., nosebleeds, blood in sputum) and in patients who have a significant risk of bleeding.

Cautions and Considerations Because bevacizumab interferes with normal wound healing, this medication must not be given to patients within four weeks of a surgical procedure.

Lenalidomide and thalidomide are reproductive toxins and should not be handled by healthcare personnel who are pregnant, possibly pregnant, or trying to conceive. Because of the high risk for reproductive toxicity, the prescribing and dispensing of these agents is strictly regulated. Prescribers, patients, and pharmacies must be registered with the manufacturers of these agents in order to access these drugs.

Drug Interactions Angiogenesis inhibitors may decrease the effectiveness of live vaccines and co-administration is not recommended. Additionally, the adverse effects of other immunosuppressants may be enhanced by angiogenesis inhibitors.

Bevacizumab may increase the cardiotoxic side effects of anthracyclines and the adverse effects of clozapine, irinotecan, sorafenib, and sunitinib.

Lenalidomide may increase the serum concentrations of digoxin. Erythropoiesis-stimulating agents may increase the risk of thromboembolism when used with lenalidomide.

Thalidomide may cause central nervous system depression and can enhance the depressant effects of other drugs that act on the central nervous system.

Monoclonal Antibodies

A **monoclonal antibody** is an antibody that has been developed from a single type of immune cell that was cloned from a parent cell. These antibodies are directed against a specific marker or antigen on target cells. Monoclonal antibodies are developed from a variety of sources, including mouse, bacterial, and human cell lines. Some of these medications designed to target specific markers on tumor cells have a limited range of activity.

Trastuzumab (Herceptin) is a monoclonal antibody developed to target the HER2/neu receptor commonly found on breast cancer cells. However, this drug does not have as much activity in treating other types of tumors.

Rituximab (Rituxan) was developed to treat non–Hodgkin's lymphoma and, therefore, targets a specific marker (CD20) on B lymphocytes. Because lymphocytes are active in various immunologic diseases, such as rheumatoid arthritis, rituximab has become a mainstay in treating many nonmalignant conditions by using the same mechanism of action—targeting CD20.

Cetuximab (Erbitux) and **panitumumab (Vectibix)** are monoclonal antibodies that target the epidermal growth factor receptor (EGFR), a growth factor receptor present on many types of cancer cells. Cetuximab has shown potential in treating head and neck, colon, lung, and pancreatic cancers. Panitumumab is used to treat colon and rectal cancers.

Because monoclonal antibodies are frequently derived from animal sources, these medications can cause allergic reactions, such as a fever, chills, and flushing. Infusion reactions with rituximab and cetuximab can be prevented by premedicating patients with acetaminophen, diphenhydramine, or, possibly, corticosteroids. More serious allergic reactions, such as **anaphylaxis**, necessitate a change in therapy.

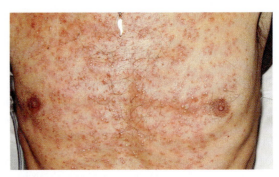

A skin rash is a known side effect of therapies that target epidermal growth factor receptors, such as cetuximab and erlotinib.

Contraindications

Specific contraindications to monoclonal antibodies have not been determined.

Cautions and Considerations Many targeted anticancer therapies cause acne-like skin reactions. Sometimes, the rash that appears from the use of targeted therapies is a sign that the treatment is working. For example, patients who develop a rash while receiving cetuximab generally have a better response to treatment than those who do not develop a rash. These rashes can usually be managed with topical creams and antibiotic gels. On some occasions, the rash may be so severe that treatment must be stopped.

Drug Interactions Trastuzumab can intensify the adverse cardiac side effects with anthracyclines. It may increase the adverse effects of other immunosuppressants. Paclitaxel may increase trastuzumab concentrations.

The risk of serious infections is increased when rituximab is used with tocilizumab.

Panitumumab may increase the photosensitizing effects of porfimer and verteporfin.

Cetuximab does not have known drug interactions.

Signal Transduction Inhibitors

Certain targeted anticancer therapies were developed to affect the molecular abnormalities associated with specific tumor types. **Signal transduction inhibitors** are included in this category and were designed to target tumor cell receptors. Typically, these medications are small molecule oral agents that block or prevent communication and intracellular functions related to tumor growth and proliferation.

There are many types of signal transduction inhibitors being used and developed for cancer treatment. **Imatinib (Gleevec)** and **dasatinib (Sprycel)** were developed to target a specific chromosomal mutation associated with chronic myelogenous leukemia (CML). This type of cancer can be fatal if it is not managed in the early stage of the disease. These drugs have revolutionized the way CML is treated, and patients on oral therapy can maintain their disease state for many years without the risk of disease progression. However, because imatinib and dasatinib work against the specific abnormality associated with CML, these drugs have not been very useful in the treatment of other types of cancer. Newer agents in this same category of drugs include **nilotinib (Tasigna)** and **bosutinib (Bosulif)**.

As previously mentioned, targeted anticancer therapies are generally better tolerated than traditional chemotherapy drugs. The side effects associated with signal transduction inhibitors vary greatly, depending on the specific target of the agent.

Edema, or the swelling of tissues caused by excessive fluid retention, is one side effect of some of these agents. In addition, many signal transduction inhibitors can cause hypertension and changes in normal cardiac conduction. Medications used to treat CML can cause mild bone marrow suppression.

Contraindications There are no specific contraindications for signal transduction inhibitors. In general, there is limited experience in using these agents during pregnancy. Patients who become pregnant while taking a signal transduction inhibitor must consult with their obstetrics/gynecology practitioner and medical oncologist to discuss the potential risks and benefits of continuing the agent during pregnancy.

Cautions and Considerations Pharmacy technicians should have a heightened awareness of the potential for drug interactions during signal transduction inhibitor therapy. Prescription drugs as well as OTC and herbal or supplemental therapies have been shown to decrease the effectiveness of these agents. For example, histamine blockers or proton pump inhibitors used for stomach acid suppression, such as famotidine or omeprazole, can decrease the absorption of dasatinib. Certain herbal therapies, such as St. John's wort, can decrease the efficacy of imatinib. Agents that interfere with the activity of these signal transduction inhibitors put patients at risk for disease progression. Other drug interactions can result in toxicity of these targeted anticancer therapies. Therefore, when pharmacy technicians are updating the patient's medical profile, they should inquire about the use of herbal therapies.

Patients who are taking oral signal transduction inhibitors to treat CML must continue their therapy without interruption to avoid progression to the accelerated phase of this disease.

Drug Interactions Immunosuppressants may decrease the efficacy of live vaccines. Coadministration is not recommended.

Bosutinib is a major substrate of CYP 3A4; drugs that inhibit CYP 3A4 will increase bosutinib levels, and drugs that induce CYP 3A4 will decrease bosutinib levels. Antacids may decrease bosutinib levels.

Dasatinib increases the QT interval and can enhance the effects of other drugs that increase the QT interval. Acetaminophen may enhance the liver toxicities associated with dasatinib. Dasatinib may increase the anticoagulant effects of drugs with antiplatelet activity. Proton pump inhibitors may decrease the concentration of dasatinib.

Imantinib is a major substrate of CYP3A4; drugs that inhibit CYP3A4 will increase imantinib levels, and drugs that induce CYP3A4 will decrease imantinib levels. Imantinib's liver toxicity side effect may be enhanced by acetaminophen. Concentrations of warfarin may be increased by imantinib.

Nilotinib is a major substrate of CYP3A4; drugs that inhibit CYP3A4 will increase nilotinib levels, and drugs that induce CYP3A4 will decrease nilotinib levels.

Miscellaneous Targeted Therapies

Vitamin A is available in a prescription form (**Vesanoid**) for the treatment of acute promyelocytic leukemia. Vesanoid should only be used by experienced providers, and patients should be under strict provider supervision. Other vitamin A supplements should not be used at the same time because of the increased risk of toxicity.

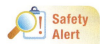

Investigational Therapies

Because knowledge of the causes of cancer is rapidly evolving, cancer therapy is a highly progressive field of research. Cancer researchers are constantly studying new approaches to improve cancer treatment outcomes. For many types of cancer, there are no curative therapies available. Even for cancers in which therapeutic options are plentiful, patients may not respond to currently available treatment options. As a result, many patients with cancer seek treatment with investigational drug therapies.

Investigational drugs are medications that are not yet approved by the US Food and Drug Administration (FDA) but are being studied as part of a clinical research program. There are thousands of clinical trials available to patients with all different stages and types of cancer. Healthcare personnel might suggest to their patients that they discuss with their physicians what clinical trial options are available within their healthcare system. Patients who are interested in investigational therapies for cancer can also conduct their own research on the Internet. For example, the National Cancer Institute provides information on clinical trials online: http://Pharmacology6e.ParadigmCollege.net/CancerClinicalTrials.

Web

Lastly, some investigational therapies for cancer may be approved for commercial use in another country or are currently under investigation for treatment of very rare or uncommon diseases. Frequently, these agents are made available to patients via expanded access or "compassionate use" approval. In this situation, the FDA allows the use of a particular investigational agent for a specific disease outside of a clinical trial. This type of approval is granted on a case-by-case basis and only in treatment of a serious medical illness or life-threatening condition. Institutional policies on how **expanded access drugs** are handled may vary, so healthcare personnel who work with these medications should ensure that all local and institutional requirements are met before initiating therapy with these agents.

Handling of Chemotherapy Agents

Individuals involved in the handling of chemotherapy risk possible accidental exposure to these hazardous agents and potential long-term effects as a result. Methods of possible accidental exposure include the following:

- inhalation, which can occur when (1) capsules or tablets are opened, broken, or crushed, or (2) hazardous drugs are prepared without adequate respiratory protection
- ingestion, which can occur when individuals are (1) eating or drinking in areas where hazardous drugs are stored or prepared, (2) placing food on contaminated surfaces, or (3) touching food or their mouths with contaminated hands
- injection, which can occur when healthcare personnel have a needlestick injury during the preparation of a chemotherapy agent
- topical absorption via the skin and/or eyes, which can occur when (1) handling oral or injectable chemotherapy agents without donning personal protective equipment (PPE), and (2) being exposed to accidental powder or liquid spillage from broken vials or leaky IV bags

Many pharmacy technicians, especially those working in a hospital setting, occasionally handle hazardous drugs (HDs), especially in compounding nonsterile and sterile medications. Others specialize in hazardous or nuclear compounding.

Recent studies have shown that even those handling the toxic agents in receiving and delivery of ingredients and final products experience more exposure than was previously known.

USP <800> outlines requirements for receipt, storage, mixing, preparing, compounding, dispensing,and administration of hazardous drugs to protect the patient, healthcare personnel, and the environment. USP Chapter <800> must be fully implemented by institutions doing hazardous compounding by July 1, 2018.

According to USP <800>, personnel in a hospital or compounding facility who come into any level of contact with HDs require specialized equipment, training, protective clothing, and procedures for the handling, preparation, and disposal of these substances. Hospitals are required to develop written policies and procedures for each aspect of HD use to be in compliance with the USP and the Joint Commission, as well as state and federal regulations.

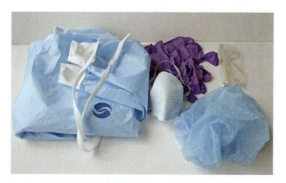

Typical PPE includes a single-use gown; sterile, nitrile chemotherapy gloves; chemotherapy safety glasses; a hair cover; and a disposable respirator.

Personal Protective Equipment

Personal protective equipment (PPE) should be used at all times when handling both oral and injectable hazardous drugs. PPE protects the handler from being exposed to hazardous drugs or their residue (if left on the outside of vials, bottles, or IV bags). PPE also serves as product protection by keeping contaminants, such as lint or bacteria, from the skin of the handler. PPE includes the following garments:

- shoe covers
- a disposable gown made of material that is impermeable to fluid
- sterile chemotherapy gloves
- chemotherapy safety glasses
- a hair cover
- a disposable respirator

Hazardous drug compounding has additional PPE requirements to meet standards set by the National Institute for Occupation Safety and Health, which include:

- a non-permeable sterile gown
- hair and shoe covers
- eye and face protection (goggles and shields)
- a special hazardous face mask with respiratory protection (a surgical mask is insufficient)
- two pairs of sterile chemotherapy gloves

The hazardous compounding PPE should be worn by a pharmacy technician when handling HDs, receiving or transporting intact or broken supplies, stocking and inventory control of the compounding area, nonsterile or sterile compounding, collecting and disposing of compounding waste, routine cleaning, and managing spills.

Before leaving the hazardous drug preparation area, all disposable protective garb must be discarded in a sealable bag in a specially marked container.

Spill Kits

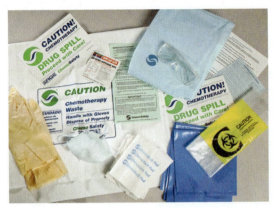

A chemotherapy spill kit is used to clean up chemotherapy spills.

Individuals working with hazardous drugs should be trained to clean up small accidental spills to reduce exposure to hazardous drugs. To help with this task, healthcare personnel should have access to **spill kits** in all areas where hazardous drugs are prepared, administered, or transported. All cleanup supplies must be placed in sealed plastic bags and disposed of in appropriately labeled chemotherapy waste containers. Large spills may need to be cleaned up by the **hazardous materials (hazmat)** team.

In addition, every institution that prepares, dispenses, or administers hazardous medications is required to have a hazardous drugs communication program to identify drugs that require special handling and to outline the protocol for managing spills and other accidental exposure. Pharmacy technicians should consult the Policy and Procedures (P&P) manual of their facility to learn these hazardous drug handling requirements.

If an accidental spill occurs, personnel should refer to **Safety Data Sheets (SDSs)**—formerly referred to as Material Safety Data Sheets—to guide the cleanup process (see Figure 16.4). SDSs are available from manufacturers for all potentially hazardous drugs and chemical products. These sheets identify the drug or chemical and include its potential hazards, handling and storage requirements, first aid measures for accidental exposure, and other critical information. There are a variety of Internet resources for obtaining SDSs for pharmaceutical products. Workplaces that handle hazardous drugs such as chemotherapy agents should keep copies of SDSs on file or have an established Internet link for each product they carry so that easy reference is possible when needed.

FIGURE 16.4
Safety Data Sheet

The Occupational Safety & Health Administration requires chemical manufacturers to provide SDSs for all hazardous chemical products.

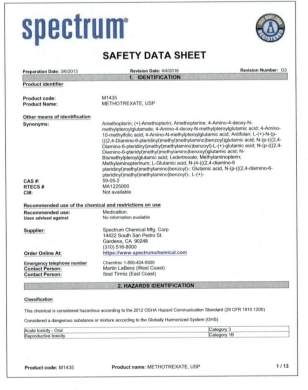

Preventing Chemotherapy-Related Medication Errors

Chemotherapy-related medication errors can occur at any step in processing an order. **Prescribing errors** occur when prescribers make an error in the order for a chemotherapy agent. **Transcription errors** occur when an order for a written chemotherapy order is incorrectly transcribed into the dispensing or computer system. (Transcription errors are virtually eliminated by the use of computerized provider order entry systems for chemotherapy drugs.) **Preparation errors** occur when a chemotherapy agent is prepared incorrectly.

Chemotherapy Preparations

Pharmacy technicians can help prevent multiple types of errors, including:

- errors in calculations: by double-checking every calculation and verifying that the correct concentration of the drug on hand was chosen
- errors in pharmacist order entry: by comparing the final product label to the original physician order for verification of drug, dose, administration schedule, route, and duration of therapy
- errors in dosing: by ensuring adherence to specific manufacturer-provided drug warnings
- errors in administration route: by using a syringe overwrap (provided by the manufacturer) for vincristine and vinblastine to draw attention to the fact that giving these drugs by the IT route is lethal for the patient.

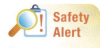

Inventory and Storage Measures to Prevent Chemotherapy Errors

Several chemotherapy drugs have look-alike, sound-alike names or have similar packaging. To prevent inadvertent chemotherapy product mix-ups, healthcare personnel must implement storage and handling measures, such as:

- not storing look-alike, sound-alike drugs next to each other
- affixing look-alike, sound-alike labels to certain medication containers
- using color-coded and/or labeled storage bins
- following manufacturers' warnings on hazardous drug products
- noticing tall man lettering on medication labels (e.g., CISplatin versus CARBOplatin, vinCRIStine versus vinBLAStine). In tall man lettering, the differing parts of two similar words are emphasized using capital letters (see Figure 16.5).

FIGURE 16.5 Carboplatin Medication Label

The medication label for carboplatin uses tall man lettering to avoid confusion with another chemotherapy drug with a similar name: cisplatin.

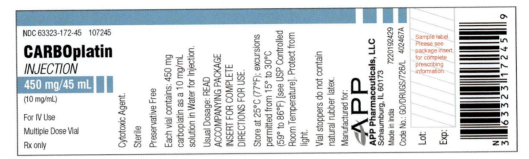

Complementary and Alternative Therapies

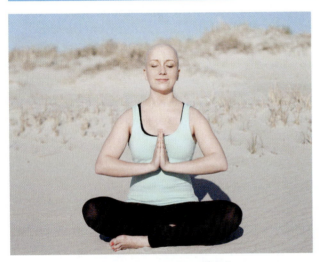

Meditation can help improve quality of life for cancer patients.

Many patients feel a loss of control when they are diagnosed with cancer or when their disease progresses. Consequently, some patients seek nontraditional or alternative approaches for treatment of their disease. Others simply prefer nontraditional therapies because of their holistic lifestyle or fundamental belief system. Although many herbal, supplemental, and complementary therapies are harmless, some are associated with significant toxicity and/or have the potential to negatively interact with traditional cancer treatments. In general, there is little scientific evidence to support many of the claims that are made for the curative potential of such supplemental and herbal therapies for cancer; however, some agents may provide effective symptom relief. Pharmacy technicians should encourage patients to discuss these agents with their oncology health professionals to determine if these medications are safe to use with their current cancer therapies.

Meditation and guided imagery may improve the quality of life of patients with cancer. These techniques may improve mood, sleep quality, and stress related to cancer treatment. Neither should be used a sole treatment; they should be used in addition to other therapies.

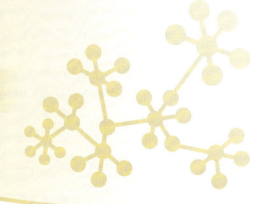

CHAPTER SUMMARY

Cancer and Its Development

- Cancer is a group of diseases characterized by the uncontrolled growth of dysfunctional cells.

- Oncogenes (promoters of cancer formation) and tumor suppressor genes (down-regulators of cancer cells) play a major role in cancer.

- Tumor cells proliferate rapidly, and during the exponential phase, the tumor is most sensitive to chemotherapy agents. A tumor burden is the number of cells or the size of the tumor tissue. The smaller the tumor burden, the more effective chemotherapy will be.

Treatments for Cancer

- Treating cancer involves aggressive and rigorous therapy within multiple modalities, including surgery, radiation therapy, immunotherapy, and chemotherapy. These treatments may be used alone or together to treat cancer.

- Chemotherapy may be described as primary, adjuvant, or palliative. Chemotherapy drugs are designed to interfere with the cell cycle at different points and have a narrow window between safe, therapeutic use and the potential for great toxicity.

Chemotherapy Drugs

- Many factors affect tumor response to chemotherapy drugs.

- To decrease the potential for treatment resistance, combination chemotherapy is usually administered.

- Cell cycle–specific drugs work on various parts of the cell cycle: when the cell prepares to divide, when the cell divides, and when the cell enlarges and makes new proteins.

- Cytotoxic drugs work by interfering with some normal processes of cell proliferation.

- Alkylating agents, antimetabolites, topoisomerase inhibitors, and antimicrotubule agents are the main categories of cytotoxic drugs.

- Cytotoxic drugs cause numerous side effects related to normal cell function, including bone marrow suppression, alopecia, nausea, vomiting, and mucositis.

- Hormonal drug therapies include antiestrogens, antiandrogens, and LHRH agonists.

- Hormonal drugs target the hormonal agent that is contributing to the growth of the specific type of tumor. These therapies block the activity of that hormone.

- Targeted anticancer therapies (angiogenesis inhibitors, monoclonal antibodies, and signal transduction inhibitors) are relatively new agents in the arsenal of cancer-fighting drugs.

- Targeted anticancer therapies have some serious and unusual side effects, they typically offer patients a much more direct treatment for their cancer.

- Investigational therapies are also used for certain patients with cancer. Although not yet approved by the FDA, these therapies are used when no curative treatment regimens are available or when a patient is not responding to currently available treatment options.

Handling and Administration of Chemotherapy Agents

- All individuals who handle or administer chemotherapy medications must don PPE and have access to spill kits and SDSs.

- There are many hazardous drug requirements with the new USP <800> guidelines.

- Safety measures for the storage and handling of these toxic agents must be implemented, including separate storage areas for look-alike, sound-alike drugs; the application of labels to call attention to look-alike, sound-alike medications; and the use of color-coded storage bins.

Preventing Chemotherapy-Related Medication Errors

- Pharmacy technicians should be alert to tall man lettering and to the manufacturers' warnings on hazardous drug products.

Complementary and Alternative Therapies

- Patients should talk to their oncology healthcare providers to discuss complementary and alternative therapies.

adjuvant chemotherapy the treatment of residual cancer cells after removal or reduction of the tumor by surgery

adjuvant radiation therapy radiation therapy that is used in conjunction with surgery to "clean up" areas of residual tumor

administration error when a chemotherapy agent is administered incorrectly

alkylating agents oldest category of traditional cytotoxic drugs

alopecia hair loss

anaphylaxis an allergic reaction

angiogenesis inhibitors drugs that prevent tumor cells from building blood vessels that will supply the tumor with vital nutrients

anthracyclines a large category of topoisomerase II inhibitors

antiandrogens drugs that block the activity of testosterone at the receptor level

antiestrogens drugs commonly used to treat breast cancer

antimetabolites drugs that work in the synthesis phase of the cell cycle

antimicrotubule agents drugs that interfere with the formation and function of microtubules

apoptosis programmed cell death

aromatase inhibitors drugs that block the effects of estrogen by preventing synthesis of estrogen in the body

asparagine an amino acid that is needed for leukemia cells to proliferate

bone marrow suppression decreased production of blood cells, and increased risk of infections and bleeding

cancer a group of diseases characterized by the uncontrolled growth of dysfunctional cells

cardiac toxicity heart damage that may be a result of certain drugs

carmustine (BCNU) a chemotherapy agent with the ability to penetrate the central nervous system, so it can be used in the treatment of brain tumors

cell cycle the process by which both normal cells and cancer cells divide

cell cycle–specific drugs drugs that exert their effects on rapidly dividing cancer cells

cell kill hypothesis predominant hypothesis applied in cancer treatment; presumes that each cycle of chemotherapy kills a certain percentage of cancer cells

chemotherapy the modality of administering drugs to treat cancer

cisplatin an alkylating agent that is used to treat many diseases including lung, ovarian, and bone cancers

combination chemotherapy regimen designed to include drugs proven to work against the tumor being treated, and having nonoverlapping toxicities and different mechanisms of action

conjunctivitis inflammation of the eye

curative an act or treatment intending to cure an illness

cyclophosphamide an alkylating agent that plays an important role in treating lymphomas, leukemias, and breast cancer

cytotoxic drugs drugs that interfere with some normal process of cell function or proliferation

"drivers" of cancer genetic alterations that promote cancer progression

edema swelling of tissues caused by excessive fluid retention

expanded access drugs the means by which investigational drugs are made available

extravasation an infusion leak under the skin during administration

folinic acid (leucovorin) a by-product of dihydrofolate reductase that helps prevent harmful effects of certain chemotherapy drugs

gemcitabine an antimetabolite drug used to treat lung and pancreatic cancers

gynecomastia enlargement of the breasts in males

hazardous materials (hazmat) a material that can be dangerous to life or environment; usually requires a special procedure for cleanup

hemorrhagic cystitis damage to and bleeding of the urinary bladder

hypertension high blood pressure

ileus a condition in which GI motility is severely reduced

immune checkpoint inhibitors used in therapies to prevent immune cells from being turned off by cancer cells.

immunotherapy a type of cancer treatment that stimulates the immune system to stop or slow the growth of cancer cells

intercalating agents chemotherapy drugs that work by inserting themselves into strands of DNA

intrathecal (IT) administration to administer drugs directly into the CNS via a lumbar puncture or spinal tap

investigational drugs a drug used in clinical trials that has not yet been approved by the FDA for use in the general population, or a drug used for nonapproved indications

leucovorin rescue using folinic acid to prevent damage to normal cells when using chemotherapy drugs that prevent cells from using folic acid

liposomal products anthracycline drugs that have been prepared in lipid formulations

lomustine agent with the ability to penetrate the CNS and used in the treatment of brain tumors

luteinizing hormone-releasing hormone (LHRH) agonists drugs given to patients with hormone-sensitive tumors

luteinizing hormone-releasing hormone (LHRH) hormone that stimulates the production of both male and female reproductive hormones

margin the area of normal tissue around the site of a tumor

mechlorethamine an alkylating agent identified as having anticancer activity

melanoma a frequently fatal type of skin cancer

mercaptopurine antimetabolite drug that interferes with cell synthesis

mesna bladder-protective medication

metastasis the process of a tumor having spread from its primary site to other parts of the body

methotrexate drug used to treat leukemia, bone cancer, breast cancer, and lymphomas

microtubules part of a cell that maintains shape and structure

monoclonal antibody an antibody developed from a single type of immune cell that was cloned from a parent cell

monoclonal to originate from a single cell

mucositis inflammation and ulceration of the mucous membranes

mutagenic having the ability to cause changes in genetic material

negative margin the absence of tumor cells

neoadjuvant chemotherapy chemotherapy used to shrink the tumor so it can be safely and completely removed with surgery

nitrosoureas drugs with the ability to penetrate the CNS and used in the treatment of brain tumors

nucleotides the structural components of DNA and RNA

oncogenes genes that promote cancer formation

ototoxicity damage to the nerves that affect hearing

palliative chemotherapy treatment of uncurable cancer

palmar-plantar erythema (hand-foot syndrome) painful sloughing and peeling of the skin on the palms of the hands and soles of the feet

pemetrexed an antimetabolite drug that is critical to the treatment of certain types of lung cancer

peripheral neuropathy extremely painful damage to the nerves that affect the hands and feet

personal protective equipment (PPE) equipment to be worn at all times when handling both oral and injectable hazardous drugs

preparation error when a chemotherapy agent is prepared incorrectly

prescribing error when a prescriber makes an error in the order for a chemotherapy agent

primary chemotherapy the initial treatment of cancer with chemotherapy

proto-oncogenes genes that code for growth factors or their receptors

pulmonary fibrosis lung toxicity

radiation therapy the use of external beam radiation delivered from a machine outside the body to the site of a tumor

resected tumors that are localized and can be surgically removed

Safety Data Sheet (SDS) the guide for a drug cleanup process

secondary cancers additional cancers in conjunction with the first cancer the patient was trying to cure

signal transduction inhibitors drugs designed to target tumor cell receptors

spill kits equipment used where hazardous drugs are prepared, administered, or transported

synergistic effect when a combination of drugs have an enhanced response because the agents work together to amplify the individual effects of each drug

targeted anticancer therapies drug therapies directed at specific molecular entities required for tumor cell development, proliferation, and growth

taxanes antimicrotubule drugs that are derived from the bark and needles of yew trees

threshold dose the lifetime cumulative dose limit for a drug

topoisomerase I enzymes enzymes that produce single-strand DNA breaks

topoisomerase I inhibitors inhibitors used to treat cancer

topoisomerase II enzymes enzymes that produce double-strand DNA breaks

topoisomerase II inhibitors drugs that inhibit topoisomerase activity by inserting themselves into strands of DNA

transcription error when an order for a written chemotherapy order is incorrectly transcribed into the dispensing or computer system

tumor burden the number of cancer cells or the size of the tumor tissue

tumor cell proliferation the exponential rate of growth early on in tumor development

tumor suppressor genes genes that turn off or downregulate the proliferation of cancer cells

vesicants drugs that can cause extravasation injury

vinca alkaloids antimicrotubule drugs derived from periwinkle plants

DRUG LIST

Chemotherapy and Cytotoxic Drugs

Alkylating Agents
bendamustine (Treanda)
busulfan (Myleran)
carboplatin (Paraplatin)
carmustine (BCNU)
chlorambucil (Leukeran)
cisplatin (Platinol)
cyclophosphamide (Cytoxan)
dacarbazine
ifosfamide (Ifex)
lomustine (Gleostine)
mechlorethamine (Mustargen)
melphalan (Alkeran)
oxaliplatin (Eloxatin)
procarbazine (Matulane)
temozolomide (Temodar)

Antimetabolites
capecitabine (Xeloda)
cladribine (Cytosar-U)
clofarabine
cytarabine
fludarabine (Fludara)
fluorouracil (Adrucil)
gemcitabine (Gemzar)
hydroxyurea (Droxia, Hydrea)
mercaptopurine (Purinethol)
methotrexate (various brands)
pemetrexed (Alimta)

Topoisomerase Inhibitors
daunorubicin (Cerubidine, Daunomycin)
doxorubicin (Adriamycin)
epirubicin (Ellence)
etoposide (VePesid)
idarubicin (Idamycin)
irinotecan (Camptosar)
mitoxantrone (Novantrone)
teniposide
topotecan (Hycamtin)

Antimicrotubule Agents
docetaxel (Taxotere)
eribulin

paclitaxel (Taxol)
vinblastine (Velban)
vincristine (Oncovin)
vinorelbine (Navelbine)

Vesicant Drugs
daunorubicin (Cerubidine, Daunomycin)
doxorubicin (Adriamycin)
epirubicin (Ellence)
idarubicin (Idamycin)
mechlorethamine (Mustargen)
mitomycin
vinblastine (Velban)
vincristine (Oncovin)
vinorelbine (Navelbine)

Miscellaneous Cytotoxic Drugs
asparaginase
bleomycin

Hormonal Drug Therapies

Antiestrogens
anastrazole
exemestane
letrozole
tamoxifen

Antiandrogens
abiraterone
bicalutamide
enzalutamide
flutamide

LHRH Agonists
goserelin (Zoladex)
leuprolide (Lupron)

Targeted Anticancer Therapies

Angiogenesis Inhibitors
bevacizumab (Avastin)
lenalidomide (Revlimid)
thalidomide (Thalomid)

Monoclonal Antibodies
cetuximab (Erbitux)
panitumumab (Vectibix)
rituximab (Rituxan)
trastuzumab (Herceptin)

Signal Transduction Inhibitors
axitinib (Inlyta)
bosutinib (Bosulif)
dasatinib (Sprycel)
erlotinib (Tarceva)
imatinib (Gleevec)
nilotinib (Tasigna)
sorafenib (Nexavar)
sunitinib (Sutent)

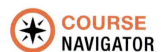

COURSE NAVIGATOR

Access interactive chapter review exercises, practice activities, flash cards, and study games.

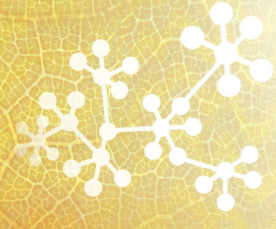

17

Vitamins, Electrolytes, Nutrition, Antidotes, and Bioterrorism

Learning Objectives

1 Describe how the body uses vitamins and electrolytes.

2 Define obesity.

3 Describe the prescription treatments for obesity.

4 Compare and contrast enteral and parenteral nutrition, including its purposes, ingredients, stability, and complications.

5 List the antidotes used to treat occurrences of poisoning.

6 Understand the importance of the emergency cart, its supplies, and its maintenance.

7 Describe the role of the pharmacy technician in the event of a bioterrorist attack.

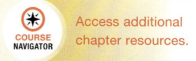

Access additional chapter resources.

Consumption of food and other nondrug substances has far-reaching effects on the health of the human body. Food contains vitamins, minerals, and other nutrients that maintain body function and aid in disease prevention and treatment. Electrolytes such as sodium regulate electrical activity in the body and need to be kept in balance with body fluids. Plant substances such as herbs can affect the body, and many of them have medicinal applications. Ingesting certain substances can result in poisoning, causing critical states and necessitating the use of lavage measures, antidotes, and supportive therapy. Due to disasters like Hurricane Katrina and the outbreak of Ebola, recent improvements have been made in dealing with life-threatening diseases and emergencies. The pharmacy technician plays an important role in emergency situations by understanding a hospital emergency system and the use and maintenance of the emergency carts. Furthermore, pharmacy technicians are trained to be primary responders in the event of a bioterrorist attack.

Vitamins

Vitamins are organic substances that are necessary for normal metabolic functioning but that are not synthesized in the body in sufficient amounts. Usually a vitamin is a **coenzyme** (a chemical other than a protein needed by an enzyme to assist in performing a metabolic function) or is converted to a coenzyme in the body. Vitamins are naturally present in many foods and can be supplemented artificially. If dietary intake of any of these substances is inadequate, a deficiency results and can lead to serious illness.

Vitamins are classified as either fat-soluble or water-soluble and serve different purposes throughout the body. Table 17.1 lists the main vitamins needed to maintain a baseline of health.

Fat-Soluble Vitamins

Fat-soluble vitamins are absorbed with dietary fats and are maintained in stores by the body, mainly in the liver. Deficiency develops only after several months of restricted intake. It is possible to ingest too much of a fat-soluble vitamin, which can result in toxic levels in the body. The fat-soluble vitamins include vitamins A, D, E, and K.

Vitamin A

Vitamin A is a family of compounds referred to as retinoic acids and can be found in two forms: provitamin A **carotenoids** such as beta-carotene, and preformed vitamin A such as **retinol**, retinal, retinoic acid, and retinyl esters. Vitamin A is needed for vision, growth, bone formation, reproduction, immune system function, and skin health.

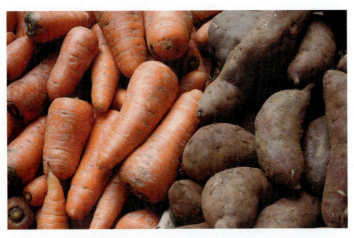

Carrots and sweet potatoes are rich sources of beta-carotene. In fact, the compound beta-carotene gives these vegetables their orange color.

Provitamin A carotenoids must be metabolized into active vitamin A via a highly regulated process. Provitamin A carotenoids can be found in green leafy vegetables; sweet potatoes; and carrots. Because the conversion to active vitamin A is regulated on an as-needed basis by the body, excessive intake of provitamin A is unlikely to cause toxicity.

Preformed vitamin A is a more active form and is found mostly in animal sources and supplements. Butter, egg yolk, kidney, and liver are common food sources of preformed vitamin A. Absorption and storage of preformed vitamin A are efficient, but toxicity can occur if excessive quantities are ingested.

Indications for Vitamin A Supplementation Vitamin A supplements are used primarily to treat deficiency. Deficiency is rarely seen in the United States, but it is the third most common nutritional deficiency in the world. Vitamin A deficiency may result in **keratomalacia**, a softening and ulceration of the cornea of the eye.

Signs and symptoms of keratomalacia include skin rash, corneal degeneration, night blindness, and dry eyes. Other manifestations of vitamin A deficiency include poor bone growth, dermatologic problems, and weakened immune system.

Vitamin A is also used to treat cataracts and reduce complications of human immunodeficiency virus (HIV), measles, and malaria.

TABLE 17.1 Vitamins

Vitamin	Function in Human Body	Vitamin Type
A (carotenoid, retinol)	Bones, skin, eyes, reproduction	Fat-soluble
B_1 (thiamine)	Metabolism, mental, cardiac	Water-soluble
B_2 (riboflavin)	Hair, skin, nails	Water-soluble
B_3 (niacin)	Cholesterol levels, brain cells, skin, bowel	Water-soluble
B_5 (pantothenic acid)	Growth, normal physiological functions and energy production	Water-soluble
B_6 (pyridoxine)	Nerves	Water-soluble
B_7 (biotin)	Hair, energy production, growth	Water-soluble
B_9 (folic acid)	Red blood cells, depression	Water-soluble
B_{12} (cobalamin)	Red blood cells	Water-soluble
C (ascorbic acid)	Immunity	Water-soluble
D (calciferol)	Bones	Fat-soluble
E (tocopherol)	Eyes, immunity, dementia	Fat-soluble
K (phylloquinone, phytonadione)	Blood clotting	Fat-soluble

Vitamin A Toxicity Excessive intake of vitamin A, usually from ingestion of pre-formed vitamin A, may cause toxicity. Signs and symptoms of vitamin A toxicity include nausea, vomiting, vertigo, blurry vision, hair loss, headache, irritability, skin peeling, and bone and liver problems.

Vitamin A can be highly teratogenic, especially in the first trimester of pregnancy, and can lead to spontaneous abortions and fetal malformations.

The United States Department of Agriculture (USDA) suggests a recommended daily allowance (RDA) of 750 mcg (as retinol activity equivalents) of vitamin A during pregnancy. Doses in excess of this allowance are contraindicated in pregnant women.

Vitamin D

Vitamin D, or **calciferol**, was first identified in the early twentieth century as a vitamin and is now recognized also as a hormone. Vitamin D and its metabolites play an important role in maintaining calcium and phosphate levels in the body. There is evidence to suggest that vitamin D plays a role in insulin resistance, obesity, metabolic syndrome, and various cancers.

Vitamin D has two major forms: ergocalciferol (vitamin D_2) and cholecalciferol (vitamin D_3). **Ergocalciferol** is largely human made and added to foods. **Cholecalciferol** is synthesized in the skin in response to sunlight and can be consumed in the diet through the intake of animal-based foods. Sunlight usually provides 80%–90% of the body's vitamin D stores. Both forms of vitamin D are made commercially and can be found in dietary supplements or fortified foods.

There are few naturally occurring food sources of vitamin D. These sources include fatty fish, fish liver oil, and egg yolks.

Indications for Vitamin D Supplementation Vitamin D is used to treat **rickets**, a childhood disease in which a lack of vitamin D results in bone softening and muscle weakness. A hallmark of rickets is bowlegs. Vitamin D can also be used to treat **osteomalacia**, a bone disorder that presents as bone pain, muscle weakness, difficulty walking, and bone fractures.

Vitamin D Toxicity Excessive intake of vitamin D can lead to toxicity. Signs and symptoms of vitamin D toxicity include high blood calcium levels, kidney stones, nausea, vomiting, thirst, increased urination, muscle weakness, and bone pain.

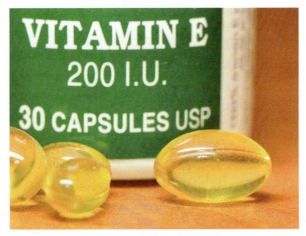

Vitamin E supplements are typically in capsule form.

Vitamin E

The physiologic role of **vitamin E**, or **tocopherol**, is still being defined, but it is thought to work as an antioxidant. Vitamin E is found in a variety of food products including oils, meat, eggs, and green leafy vegetables. The form that is best known for its role in human health, alpha-tocopherol, is abundant in olive oil and sunflower oil. Gamma-tocopherol can be found in soybean oil and corn oil.

Indications for Vitamin E Supplementation Vitamin E deficiency rarely occurs except in cases of specific genetic or malabsorption disorders. Vitamin E deficiency can cause neuromuscular disorders, fragile red blood cells (RBCs), and hemolysis, and it may be treated with supplementation.

Laboratory studies support the use of vitamin E in the treatment of macular degeneration and Alzheimer's disease. Vitamin E also has been shown to reduce the risk of some cancers and dementia and to improve immune system function. Other indications for the use of vitamin E include diabetic retinopathy and cardiovascular disease. Topical use of vitamin E can improve skin health, healing, and hydration.

Vitamin E Toxicity Very high doses of vitamin E may result in bleeding or stroke.

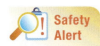

Safety Alert

Patients who are taking warfarin, a common anticoagulant, need to monitor their intake of foods rich in vitamin K. These foods include green leafy vegetables, green onions, and avocados. Most patients can consume these foods as long as they keep their intake consistent.

Vitamin K

Vitamin K functions as a coenzyme for the hepatic production of blood clotting factors and for bone metabolism. Dietary forms of vitamin K (**phylloquinone** and **phytonadione**) are found in green leafy vegetables such as spinach, broccoli, and brussels sprouts, and in fats such as plant oils and margarine.

Indications for Vitamin K Supplementation Vitamin K deficiency is rare in otherwise healthy adults. Signs and symptoms of vitamin K deficiency usually are associated with impaired coagulation (such as easy bruising, mucosal bleeding, or blood in the urine

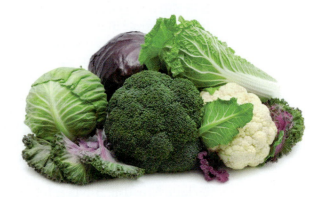

Vitamin K can be found naturally in many commonly consumed vegetables including broccoli, cabbage, and kale.

or stool). Therefore, vitamin K is administered in situations where blood clotting is desired. One of these situations is the reversal of warfarin, a common anticoagulant.

Another indication for the administration of vitamin K is in cases of deficiency caused by drug therapy (for example, salicylates, sulfonamides, quinine, quinidine, and broad-spectrum antibiotics). Vitamin K injection may also be administered to neonates suffering from a deficiency.

Vitamin K Toxicity Vitamin K toxicity is rare. Signs of toxicity include anemia and jaundice.

Water-Soluble Vitamins

Water-soluble vitamins (the B complex and vitamin C) are present in extracellular fluids, which are readily excreted by the kidneys. Because these vitamins are not stored in the body and the kidneys rapidly remove any excess, a deficiency quickly becomes apparent if dietary sources are inadequate, but an overdose is unlikely to be as serious as with fat-soluble vitamins.

Vitamin B$_1$

Vitamin B$_1$, or **thiamine**, is an important coenzyme involved in carbohydrate metabolism. It also plays a role in nerve impulse propagation. Thiamine is found in food products such as yeast, legumes, pork, rice, and cereals. However, thiamine is denatured at high temperatures, and cooking, baking, canning, and pasteurization can destroy it.

Indications for Vitamin B$_1$ Supplementation Thiamine supplements are used to treat vitamin B$_1$ deficiency. Signs and symptoms of vitamin B$_1$ deficiency include impaired memory, lactic acidosis, visual disturbances, and mental status changes. Thiamine deficiency is most common during pregnancy and in **Wernicke-Korsakoff syndrome**, which can occur in patients who abuse alcohol. Patients with known alcohol abuse may be given thiamine supplements when hospitalized to combat symptoms of alcohol withdrawal. In addition, thiamine supplements are used to treat patients who have **beriberi**, a disease that results from a diet low in vitamin B$_1$. Beriberi presents with numbness and tingling, edema, and heart failure.

Vitamin B$_2$

Vitamin B$_2$, or **riboflavin**, is a coenzyme involved in tissue respiration and normal cell metabolism. Riboflavin is found in many foods such as cereal, green vegetables, milk, and some meats. It is also made in the intestines by bacteria.

Indications for Vitamin B$_2$ Supplementation Riboflavin is typically used to treat vitamin B$_2$ deficiency, but it can also be used in doses of 400 mg a day to decrease migraine headaches. Signs of vitamin B$_2$ deficiency include mucositis, skin rash, cracked lips, photophobia, tearing, poor vision, poor wound healing, and anemia.

Vitamin B$_3$

Vitamin B$_3$, or **niacin**, is essential for reactions in the body that produce **adenosine triphosphate (ATP)**, a critical molecule in cellular energy production. The two most common forms of niacin are nicotinic acid and nicotinamide. Niacin also helps regulate the production and activity of cholesterol molecules in the blood. Vitamin B$_3$ is found in yeast, peanuts, peas, beans, whole grains, potatoes, and lean meats.

Indications for Vitamin B$_3$ Supplementation Niacin is most frequently used to treat patients with **dyslipidemia**, a condition signified by elevated total or low-density lipoprotein (LDL) cholesterol levels or low levels of high-density lipoprotein (HDL) cholesterol. Niacin lowers triglycerides and LDL levels and raises HDL levels. The dose required for these effects is at least 1,200–1,500 mg a day.

In addition, niacin supplements are used to treat vitamin B$_3$ deficiency. This deficiency may result from the use of certain medications such as isoniazid, 5-fluorouracil, pyrazinamide, 6-mercaptopurine, hydantoin, ethionamide, phenobarbital, azathioprine, and chloramphenicol.

A deficiency of vitamin B$_3$ may result in **pellagra**, a disease that presents with hyperpigmented rash in areas of exposed skin, red tongue, swelling of the mouth and tongue, diarrhea, sensitivity to light, and neurologic symptoms such as insomnia, anxiety, and disorientation. Pellagra often develops in patients who have certain gastrointestinal (GI) diseases or alcoholism.

Vitamin B$_5$

Vitamin B$_5$, or **pantothenic acid**, is a precursor to coenzyme A. Coenzyme A has an important role in the synthesis of many molecules, such as vitamins A and D, cholesterol, steroids, heme, fatty acids, amino acids, and proteins. Vitamin B$_5$ is found in whole grains, potatoes, chicken, beef, egg yolk, liver, kidney, broccoli, and milk. Pantothenic acid can also be produced by bacteria in the colon.

Indications for Vitamin B$_5$ Supplementation Pantothenic acid supplements are usually used to treat vitamin B$_5$ deficiency. Signs of deficiency include paresthesia, dysesthesia, fatigue, malaise, headache, insomnia, vomiting, and abdominal cramps.

Vitamin B$_6$

Vitamin B$_6$, or **pyridoxine**, is converted in the body to the coenzymes responsible for amino acid metabolism. Common forms include pyridoxine, pyridoxal, and pyridoxamine. Pyridoxine and pyridoxamine are predominantly found in plant-based foods such as vegetables, whole grains, and nuts. Pyridoxal is most commonly derived from animal source foods, though cooking, processing, and storage can reduce vitamin B$_6$ levels by up to 50%.

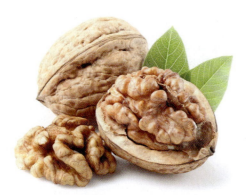

Walnuts are a rich source of pantothenic acid.

Indications for Vitamin B$_6$ Supplementation Pyridoxine is used to treat and prevent vitamin B$_6$ deficiency. Dermatitis may be present in patients with pyridoxine deficiency. Other side effects include neuropathy, weakness, dizziness, and anemia.

Vitamin B$_7$

Vitamin B$_7$, or **biotin**, a coenzyme involved in metabolism, plays an essential role in many processes including cell replication. Biotin can be found in a variety of plants (particularly peanuts and green leafy vegetables), liver, egg yolk, soybeans, and yeast.

Indications for Vitamin B$_7$ Supplementation Biotin supplements are taken for vitamin B$_7$ deficiency. Signs of deficiency include skin rash, hair loss, change in hair color, depression, tiredness, hallucinations, and numbness and tingling. Biotin deficiency is typically associated with altered absorption, such as short bowel syndrome.

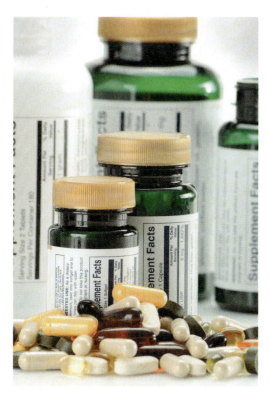

Self-medicating with large doses of vitamins can cause problems. A well-balanced diet is the best way to ensure good health.

Consumption of large quantities of raw egg whites can also lead to biotin deficiency.

Vitamin B$_9$

Vitamin B$_9$, also known as **folic acid** or **folate**, plays a major role in intracellular metabolism and the breakdown of **homocysteine**, an amino acid associated with cardiovascular disease. It is also involved in the production of the neurotransmitter serotonin. Folic acid is frequently added to foods but is naturally found in green leafy vegetables, fruits, cereals, grains, and red meat.

Indications for Vitamin B$_9$ Supplementation Folic acid supplements are used to treat vitamin B$_9$ deficiency. Signs of deficiency include anemia, diarrhea, and a swollen or painful tongue. A lack of vitamin B$_9$ also has a deleterious effect on the cardiovascular system and is associated with a higher risk of coronary heart disease, stroke, and peripheral vascular disease.

Deficiencies in folic acid cause anemia and neural tube defects in a developing fetus. Consequently, folic acid supplements are highly recommended for all women who are pregnant or planning to get pregnant. Taking folic acid can greatly reduce the incidence of some birth defects.

Vitamin B$_9$ supplements are also used to reduce homocysteine levels in patients with end-stage kidney disease. Other uses include treatment for chronic fatigue syndrome, depression, and vitiligo.

Vitamin B$_{12}$

Vitamin B$_{12}$, or **cobalamin**, is a coenzyme necessary for cell reproduction, normal growth, and RBC production. It is found in fish, milk, bread, and meat. Intestinal absorption of vitamin B$_{12}$ requires intrinsic factor, which is produced in the stomach. Patients who have undergone a gastrectomy will need to take lifelong vitamin B$_{12}$ injections because they are unable to produce intrinsic factor.

Indications for Vitamin B$_{12}$ Supplementation Vitamin B$_{12}$ deficiency takes a long time to develop and is easily treated with supplements. It is most common in older adults and strict vegetarians. Signs of B$_{12}$ deficiency include anemia, swollen or painful tongue, and nerve pain and degeneration.

Other indications for cobalamin supplements are pernicious anemia and end-stage renal disease.

Vitamin C

Vitamin C, or **ascorbic acid**, is best known for its role in immune system function and as an antioxidant. **Antioxidants** are thought to be protective substances that can prevent cell damage caused by free radicals. Vitamin C is found in citrus fruits, tomatoes, potatoes, Brussels sprouts, cauliflower, broccoli, strawberries, blueberries, cabbage, and spinach.

Indications for Vitamin C Supplementation Small doses (100–250 mg a day) of vitamin C supplements are used to treat deficiency. Signs of deficiency include poor wound healing, fatigue, and depression. Vitamin C is most effective for treating a severe deficiency known as **scurvy**, a disease rarely seen in the United States. Scurvy presents with fatigue, anemia, hemorrhage, nosebleeds, spongy gums, and enlargement of hair follicles. Other indications for vitamin C supplements are macular degeneration, seasonal allergies, poor iron absorption, and protein metabolism in premature infants.

Many individuals also take large doses of vitamin C supplements (1–3 g a day) to prevent illness, such as the common cold, with some individuals taking the vitamin as part of their drug regimen for prevention of cancer, atherosclerosis, and sunburn. However, they should be aware that high doses of supplemental vitamin C may increase their risk for kidney stones.

Fluids, Electrolytes, and Acid-Base Balance

Fluids and electrolytes are highly related and dependent on each other. A change in one component usually causes subsequent changes to the other. Electrolytes are solutes dissolved in a solvent, usually water. Water moves from areas of low solute concentration to areas of high solute concentration in an attempt to maintain equilibrium. Thus, fluids and electrolytes move around the body in relation to each other. A loss of fluids in one area of the body prompts a shift in fluids from another area to replace what was lost. During this shift, electrolytes are exchanged in an effort to balance the concentration of solutes between fluid compartments of the body.

Fluids

Body fluids are divided into two compartments: **intracellular** (inside cells) and **extracellular**. Intracellular fluid is found inside cells while extra cellular fluid is found in interstitial spaces between cells or in the intravascular space (i.e., lymph and plasma). Body fluids are in equilibrium across the capillary walls. In fact, the chemical and physical processes that proceed in an effort to maintain equilibrium are some of the most important processes in the human body.

The human body consists of 40%–70% water by weight and varies between men and women. Figure 17.1 shows the average percentage of body weight that is made up of water in adult men and women. The difference is due to skeletal weight and the inverse relation of water to adipose tissue.

The percentage of body water (that is, fluid levels) varies according to conditions, weight, sex, and age. Fatty tissue holds little water. Therefore, the proportion of water in obese persons may be as little as 55%, whereas in lean, well-muscled persons it may be as much as 70%. Women generally have more fat than men; therefore, they have proportionally less body water. The body loses water as it ages. Newborns may have as much as 75% or more water by weight; older adults may have 60% or less.

Water deficits are caused by loss of body fluids as a result of such conditions as vomiting, diarrhea, edema, and excessive sweating from fever; large urine output; and acute weight loss (more than 5% of body weight). A water deficit can cause dry skin and mucous membranes, longitudinal wrinkling of the tongue, hypotension, tachycardia, and lowered body temperature. A loss of 25% of body water can lead to death.

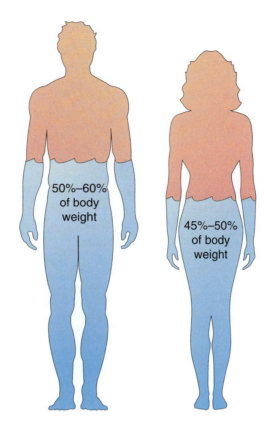

50%–60% of body weight

45%–50% of body weight

Fluids and Solutions

IV fluid products are used to replace fluids and electrolytes lost through dehydration, and parenteral nutrition solutions are used to supply essential trace minerals. Parenteral nutrition solutions are also used as a liquid vehicle for administering IV drug therapy. IV fluids can be categorized by tonicity or content (i.e., colloids versus crystalloids).

Tonicity refers to the concentration of a solute (dissolved substance) in a solvent (liquid vehicle, such as water) and how that concentration affects the movement of water across membranes. The concept of tonicity refers only to molecules, such as ions and electrolytes, that do not move easily across membranes. Fluid and electrolyte products have labeled concentrations in grams of solute per 100 mL of solvent, which is displayed as percent concentration.

Another related concept that affects tonicity is **osmolarity**. Osmolarity refers to the concentration of all molecules, both those that move across membranes and those that do not, in a set volume of fluid. Osmolarity is measured in milliosmoles (mOsm) per liter (L). The osmolarity of plasma is approximately 275–300 mOsm/L.

Types of Fluids and Solutions

Isotonic solutions have a concentration similar to blood plasma. Isotonic fluid products replace daily fluid and electrolyte loss and prevent dehydration. When administered by IV solution, an isotonic solution maintains the normal balance between the vascular volume and interstitial spaces. Isotonic solutions are sometimes referred to as maintenance solutions. The most common isotonic IV solution used is normal saline (0.9% NaCl). Figure 17.2 shows what can happen when cells in the blood or body are exposed to solutions that are not isotonic.

FIGURE 17.2
Tonicity Effects on Cells in Solution

Body cells can be bathed with isotonic solution without a net change between intracellular and extracellular concentrations. Hypertonic solutions cause water to flow out of the cells while hypotonic solutions cause a net flow of water into the the cells.

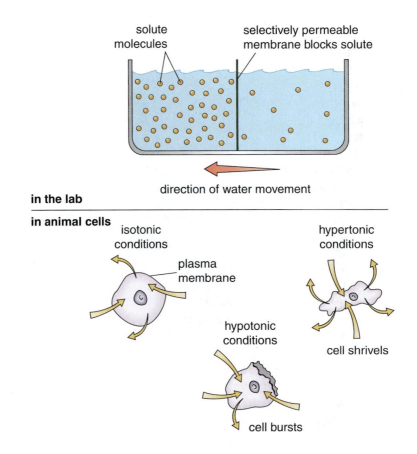

in the lab

in animal cells

Work Wise

A 0.9% NaCl solution is often called "NS" which is an abbreviation for normal saline. Dextrose containing solutions are often abbreviated as "D" plus its percentage. For example, dextrose 5% in sterile water is often called "D5." A commonly used crystalloid solution is dextrose 5% in 0.45% NaCl. This is usually referred to as "D5, half NS."

Hypertonic solutions contain a higher concentration of solute than bodily fluids. The osmolarity of these products is usually over 350 mOsm/L. Hypertonic solutions are used when urgent sodium replenishment is needed as part of hydration. They are indicated for severe sodium depletion from excess sweating, vomiting, or diarrhea. They are also used to treat excessive water intake, overuse of enemas or irrigating solutions (during surgery), and when sodium-free fluids and electrolyte products have been used for fluid replacement. Cells placed in a hypertonic solution shrivel and shrink as water passes out of the cell membrane (see Figure 17.2).

Hypotonic solutions contain a lower concentration of solute than bodily fluids. The osmolarity of these products is usually less than 280 mOsm/L. Hypertonic solutions treat dehydration by diluting the concentration of particles within the bloodstream, which decreases the osmolarity. Water leaves the blood and enters interstitial and intracellular spaces. Cells placed in a hypotonic solution swell and burst as water rushes into the cell. Hypotonic solutions are commonly referred to as hydrating solutions, because they are used to correct dehydration.

Crystalloid IV solutions contain electrolytes, and **colloid solutions** contain proteins and other large molecules (such as fats).

Crystalloid solutions contain small ions and molecules. They are used to replace lost fluid and treat dehydration. Crystalloid solutions are used on a daily basis as a liquid vehicle for administering IV drugs. Both normal saline and dextrose in water are crystalloid solutions. Dextrose is desirable when a patient has need for caloric energy (such as in malnutrition) or when glucose levels are low. Table 17.2 contains examples of common crystalloid solutions along with their associated osmolarity.

1,000 ml

Lactated Ringer's and 5% Dextrose®

Injection

Lactated Ringer's is a crystalloid solution that is often used in combination with 5% dextrose.

Molecules in colloid products are so large that they do not quickly or easily move from the bloodstream to surrounding tissues. In that way, colloids act similarly to hypertonic solutions. They increase the osmolarity of blood plasma, which pulls fluid from interstitial spaces. Colloid solutions are commonly referred to as blood volume expanders. Examples of colloid solutions include albumin, dextran, and blood itself.

Hypertonic solutions must be administered slowly and monitored closely. If given too quickly, the mass exodus of fluid from vital tissues can cause damage. Resulting fluid overload inside the blood vessels can cause heart failure.

Hypotonic solutions must also be used with caution. If administered too quickly, fluid will shift into the cerebral compartment and cause increased intracranial pressure and brain damage.

Contraindications Solutions that contain sodium chloride are contraindicated in patients with hypertonic uterus, hypernatremia, and fluid retention. Solutions that contain dextrose are not for use in patients with hypersensitivity to corn or corn products; delirium tremens and dehydration; and anuria. Albumin solutions are contraindicated in severe anemia and cardiac failure. Hetastarch solutions should not be used in patients with renal failure with oliguria or anuria, fluid overload, bleeding or coagulation disorders, critical illness, and severe liver disease. Hypertonic solutions should not be used in patients with intracranial or intraspinal hemorrhage.

Cautions and Considerations Hypertonic solutions can be quite irritating and corrosive to tissues and blood vessels. They must be administered via a central IV line (i.e., surgically inserted into a port in a central vein), not a peripheral IV line placed in the arm or hand.

Sterile water for injection is a product available in the pharmacy. It is used for diluting other IV drugs or fluids and should never be administered by itself. Injecting or administering pure water through an IV line causes mass hemolysis as water rushes from the plasma into red blood cells, quickly bursting them. Hemolysis destroys the blood and releases intracellular material in mass amounts, resulting in death.

TABLE 17.2 Common Crystalloid Solutions

Tonicity	Solution	Osmolarity (mOsm/L)
Hypotonic (hydrating) solutions	0.45% NaCl (½ NS)	155
	Dextrose 2.5% in sterile water (D2.5W)	140
Isotonic solutions	Dextrose 2.5% in 0.45% NaCl (D2.5W in ½ NS)	280
	Dextrose 5% in sterile water (D5W)	300
	0.9% NaCl (normal saline [NS])	310
	Lactated Ringer's solution (LR)	275
Hypertonic solutions	Dextrose 5% in 0.45% NaCl (D5W in ½ NS)	405
	Dextrose 5% in 0.9% NaCl (D5W in NS)	560
	Dextrose 10% in sterile water (D10W)	600
	3, 5, 14.6, and 23.4% NaCl concentrates	Varies

Electrolytes

Electrolytes are molecular compounds that form ions when dissolved in water. Because water forms the majority of body fluid, electrolytes exist throughout the body as positively or negatively charged ions. For example, sodium chloride (table salt) dissociates into sodium (Na^+) and chloride (Cl^-) when dissolved in water. Positively charged ions are called **cations**, and negatively charged ions are **anions**. Important cations in the body are sodium (Na^+), potassium (K^+), calcium (Ca^{2+}), and magnesium (Mg^{2+}). Important anions include chloride (Cl^-), bicarbonate (HCO_3^-), and, at times, phosphate (PO_4^-). The concentration of electrolytes is measured in **milliequivalents (mEq)** per liter (L). Electrolytes are present in both intracellular and extracellular fluid, though in differing concentrations, depending on the ion. Specific ion pumps (e.g., sodium-potassium ion pumps) and channels (e.g., chloride channels) in cellular membranes maintain these concentrations.

Water passively moves across cellular membranes by **osmosis** to maintain the overall equilibrium in concentration of total molecules on both sides. If a solute (for example, an ion) is added to one side of the membrane, water moves to that side to keep the concentration constant on both sides. More often than not, the concentration of intracellular and extracellular fluid remains constant.

Sodium (Na^+)

Sodium is the primary cation of extracellular fluid. Sodium has a variety of crucial functions, including retaining fluid in the body, generating and transmitting nerve impulses, maintaining acid-base balance, regulating enzyme activities, and regulating the osmolarity and electroneutrality of cells. The kidneys are responsible for maintaining normal sodium concentrations in plasma and other body fluids. The average diet provides sufficient sodium to meet the body's requirements.

Hyponatremia is low sodium concentration, and **hypernatremia** is elevated sodium concentration relative to normal range. Hyponatremia is related to sodium loss or a relative excess of water in the extracellular space. It can be caused by excessive water intake, overuse of salt-wasting diuretics, adrenal gland insufficiency, and kidney or liver failure. Low sodium concentrations can also occur with fluid loss caused by excessive sweating or vomiting. Hypernatremia can be caused by dehydration from lack of fluid intake, diarrhea, and deficiency of antidiuretic hormone. Heart disease and kidney failure can also cause hypernatremia.

Potassium (K^+)

Potassium is the primary cation of intracellular fluid. Potassium is important in the regulation of the acid-base balance and water balance of the body, in protein synthesis and carbohydrate metabolism, in muscle building, and in the function of the nervous system.

Hypokalemia is a condition of lower than the normal potassium concentration. Potassium can be lost through overuse of potassium-wasting diuretics, vomiting or gastric suctioning, or excessive urine output. Signs of hypokalemia include reduced muscle tone (decreased reflexes), weakness, confusion, drowsiness, depression, low blood pressure, and cardiac arrhythmias. **Hyperkalemia** results from an increase in potassium levels. High potassium is a dangerous condition because cardiac function and contractility are greatly affected. Cardiac arrest can occur when potassium levels are too high. Hyperkalemia can be caused by kidney failure, diarrhea, excessive use of

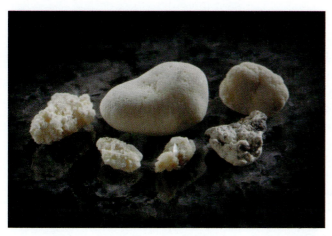
Kidney stones, as seen in this picture, may be a result of high calcium levels.

potassium-sparing diuretics, Cushing's syndrome, severe burns, and septic shock (severe systemic infection). Signs and symptoms include depressed breathing, diarrhea, nausea, vomiting, irritability, confusion, anxiety, intestinal upset, and cardiac arrhythmias.

Calcium (Ca²⁺)

Calcium is important in bone formation and dynamics, muscle contraction, and blood coagulation. When a patient's blood test shows low calcium, their albumin levels should be checked. Low albumin often results in low calcium levels, because calcium is highly bound to this protein.

Hypocalcemia is a depletion in calcium levels in the body. Low calcium can be caused by insufficient calcium intake or parathyroid disease. Signs and symptoms of hypocalcemia include hyperexcitability of nerves and muscle contraction (tetany). Muscle spasms and seizures and even death can occur. **Hypercalcemia** is an excess of calcium in the blood. It can be caused by excessive intake of calcium supplements and by some cancerous tumors. When calcium levels are high, crystals form in the urine and cause kidney stones.

Magnesium (Mg²⁺)

Magnesium is the second most abundant cation in intracellular fluids. Most magnesium is found in bones and within cells. Many body enzymes and enzyme systems need magnesium for activation. Magnesium helps maintain normal nerve and muscular function, the transmission of impulses across neuromuscular junctions, and steady heart rhythms.

Hypomagnesemia is a depletion of magnesium in the body. Magnesium can be lost through alcohol abuse, pregnancy-induced hypertension, or drug therapy that causes increased magnesium excretion. Digoxin, estrogen, and diuretics can deplete magnesium. Signs and symptoms of hypomagnesemia include muscle cramps, confusion, hypertension, tachycardia, arrhythmias, tremors, hyperactive reflexes, hallucinations, and seizures. **Hypermagnesemia** is too much magnesium in the body. It can be caused by renal failure, an overdose of IV magnesium infusion, or the use of enemas containing magnesium. Symptoms of hypermagnesemia may not immediately be apparent to patients. Signs include reduced deep tendon reflexes and changes in cardiac function.

Chloride (Cl⁻)

In the body, **chloride** functions to transport carbon dioxide, form hydrochloric acid in the stomach, retain potassium, and maintain osmolarity of the cells. An excess or deficiency of chloride mainly effects the acid-base balance in the body.

Hypochloremia is a depletion of chloride in the body, and **hyperchloremia** is an excess of chloride. Hypochloremia can be caused by loss of fluid from excessive production of urine or sweat and from gastric suctioning. Some diuretics also deplete chloride. Hyperchloremia can be caused by diarrhea, kidney disease, or diabetes insipidus.

Phosphate (PO$_4^-$)

Phosphate is an anion that plays an important role in energy production within cells. Without sufficient phosphate, normal cell function is not possible. Phosphate is commonly counterbalanced with calcium in the bloodstream. Excessive intake of phosphate can deplete calcium levels and affect bone health.

Hypophosphatemia is a drop in phosphate in the bloodstream. It can be caused by anorexia or severe malnutrition. Signs and symptoms include weakness, respiratory failure, heart failure, hemolysis, and rhabdomyolysis (mass muscle tissue breakdown). **Hyperphosphatemia** can be caused by tumor lysis syndrome (a condition that can occur when receiving chemotherapy drugs for large cancer tumors), rhabdomyolysis (massive muscle breakdown), lactic acidosis, or diabetic ketoacidosis. Taking bisphosphonates or too much vitamin D, or overusing bowel prep products containing phosphate can also cause hyperphosphatemia. Symptoms of hyperphosphatemia are not always apparent to patients but often include kidney damage or failure.

Electrolyte Replacement

Electrolytes are most commonly prescribed for patients who already have an electrolyte deficiency, or if a deficiency is anticipated. They are seldom administered in high doses to prevent disease, as is commonly the case with vitamins. Large quantities of electrolytes can be harmful.

Electrolytes in body fluids can be replaced in a variety of ways. In parenteral nutrition (discussed later in this chapter), electrolyte solutions are combined with carbohydrates, proteins, and fats in large-volume bags and infused through an IV line. In some cases, correcting the underlying cause for an imbalance is enough to correct an abundance or a deficiency of a particular electrolyte. In other cases, replacement or supplementation is needed. When depletion is mild, replacement be achieved by changing the diet to include the absent mineral or taking an oral supplement. For instance, athletes use sports drinks to replenish fluids and electrolytes lost from sweating. Oral liquid electrolyte mixtures are available over-the-counter (OTC) to treat mild dehydration from vomiting or diarrhea (see Table 17.3). These products are generally safe to use because they contain only small amounts of electrolytes.

When immediate correction is needed or severe deficiencies exist, IV electrolyte products are used. Electrolytes are added to IV fluids, such as normal saline or dextrose in water, and administered. Laboratory results are used to guide therapy. Dosing must be individualized depending on the reason for the electrolyte imbalance and fluid status of the patient.

Oral potassium supplements are typically used to replace potassium lost from diuresis. Some diuretics deplete potassium, so patients must take a potassium supplement while on those drug therapies. Doses are individualized to patients. Intravenous potassium solutions should be diluted to a concentration no greater than 100 mEq/L. More concentrated solutions may cause **phlebitis** (irritation of the vein), and rapid infusions can result in lethal cardiac arrhythmias. Klor-Con is a brand name for oral potassium and is commonly used by patients who take diuretics.

Common side effects of high potassium levels include nausea, vomiting, diarrhea, and abdominal pain. In some cases, potassium supplements have been associated with GI ulceration. At a minimum, they can be irritating to the GI tract. Patients should take oral potassium products with a full glass of water to reduce these effects. Effervescent powder products should be mixed with plenty of water to prevent stomach and intestinal irritation. Taking potassium supplements with food may also decrease stomach upset.

TABLE 17.3 Common Oral Liquid Electrolyte Mixtures

Product	Electrolyte Content	Other Content
Infalyte	Na, K, Cl	Rice syrup
Naturalyte	Na, K, Cl	Dextrose
Pedialyte	Na, K, Cl	Dextrose
Pedialyte Freezer Pops	Na, K, Cl	Dextrose
Rehydrate	Na, K, Cl	Dextrose

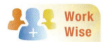

Work Wise

Potassium supplementation is used for a variety of reasons. You may find other healthcare providers refer to potassium supplements as "K" and potassium chloride supplements as "KCL."

Other than treating a deficiency, oral magnesium products have been used with some controversy in people with heart disease and diabetes. Magnesium sulfate is commonly used to treat preeclampsia and eclampsia. It is administered intravenously for acute prevention of uterine contractions in preterm labor.

Common side effects of magnesium supplements include diarrhea. Taking magnesium supplements with food can decrease this effect. Over time, this effect usually decreases.

Phosphorus products are used primarily in cases of malnourishment. Some patients do not acquire sufficient phosphorus because they have GI absorption abnormalities.

Common side effects of phosphate-containing supplements include stomach upset or diarrhea. Over time, these effects usually subside. Phosphorus supplements have also been associated with kidney stones. Patients should seek medical attention if they have back or flank pain and/or difficult or painful urination, especially if associated with nausea and vomiting. These can be signs of kidney stone formation.

Oral calcium products are used to prevent and treat bone loss from osteoporosis, rickets (which may be caused from calcium deficiency or vitamin D deficiency), and osteomalacia. They are also used for tetany. Calcium products are listed in Table 17.4. They are absorbed more efficiently when taken with vitamin D.

Common side effects of calcium supplementation include constipation. Taking calcium supplements with food and drinking plenty of water may diminish occurrences of constipation. If hypercalcemia occurs, kidney stones can form. Patients should seek medical attention if they have back or flank pain and/or difficult or painful urination, especially if associated with nausea and vomiting. These can be signs of kidney stone formation. Various calcium salts are used for different purposes. Five calcium salts currently in use are calcium chloride, calcium carbonate, calcium citrate, calcium acetate, and calcium gluconate.

Calcium chloride is the fastest of the calcium salts to diffuse into the bloodstream, so it is the salt primarily used in cardiac emergencies. It moderates nerve and muscle performance through regulation of the action potential excitation threshold. If infused directly into an IV line or mixed in too high a concentration with phosphate, calcium will precipitate. IV is the only available dosage form of calcium chloride.

Calcium carbonate (Caltrate, Os-Cal, Tums) is typically used as an antacid and is sold under many brand names, such as Tums. It is also used as a dietary supplement to prevent a negative calcium balance. Calcium carbonate is taken only by mouth. Calcium cannot penetrate bone without the aid of vitamin D, so most of these supplements have vitamin D added to them.

TABLE 17.4 Common Electrolyte Replacement Products

Generic (Brand)	Pronunciation	Dosage Form	Dispensing Status
Sodium			
sodium chloride (Slo-Salt, Sustain)	SOE-dee-um KLOR-ide	IV solution, injectable concentrate 14.6%, 23.4%, tablet	Rx
sodium phosphate*	SOE-dee-um FOS-fate	Injectable concentrate, oral solution, rectal solution, tablet	Rx, OTC
Potassium			
potassium acetate	poe-TASS-ee-um AS-e-tate	IV additive (diluted to 40–80 mEq/L)	Rx
potassium chloride (K-Dur, K-Lor, K-Lyte, Klor-Con, Micro-K) (varying strengths, 8–25 mEq per dose)	poe-TASS-ee-um KLOR-ide	IV additive, tablet, capsule, liquid, effervescent powder	Rx
potassium phosphate*	poe-TASS-ee-um FOS-fate	IV additive	Rx
Calcium			
calcium acetate (Eliphos, PhosLo, Phoslyra)	KAL-see-um AS-e-tate	Capsule, oral solution, tablet	Rx, OTC
calcium carbonate (Caltrate, Os-Cal, Tums)	KAL-see-um KAR-bo-nate	Tablet, suspension	OTC
calcium chloride	KAL-see-um KLOR-ide	Injection	Rx
calcium citrate (Calcitrate)	KAL-see-um SI-trate	Tablet	OTC
calcium gluconate	KAL-see-um GLOO-koh-nate	Capsule, injection, tablet	OTC
calcium lactate (Cal-Lac)	KAL-see-um LAK-tate	Capsule, tablet	OTC
Magnesium			
magnesium chloride (Chloromag)	mag-NEE-zhum KLOR-ide	Solution for injection, tablet	Rx
magnesium gluconate (Mag-G, Magtrate, Magonate)	mag-NEE-zhum GLOO-koh-nate	Tablet, liquid	OTC
magnesium lactate (Mag-Tab)	mag-NEE-zhum LAK-tate	Tablet	OTC
magnesium oxide (Mag-Cap, Mag-Ox, Maox, Uro-Mag)	mag-NEE-zhum OX-side	Capsule	OTC
magnesium sulfate (Mag-200)	mag-NEE-zhum SUL-fate	Capsule, solution for injection	Rx, OTC
Phosphate			

*Phosphate containing products are listed by the cation salts.

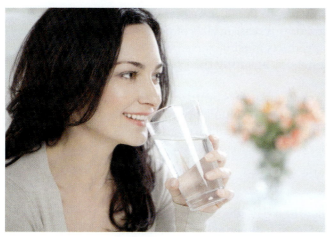

Many oral electrolyte supplements, such as potassium chloride, should be taken with a full glass of water.

Calcium citrate (Calcitrate) is better absorbed than other calcium products. It should be given in combination with vitamin D to build bones. It should be taken in two or three doses separated by six hours each.

Calcium acetate (Eliphos, PhosLo, Phoslyra) is used to control hyperphosphatemia in end-stage renal failure. It binds to the phosphorus in the GI tract more efficiently than other calcium salts. This efficient binding is due to its lower solubility and subsequent reduced absorption and increased formation of calcium phosphate. It can be administered as a capsule, tablet, or injection.

Calcium gluconate is used to prevent negative calcium balances. It moderates muscle and nerve performance and allows normal cardiac function. It is used in total parenteral nutrition and can be taken orally or parenterally.

Contraindications Contraindications to sodium chloride include hypertonic uterus, hypernatremia, and fluid retention.

Potassium replacements are contraindicated in hyperkalemia and diseases where high potassium levels may be encountered. Solid potassium dosage forms are contraindicated in patients who may have delay or arrest in passage through the gastrointestinal tract.

Calcium chloride is contraindicated in digoxin toxicity. The gluconate form of calcium should not be used in patients with ventricular fibrillation, hypercalcemia, and also should not be used concomitantly with ceftriaxone in neonates. Calcium lactate is contraindicated in hypercalcemia and ventricular fibrillation. Calcium carbonate and citrate do not have contraindications.

Magnesium chloride is contraindicated in kidney impairment, myocardial disease, and coma. The gluconate and lactate forms of magnesium have no contraindications.

Phosphate replacements are contraindicated in hyperphosphatemia and hypocalcemia. Potassium phosphate is contraindicated in hyperkalemia.

Safety Alert

The Institute of Safe Medication Practices publishes a list of high-alert medications that may cause significant patient harm when used in error. Potassium chloride for injection is included on this list. Errors in injectable potassium chloride administration can cause heart abnormalities and even death.

Cautions and Considerations Most electrolyte products cannot be used in patients with kidney failure or impairment. If they are used in these cases, they must be monitored closely. Patients with kidney problems should notify their healthcare providers before taking an electrolyte supplement.

Injectable potassium products must be diluted before administration. Potassium is diluted and added to a large-volume IV solution, then mixed well before administration. Such infusions must also be administered slowly because they can be irritating to the veins and painful for the patient. Usually, 40 mEq of potassium are added to 1 L IV fluid. The maximum safe concentration is 80 mEq/L.

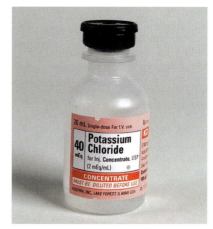

Vials of potassium have black tops to help alert healthcare providers to dilute it prior to administration.

Administering too much potassium can be fatal because it will interfere with heart function and cause cardiac arrest. For this reason, vials of potassium concentrate have black tops. Injectable potassium products must be mixed well, so that the entire IV bag has a consistent concentration. Fully agitating the IV bag once potassium is added will help ensure consistent mixing.

Calcium and phosphate salts cannot always be mixed in the same IV bags. They can chelate, or bond chemically to form an insoluble precipitate. The precipitate appears as small white specks or lumps of material within the bag. If infused through an IV, the precipitate clogs capillaries and has severe adverse effects for the patient.

Acid-Base Balance

Acidosis occurs when extracellular fluid (i.e., blood) contains excess **hydrogen ions** (commonly from an abundance of carbon dioxide), which causes the blood pH to drop below the normal range. **Metabolic acidosis** occurs when excess acid is produced, bicarbonate is lost (such as with diarrhea), or the kidneys do not excrete enough acid. **Respiratory acidosis** results from slow breathing and retention of carbon dioxide in the blood.

Alkalosis is typically caused by a loss in hydrogen ions, producing a relative increase in bicarbonate, which increases blood pH. Hydrogen ions can be lost from the GI tract (e.g., by vomiting) or in urine. **Metabolic alkalosis** takes place when excess acid is excreted via the kidneys (such as in over diuresis) or acid is lost from the stomach (either from vomiting or gastric suction). **Respiratory alkalosis** occurs when breathing becomes more rapid, and more carbon dioxide is exhaled and eliminated from the blood.

When either a metabolic or respiratory process is contributing to an acid-base imbalance, the other pathway makes adjustments for it. Correction in pH can occur quickly with respiratory changes, but metabolic correction takes time. In either case, drug therapy may be needed to address the imbalance if severe or urgent.

Acidifying and Alkalinizing Agents

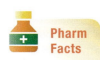

Pharm Facts

Sodium bicarbonate (baking soda), sometimes used to correct acid-base imbalances, can be found in the pharmacy and at the grocery store. When combined with moisture and an acidic ingredient in baking, sodium bicarbonate produces bubbles of carbon dioxide. This helps baked goods to rise.

Some electrolyte products are used primarily for their acidic or basic properties in acidosis or alkalosis rather than for electrolyte deficiencies. Acidic electrolyte products are used to treat alkalosis, and basic products are used to treat acidosis (see Table 17.5).

Ammonium chloride is an acidic substance used for hypochloremia and metabolic alkalosis. It is typically administered in doses of 100–200 mEq mixed with 500–1,000 mL normal saline and then infused slowly over approximately three hours. This infusion prompts the kidneys to use ammonium in place of sodium in excretion processes. Less sodium is then available to combine to make sodium bicarbonate.

Sodium bicarbonate is a basic substance used as an antacid for heartburn and acid indigestion, a systemic alkalinizer for treating metabolic acidosis, and a urinary alkalinizer when treating hemolytic emergencies and drug overdoses (i.e., salicylates and lithium). When used as an antacid, adult patients take 325–2,000 mg one to four times daily. The oral powder is administered by mixing ½ teaspoonful in half a glass (120 mL) of water and drinking as often as every two hours. When used as an oral systemic alkalinizer, 1,000–2,000 mg are dissolved in 1–2 L of water and consumed within one hour. When using the IV form for systemic alkalinization, 2–5 mEq/kg are given over four to eight hours, which allows the blood pH to be adjusted upward gently. A urinary alkalinizer, the dose is six 650 mg tablets initially, and then two to four tablets every four hours under supervision of a physician.

TABLE 17.5 Common Acidifying and Alkalinizing Products

Generic Drug	Pronunciation	Dosage Form	Dispensing Status
Acidifying Agent			
Ammonium chloride	a-MONE-ee-yum KLOR-ide	Injection	Rx
Alkalinizing Agent			
Sodium bicarbonate	SOE-dee-um bye-KAR-bo-nate	Injection	Rx

Close supervision and monitoring must accompany use of any acidifying or alkalinizing agent to prevent overcorrections in pH. Most side effects are related to overshooting pH goals. Excess ammonium chloride can result in ammonium toxicity. Patients must be watched for pallor, sweating, retching, irregular breathing, changes in heart rate, twitching, and convulsions. If left untreated, coma and death could occur. Excess sodium bicarbonate can result in sodium toxicity, which causes fluid overload. Renal function and cardiac function are impaired when sodium and water retention occur.

Sodium bicarbonate is a hypertonic solution that can cause extravasation (ulceration of local tissue at the injection site). As is true of chemical burns, this process causes tissue necrosis (death) and skin sloughing. To prevent extravasation, any pain experienced during infusion should be given prompt attention and treatment.

Contraindications Ammonium chloride is contraindicated in severe liver or kidney dysfunction. Contraindications to sodium bicarbonate include alkalosis, hypernatremia, severe pulmonary edema, hypocalcemia, and unknown abdominal pain.

Cautions and Considerations The concentrations and rates of infusion must be precise to prevent adverse effects. For instance, the maximum concentration of ammonium chloride when mixed should be 1%–2%. The maximum infusion rate of ammonium chloride is 5 mL/min to prevent venous irritation and ammonium toxicity. For this same reason, sodium bicarbonate is typically given slowly. In these cases, healthcare providers must be very attentive to signs of extravasation. Controlled infusion rates and frequent laboratory tests are necessary to prevent dramatic swings in pH and allow for gradual, safe correction of acidosis or alkalosis situations.

Nutritional Disorders

Nutrition is an important component of health and wellness. When an individual receives too much or too little of the daily caloric, protein, or micronutrient needs for his or her age and size, overnutrition (obesity) or undernutrition (malnutrition) can result. Both obesity and malnutrition can have negative health impacts and result in higher morbidity and mortality. According to the World Health Organization, global obesity has more than doubled since 1980, and more than 1.9 billion adults were overweight in 2014. Once a problem associated with high-income countries, obesity is now on the rise in low- and middle-income countries. In fact, most of the world's population lives in countries where being overweight kills more people than being underweight. Malnutrition, however, is still a major concern. It is estimated that malnutrition contributes to more than one-third of child deaths worldwide.

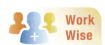

Obesity

Obesity is a condition characterized by the excessive accumulation and storage of fat in the body. Obesity is a major healthcare concern. The Centers for Disease Control and Prevention (CDC) estimates that in 2010, nearly 70% of adults and 32% of children in the United States were overweight. The CDC also reports that more than one-third of the population in the United States is obese. This statistic has climbed over the past few decades. Figure 17.3 illustrates obesity prevalence throughout the United States.

Environmental factors that contribute to obesity include leading a sedentary lifestyle, having a readily available food supply, and consuming increased amounts of fats and refined sugars and decreased amounts of fruits and vegetables. In the United States, these environmental factors are readily apparent. Food portions are larger than those in other industrialized countries, and the lifestyle of many individuals has become sedentary, as technology has taken over many manual labor tasks.

Genetics is a major factor in obesity and the distribution of body fat. For instance, obesity among first-degree relatives (parents and siblings) is a strong predictor of obesity in adulthood.

Physiologic factors affect appetite control. Peptides such as leptin and incretins as well as neurotransmitters such as serotonin, norepinephrine, and dopamine are involved in **satiety**, the sensation of feeling full and satisfied. As weight and adipose (fat) tissue accumulate, it is thought that the normal release and sensitivity to these hormones and neurotransmitters are affected. Other physiologic contributors include medical conditions such as hypothyroidism and Cushing's syndrome. Certain drugs, such as corticosteroids, also cause fat redistribution and appetite changes that foster weight gain.

FIGURE 17.3
CDC Obesity Prevalence Map

According to the CDC, the prevalence of obesity in the United States varies from state to state. The causes of obesity are multifactorial and not fully understood. Environmental, genetic, physiologic, and psychological factors all contribute in different ways to the development of obesity.

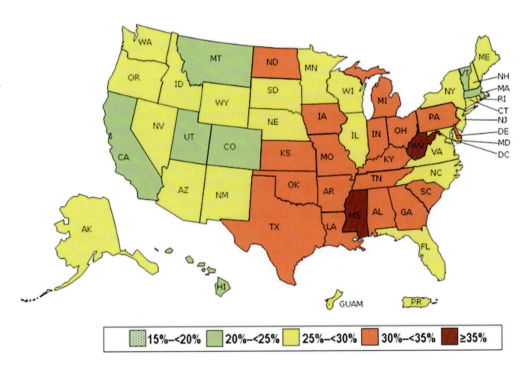

15%–<20% 20%–<25% 25%–<30% 30%–<35% ≥35%

Obesity is associated with serious health risks and mortality (see Table 17.6). **Centrally distributed fat** is adipose tissue that accumulates in the abdominal area, rather than in the hips, thighs, or buttocks. This kind of fat distribution is linked to heart disease and diabetes. Obese people also have greater rates of depression and psychological disturbances. Consequently, preventing and treating obesity is an important effort within health care. Reducing body weight has been shown to reduce morbidity and mortality in overweight and obese patients.

The preferred treatment for obesity is lifestyle intervention, a combination of diet and exercise, and behavior modification. Initial treatment should create a caloric deficit by reducing caloric intake and/or increasing caloric expenditure. Patients who restrict caloric intake and also perform physical activity will lose weight. Some individuals find these interventions difficult. Changes must be permanent to keep off lost weight. Consequently, providing products and services for weight loss and physical fitness is a billion-dollar industry.

Special diets tend to restrict specific components of nutrition to achieve weight loss. Popular weight loss programs include those that restrict the intake of carbohydrates, fats, or both. These programs are not often sustainable because they do not represent a balanced way to eat that ensures adequate nutrition in the long term. The most successful and healthy diets are those that restrict caloric intake while maintaining a proper balance of nutrients.

Some patients are candidates for more aggressive therapy options. Medications and surgical intervention can achieve significant weight loss. Surgical options are collectively referred to as **bariatric surgery** and include (1) restrictive procedures (**laparoscopic** or **gastric banding**) that effectively make the stomach smaller and prevent excess food intake, and (2) malabsorptive techniques (**gastric bypass**) that bypass parts of the intestine, thus preventing nutrients from being fully absorbed. Whether surgical or drug therapy is chosen for weight loss, patients must first meet specific criteria. Usually, surgical methods are limited to patients with a body mass index (BMI) of 40 or higher. Some patients with a BMI of 30 or higher will be considered candidates for surgery if they have comorbid health conditions (see Table 17.6).

TABLE 17.6 Comorbid Conditions of Obesity

Breast and colon cancer	Hypertension
Congestive heart failure	Inflammatory disorders
Coronary artery disease	Obstructive airway disease
Degenerative bone and joint disease	Osteoarthritis
Depression	Polycystic ovarian syndrome
Eating disorders	Pulmonary hypertension
Gallbladder inflammation	Skin tags, stretch marks, and other dermatologic problems
Gastroesophageal reflux disorder	Sleep apnea
Hiatal hernia	Stroke
High cholesterol	Type 2 diabetes

Lipase Inhibitors

Medications that are commonly used to treat obesity are lipase inhibitors. As the name suggests, **lipase inhibitors** work by binding to gastric and pancreatic lipase enzymes in the intestines, thereby preventing the enzymes from breaking down fats into a form that can be absorbed. Fat then passes through the intestines and out of the rectum, where it is excreted in stool. Orlistat, a commercially available lipase inhibitor, is available over the counter and by prescription. It is taken three times a day with each meal that contains fat (see Table 17.7).

Common side effects of orlistat include fatty or oily stools, fecal incontinence or urgency, gas, and diarrhea. These effects may decrease over time. Patients can reduce or prevent these effects by limiting fat intake to less than 30% of total calories. If not, they may find the side effects become intolerable.

Contraindications Orlistat is contraindicated in chronic malabsorption syndrome, cholestasis, and pregnancy.

Cautions and Considerations Because orlistat interferes with the absorption of fat, it can also prevent absorption of fat-soluble vitamins. Patients should take multivitamin supplements to combat potential vitamin deficiencies.

Drug Interactions Orlistat may decrease concentrations of amiodarone, anticonvulsants, cyclosporine, levothyroxine, multivitamins, and vitamin D analogs. Warfarin levels may be increased by orlistat.

TABLE 17.7 Lipase Inhibitors

Generic (Brand)	Pronunciation	Dosage Form	Dispensing Status
orlistat (Alli)	OR-li-stat	Capsule	OTC
orlistat (Xenical)	OR-li-stat	Capsule	Rx

Sympathomimetic Drugs

One class of drugs used to treat obesity, **sympathomimetics**, stimulates the central nervous system (CNS), much as amphetamines do. These medications are used with exercise, behavior modification, and reduced caloric intake to produce weight loss in patients with a BMI of 30 or higher (or over 27 with the presence of other risk factors, such as high blood pressure, diabetes, or high cholesterol). The sympathomimetics stimulate dopamine and norepinephrine and prevent the reuptake of serotonin. Increased neurotransmitter levels signal a sense of satiety. In effect, patients do not feel as hungry. Fast-acting dosage forms are taken 30 minutes to 1 hour prior to eating, and long-acting forms are taken once a day (see Table 17.8).

Common side effects of sympathomimetics are headache, stomachache, insomnia, nervousness, tachycardia, and irritability. Taking these medications in the morning may help reduce insomnia, but other effects can be limiting if they are bothersome. Sympathomimetics can also cause dry mouth, difficulty urinating, and constipation. Patients with urinary problems should not take these medications, and drinking plenty of water can help with these effects. In men, sympathomimetics can cause impotence. Patients should discuss the risks versus benefits of sympathomimetics with their healthcare practitioners.

TABLE 17.8 Common Sympathomimetic Drugs

Generic (Brand)	Pronunciation	Dosage Form	Dispensing Status
benzphetamine (Didrex, Regimex)	benz-FET-ah-meen	Tablet	C-III
diethylpropion	dye-eth-ill-PROE-pee-on	Tablet	C-IV
phendimetrazine (Bontril)	fen-di-MEH-tra-zeen	Capsule, tablet	C-III
phentermine (Adipex-P, Suprenza)	FEN-ter-meen	Capsule, tablet	C-IV
Combination Product			
phentermine-topiramate (Qsymia)	FEN-ter-meen toe-PEER-i-mate	Capsule	C-IV

A possible side effect of sympathomimetics is **serotonin syndrome**, a condition causing a dangerous rise in blood pressure and heart rate. Other symptoms include agitation, confusion, twitching and shivering. Serotonin syndrome is a serious health condition and can even result in death.

Contraindications The sympathomimetics are contraindicated in patients with coronary heart disease, high blood pressure, hyperthyroidism, and in patients with a history of drug abuse.

Cautions and Considerations All CNS stimulants are controlled substances and have addiction and abuse potential. Patients must be informed that a new prescription is needed each time they need a refill.

Drug Interactions Sympathomimetics may enhance the analgesic effect of opioids. They may decrease the sedative effects of antihistamines and drugs for insomnia. Sympathomimetics may increase blood pressure and may enhance the hypertensive effects of other drugs (such as linezolid and monoamine oxidase inhibitors [MAOIs]). Lithium may decrease the stimulatory effects of sympathomimetics.

Serotonin Agonists

Serotonin is a neurotransmitter that can affect mood, social behavior, sleep, memory, sexual desire, and appetite and digestion. It is manufactured in the brain and intestines and generally signals satiety in animals and human beings. **Serotonin agonists** activate serotonin receptors and therefore reduce appetite and food intake.

Lorcaserin (Belviq), the serotonin agonist available in the United States, may be used in addition to a reduced calorie diet and exercise regimen in patients with a BMI of 30 or higher (or 27 or higher with the presence of other risk factors, such as high blood pressure, diabetes, or high cholesterol). Lorcaserin is taken twice a day, with or without food (see Table 17.9).

Common side effects of serotonin agonists include headache, upper respiratory infection, back pain, dizziness, and nausea.

Contraindications Lorcaserin is contraindicated in pregnancy and in patients with renal dysfunction.

Cautions and Considerations Lorcaserin-induced weight loss may pose risks in patients who are taking oral medications to treat type 2 diabetes. In these patients, weight loss may increase the risk for hypoglycemia; therefore, dose reduction of diabetes medications may be warranted. Lorcaserin should not be continued if it is not effica-cious, meaning it should be discontinued in patients who do not lose 5% of their body weight after 12 weeks of drug therapy.

Drug Interactions Serotonin syndrome is a risk with serotonin agonist use. Lorcaserin should not be used in combination with medications that increase serotonin activity. For example, many types of antidepressants, such as selective serotonin reuptake inhibitors (SSRIs), serotonin-norepinephrine reuptake inhibitors (SNRIs), bupropion, tricyclic antidepressants (TCAs), and MAOIs should not be taken concurrently with lorcaserin.

TABLE 17.9 Serotonin Agonist

Generic (Brand)	Pronunciation	Dosage Form	Dispensing Status
lorcaserin (Belviq)	lor-ca-SER-in	Tablet	C-IV

Glucagon-Like Peptide Receptor Agonists

Glucagon-like peptide is a gastric hormone that stimulates glucose-dependent insu-lin secretion and inhibits glucagon release and gastric emptying. It acts as a regulator of appetite and caloric intake. **Glucagon-like peptide receptor agonists** act similarly to endogenous glucagon-like peptide, and there is evidence to suggest these medica-tions decrease body weight through decreased caloric intake. **Liraglutide (Saxenda)**, a glucagon-like peptide receptor agonist, is indicated as an adjunct therapy to a reduced calorie diet and increased physical activity for long-term weight management in adults with a BMI of 30 or higher (or 27 or higher with the presence of other risk factors, such as high blood pressure, diabetes, or high cholesterol). Liraglutide is approved by the FDA and is available as a solution for subcutaneous injection (see Table 17.10).

Liraglutide may cause nausea, hypoglycemia, diarrhea, constipation, vomiting, headache, decreased appetite, dyspepsia, fatigue, dizziness, abdominal pain, and increased lipase activity.

Contraindications Liraglutide is contraindicated in patients with a personal or family history of medullary thyroid carcinoma or multiple endocrine neoplasia type 2. Liraglutide should not be used by pregnant patients.

Cautions and Considerations Because liraglutide can cause insulin secretion, it should be used cautiously with other secretagogues. There may be an increased risk of thyroid tumors with use, and patients should be counseled about their symptoms. Liraglutide has been associated with acute pancreatitis and gallbladder disease. Patients should discontinue use if either of these conditions is suspected or confirmed.

TABLE 17.10 Glucagon-Like Peptide Receptor Agonist

Generic (Brand)	Pronunciation	Dosage Form	Dispensing Status
liraglutide (Saxenda)	LIR-a-GLOO-tide	Solution for injection	Rx

Malnutrition

Malnutrition is a lack of adequate nutrient intake to supply basic metabolic needs. It can be related to an overall lack of calorie or protein consumption, or it may be associated with a deficiency in a specific micronutrient (for example, a vitamin or mineral). Malnutrition is most prevalent in underdeveloped countries. Children living in these poorer nations are especially vulnerable to malnutrition. They often develop **marasmus**, a chronic condition caused by inadequate caloric and protein intake over a prolonged period. Wasting of muscle and fat tissue is observed, a condition known as **cachexia**. Individuals in these underdeveloped countries are also at risk for **kwashiorkor**, a condition in which caloric intake is adequate but protein intake is deficient. These patients, paradoxically, usually appear well nourished because heightened metabolic rates break down protein stores but leave adipose tissue intact. However, patients may accumulate fluid in the abdomen, hands, face, and feet.

In the United States, malnutrition is most often encountered in the inpatient setting, where it is associated with disease states, acute illness, and even drug therapy. Some causes for malnutrition include the following:

- anorexia
- food allergies or intolerance
- chronic infection or inflammatory conditions
- cancer
- endocrine disorders
- pulmonary disease
- cirrhosis of the liver
- renal failure
- nausea, vomiting, or diarrhea
- trauma, burns, or sepsis
- inflammatory bowel disease, Crohn's disease, or short bowel syndrome
- inadequate parenteral or enteral nutrition
- psychiatric or psychological conditions

Signs of malnutrition include weight loss, skin changes (too dry, shiny, or scaly), hair loss, fatigue, poor wound healing, pallor (pale skin), sunken eyes, dry mouth and eyes, visible loss of muscle mass, and fluid accumulation in the abdomen or around the ankles and tailbone.

An individual cannot go longer than 7 to 10 days without food or nutrition; malnutrition will ensue and negatively affect health outcomes. When a patient cannot be fed normally, nutrition must be supplied by alternative methods. Enteral nutrition and parenteral nutrition are artificial ways to feed patients that do not involve swallowing.

Enteral Nutrition

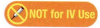

Enteral nutrition is a method of feeding a patient liquid nutrients through a tube inserted into the GI tract. The tube can be inserted manually or surgically. A nasogastric (NG) tube is manually inserted. A gastrostomy (G) tube and a jejunostomy (J) tube are placed surgically in the stomach and jejunum, respectively (see Figure 17.4). A liquid nutrient formula is injected through the tube, either in bolus doses to mimic eating a meal or continuously with an enteral pump.

FIGURE 17.4
Enteral Feeding Tube Sites

NG tubes are uncomfortable for patients, so such tubes are suitable for only short-term use. If enteral feeding is necessary for more than a few days, a G tube or J tube will be placed surgically.

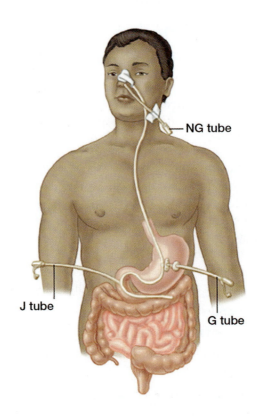

NG tube

J tube

G tube

Pharm Facts

An NG tube, also known as a Levin tube, is made from lightweight polyurethane material.

Indications for enteral feeding include bowel obstruction, short bowel syndrome, and Crohn's disease. Patients in long-term care who are unable to swallow foods voluntarily because of a severe stroke or prolonged coma may have an enteral feeding tube to maintain a patient's hydration status.

Specialized enteral feeding products are available for specific conditions, so patients must be matched with appropriate formulas. Healthcare personnel should never administer enteral nutrition through an intravenous (IV) line. These preparations are neither sterile nor formulated for that use. Enteral feeding is preferred to parenteral feeding because it keeps the GI tract functional and prevents abdominal infections. Various enteral feeding products are highlighted in Table 17.11.

TABLE 17.11   Most Commonly Used Enteral Nutrition Formulations

Enteral Feeding	Population Receiving
Fibersource HN, Jevity Plus, Probalance	Patients with high nitrogen needs, noninjured patients, nursing home patients
Fibersource, Jevity, Ultracal	Patients with intact GI tracts who are unable to eat for various reasons
Isosource VHN, Promote, Replete	Patients with very high nitrogen needs, trauma victims, burn victims
Magnacal Renal, Nepro, Novasource Renal	Renal patients on dialysis
Impact, Impact Glutamine, Perative	Immunocompromised patients, abdomen trauma victims, seriously ill patients
Choice DM, Glucerna, Resource Diabetic	Diabetic patients

Parenteral Nutrition

Parenteral nutrition (PN; often referred to as **total parenteral nutrition [TPN]**) is provided by feeding a patient through an IV line. TPN is used when the digestive tract cannot be used for nutrient absorption. Indications for TPN include severe burns, intolerance to enteral feeding, anorexia nervosa (refusal to eat), pancreatitis, severe gallbladder disease, inflammatory bowel disease, and severe diarrhea. TPN may also be necessary in pregnancy, acquired immunodeficiency syndrome (AIDS), and cancer.

TPN carries risks for complications. TPN is complex in that it supplies all the fluids, electrolytes, nutrients (carbohydrates, proteins, and fats), vitamins, and minerals that a patient needs intravenously. If an essential nutrient or trace element is not included, a patient can easily become nutritionally deficient or imbalanced. Regular laboratory monitoring is necessary to guide TPN therapy and protect against infection. Special care must be taken when adding trace minerals to a TPN formula because of the heightened risk of underdosing or overdosing these elements.

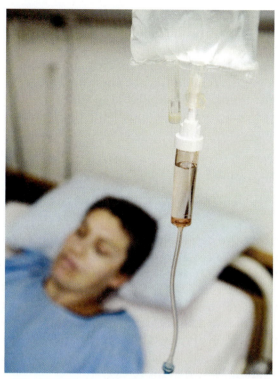

Parenteral nutrition is administered intravenously.

Complications of Parenteral Nutrition Patients may experience various complications as a result of PN, including the following:

- acid-base imbalance
- dehydration
- elevated serum triglycerides
- failure to induce anabolism
- high serum lipid concentrations
- hyperammonemia
- hyperglycemia or hypoglycemia
- hypoalbuminemia
- imbalance of electrolytes
- liver toxicity

Even patients without diabetes may show increased blood sugar levels when on PN; therefore, insulin may be added to the solution even for patients without diabetes.

Infections are frequently a problem for patients receiving parenteral nutrition. PN solutions are rich in nutrients and therefore capable of hosting many types of bacteria and fungi. Aseptic technique should be used in the preparation of parenteral products, and the solution should be tested for microbial growth. The area around the central line should be inspected for infection often; the line may need to be removed and replaced in the case of infection. PN may be discontinued in the case of line infection and sometimes reformulated when restarted.

Preparing Parenteral Nutrition Solutions PN solutions are formulated to ensure adequate absorption of nutrients from circulation, providing fluids, carbohydrates, and protein while maintaining osmolarity.

Two types of PN solutions are available: (1) a solution that contains lipids in addition to amino acids and dextrose, known as a **total nutrient admixture (TNA)** or a **three-in-one**; and (2) a solution that does not contain lipids but includes amino acids and dextrose (a **two-in-one**). Both three-in-one and two-in-one solutions have electrolytes added. The three-in-one formula offers the following advantages:

- lower cost of preparation and delivery
- less nursing time needed for administration
- potentially reduced risk of sepsis with fewer points of entry of the administration line

The three-in-one formulations also have two disadvantages. First, the risk of IV line occlusion is greater and larger filters must be used. Larger filters lead to less microbial elimination. Second, if precipitation of the electrolytes occurs, it cannot be seen because of the opacity of lipid formulations.

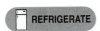

With either type of PN solution, the electrolytes are added to the mixture during initial preparation, but the vitamins are always added just before administration. This mixture is usually stable for 24 hours after addition of the vitamins. Both types of PN solution may remain at room temperature for 24 hours (usually a parenteral bag is hung this long). Otherwise the solution is always stored in the refrigerator.

When mixing a three-in-one PN, electrolytes should be added carefully. **Pooling** saves considerable time, but this method is controversial because precipitation is more common when it is used. In pooling, all the electrolytes except phosphate are put into a small-volume parenteral bag and then transferred into each batch. Cysteine is sometimes added to prevent precipitation of the electrolytes. If pooling is used, the phosphates must be separate from the calcium and magnesium. The phosphates should be injected into the bag first; next, the amino acids, dextrose, lipids, and water should be added; and then the pooled electrolytes are added. When the PN is mixed in this way, precipitation is very unlikely to occur.

Solutions that contain lipids should be carefully inspected in the pharmacy and before infusion for **cracking**, or separation. Cracking can be demonstrated by adding hydrochloric acid to the PN solution. The result is a distinct separation of the oil that is easily visible.

To provide all nutrients intravenously, PN solutions must contain a large number of components in a relatively small volume of fluid. The possibility of component interactions and microprecipitation is quite high and must be considered when mixing each batch. Solutions that do not contain lipids should be inspected during preparation against both black and white backgrounds with proper lighting. All bags with precipitates should be discarded. It is advantageous to look for particulate matter before adding insulin or albumin, because particles can be removed by passing the mixture through a filter into another bag, but albumin and insulin cannot pass through microfilters.

Calcium and phosphorus are the electrolytes that cause the most problems with precipitation. The phosphate ion should always be added to the bag first and mixed thoroughly with other ingredients. After the PN solution is mixed, the calcium ion is added with constant swirling. Calcium chloride should not be used; calcium gluconate is preferred. The sulfate salt is the preferred form for magnesium. The actual concentration of magnesium depends on the amount of calcium, because both destabilize the lipid emulsion.

Safety Alert

All IV products must be labeled with beyond use dates.

Table 17.12 lists the recommended multivitamin additions for PN. These come in one bottle and are added to the PN as close to the time of administration as possible because vitamins degrade more rapidly than other components. Tables 17.13 and 17.14 list other additions that may vary according to the product.

TABLE 17.12 Recommended Multivitamin Additions for PN

Vitamin	Pronunciation	Daily Adult Dose
Ascorbic acid (vitamin C)	a-SKOR-bik AS-id	60 mg
Biotin (vitamin B_7)	BYE-oh-tin	150 mcg
Cyanocobalamin (vitamin B_{12})	sye-an-oh-koe-BAL-a-min	2 mcg
Ergocalciferol (vitamin D_2)	er-goe-kal-SIF-e-rawl	200 mg
Folic acid (vitamin B_9)	FOE-lik AS-id	180 mcg
Niacin (vitamin B_3)	NYE-a-sin	15 mg
Pyridoxine (vitamin B_6)	peer-i-DOX-een	1.6 mg
Retinol (vitamin A)	RE-tin-awl	800 mg
Riboflavin (vitamin B_2)	RYE-boe-flay-vin	1.3 mg
Thiamine (vitamin B_1)	THYE-a-min	1.1 mg
Tocopherol (vitamin E)	to-KOF-er-awl	12 mg

TABLE 17.13 Recommended Trace Element Additions for TPN

Vitamin	Daily Adult Dose
Chromium	10–15 mcg
Copper	0.5–1.5 mg
Manganese	0.15–0.80 mg

TABLE 17.14 Standard per Liter Additions for TPN

Additive	Amount per Liter
Acetate	Limited by cation
Calcium	9 mEq
Chloride	Limited by cation
Insulin, regular	30 units (dependent on blood glucose level)
Magnesium	12 mEq
Phosphate	21 mEq
Potassium	80 mEq
Sodium	Patient tolerance
Zinc	2.5–4.0 mg

After the PN solution is mixed and given a final inspection, each batch should be clearly labeled with the patient's name, address or hospital unit, solution name, concentration and volume, and additives. Instructions for the additives, such as vitamins, should be given on the label, and a beyond use date must be included on any IV product. In many practice settings, it is the pharmacy technician who mixes PN solutions, which are then checked by the pharmacist and sent out to the patient.

Poisons and Antidotes

Prevention of accidental poisoning should be a major concern of healthcare professionals. More than two-thirds of accidental poisonings occur in children under six years of age, and in many of these cases the child ingests compounds meant for household use. Drugs in particular present a danger to children. The following are the drugs that cause the most childhood poisonings:

- Iron tablets are the leading cause of fatal poisonings in children.
- Tricyclic antidepressants are extremely toxic in children. Small amounts can cause heart arrhythmias, seizures, and shock.
- Calcium channel blockers are becoming a major problem; they lead to low blood pressure and heart failure.
- Opiates (even diphenoxylate in Lomotil) can cause respiratory failure.
- Aspirin poisoning is down dramatically because of childproof caps and the increased use of nonaspirin OTC pain relievers. Symptoms of aspirin poisoning include tinnitus, nausea, and vomiting. Nausea and vomiting occur with doses greater than 150 mg/kg.
- Alcohol is often overlooked, but small amounts can cause low blood sugar, coma, and seizures. Some mouthwashes contain enough alcohol to harm a child.

Poisoning also frequently occurs among older persons who mistake household chemicals for medication. It also happens as a result of occupational exposure to harmful chemicals.

Ingestion is the most common route of poisoning. Once a toxic substance is ingested, there are two concerns: (1) eliminating it from the patient's GI tract to prevent absorption, and (2) diminishing the effects of the dose absorbed. In addition, **supportive therapy** consists of establishing the airway and performing cardiopulmonary resuscitation (CPR); maintaining body temperature, nutritional status, and fluid and electrolyte balance; and preventing circulatory collapse, hypoglycemia, uremia, and liver failure.

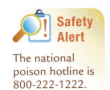

Safety Alert

The national poison hotline is 800-222-1222.

Decontamination

The first step when a patient has ingested poison is to remove as much of the ingested poison as possible, a process called **decontamination**. For orally ingested drugs, this means emptying the stomach, administering an adsorbent (such as activated charcoal), or catharsis (vomiting). Decontamination should be considered when a sufficient amount of a potentially toxic substance has been ingested within a specific time.

The patient's stomach may be emptied by inducing vomiting or by a **gastric lavage**, commonly known as a stomach pump, a procedure to wash out or irrigate a patient's stomach. This procedure involves passing a tube into the stomach, pumping warm water or saline in, and pumping stomach contents out until the fluid withdrawn is clear. Gastric lavage should not be used, and vomiting should not be induced, if the poison is corrosive or volatile. Gastric lavage should not be performed if 60 minutes or more have elapsed since ingestion. For patients in coma, convulsing, or with no gag reflex, a tube should first be passed into the patient's trachea to ensure an open airway.

Activated charcoal has become the primary emergency room treatment for preventing absorption of poison from the GI tract. It is administered as a powder dispersed in water. Like gastric lavage, activated charcoal should not be used for patients at risk for aspiration.

Cathartics are used with activated charcoal to further decrease the absorption of the ingested agent. Speeding the travel and elimination of gastric contents decreases the likelihood of absorption. Saline cathartics, such as magnesium sulfate and magnesium citrate, or hyperosmotic cathartics, such as sorbitol, are the agents of choice.

Pharmacologic Antagonists (Antidotes)

Usually, it is not possible to eliminate the poison completely, so if possible, three additional steps are taken to diminish the effective dose of the ingested absorbed poison:

1. Supportive care, or treating the patient's symptoms, is a major part of therapy. This may include keeping the patient's airway patent, treating high or low blood pressure, and correcting arrhythmias.
2. Pharmacologic antagonists (specific antidotes) are given to counteract the effects of the poison.
3. Dialysis and exchange transfusion are needed if the patient has ingested a very large dose of a water-soluble poison. Dialysis and exchange transfusion are contraindicated if the patient has ingested a fat-soluble, protein-bound, or tissue-bound substance.

An **antidote** is a drug that reduces the harmful effects of a poison. Some antidotes are chelating agents. A **chelating agent** is an organic molecule that chemically bonds to a metal ion, which prevents the ion from interacting with biological molecules as it circulates through the body and is eventually removed through the kidney or the liver. Table 17.15 lists the most commonly used antidotes.

Acetylcysteine (Acetadote) is used for acetaminophen overdose.

Atropine is used in poisoning from cholinergic agents to treat drug-induced bradycardia.

A cyanide antidote kit contains amyl nitrite inhalers, sodium nitrite ampules for injection, and sodium thiosulfate ampules for injection.

Dapsone may be useful in tissue disorders caused by spiders or insects, such as bites from the brown recluse spider. It is also used in the treatment of leprosy.

Deferoxamine (Desferal) is a chelator for ferric iron and is used in acute iron poisoning.

Digoxin immune Fab (Digibind, DigiFab) is used to treat life-threatening digoxin overdose, referred to as "dig toxicity." It is often used to treat chronic ingestions leading to toxic steady-state concentrations, or for acute ingestions of digoxin in children.

TABLE 17.15 Most Commonly Used Antidotes

Generic (Brand)	Pronunciation	Dosage Form	Dispensing Status	Chemical It Binds To or Reverses
acetylcysteine (Acetadote)	a-se-teel-SIS-teen	Injection, oral liquid	Rx	Acetaminophen
activated carbon, charcoal (many)	AK-ti-vay-ted KAR-bon	Oral liquid	OTC	Contaminants in the GI tract
amyl nitrite (none)	AY-mil NYE-trite	Solution for inhalation	Rx	Cyanide
antivenin (various products available)	an-tye-VEN-in	Injection	Rx	Snake bites
atropine (none)	AT-roe-peen	Injection	Rx	Cholinergic agents
Centruroides immune F(ab')$_2$ (equine) (Anascorp)	sen-tra-ROY-dez i-MYUN fab too E-kwine	Injection	Rx	Scorpion stings
dapsone (none)	DAP-sone	Tablet	Rx	Spider bites
deferoxamine (Desferal)	dee-fer-OX-a-meen	Injection	Rx	Iron
digoxin immune Fab (Digibind, DigiFab)	di-JOX-in im-MYOON FAB	Injection	Rx	Digoxin, digitoxin
dimercaprol (BAL in Oil)	dye-mer-KAP-role	Injection	Rx	Lead, arsenic, mercury, gold, bismuth, chromium, nickel, copper
edetate calcium disodium (Calcium Disodium Versenate)	ED-e-tate KAL-see-um dye-SOE-dee-um	Injection	Rx	Lead
flumazenil (Romazicon)	floo-MAZ-e-nil	Injection	Rx	Benzodiazepines
fomepizole (Antizol)	foe-MEP-i-zole	Injection	Rx	Ethylene glycol, methanol
glucagon (GlucaGen)	GLOO-ka-gon	Injection	Rx	Insulin, beta blockers, possibly calcium channel blockers
methylene blue (Urolene Blue)	METH-i-leen BLOO	Injection	Rx	Cyanide
naloxone (Narcan)	nal-OX-one	Injection	Rx	Narcotics
octreotide (Sandostatin)	ok-TREE-oh-tide	Injection	Rx	Oral sulfonylureas
penicillamine (Cuprimine, Depen Titratabs)	pen-i-SIL-a-meen	Capsule, tablet	Rx	Copper, zinc, mercury, lead
phentolamine (Regitine)	fen-TOLE-a-meen	Injection	Rx	Extravasation caused by IV norepinephrine
physostigmine (none)	fye-zoe-STIG-meen	Injection	Rx	Atropine and other belladonna alkaloids
phytonadione, vitamin K (AquaMEPHYTON, Mephyton)	fye-toe-na-DYE-one	Injection, tablet	Rx	Warfarin
polyethylene glycol (GoLYTELY, HalfLytely, MiraLax)	pol-ee-ETH-il-een GLYE-kawl	Oral liquid	Rx	Contaminants in the GI tract
pralidoxime (Protopam)	pral-i-DOX-eem	Injection	Rx	Organophosphates
protamine sulfate (none)	PROE-ta-meen SUL-fate	Injection	Rx	Heparin

pyridoxine, vitamin B$_6$	peer-i-DOX-een	Injection, tablet	OTC, Rx	Isoniazid (INH), hydralazine
sodium nitrite (none)	SOE-dee-um NYE-trite	Injection	Rx	Cyanide
sodium nitrite-sodium thiosulfate (Nithiodote)	SOE-dee-um NYE-trite/SOE-dee-um thye-oh-SUL-fate	Injection	Rx	Cyanide
sodium thiosulfate (Versiclear)	SOE-dee-um thye-oh-SUL-fate	Injection	Rx	Arsenic, cyanide

Safety Alert

Diprolene, dantrolene, and dapsone can be easily confused.

Dimercaprol, also called **British Anti-Lewisite** or **BAL in Oil**, forms a stable chelate with lead, arsenic compounds (such as lewisite, a chemical weapon used in World War II), mercury compounds, gold salts, bismuth, chromium, nickel, and copper. It also reactivates enzymes shut down by these metals.

Edetate calcium disodium (Calcium Disodium Versenate) is a chelating agent for injection that enhances the mobilization and excretion of lead from the body.

Fomepizole (Antizol) is a competitive inhibitor for the metabolism of methyl alcohol and ethylene glycol. It is used to reverse ethylene glycol and methanol toxicity. It forms a complex with and inactivates alcohol dehydrogenase, thus preventing the formation of formaldehyde and the other toxic metabolites of the alcohols. Fomepizole is diluted in normal saline and dextrose and is stable for at least 48 hours when refrigerated. The solution may become solid in the bottle, and in this case, it should be warmed by rotating it in the hand or running it under warm water.

Glucagon (GlucaGen) is an antidote for hypoglycemia.

Methylene blue (Urolene Blue) is used to treat cyanide poisoning.

Naloxone (Narcan) reverses opioid respiratory depression.

Octreotide (Sandostatin) is an analog of somatostatin. It is used to counteract oral sulfonylureas.

Penicillamine (Cuprimine, Depen Titratabs) is a chelator of copper, zinc, mercury, and lead. It promotes the excretion of these metals in the urine.

Phentolamine (Regitine) is an injectable product used for extravasation caused by IV norepinephrine.

Pralidoxime (Protopam) is an acetylcholinesterase reactivator used for acetylcholinesterase-inhibiting agents (organophosphates), such as certain pesticides (parathion or malathion) and nerve gases used in chemical warfare. It is given after atropine in life-threatening situations.

Protamine sulfate is the antidote for heparin overdose. It forms a stable complex with heparin, neutralizing its anticoagulant effects.

Physostigmine is a cholinesterase inhibitor used to reverse toxic effects of drugs that block acetylcholine receptors (e.g., atropine and other belladonna alkaloids).

Phytonadione (AquaMEPHYTON, Mephyton) is vitamin K (previously discussed in this chapter), which promotes formation of clotting factors; it is an antagonist for warfarin.

Pyridoxine (vitamin B$_6$) releases glycogen stored in the liver and muscles. Pyridoxine acts as an antidote to isoniazid, hydralazine, and cycloserine toxicity.

Sodium nitrate and **sodium thiosulfate (Versiclear)**, whether used separately or together, help the body safely excrete cyanide in the urine. These medications are stored in the refrigerator and administered by IV. They must be protected from light. The drugs are administered via slow IV injection—the sodium nitrite first, then the sodium thiosulfate. If symptoms return, both may be administered again at half the original dose. The patient must be monitored for at least 24–48 hours. Cyanide levels may be used to determine dose.

Antivenins

An **antivenin** is a material used to treat poisoning by animal venom. Antivenin is produced by injecting a host, often an animal, with venom, which produces very high levels of circulating antibodies that are then harvested and used for treatment. The dose required to fight the animal venom may be large. A high percentage of patients experience serum sickness (an immune reaction to a foreign protein) from the antivenin.

Antivenin was originally developed to treat bites from two species of North American rattlesnakes (a type of pit viper). This antivenin has been shown to be clinically effective against venoms of all pit vipers, whose bites are deadly. The drug must be on hand at the time of the emergency, together with epinephrine 1:1,000, IV antihistamine, and hydrocortisone. First, a very small dose of the antivenin is pretested, and, if a reaction occurs, the value of giving the antivenin must be weighed against the risk of reaction.

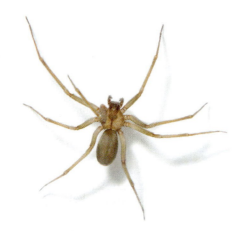
Brown recluse spider bites may require antivenin therapy.

In North America, the two most common bites from poisonous spiders are those from black widow and brown recluse spiders. Most healthy adults will survive the bite of a black widow spider with only supportive care. However, antivenin is indicated for patients under 12 years of age and for those older than 65 years with medical problems such as hypertension and cardiovascular disease. For a brown recluse spider bite, some physicians prescribe **dapsone** in an attempt to preserve the skin around the bite. Dapsone is a sulfone antimicrobial. It causes photosensitivity, and the physician should be notified if persistent sore throat, fever, malaise, or fatigue occurs.

Centruroides antivenom (Anascorp) is approved for stings by *Centruroides* scorpions. In some cases, these stings can become life-threatening. Anascorp is made from the plasma of horses that are immune to the scorpion's venom. Each vial is reconstituted with 5 mL normal saline, then mixed in 50 mL bags for infusion. The initial dose is three vials administered every 30 to 60 minutes as needed. It is administered over 10 minutes.

Many hospitals do not even carry antivenins, because they are so expensive and so rarely used. But when they are needed, there is little time to get them. Hospitals usually must call each other to find the needed material. If a hospital pharmacy does stock an antivenin, the technician should create a kit containing the antivenin and other drugs that must be administered with it. This kit will go up automatically when the order is written for the antivenin. The technician is responsible for maintaining this kit and putting a system in place to check the dates of the medications on a regular basis.

Emergency Procedures

The emergency procedures to deal with the conditions that may lead to sudden death are to stabilize the patient at the scene and then transport to a site of continuing care. Basic life support involves measures to prevent circulatory or respiratory arrest or provide external support for circulation and respiration if they have failed. Advanced cardiac life support ensures ready access to adjunctive equipment to support ventilation, give IV infusions, administer drugs, and provide cardiac monitoring, defibrillation, arrhythmic control, and postresuscitation care. The objectives of basic life support are to:

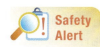
- correct hypoxia,
- reestablish spontaneous circulation,
- optimize cardiac function,
- suppress sustained ventricular arrhythmias,
- correct acidosis,
- relieve pain, and
- treat congestive heart failure.

A patient in asystole has a flat electrocardiogram (ECG) tracing. Various terms are used to categorize the causes of death. **Sudden cardiac death** is death that occurs within 24 hours of the onset of illness or injury. Most patients have no symptoms immediately before collapse. The aim of treatment is to prevent ventricular fibrillation or to treat the arrest itself.

Sudden arrhythmic death is the loss of consciousness and pulse without prior circulatory collapse. It is *not* preceded by circulatory impairment, but it may be preceded by chronic heart failure. Death results from ventricular fibrillation associated with myocardial infarction (MI), transient myocardial ischemia, and underlying myocardial abnormalities (usually from previous MI).

Myocardial failure is a gradual circulatory failure and collapse before loss of pulse. It is due to hemorrhage, trauma, infarction, stroke, or respiratory failure.

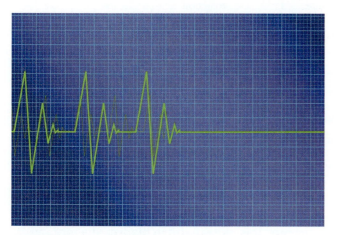

Code Blue emergency procedures are set in motion when life-threatening situations arise.

The American Heart Association has recommended guidelines for use of oxygen. The aim is to increase the oxygen level in the blood, thereby raising levels in organs and tissues. Indications include acute chest pain due to suspected or confirmed heart attack, suspected hypoxia of any cause, and cardiopulmonary arrest.

Hospitals use a system of codes to alert staff of various emergency situations. A **Code Blue** is initiated when a patient is in a life-threatening situation, such as when a patient's heart has stopped or breathing has ceased. In response to a Code Blue alert, emergency hospital personnel respond with appropriate emergency procedures.

Drugs Used for Emergency Procedures

Table 17.16 presents the most commonly used agents for cardiac emergencies.

Adenosine (Adenocard) is an antiarrhythmic used in tachycardia. It works by slowing conduction and restoring normal sinus rhythm. Adenosine should be administered by rapid bolus. **Amiodarone (Cordarone, Nexterone, Pacerone)** is an antiarrhythmic agent that inhibits adrenergic stimulation, prolongs the action potential and refractory period in myocardial tissue, and decreases atrioventricular conduction and sinus node function. During a Code Blue emergency, amiodarone may be mixed and infused in a plastic container. If the patient is put on a continuous infusion or drip, however, it must be mixed in a glass container unless the hospital uses polyolefin bags. It is incompatible with most drugs and must be protected from light.

TABLE 17.16 Drugs Recommended by Advanced Cardiac Life Support Guidelines for Cardiac Emergencies and Blue-Alert Carts

Generic (Brand)	Pronunciation	Dosage Form	Dispensing Status
adenosine (Adenocard)	a-DEN-oh-seen	Injection	Rx
amiodarone (Cordarone, Nexterone, Pacerone)	am-ee-OH-da-rone	Injection	Rx
atropine (none)	A-troe-peen	Injection	Rx
calcium chloride (none)	KAL-see-um KLOR-ide	Injection	Rx
dextrose 50% (none)	DEX-trohs	Injection	Rx
diltiazem (Cardizem)	dil-TYE-a-zem	Injection	Rx
dobutamine (Dobutrex)	doe-BYOO-ta-meen	Injection	Rx
dopamine (Intropin)	DOE-pa-meen	Injection	Rx
epinephrine (Adrenalin)	ep-i-NEF-rin	Injection	Rx
etomidate (Amidate)	e-TOM-i-date	Injection	Rx
flumazenil (Romazicon)	FLOO-may-ze-nil	Injection	Rx
ibutilide (Corvert)	i-BYOO-ti-lide	Injection	Rx
lidocaine (none)	LYE-doe-kane	Injection	Rx
magnesium sulfate (Mag-200)	mag-NEE-zee-um SUL-fate	Injection	Rx
naloxone (Evzio, Narcan)	nal-OX-one	Injection	Rx
norepinephrine (Levophed)	nor-ep-i-NEF-rin	Injection	Rx
procainamide (Pronestyl)	proe-KANE-a-mide	Injection	Rx
vasopressin (none)	vay-soe-PRES-in	Injection	Rx
verapamil (Calan, Verelan)	ver-AP-a-mil	Injection	Rx

Atropine blocks vagus nerve stimulation, which slows the heart, allowing the sympathetic system to speed the heart rate. It is most useful in bradycardia for rates less than 60 beats per minute and in atrioventricular nodal block. However, atropine increases oxygen demand on the heart during arrhythmias and hypotension.

Calcium chloride is used for cardiac resuscitation necessitated by hypocalcemia, hyperkalemia, calcium channel blocker overdose, or beta blocker overdose.

Dextrose 50% is indicated for diabetic coma.

Diltiazem (Cardizem) is used for atrial fibrillation or flutter and paroxysmal supraventricular tachycardia.

Dobutamine (Dobutrex) is a beta-1 selective sympathomimetic adrenergic agonist. It increases heart rate with little action on beta-2 or alpha receptors. Dobutamine is used to increase cardiac output in the short-term treatment of patients who have a very weak heartbeat because of organic heart disease, cardiac surgical procedures, or acute myocardial infarction. It is compatible with dopamine, epinephrine, isoproterenol, and lidocaine. The drug is stable for 48 hours after mixing if refrigerated and for six hours if not refrigerated. It may turn slightly pink, but this color change does not indicate a significant loss of potency.

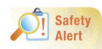

Safety Alert

In an emergency situation it would be very easy to confuse dobutamine and dopamine. Be sure they are not stored side by side on the emergency cart or box.

Dopamine (Intropin) increases blood pressure by causing constriction of peripheral vessels while maintaining blood flow to internal organs and kidneys. It is used to support blood pressure. Dopamine is also used as adjunctive treatment of left ventricular failure secondary to acute myocardial infarction, and in shock from sympathomimetic amines.

Epinephrine (Adrenalin) is one of the most commonly used agents in cardiopulmonary arrest. A strong heart stimulant, it increases contractility and excitability. It is used in any form of cardiopulmonary standstill and helps to convert fine ventricular fibrillations to a coarser form that is easier to defibrillate. Epinephrine must be used cautiously in the presence of liver disease, low cardiac output, or allergy.

Etomidate (Amidate) is used to calm the patient and prevent resistance to intubation. Another anesthetic inducer may be used, but, if the patient must be intubated to begin breathing again, the process is easier if some form of anesthesia is available. Etomidate acts very quickly and is safe enough to be used in children.

Flumazenil (Romazicon) is used for benzodiazepine overdoses.

Ibutilide (Corvert) is used for acute termination of atrial fibrillation or flutter. It prolongs the action potential in cardiac tissue. It is stable for 24 hours at room temperature and for 48 hours if refrigerated.

Lidocaine stabilizes ventricular arrhythmias and can be administered intravenously, intraosseiously, and endotracheally.

Magnesium sulfate (Mag-200) is used to treat cardiac arrhythmias and prevent seizures. It slows the rate of sinoatrial node impulse formation and prolongs conduction time.

Naloxone (Narcan) is used to reverse narcotic overdose.

Norepinephrine (Levophed) causes increased contractility and heart rate as well as vasoconstriction, thereby increasing systemic blood pressure and coronary blood flow.

Procainamide (Pronestyl) increases the fibrillation threshold and prevents recurrence; it is used to suppress arrhythmias not responsive to lidocaine or in lidocaine allergy. It is not used in ventricular fibrillation because of the slow onset of activity. This drug can cause hypotension, ECG changes, and kidney disease.

Vasopressin is an antidiuretic hormone that may be used in code-blue scenarios. It is usually used in the treatment of ventricular fibrillation or pulseless ventricular tachycardia.

Verapamil (Calan, Verelan) is a calcium channel blocker (slows the movement of calcium ions through slow channels). It slows sinoatrial node action, slows atrioventricular node conduction, and dilates coronary artery smooth muscle. It is used in atrial fibrillation and/or flutter that result in fast ventricular rates. Use of this drug may result in hypotension and heart block.

Bioterrorism

Bioterrorism is an attack or threatened attack by terrorists whereby the weapons are biologic agents and emerging infectious diseases. Potential biologic agents include both microorganisms and toxins. Disease-causing microorganisms may **propagate** (grow and spread) either in the environment or in a living host. **Toxins** are the product of living organisms, including those derived from plants, bacteria, or fungi. The major difference between toxins and microorganisms is that toxins do not reproduce.

The threat posed by biologic agents, particularly bacteria and viruses, is increased by the fact that, once they are released, containment is very difficult and potentially impossible. For obvious security reasons, limited information is available as to how a bioterrorism attack would be dealt with by government and emergency preparedness officials. Although a bioterrorism attack could potentially be unlike any disaster that the response community has faced before, it would likely present many of the same challenges as a natural disaster.

Biologic Agents with Potential for Bioterrorism

Among the diseases that might be used in a bioterrorist attack are anthrax, plague, tularemia, and smallpox. As a member of the response team, the pharmacy technician will have several important responsibilities in dealing with an outbreak.

Before dispensing medications to treat or prevent an outbreak, it will be important to identify patient allergies. This will be a role for the pharmacy technician. Technicians will document drug allergies and dispense drugs. Keeping records of who receives which drugs will be a massive task, and one that pharmacy technicians are well-equipped to perform.

Anthrax

Anthrax is caused by the bacterium *Bascillus anthracis*. Disease occurs when anthrax spores are introduced to an individual either subcutaneously or via inhalation. There are three forms of anthrax: cutaneous, inhalation, and oropharyngeal/gastrointestinal. Anthrax is treated with antibiotics (usually ciprofloxacin or doxycycline). A vaccine is available for anthrax; once a person is exposed, the vaccine may be administered.

Plague

Plague is caused by the bacterium *Yersinia pestis*. People are infected with plague by bites from infected fleas, scratches or bites from infected animals, and exposure to infected humans. Infection can also be introduced directly into the lungs through inhalation. There are three forms of plague: bubonic, septicemic, and pneumonic. Plague is extremely contagious in any form. Antibiotics would be dispensed to the population as both prophylaxis and treatment.

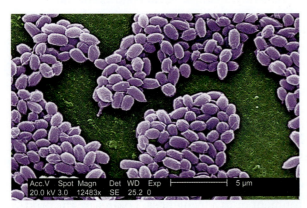 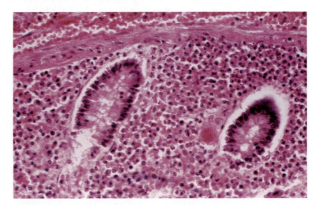

These images show anthrax bacteria at medium (left) and high (right) magnification.

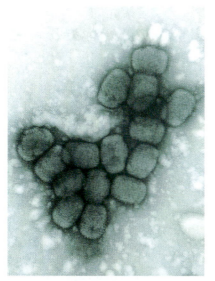

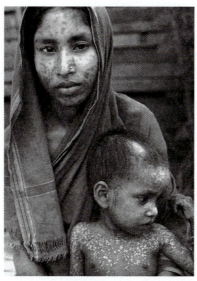

Tularemia

Tularemia is caused by *Francisella tularensis* bacteria and is not contagious, but it is useful as a biological weapon because its effects are debilitating and only a few organisms are required to cause an infection. There are six forms of tularemia: ulceroglandular, oculoglandular, oropharyngeal, typhoidal, pneumonic, and septic. In the event of an attack in which tularemia is dispersed, antibiotics would be dispensed. An investigational vaccine is available, but its use is restricted to high-risk groups.

Smallpox was responsible for millions of deaths throughout history. These photos show smallpox virus under high magnification (left) and victims with the conspicuous blisters (right).

Smallpox

Smallpox is caused by the virus *Variola major*. Even though smallpox was eradicated in 1979, stocks of this virus still exist. In the event of exposure, vaccination should be given within one to four days. Care would be simply supportive.

While smallpox is no longer prevalent in developed nations, it is important to know that viruses such as smallpox are stored in locations around the globe, especially in research institutions. These stores are protected with high levels of security.

Viral Hemorrhagic Fevers

Viral hemorrhagic fevers are caused by a diverse group of viruses. The mode of transmission, clinical course, and mortality of these illnesses vary with the specific virus, although most natural outbreaks have involved the Ebola and Marburg viruses. Ribavirin (Rebetol, Virazole) is under investigation as a potential treatment for these viruses. However, treatment is mainly supportive. Hemorrhage should be treated with the usual blood products. Disseminated intravascular coagulation with complications of ischemia may be treated with heparin. Resulting infections should be aggressively managed.

Toxins

Botulinum toxin is a neurotoxin that is produced by the bacterium *Clostridium botulinum*. Botulin toxin blocks the release of acetylcholine at the neuromuscular junction and at receptors in the autonomic nervous system, resulting in muscular paralysis. As a biological weapon, it may be spread by ingestion, inhalation, or injection. It is treated with an antitoxin.

Ricin is a toxin that is derived from the castor bean. It acts by disabling the molecular machinery for protein synthesis. There is no known treatment and no antidote, but a vaccine has been developed. Ricin is easy to produce in large amounts. If a person is exposed to as little as 3 mcg by inhalation or injection, it can be lethal. If ricin is ingested, charcoal lavage should be used; contaminated patients should have their clothes removed and be decontaminated prior to treatment.

The Role of the Pharmacy Technician

The US government has a supply of antibiotics and vaccines to be used in the event of a bioterrorism emergency. As mentioned, if a bioterrorist attack occurs, the pharmacy technician would play a very important supportive role. In that event, healthcare providers would need to be aware of unusual symptoms in a group of people. Dispensing drugs, maintaining patient profiles, and documenting patient allergies would be critical components of the response to a bioterrorist attack, which would place pharmacy technicians on the front line of defense.

Complementary and Alternative Therapies

While bacteria and other microorganisms are often thought of as harmful, many microorganisms are needed to help the body function. For example, the normal bacteria of the intestinal tract helps digest food, destroy harmful microorganisms, and even produce vitamins. When normal bacteria levels are altered, patients may experience health consequences. Sometimes **probiotics**, which are live microorganisms ingested for health benefits, are used to maintain or restore normal bacteria in the body. There are various probiotic formulations available (see Table 17.17 for more information).

Researchers are studying the efficacy of probiotics for various health disorders. They are commonly used for gastrointestinal disorders such as irritable bowel syndrome and diarrhea. Probiotics may also be used for dermatologic conditions such as eczema, genitourinary disorders such as vaginal infections, and allergies.

Probiotics are generally safe for individuals. However, as they contain live microorganisms, probiotics should not be used in patients with compromised immune systems. Common side effects include stomach upset and eructation (burping).

TABLE 17.17 **The Most Common Probiotic Products**

Probiotic	Species	Form	Use
Acidophilus (generic)	*Lactobacillus acidophilus*	Capsule, liquid, powder, suppository	Diarrhea, vaginitis
Activia	*Bifidobacterium animalis*	Yogurt	Constipation
Align	*Bifidobacterium infantis*	Capsule	Irritable bowel syndrome
Culturelle	*Lactobacillus GG*	Capsule	Diarrhea
Flora-Q	*Lactobacillus acidophilus, Bifidobacterium, L. paracasei, Streptococcus thermophilus*	Capsule	Irritable bowel syndrome
Lactinex	*Lactobacillus acidophilus, L. helveticus*	Tablet, granules	Diarrhea, cold sores

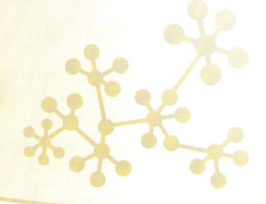

CHAPTER SUMMARY

Vitamins

- Vitamins are classified as water-soluble or fat-soluble. The B vitamins and vitamin C are water-soluble; vitamins A, D, E, and K are fat-soluble.

- Vitamin supplementation may be necessary to treat or prevent certain medical conditions.

- It is possible to oversupplement fat-soluble vitamins; it is less likely to oversupplement water-soluble vitamins.

Fluids, Electrolytes, and Acid-Base Balance

- Water is the major constituent of living cells. Body fluids are divided into two compartments, intracellular and extracellular.

- Water deficits are caused by loss of body fluids as a result of such conditions as vomiting, diarrhea, edema, and excessive sweating from fever; high urine output; and acute weight loss of more than 5% of body weight. Water loss can cause dryness of skin and mucous membranes, longitudinal wrinkling of the tongue, hypotension, tachycardia, and lowered body temperature. A loss of 25% of body water can result in death.

- An isotonic solution has the same level of particles, and thus the same tonicity, as body fluids.

- Sodium is the primary cation of extracellular fluid.

- Potassium is the primary cation of intracellular fluid.

- Calcium is associated with bone formation and dynamics, muscle contraction, and blood coagulation.

- Each calcium salt has a specific use.

- Hydrogen ions regulate the acidity or alkalinity of body fluids.

Nutritional Disorders

- Obesity is a major health concern and is a condition characterized by the excessive accumulation and storage of fat in the body.

- Lipase inhibitors, sympathomimetic drugs, serotonin agonists, and glucagon-like peptide receptor agonists may be used in appropriate patients for obesity.

- Malnutrition is a lack of adequate nutrient intake to supply basic metabolic needs.

- Enteral formulas, which are introduced through a tube directly into the stomach or small intestine, are preferred to feeding by vein (parenteral nutrition) because the lower abdomen continues to function. The pharmacy technician should always label enteral preparations so that they are not confused with intravenous preparations.

- The advantages of three-in-one formulations are lower costs of preparation and delivery, less nursing time needed for administration, and potentially reduced risk of sepsis with fewer points of entry of the administration line.

- The disadvantages of three-in-ones are their short stability and the inability to see precipitates if they occur.

Poisons and Antidotes

- The drugs that cause the most childhood poisonings are iron tablets, tricyclic antidepressants, calcium channel blockers, opiates, aspirin, and alcohol.

- Once a poison is ingested, there are two concerns: (1) removing it from the GI tract before it can be absorbed, and (2) diminishing the effects of poison that has been absorbed.

- Activated charcoal has become the primary emergency room treatment to prevent absorption of poison from the GI tract.

Emergency Procedures

- The pharmacy technician is responsible for keeping the alert carts/boxes stocked. All medications must be kept up to date. An out-of-date medication could cost someone his or her life.

- Advanced cardiac life support guidelines should be followed when determining which drugs will be on a blue-alert cart.

Bioterrorism

- Bioterrorism may include biologic agents and emerging infectious diseases.

- Possible diseases that could be used in a bioterrorist attack include anthrax, plague, tularemia, and smallpox among others. The response to an attack would include measures for containment, vaccination, treatment, and supportive care.

- The pharmacy technician would be a primary responder responsible for dispensing drugs appropriately and maintaining patient profiles.

acidosis a blood pH below 7.35; a metabolic condition due to excessive loss of bicarbonate or sodium

activated charcoal a decontamination agent that is used to prevent absorption of poison from the GI tract

adenosine triphosphate (ATP) a critical molecule in cellular energy production

alkalosis a blood pH above 7.45; a metabolic condition due to excessive loss of potassium or chloride

ammonium chloride the chloride salt of ammonium

anions negatively charged ions

antidote a drug that counters the harmful effects of a poison

antioxidants substances that can prevent cell damage caused by free radicals

antivenin a material used in treatment of poisoning by animal venom

ascorbic acid known as vitamin C

bariatric surgery surgical options to achieve significant weight loss

beriberi a condition associated with thiamine deficiency that presents with numbness, tingling, edema, and heart failure

bioterrorism an attack or threatened attack by terrorists whereby the weapons are biologic agents and emerging infectious diseases

botulinum toxin neurotoxin that blocks the release of acetylcholine at the neuromuscular junction, resulting in muscular paralysis

cachexia a condition when muscle and fat tissue wastes away

calciferol the collective name of the D vitamins

calcium citrate the citrate salt of calcium

cations positively charged ions

centrally distributed fat adipose tissue that accumulates in the abdominal area rather than in the hips, thighs, or buttocks

chelating agent a drug that bonds to a metal ion to prevent it from reacting with biological compounds

cholecalciferol another name for vitamin D_3

Code Blue a system to communicate that a patient is in a life-threatening situation

coenzyme a chemical other than a protein that is needed to assist an enzyme in performing a metabolic function

colloids components of a crystalloid IV solution made up of proteins and other large molecules

cracking separation of lipid from a parenteral nutrition solution

crystalloid an IV solution containing electrolytes

cobalamin also known as vitamin B_{12}; a coenzyme necessary for cell reproduction and normal growth

decontamination removal of ingested poison

dyslipidemia an abnormal amount of lipids in the blood

electrolyte a substance that dissociates into ions in solution and is thus capable of conducting electricity

enteral nutrition feeding a patient liquid food through a tube that leads to the gastrointestinal system

extracellular refers to substances outside cells

fat-soluble vitamins vitamins that are absorbed along with dietary fat and are maintained in large stores by the body; vitamins A, D, E, and K

folic acid (folate) also known as vitamin B_9; plays a role in intracellular metabolism

gastric banding laparoscopic surgery; a restrictive procedure of weight loss surgery

gastric bypass surgery procedure that bypasses parts of the intestine to prevent nutrients from foods being fully absorbed

gastric lavage a procedure to wash out or irrigate the patient's stomach; commonly known as a *stomach pump*

glucagon-like peptide gastric hormone that stimulates glucose-dependent insulin secretion; inhibits glucagon release and gastric emptying

glucagon-like peptide receptor agonists medications that decrease body weight through decreased caloric intake

homocysteine an amino acid associated with cardiovascular disease

hypercalcemia an excess of calcium in the blood

hyperchloremia an excess of choride

hyperkalemia a condition of higher than normal potassium

hypermagnesemia when magnesium levels in the body are too high

hypernatremia elevated sodium concentration relative to the normal range

hyperphosphatemia caused by tumor lysis syndrome; too much phosphate in a patient's system

hypertonic solution a solution with a higher concentration of particles than body fluids contain

hypocalcemia a depletion in calcium levels in the body

hypochloremia a depletion of chloride in the body

hypokalemia a condition of lower than normal potassium

hypomagnesemia a depletion of magnesium in the body

hyponatremia low sodium concentration relative to the normal range

hypophosphatemia a drop in phosphate in the bloodstream

hypotonic solution a solution with a lower concentration of particles than body fluids contain

intracellular refers to substances inside cells

isotonic solution a solution with the same level of particles, and thus the same tonicity, as body fluids

IV fluid products used to replace fluids and electrolytes lost through dehydration

keratomalacia softening and ulceration of the cornea of the eye

kwashiorkor a condition in which caloric intake is adequate but protein intake is deficient

lipase inhibitors agents that bind to gastric and pancreatic lipase enzymes in the intestines, preventing enzymes from breaking down fats to be absorbed

malnutrition any disorder of nutrition

marasmus a chronic condition caused by inadequate caloric and protein intake over a prolonged time

metabolic acidosis when excess acid is produced, bicarbonate is lost, or kidneys do not excrete enough acid

metabolic alkalosis when excess acid is excreted via the kidneys

milliequivalents (mEq) unit commonly used to measure electrolytes

obesity a condition characterized by excessive accumulation and storage of fat in the body

osmolarity the concentration of all molecules in a set volume of fluid

osmosis process by which water passively moves across cellular membranes

osteomalacia demineralization and weakening of the skeleton; caused by a deficiency of vitamin D in adults

parenteral nutrition (PN) feeding a patient by supplying a nutrient solution through a vein

pellagra a disease that presents with hyperpigmented rash in areas of exposed skin, swelling of the mouth and tongue, diarrhea, and anxiety; develops in patients with GI diseases or alcoholism

phlebitis inflammation of the vein

phosphate an anion that plays a role in energy production within cells

phytonadione vitamin K_1

pooling a time-saving process used when preparing a three-in-one TPN, in which all electrolytes except phosphate are put into a small-volume parenteral bag and then transferred into each batch

probiotic live microorganisms ingested for health benefits

propagate reproduce

respiratory acidosis a form of acidosis resulting from slow breathing and retention of carbon dioxide in the blood

respiratory alkalosis when breathing becomes more rapid and more carbon dioxide is exhaled and eliminated from the blood

rickets a childhood disease in which a lack of vitamin D results in bone softening and muscle weakness

ricin a toxin derived from the castor bean that acts by disabling the molecular machinery for protein synthesis

satiety the sensation of feeling full and satisfied

scurvy a disease rarely seen in the United States, indicative of severe lack of vitamin C

serotonin a neurotransmitter that can affect mood, social behavior, sleep, memory, sexual desire, and appetite/digestion

serotonin agonists agents that activate serotonin receptors to reduce appetite and food intake

serotonin syndrome a possible serious side effect of sympathomimetics; condition causing a dangerous rise in blood pressure and heart rate

sodium bicarbonate the bicarbonate salt of sodium

sudden cardiac death death that occurs within 24 hours of the onset of illness or injury

supportive therapy therapy for poisoning that consists of establishing the airway and providing cardiopulmonary resuscitation (CPR); maintaining body temperature, nutritional status, and fluid and electrolyte balance; and preventing circulatory collapse, hypoglycemia, uremia, and liver failure

sympathomimetics drugs to treat obesity that stimulate the central nervous system as much as amphetamines

three-in-one see total nutrient admixture

tocopherol one of the alcohols that constitute vitamin E

tonicity the relationship of a solution to the body's own fluids; measured by determining the number of dissolved particles in a solution

total nutrient admixture (TNA) an amino acid–dextrose–lipid formulation used for parenteral nutrition; often called a *three-in-one*

total parenteral nutrition (TPN) an IV solution that provides long-term nutritional support, feeding a patient through the veins only

toxin the product of living organisms, including those derived from plants, bacteria, or fungi

two-in-one a formulation for parenteral nutrition that contains only amino acids and dextrose

vitamin an organic substance that is necessary for the normal metabolic functioning of the body but that the body does not synthesize, so it must be obtained from food

water-soluble vitamins vitamins that are excreted in the urine and are not stored in the body; vitamin C and the B vitamins

Wernicke-Korsakoff syndrome a syndrome where thiamine deficiency is present and occurs in patients who abuse alcohol

DRUG LIST

Vitamins

A (carotenoid, retinol)
B_1 (thiamine)
B_2 (riboflavin)
B_3 (niacin)
B_5 (pantothenic acid)
B_6 (pyridoxine)
B_7 (biotin)
B_9 (folic acid)
B_{12} (cobalamin)
C (ascorbic acid)
D (cholecalciferol, ergocalciferol)
E (tocopherol)
K (phylloquinone, phytonadione)

Electrolytes

calcium, Ca^{2+}
chloride, Cl^-
hydrogen ions, H^{+9}
magnesium, Mg^{2+}
potassium, K^+ (Klor-Con)
sodium, Na^{1+}

Lipase Inhibitors

orlistat (Alli, Xenical)

Sympathomimetic Drugs

benzphetamine (Didrex, Regimex)
diethylpropion
phendimetrazine (Bontril)
phentermine (Adipex-P, Suprenza)

Serotonin Agonist

lorcaserin (Belviq)

Glucagon-like Peptide Receptor Agonist

liraglutide (Saxenda)

Enteral Nutrition Formulations

Choice DM
Fibersource
Fibersource HN
Glucerna
Impact
Impact Glutamine
Isosource VHN
Jevity
Jevity Plus
Magnacal Renal
Nepro
Novasource Renal
Perative
Probalance
Promote
Replete
Resource Diabetic
Ultracal

Antidotes

acetylcysteine (Acetadote)
activated carbon, charcoal
amyl nitrite
antivenin
atropine
centruroides antivenom (Anascorp)
dapsone
deferoxamine (Desferal)
digoxin immune Fab (Digibind, DigiFab)
dimercaprol, British Anti-Lewisite
    (BAL in Oil)
edetate calcium disodium (Calcium
    Disodium Versenate)
flumazenil (Romazicon)
fomepizole (Antizol)
glucagon (GlucaGen)
methylene blue (Urolene Blue)
naloxone (Narcan)
octreotide (Sandostatin)
penicillamine (Cuprimine, Depen Titratabs)
phentolamine (Regitine)
physostigmine
phytonadione, vitamin K
    (AquaMEPHYTON, Mephyton)
polyethylene glycol (GoLYTELY, HalfLytely,
    MiraLax)
pralidoxime (Protopam)
protamine sulfate

pyridoxine (vitamin B_6)
sodium nitrite
sodium thiosulfate (Versiclear)

Code Blue Emergencies

amiodarone (Cordarone, Nexterone, Pacerone)
atropine
calcium chloride
dextrose 50%
digoxin (Lanoxin)
diltiazem (Cardizem)
dobutamine (Dobutrex)
dopamine (Intropin)
epinephrine (Adrenalin)
etomidate (Amidate)
flumazenil (Romazicon)
ibutilide (Corvert)
lidocaine
magnesium sulfate (Mag-200)
naloxone (Narcan)
norepinephrine (Levophed)
procainamide (Pronestyl)
vasopressin
verapamil (Isoptin)

Probiotics

Acidophilus
Activia
Align
Culturelle
Flora Q
Lactinex

Black Box Warnings

acetylcysteine (Acetadote, Mucomyst)
amiodarone (Cordarone)
dopamine (Intropin)
edetate calcium disodium (Calcium Disodium Versenate)
flumazenil (Romazicon)
ibutilide (Corvert)
norepinephrine (Levophed)
penicillamine (Cuprimine, Depen Titratabs)
phytonadione, vitamin K (AquaMEPHYTON)
procainamide (Pronestyl)
protamine sulfate
sodium nitrite
sodium nitrite-sodium thiosulfate (Nithiodote)
sodium thiosulfate (Versiclear)

Medication Guide

amiodarone (Cordarone, Nexterone, Pacerone)

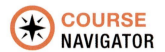
COURSE NAVIGATOR

Access interactive chapter review exercises, practice activities, flash cards, and study games.

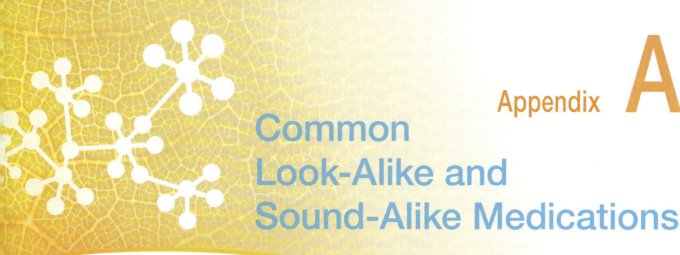

Common Look-Alike and Sound-Alike Medications

While manufacturers have an obligation to review new trademarks for error potential before use, there are some actions that prescribers, pharmacists, and pharmacy technicians can do to help prevent errors with products that have look- or sound-alike names. The Institute for Safe Medication Practices (ISMP) provides several types of tools that are designed to prevent dispensing errors. These include the following recommended actions as well as a list of look-alike and sound-alike drugs.

- **Use electronic prescribing** to prevent confusion with handwritten drug names.
- **Encourage physicians to write prescriptions that clearly specify the dosage form, drug strength, and complete directions.** They should include the product's indication on all outpatient prescriptions and on inpatient *prn* orders. With name pairs known to be problematic, reduce the potential for confusion by writing prescriptions using both the brand and generic name. Listing both names on medication administration records and automated dispensing cabinet computer screens also may be helpful.
- **Whenever possible, determine the purpose of the medication** before dispensing or administering it. Many products with look-alike or sound-alike names are used for different purposes.
- **Accept verbal or telephone orders only when truly necessary.** Require staff to read back all orders, spell the product name, and state its indication. Like medication names, numbers can sound alike, so staff should read the dosage back in numerals (eg. "one five" for 15 milligrams) to ensure clear interpretation of dose.
- **When feasible, use magnifying lenses and copyholders** under good lighting to keep prescriptions and orders at eye level during transcription to improve the likelihood of proper interpretation of look-alike product names.
- **Change the appearance of look-alike product names** on computer screens, pharmacy and nursing unit shelf labels, and bins (including automated dispensing cabinets), pharmacy product labels, and

medication administration records by highlighting, through bold face, color, and/or capital letters, the parts of the names that are different (e.g., hydr**OXY**zine, hydr**ALA**zine). These are called "tall man" letters.

- **Install a computerized reminder** (also placed on automated dispensing cabinet screens) for the most serious confusing name pairs so that an alert is generated when entering prescriptions for either drug. If possible, make the reminder auditory as well as visual.

- **Affix "name alert" stickers** in areas where look-alike or sound-alike products are stored (available from pharmacy label manufacturers).

- **Store products with look-alike or sound-alike names in different locations.** Avoid storing both products in the fast-mover area. Use a shelf sticker to help locate the product that is moved.

- **Continue to employ an independent check in the dispensing process** (one person interprets and enters the prescription into the computer and another reviews the printed label against the original prescription and the product).

- **Open the prescription bottle or the unit dose package in front of the patient** to confirm the expected product appearance and review the indication. Caution patients about error potential when taking products that have a look-alike or sound-alike counterpart. Take the time to fully investigate the situation if a patient states he or she is taking an unknown medication.

- **Monitor reported errors caused by look-alike and sound-alike medication names** and alert staff to mistakes.

- **Look for the possibility of name confusion when a new product is added to the formulary.** Have a few clinicians handwrite the product name and directions, as they would appear in a typical order. Ask frontline nurses, pharmacists, technicians, unit secretaries, and physicians to view the samples of the written product name as well as pronounce it to determine if it looks or sounds like any other drug product or medical term. It may be helpful to have clinicians first look at the scripted product name to determine how they would interpret it before the actual product name is provided to them for pronunciation. Once the product name is known, clinicians may be less likely to see more familiar product names in the written samples. If the potential for confusion with other products is identified, take steps to avoid errors as listed below.

- **Encourage reporting of errors** and potentially hazardous conditions with look-alike and sound-alike product names and use the information to establish priorities for error reduction. Also maintain awareness of problematic product names and error prevention recommendations provided by ISMP (www.ismp.org and also listed on the quarterly *Action Agenda*), FDA (www.fda.gov), and United States Pharmacopoeia (USP; www.usp.org).

Web

- **Review any look-alike and sound-alike drug name pairs in use at your practice location.** Go to ISMP's website to review these medications, available at http://Pharmacology6e.ParadigmCollege.net/ConfusedDrugNames. Decide what actions might be warranted to prevent medication errors. Stay current with alerts from ISMP, FDA, and USP in case new problematic name pairs emerge.

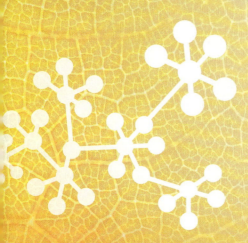

Common Pharmacy Abbreviations and Acronyms

The abbreviations with red lines through them are ones that are still in use but are discouraged by Institute for Safe Medication Practices (ISMP). The ISMP recommends the use of the correct words instead. Many of these discouraged abbreviations are also on the Joint Commission's Official "Do Not Use" List of Abbreviations.

Abbreviation	Meaning
A-B-C	
aaa	apply to affected area
ACA	Affordable Care Act (Patient Protection and Affordable Care Act)
~~ac; a.c.; AC~~	before meals
ACE	angiotensin-converting enzyme inhibitors
ad; a.d.; AD	right ear
ADD	attention-deficit disorder
ADH	antidiuretic hormone
ADHD	attention-deficit hyperactivity disorder
ADME	absorption, distribution, metabolism, and elimination
ADR	adverse drug reaction
AIDS	acquired immune deficiency syndrome
AM; a.m.	morning
ANDA	Abbreviated New Drug Application
APAP	acetaminophen; Tylenol
AphA	American Pharmacy Association
ARBs	angiotensin receptor blockers
~~as; a.s.; AS~~	left ear
ASA	aspirin
~~au; a.u.; AU~~	both ears; each ear
b.i.d.; BID	twice daily
BMI	Body Mass Index
BP	blood pressure
BUD	beyond-use date
°C	degrees centigrade; temperature in degrees centigrade
Ca^{++}	calcium

Abbreviation	Meaning
Cap, cap	capsule
CDC	Centers for Disease Control and Prevention
CF	cystic fibrosis
CHF	congestive heart failure
CNS	Central Nervous System
COPD	chronic obstructive pulmonary disease
CPR	cardio pulminary resuscitation
CSP	compounded sterile preparation
CV	cardiovascular
D-E-F	
D_5; D_5W; D5W	dextrose 5% in water
D_5 ¼; D5 1/4	dextrose 5% in ¼ normal saline; dextrose 5% in 0.225% sodium chloride
D_5 ⅓; D5 1/3	dextrose 5% in ⅓ normal saline; dextrose 5% in 0.33% sodium chloride
D_5 ½; D5 1/2	dextrose 5% in ½ normal saline; dextrose 5% in 0.45% sodium chloride
D_5LR; D5LR	dextrose 5% in lactated Ringer's solution
D_5NS; D5NS	dextrose 5% in normal saline; dextrose 5% in 0.9% sodium chloride
DAW	dispense as written
~~DC; d/c~~	discontinue
D/C	discharge
DCA	direct compounding area
Dig	digoxin
disp	dispense
EC	enteric-coated
Elix	elixir
eMAR	electronic medication administration record
EPO	epoetin alfa; erythropoietin
ER; XR; XL	extended-release
°F	degrees Fahrenheit; temperature in degrees Fahrenheit
$FeSO_4$	ferrous sulfate; iron
G-H-I	
g, G	gram
gr	grain
GI	gastrointestinal
GMP	good manufacturing practice
gtt; gtts	drop; drops
h; hr	hour
HC	hydrocortisone
HCTZ	hydrochlorothiazide
HIPAA	Health Insurance Portability and Accountability Act
HIV	human immunodeficiency virus
HMO	Health Maintenance Organization
HRT	hormone replacement therapy

Abbreviation	Meaning
~~h.s.~~; ~~HS~~	bedtime
IBU	ibuprofen; Motrin
ICU	intensive care unit
IM	intramuscular
IND	Investigational New Drug Application
Inj	injection
IPA	isopropyl alcohol
ISDN	isosorbide dinitrate
ISMO	isosorbide mononitrate
ISMP	Institute for Safe Medication Practices
IV	intravenous
IVF	intravenous fluid
IVP	intravenous push
IVPB	intravenous piggyback
J-K-L	
K; K+	potassium
KCl	potassium chloride
kg	kilogram
L	liter
LAFW	laminar airflow workbench; hood
lb	pound
LD	loading dose
LVP	large-volume parenteral
JCAHO	Joint Commission on the Accreditation of Healthcare Organizations
M-N-O	
Mag; Mg; MAG	magnesium
MAR	medication administration record
mcg	microgram
MDI	metered-dose inhaler
MDV	multiple-dose vial
mEq	milliequivalent
mg	milligram
~~MgSO~~$_4$	magnesium sulfate; magnesium
mL	milliliter
mL/hr	milliliters per hour
mL/min	milliliters per minute

Abbreviation	Meaning
MMR	measles, mumps, and rubella vaccine
MRSA	methiciliin-resistant S. aureaus
MOM; M.O.M.	milk of magnesia
M.S.	morphine sulfate (save MS for multiple sclerosis)
MU†; mu	million units
MVI; MVI-12	multiple vitamin injection; multivitamins for parenteral administration
Na⁺	sodium
NABP	National Association of Boards of Pharmacy
NaCl	sodium chloride; salt
NDA	New Drug App
NDC	National Drug Code
NF; non-form	nonformulary
NKA	no known allergies
NKDA	no known drug allergies
NPO, npo	nothing by mouth
NR; d.n.r.	no refills; do not repeat
NS	normal saline; 0.9% sodium chloride
½ NS	one-half normal saline; 0.45% sodium chloride
¼ NS	one-quarter normal saline; 0.225% sodium chloride
NSAID	nonsteroidal anti-inflammatory drug
NTG	nitroglycerin
OC	oral contraceptive
od; o.d.; OD	right eye
ODT	orally disintegrating tablet
OPTH; OPHTH; Opth	ophthalmic
os; o.s.; OS	left eye
OTC	over the counter; no prescription required
ou; o.u.; OU	both eyes; each eye
oz	ounce
P-Q-R	
p.c.; PC	after meals
PCA	patient-controlled anesthesia
PCN	penicillin
pH	acid-base balance
PHI	protected health information
PM; p.m.	afternoon; evening
PN	paternal nutrition

Abbreviation	Meaning
PNS	peripheral nervous system
PO; po	orally; by mouth
PPE	personal protective equipment
PPI	proton pump inhibitor
PR	per rectum; rectally
PRN; p.r.n.	as needed; as occasion requires
PTSD	Post Traumatic Stress Disorder
PV	per vagina; vaginally
PVC	polyvinyl chloride
q	every
q.h.; qhour	every hour
q2h	every 2 hours
q4h	every 4 hours
q6h	every 6 hours
q8h	every 8 hours
q12h	every 12 hours
q24h	every 24 hours
q48h	every 48 hours
QA	quality assurance
QAM; qam	every morning
qDay; QD	every day
q.i.d.; QID	four times daily
QOD; Q other day; Q.O. Day	every other day
QPM; qpm	every evening
qs; qsad	quantity sufficient; a sufficient quantity to make
QTY; qty	quantity
qwk; qweek	every week
RA	rheumatoid arthritis
RDA	recommended daily allowance
Rx	prescription; pharmacy; medication; drug; recipe; take
S-T	
sig	write on label; signa; directions
SL; sub-L	sublingual
SMZ-TMP	sulfamethoxazole and trimethoprim; Bactrim
SNRI	serotonin nonrepinephrine reuptake inhibitor
SPF	sunburn protection factor

Abbreviation	Meaning
SR	sustained-release
~~SS~~; ~~ss~~	one-half
SSRI	selective serotonin reuptake inhibitor (don't use for sliding scale insulins)
STAT, Stat	immediately; now
STD	sexually transmitted disease
~~Sub-Q~~; ~~SC~~; ~~SQ~~; ~~sq~~, subcut, SUBCUT	subcutaneous
SUPP; Supp	suppository
susp	suspension
SVP	small-volume parenteral
SW	sterile water
SWFI	sterile water for injection
Tab; tab	tablet
TB	tuberculosis
TBSP; tbsp	tablespoon; tablespoonful; 15 mL
TDS	transdermal delivery system
~~t.i.d.~~; ~~TID~~	three times daily
~~t.i.w.~~; ~~TIW~~	three times a week
TKO; TKVO; KO; KVO	to keep open; to keep vein open; keep open; keep vein open (a slow IV flow rate)
TNA	Total Nutrition Admixture
TPN	total parenteral nutrition
TSP; tsp	teaspoon; teaspoonful; 5 mL
U-V-W	
~~U or u~~	unit
~~u d, UD, ut dictum~~	as directed
ung	ointment
USP	U.S. Pharmacopoeial Convention
USP-NF	U.S. Pharmacopoeia-National Forumulary <italics>
UTI	urinary tract infection
UV	ultraviolet light
VAG; vag	vagina; vaginally
Vanco	vancomycin
VO; V.O.; V/O	verbal order
w/o	without
X-Y-Z	
Zn	zinc
Z-Pak	azithromycin; Zithromax

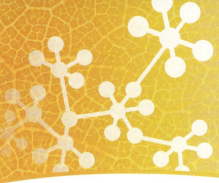

GENERIC AND BRAND NAME DRUG INDEX

Note: Page numbers followed by a *t* indicate that the reference appears in a table, and page numbers followed by a *p* indicate that the reference appears in a photo.

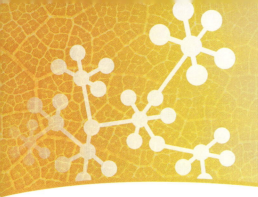

SUBJECT INDEX

Note: Page numbers followed by a *t* indicate that the reference appears in a table, page numbers followed by an *f* indicate that the reference appears in a figure, and page numbers followed by a *p* indicate that the reference appears in a photo.

inflammation
  drug therapy for, 517–521
influenza
  antiviral drugs for, 122t, 124–126
  vaccine for, 120, 148t, 149
  as viral infection, 118
influenza A, antiviral drug for, 124–126
influenza B, antiviral drug for, 124–126
inhalant anesthetics, 164–167, 165t
inhalation route, 49
inhaler
  CFC, 295
  dry-powder, 296
  HFA, 295, 296
  steps for using, 295–296
inhibition, 31, 32
injectable anesthesia, 167–171, 167t
injection
  as dosage route, 48
  needle size, 48
inscription, 42
insomnia, 237, 247
instillation, 49
Institute for Safe Medication Practices
  (ISMP), 22, 44
institutional setting, 41
insulin, 591–595, 593t, 735t
insulin secretagogues, 599–600
integrase, 127
integrase inhibitor, 140t, 141–142
integrative medicine, 12
interaction, 37
intercalating agents, 682
interferon, 120
  for multiple sclerosis, 276
international normalized ratio (INR),
  475
intracellular fluids, 714
intradermal injection, 48
intramuscular (IM) injection, 48
intraspinal injection, 48
intrathecal (IT) administration, 680
intrathecal injection, 48
intrauterine devices, 576, 576p
intravenous (IV) injection, 48
investigational drugs, 694
Investigational New Drug (IND)
  Application, 12
irritable bowel syndrome, 389
irritant receptor, 321
ischemic stroke, 486
isomer, 283
isotonic solution, 715, 717t
IV fluid, 715
IVIG, 397

J

Japanese encephalitis vaccine, 148t, 149
jaundice, 85
jock itch, 636
joints
  anatomy and physiology of,
    509–512, 510f, 511f
  gouty arthritis, 538–540

inflammation and swelling,
  517–521
osteoarthritis, 521–528, 525t
rheumatoid arthritis, 529–536, 530t
systemic lupus erythematosus,
  536–537
types of, and function, 510, 511f
Journal of Pharmacy Technology, 10

K

keratolytic agent, 628
keratomalacia, 708
kidneys
  acute kidney injury, 416–422
  aging and, 51, 52
  anatomy and physiology of,
    411–415, 412f–413f, 415f
  anemia therapies, 418–419
  assessing function of, 415
  chronic kidney disease, 416–422
  dialysis therapies, 417–419, 417f–
    418f
  supplemental therapies, 419–420
  transplant therapy, 418, 420–422
Klebsiella spp., 69t
Koch, Robert, 643
kwashiorkor, 731

L

labels, medication, 55, 55f, 56f
  right drug and, 45f
lab values, 8t
lactic acidosis, 598
lactobacilli, 402
Lactobacillus spp., 69t
laparoscopic banding, 727
latency, 119
laxatives, 381–386, 382t–383t
legend drug, 14
Legionella spp., 69t
leucovorin rescue, 680–681
leukopenia, 458
leukotriene inhibitor, 301–302, 302t
LHRH agonists, 689
lice, 639–642, 640p, 641t
lincosamides
  most commonly used, 84t
  overview of, 83–84
  side effects and dispensing issues of,
    85–86
  therapeutic uses of, 84–85
lipase, 316
lipase inhibitors, 728
lipid-lowering agents, 491–496, 491t,
  572t
lipids, 29
lipoprotein, 489–490
liposomal products, 684
Li Shizhen, 4
Lister, Joseph, 7, 643
Listeria monocytogenes, 69t
live attenuated vaccines, 145
liver enzyme lab values, 8t
loading dose, 34, 83

local anesthesia, 174–176, 175t
local effect, 35
local infection, 49
local viral infection, 119
long-acting beta agonists (LABAs),
  309–313, 310t
long-acting insulin, 591
long QT syndrome, 74
long-term persistent medications, 295
loop diuretic, 431t, 432–433
Lou Gehrig disease, 276
low-density lipoproteins (LDL), 490
low-molecular-weight heparins, 476t, 478
lungs. *See also* respiratory system
  aging and, 51
  exchange of oxygen/carbon dioxide
    in lungs, 292, 292f
  natural defense system, 306, 306f
lupus, 536–537
luteinizing hormone (LH), 556
luteinizing hormone-releasing hormone
  (LHRH), 689
luteinizing hormone-releasing hormone
  agonists, 689
Lyme disease, 88

M

macrolides, 70, 650t
  most commonly used, 84t
  overview of, 83–84
  side effects and dispensing issues of,
    85–86
  therapeutic uses of, 84–85
magnesium, 719, 735t
maintenance dose, 34
malabsorption, 316
male condom, 566–567, 566p
male reproductive system
  contraception for, 566–567
  erectile dysfunction (ED), 557–559
  hormones in transsexualism sex
    reassignment, 565–566
  male hormones and sexual dysfunc-
    tion, 556–559
  sexually transmitted diseases
    (STDs), 94–96
male-to-female (MTF) transgender
  reassignment, 565–566
malignant hyperthermia, 163–164
malnutrition, 731–736
manganese, 735t
mania, 207–208
marasmus, 731
marijuana, 199
mast cells, 293
mast cell stabilizers, 302–303, 304t
measles, mumps, rubella vaccine, 148t,
  149
medication errors
  administration errors, 697
  inventory and storage measure to
    prevent, 697
  preventing chemotherapy-related,
    697

S

Saccharomyces boulardii, 103, 104, 402
safety. *See* medication safety
Safety Data Sheets (SDSs), 696, 696*f*
salicylates, 518–520, 519*t*
saline laxatives, 385
saliva, 355
Salix alba, 541
salmonella, 373
Salmonella typhi, 69*t*
satiety, 726
saw palmetto, 435–436
scabies, 639, 642, 642*p,* 643*f*
Schedule II drugs, 180
schizophrenia, 224
Schmiedeberg, Oswald, 7
scrotal transdermal system, 556–557
scurvy, 714
seasonal affective disorder (SAD), 208
sebaceous glands, 620, 620*f*
seborrheic dermatitis, 628
secondary cancers, 677
secondary diabetes, 589
secretion, 414
sedatives, 236
seizure(s)
    causes of, 254–255
    generalized, 255*f,* 256
    overview of, 253–255
    partial, 255, 255*f*
seizure disorders, 253–267, 258*t*–261*t*
    calcium channel blockers, 258*t,*
      264–265
    GABA enhancers, 258*t,* 260*t*–261*t,*
      265–266
    glutamate inhibitors, 258*t,*
      266–267
    overview of drug therapy for,
      256–257
    sodium channel blockers, 257–264,
      258*t*–260*t*
selective aldosterone receptor antago-
    nist, 468*t*
selective estrogen receptor modulators
    (SERMs), 584
selective serotonin reuptake inhibitor
    (SSRI), 208–213, 209*t*
self-emulsifying drug delivery system
    (SEDDS), 139
Semmelweis, Ignaz Philip, 7
sepsis, antibiotics to treat, 79
serotonin, 159, 160, 729
    migraines and, 192
    schizophrenia and, 224–225
    selective serotonin reuptake inhibi-
      tor (SSRI), 208–213, 209*t*
    serotonin norepinephrine reuptake
      inhibitor (SNRI), 213–216, 213*t*
serotonin agonists, 729–730
serotonin and norepinephrine reuptake
    inhibitor (SNRI), 208, 213–216, 213*t*
serotonin receptor antagonists, 392*t,*
    393–394

serotonin syndrome, 208–209, 729
serum creatinine (SCr), 415
serum plasma lab values, 8*t*
sexually transmitted diseases (STDs)
    agents for treating, 96*t,* 97
    antibiotics for, 94–97, 96*t*
    chlamydia, 94
    gonorrhea, 94–95
    syphilis, 95–96
Shiatsu acupressure, 401
Shigella spp., 69*t*
shingles, antiviral drug for, 121
short-acting beta-agonists (SABAs),
    296–298, 297*t*
short-acting insulin, 591
side effects
    antibiotics, 71–72
    defined, 35
    noncompliance and, 56
signa, 42
signal transduction inhibitors, 690*t,*
    692–693
simple partial seizure, 255
sinoatrial (SA) node, 444, 455–457,
    455*f*–456*f*
skeletal muscles, 510, 512*f*
    anesthesia effects on, 162*t*
skin
    acne, 624–628
    anatomy and physiology, 619–620,
      620*f*
    antiseptics and disinfectants, 642*t,*
      643–645, 643*t*
    bacterial infections, 634–636
    dandruff, 633–634
    dermatitis, 628–633
    eczema, 629–633
    fungal infections, 636–638, 637*t*
    infections of, 634–639
    lice and scabies, 639–642
    photosensitivity, 623
    psoriasis, 629–633
    Rosacea, 624–628
    sun exposure and skin cancer,
      620–622
    topical corticosteroids, 630, 631*t*
    viral infections, 638–639, 639*t*
    warts, 638–639
    wrinkles, 624–628
sleep, stages of, 237
sleep disorders
    insomnia, 237
    narcolepsy, 238–239, 238*t*
    therapy for, 239–243, 247
    Z-drugs, 242–243
slow viral infection, 119
small intestines, drug absorption in,
    30–31
    grapefruit and, 36*p,* 37
smallpox, 745, 745*p*
smoking cessation, 220, 335–340
    benefits of, 336, 336*t*
    drug therapy for, 338–340

    planning to stop smoking, 337–338
    symptoms of nicotine withdrawal,
      336–337, 337*t*
smooth muscle, 510, 512*f*
sodium, 412, 718, 735*t*
sodium bicarbonate, 724–725
sodium channel blockers, 257–264,
    258*t*–260*t*
sodium-glucose linked transporter-2
    (SGLT-2) inhibitors, 601–602
solubility, 29
soluble fiber, 379–380
solutions, 49
    types of, 715–717
somatic nervous system, 158, 158*f*
somatic pain, 517
somatropin, 603–604
spacer, 295
specificity, 28
spectrum of activity, 70
SPF (sun protection factor), 621
spill kits, 695, 695*p*
spiral-shaped bacteria, 68, 68*f,* 69*t*
spirochetes, 68, 68*f,* 69*t*
squamous cell carcinoma, 621
stable angina, 447
Staphylococcus aureus, 68, 69*t,* 83, 634–635
statins, 492–493, 493*t*
status asthmaticus, 294–295
status epilepticus, 256
steatorrhea, 316
Stevens-Johnson syndrome, 73, 73*p*
stimulant laxative, 382*t*–383*t,* 385–386
Streptococcus pneumoniae, 69*t,* 83
Streptococcus pyogenes, 69*t,* 83
Streptopeptococcus, 69*t*
stress ulcer, 365–366
stretch receptor, 321
stroke, 485–489
    causes of, 486
    hemorrhagic, 486, 487
    ischemic, 486
    overview of, 485–486
    risk factors for, 487, 487*t*
    stroke management, 487–489
    types of, 486–487
subcutaneous injection, 48
sublingual route, 48
substance P, 265
substantia nigra, 269, 269*f*
sudden cardiac death, 741
sulfonamide, 68, 650*t*
    most commonly used, 73*t*
    overview of, 72–73
    side effects and dispensing issues of,
      73–74
    therapeutic uses of, 73
sulfonamides, 70
sulfonylureas, 597
sunscreen, 621, 621*f*
supportive therapy, 736
suppositories, 49
suppuration, 643

surfactant, 316
surfactant laxative, 382*t*, 384
suspensions, 49
Susrutas, 4
sweat glands, 620, 620*f*
sympathetic nervous system, 159, 159*f*
sympathomimetic drugs, 728–729, 729*t*
synergism, 37*t*
synergistic drug therapy, 86
synergistic effect, 672
syphilis, 68, 95–96
systemic effect, 35, 49
systemic lupus erythematosus, 536–537
systolic blood pressure, 466

T

tachycardia, 455, 457*t*
tachypnea, 305
tardive dyskinesia, 227
target, of hormone, 549
targeted anticancer therapies, 689–694
    angiogenesis inhibitors, 690–691, 690*t*
    monoclonal antibody, 690*t*, 691–692
    signal transduction inhibitors, 690*t*, 692–693
taxanes, 685
testes, 550*f*
testosterone, 556
testosterone patches, 557–558
tetracyclic antidepressants, 215*t*, 218
tetracycline antibiotics
    mechanism of, 70
    side effects and dispensing issues, 88
    therapeutic uses of, 87–88
therapeutic agent, 10
therapeutic effect, 35
therapeutic level, 34
therapeutic range, 33*f*, 34
thiamine, 709*t*, 711, 735*t*
thiazide diuretic, 431*t*, 434–435
thiazolidinediones (TZDs), 600–601
third-space fluid shift, 681
threshold dose, 683
thrombocytopenia, 458, 477
thrombus, 474
thymus gland, 550*f*
thyroglobulin, 550
thyroid gland, 550*f*
    anatomy and physiology of, 550–552, 551*f*, 552*f*
    hyperthyroidism, 554–555, 554*t*, 555*p*
    hypothyroidism, 552–554, 553*t*
thyroid-stimulating hormone (TSH), 550, 552*f*
thyroid storm, 554
thyrotoxicosis, 554
thyroxine (T$_4$), 550, 552*f*
tinea, 636
tinnitus, 432
T-lymphocytes, 120
tocolytic agent, 580

tocopherol, 709*t*, 710, 735*t*
Today's Technician, 10
tolerance, 36
tonic-clonic seizure, 256
tonicity, 715
tophus, 538
topical route, 46*t*, 49
topoisomerase I enzymes, 682
topoisomerase I inhibitors, 682
topoisomerase II enzymes, 682
topoisomerase II inhibitors, 682
topoisomerase inhibitors, 674*t*, 678*t*–679*t*, 682–685
total cholesterol, 490
total nutrient admixture (TNA), 734
total parenteral nutrition (TPN), 733
toxin, 743
trade name, 11
transcription errors, 697
transdermal contraceptives, 573–574
transient ischemic attack (TIA), 485
traveler's diarrhea, 373, 376–377
travel immunization clinics, 146
travel vaccines, 146
Treponema pallidum, 69*t*, 95
Trichomonas, 90
Trichomonas vaginalis, 96
tricyclic antidepressants (TCA), 178, 215*t*, 217, 572*t*
triglycerides, 490
triiodothyronine (T$_3$), 550, 552*f*
triptans, 195
T-score, 581
tuberculosis, 318–320, 319*t*
    multidrug-resistant tuberculosis (MDR-TB), 319
    overview of, 318–319
    treatment for, 319–320, 319*t*
tularemia, 745
tumor burden, 669
tumor cell proliferation, 669, 670*f*
tumor suppressor genes, 668
Type I diabetes, 588
Type II diabetes, 588–589
typhoid vaccine, 148*t*, 149

U

ulcerative colitis, 368–371
ulcers
    drug-induced, 366, 366*t*
    duodenal, 365
    gastric, 365
    H. pylori and, 366–367
    peptic, 365
    stress, 365–366
unstable angina, 447
uremia, 414
ureter, 414, 415*f*
uric acid, 538
urinary analgesics, 425
urinary bladder, 414, 415*f*
urinary incontinence, 423–424
urinary system
    aging and, 51

benign prostatic hyperplasia, 426–430, 426*f*, 427*t*
    diuretics, 430–435, 431*t*
    urinary incontinence, 423–424
    urinary tract infections (UTIs), 424–426, 425*t*
urinary tract, 423
urinary tract infections (UTIs), 72–73, 424–426, 425*t*, 436
urticaria, 36
USAN (United States Adopted Name), 11
US National Library of Medicine, 16
USP Dictionary of USAN and International Drug Names, 11
U.S. Pharmacopoeia (USP), 6

V

Vaccine Information Statement (VIS), 149–150
vaccine/vaccination
    Bacille Calmette-Guerin (BCG) vaccine, 147, 148*t*
    common, 146–150, 148*t*
    defined, 120
    difficulty in developing, 120
    diphtheria, tetanus, pertussis, 148*t*
    Haemophilus influenza B or HIB, 147, 148*t*
    Hepatitis A, 147, 148*t*, 397
    Hepatitis B, 148*t*, 397
    human papillomavirus (HPV), 147, 148*t*
    influenza, 120, 148*t*, 149
    Japanese encephalitis, 148*t*, 149
    live attenuated and inactivated, 145
    measles, mumps, rubella, 148*t*, 149
    meningococcal, 148*t*, 149
    pneumococcal, 148*t*, 149
    polio, 148*t*, 149
    rotavirus, 148*t*, 149
    schedule for, 145, 146*t*–147*t*
    travel vaccines, 146
    typhoid, 148*t*, 149
    varicella, 148*t*, 149
    viral infections and, 120–121
    yellow fever, 148*t*, 149
    zoster, 148*t*
vaginal ring, 574, 574*f*
vaginal route, 49
vaginitis, 96
vancomycin
    overview of, 82
    therapeutic uses and side effects, 82–83
vancomycin-resistant *Enterococcus* (VRE), 82, 91
variant angina, 447
varicella vaccine, 148*t*, 149
varicose veins, 496–497
vascular theory, 192
vasodilators, 462–463, 464*t*, 468*t*
vasomotor symptoms, 560
ventricular fibrillation, 457*t*